Assay	Reference Value
Special Hematology Tests (*continued*)	
Megakaryocytes	<0.1
Reticulum cells	0.3
Plasma cells	1.8
Myeloid:erythroid ratio (M:E ratio)	2.5:1.0
Donath-Landsteiner	Positive = pink or red color in test sample; no hemolysis in control tube
	Negative = no hemolysis (both tubes)
Hemoglobin F	Adults: 0.9%
	Infants > 1 yr: 2.0%
	Neonates: 70–90%
Osmotic fragility	Normal = hemolysis ends at 0.30% NaCl; beginning hemolysis should not occur over 0.45%
Sickle cell screening	Abnormal (positive) = any sickled cells
Sucrose hemolysis	Negative = <10% hemolysis
Special Stains	
Acid phosphatase in leukocytes	
Without tartrate	All leukocytes demonstrate granular sites of enzyme activity
With tartrate	An occasional granule seen in lymphocytes; all other leukocytes have no granular sites
Alkaline phosphatase	
Fast blue RR	32–182 LAP score
Fast violet B	12–180 LAP score
Esterase (alpha-naphthyl acetate esterase) in leukocytes	Positive = black granulation in monocytes
Esterase (naphthol AS-D chloroacetate esterase) in leukocytes	Positive = red granulation in cells of myelogenous (granulocytic) lineage
Glucose 6-phosphate dehydrogenase (G6PD)	Positive = incubated normal samples fluoresce
	Negative = enzyme deficient; no fluorescence or very dull fluorescence
Heinz bodies	Normal = an occasional Heinz body
Periodic acid–Schiff (PAS) in leukocytes	Positive = lymphoblasts usually exhibit coarse granules; early erythroid precursors may exhibit intense cytoplasmic granular PAS
Peroxidase (myeloperoxidase) in leukocytes	Positive = gray-black intracellular granules in neutrophils and precursors; monocytes react weakly; eosinophils stain red-orange; basophils stain blue; lymphocytes do not stain
Reticulocyte	0.5–1.5% (corrected in adults)
	2.5–6.5% (corrected in neonates)
Siderocyte	0–1% of mature red blood cells (peripheral blood)
Sudan black B	Positive = blue-black granulation in neutrophils and their precursors; monocytes less intense staining; lymphocytes do not stain
Hemostasis and Coagulation	
Activated partial thromboplastin time (APTT)	<35 sec
Prothrombin time (PT)	<10–15 sec
Antithrombin III	80–100%
Bleeding time (Ivy)	2–8 min
Clot lysis	No clot lysis before 48 hr
Clot retraction	44–64%
Ethanol gelation test	No clumping
Euglobulin lysis test	Clot lysis begins in >2 hr; complete in 4 hr
Fibrin degradation products (FDPs), or	
Fibrin split products (FSPs)	<8–10 μg/mL
Fibrin stabilizing factor	Normal dissolution in 24 hr
Fibrinogen levels	200–400 mg/dL
Fibrinogen titer	1:128–1:256
Hicks–Pitney test	Sufficient thromboplastin in 3–5 min to clot normal plasma in <13 sec
Lupus anticoagulant	Negative
Protamine sulfate	Positive = fibrin threads indicate the presence of fibrin degradation-split products
Prothrombin consumption	>20 sec
	<18 sec (abnormal)
Thrombin time	<20 sec; 8–10 sec (average)
Body Fluids	
Cerebrospinal fluid (CSF)	Clear, colorless
	Total WBC count = 0–5 WBCs $\times$ 10^6/L (conservative)
	Differential = rare to few lymphocytes
Synovial fluid	Pale yellow, clear
	Total WBC count = <2 $\times$ 10^6/L
	Differential = <25% segmented neutrophils, no crystals
Pleural, pericardial, and peritoneal fluid	Total WBC count = <1 $\times$ 10^9/L
Seminal fluid	Total sperm cells = 60–150 $\times$ 10^9/L
	Motility (fresh specimen) = >60%

*Values are expressed in Standard International (SI) units whenever applicable.
fL = femtoliters; LAP = leukocyte alkaline phosphatase; pg = picograms.

Clinical Hematology
THEORY AND PROCEDURES

3 — THIRD EDITION

Clinical Hematology
THEORY AND PROCEDURES

MARY L. TURGEON, EdD, MT(ASCP), CLS

Lorraine Snell Visiting Professor
Department of Medical Laboratory Science
Northeastern University

Clinical Adjunct Assistant Professor
Tufts University
School of Medicine
Boston, Massachusetts

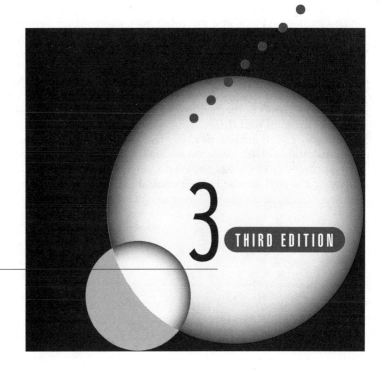

3 THIRD EDITION

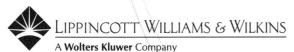

LIPPINCOTT WILLIAMS & WILKINS
A **Wolters Kluwer** Company

Philadelphia • Baltimore • New York • London
Buenos Aires • Hong Kong • Sydney • Tokyo

Acquisitions Editor: Lawrence McGrew
Assistant Editor: Holly Chapman
Project Editor: Gretchen Metzger
Senior Production Manager: Helen Ewan
Production Coordinator: Michael Carcel
Design Coordinator: Brett Mac Naughton
Indexer: Alexandra Nickerson

Edition 3

9 8 7 6 5 4 3 2 1

Library of Congress Cataloging in Publications Data

Turgeon, Mary Louise.
    Clinical hematology : theory and procedures / Mary L. Turgeon. --
3rd ed.
      p.   cm.
    Includes bibliographical references and index.
    ISBN 0-316-85623-1 (alk. paper)
    1. Hematology. I. Title.
    [DNLM: 1. Hematologic Diseases. 2. Hematology--methods.   WH
100T936c 1999]
RB145.T79   1999
616.1'5--dc21
DNLM/DLC
for Library of Congress   98-38545
                                     CIP

DEDICATION

To
Roger L. Greiger, MD

mille grazie

PREFACE

Nothing gives me more pleasure than to have completed the third edition of *Clinical Hematology*. In the decade since the original edition of the book was published, both my world and the world of the clinical laboratory have grown and forged new frontiers. Students, faculty, and working professionals on three continents have enthusiastically used *Clinical Hematology* and provided invaluable feedback.

This edition of *Clinical Hematology* capitalizes on the strengths of preceding editions and presents additional or revised information in most chapters. The biggest change in the third edition is the enlargement of the content related to anemia. Various types of anemias have been separated into individual chapters and assembled into a complete section. These chapters are presented in the same format as the other didactic chapters of the book.

Another important change in the third edition is the presentation of the latest information on hemostasis and thrombosis in two chapters. Chapter 26 presents basic knowledge including new information on the role of the endothelium, and Chapter 27 describes disorders related to hemostasis and thrombosis. Other content revisions include updated safety information in Chapter 1. Quality assurance and specimen collection facts in Chapter 2 reflect the newest thinking in the field. The most recent research findings on cytokines are described in Chapter 4. Chapter 25, Instrumentation in Hematology, contains information related to classic instrumentation, as well as updated information on more sophisticated technology. To keep readers abreast of the rapidly occurring changes in the field of medical instrumentation, Internet home page addresses of major equipment manufacturers have been included in Chapter 25. Innovative text inclusions (e.g., Body Fluid Analysis) that were introduced in the second edition have been retained for the third edition.

The pedagogy that was introduced in the original edition and has since become standard in the industry has been retained. A topical outline and behavioral objectives are presented at the beginning of each chapter. Chapter highlights and revised review questions are provided at the conclusion of each chapter. More case studies have been added to many chapters. As in the preceding editions, procedures are organized according to the format suggested by the National Commission for Clinical Laboratory Standards (NCCLS). This format introduces students to the typical procedural write-up encountered in a working clinical laboratory.

Clinical Hematology, Third Edition, is intended to fulfill the needs of students and faculty in the field of hematology for an entry-level textbook. Students in medical laboratory science (clinical laboratory technology), medical office assisting, physician assisting, and nursing, as well as working technologists in need of cross-training, are the primary audience for the book. Some portions of the book may be omitted depending upon need. Medical technologists (clinical laboratory scientists) can use the book in its entirety. Journal reading assignments or additional case studies can be used as a supplement to the text. Comments from instructors, students, and other professionals are welcome at mturgeon.1@worldnet.att.net.

Mary L. Turgeon
Boston, Massachusetts

ACKNOWLEDGMENTS

My objective in writing *Clinical Hematology, Third Edition,* continues to be to integrate basic scientific concepts, procedural theory, and clinical applications. Because the body of knowledge in hematology continues to expand, writing and revising a book that addresses the holistic needs of those in the clinical sciences continues to be a challenge. In addition, this book continues to provide me with the opportunity to learn and to share my working and teaching experience, and insight as an educator, with others.

Special thanks to Larry McGrew for his enthusiastic support of my work. Thank you to Holly Chapman and Gretchen Metzger for their efforts on my behalf.

MLT

CONTENTS

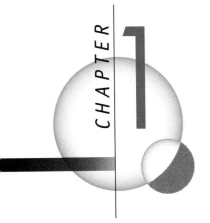

CHAPTER 1

An Introduction to Hematology

An overview of the hematology laboratory
The study of hematology
Functions of the hematology laboratory
Important laboratory practices and documents
Quality assurance in the hematology laboratory

Nonanalytical factors in quality assurance
Analysis of quantitative data
Using statistical data in the hematology laboratory
Frequency distribution
Histogram
Summary

An overview of the hematology laboratory
Quality assurance in the hematology laboratory
Using statistical data in the hematology laboratory
Bibliography
Review questions

OBJECTIVES

An overview of the hematology laboratory
- Describe the role of the medical technologist or medical technician in providing quality patient care.
- List at least four functions of the hematology laboratory.
- Describe five essential safety practices.
- Explain the basic techniques in the prevention of disease transmission.
- Explain the purpose and contents of a laboratory safety manual.
- Name the three components of the Personal Protective Equipment Standard.
- Name two essential components of the laboratory policies document.
- Describe the contents of the laboratory procedures manual.

Quality assurance in the hematology laboratory
- List and explain the eight essential nonanalytical factors in quality assurance.

- Define the terms used in describing quality assurance.
- Name the five functions of a quantitative quality control program.
- Define a variety of basic statistical terms.
- Describe the terms and state the formulas for the standard deviation, coefficient of variation, and z score.
- Describe the use of a Levey-Jennings quality control chart.
- Explain the three types of changes that can be observed in a quality control chart.
- Briefly describe computer-based control systems.

Using statistical data in the hematology laboratory
- Name the process of grouping data in classes and determining the number of observations that fall in each of the classes.
- Name and describe the most frequently used application of a histogram.

AN OVERVIEW OF THE HEMATOLOGY LABORATORY

Hematology, the study of blood, is an essential medical science. In this discipline, the fundamental concepts of biology and chemistry are applied to the medical diagnosis and treatment of various disorders or diseases related to or manifested in the blood and bone marrow.

The Study of Hematology

Basic procedures such as the complete blood cell count (CBC), which includes the measurement and examination of red blood cells (erythrocytes), white blood cells (leukocytes), and platelets (thrombocytes), and the erythrocyte sedimentation rate (ESR) frequently guide the physician in the development of a patient's differential diagnosis. The field of hematology also includes the study of hemostasis and thrombosis.

Functions of the Hematology Laboratory

Medical technologists (clinical laboratory scientists) and technicians (clinical laboratory technicians) in the hematology laboratory play a major role in patient care. The assays and examinations that are performed in the laboratory can do the following:

1. Confirm a physician's clinical impression of a possible hematological disorder
2. Establish a diagnosis or rule out a diagnosis
3. Detect an unsuspected disorder
4. Monitor the effects of radiation or chemotherapy

Although the CBC is the most frequently requested procedure, the technologist or technician must be familiar with the theory and practice of a wide variety of automated and manual tests performed in the laboratory in order to provide quality patient care.

Important Laboratory Practices and Documents

Prevention of Disease Transmission

The discovery of human immunodeficiency virus type 1 (HIV-1) generated policies from the Centers for Disease Control and Prevention (CDC) and mandated regulations by the Occupational Safety and Health Administration (OSHA) in regard to the handling of blood and body fluids. According to the CDC concept of universal precautions, all human blood and other body fluids (Table 1.1) are treated as potentially infectious for blood-borne pathogens. The term *standard precautions* has been introduced recently to underscore the fact that all bodily fluids are potentially infectious.

Universal precautions is an approach to infection control, used to prevent occupational exposures to blood-borne pathogens. It eliminates the need for separate isolation procedures for patients known or suspected to be infectious. The application of universal precautions also eliminates the need for warning labels on specimens.

The modes of transmission for HBV and HIV are similar, but the potential for transmission in the occupational setting

TABLE 1.1 **Potentially Infectious Materials**

Specific Human Fluids

Amniotic fluid

Blood

Cerebrospinal fluid

Pleural fluid

Saliva in dental procedures

Semen

Sweat

Synovial fluid

Tears

Vaginal secretions

Other Materials

Any body fluid that is visibly contaminated with blood

All body fluids in situations in which it is difficult or impossible to differentiate between body fluids

Unfixed tissue or organ (other than intact skin) form a human (living or dead)

HIV-containing cell or tissue cultures

Organ cultures or HIV-containing culture medium

Teeth

Vomitus

is greater for HBV than HIV. An occupational exposure is defined as a percutaneous injury, for example, a needle stick or cut with a sharp object, or contact by mucous membranes or nonintact skin (especially when the skin is chapped, abraded, or afflicted with dermatitis or the contact is prolonged or involving an extensive area) with blood, tissues, blood-stained body fluids, body fluids to which universal precautions apply, or concentrated virus. Blood is the single most important source of HIV and HBV exposure in the workplace. However, the most feared hazard of all, the transmission of HIV through occupational exposure, is among the least likely to occur if proper safety practices are followed. Most exposures do not result in infection. The average overall risk of developing occupationally acquired HIV in untreated exposures is 0.3%. The risk varies with the type of exposure and factors, e.g., amount of infected blood in the exposure, the length of contact with infectious material, the amount of virus in the patient's blood or body fluid or tissue at the time of exposure, and whether or not post-exposure treatment was taken (call the National AIDS Hotline, 1-800-342-2437 for current CDC recommendations regarding post exposure treatment). A total of 54 cases of occupationally acquired HIV have been documented by the CDC as of December, 1997. Another 132 health care workers are listed as possible occupational exposures. Clinical laboratory staff have the second highest rate of exposure with 16 documented and 18 possible occupational exposures. The majority of exposures are from needle sticks or cuts. Blood is the most commonly implicated infected body fluid.

Adherence to infection control precautions such as wearing gloves minimizes the risk of exposure to diseases transmitted by blood or body fluids. Masks, protective eyewear, and aprons or gowns should be worn during procedures that are likely to generate droplets of blood or other body fluids. Proper disposal of gloves and other potentially contaminated items, washing of hands after completing laboratory activities, and removal of laboratory coats before leaving the laboratory should reduce disease transmission.

In some cases, reverse isolation technique is used in order to protect the patient (e.g., burn victims) from infectious agents. Specific isolation techniques are also employed in the nursery because newborn and premature infants are at a high risk for infection.

The following are essential safety practices in the hematology laboratory.

1. Gloves should be used properly. General guidelines related to the selection and general use of gloves include the following:
   A. Use sterile gloves for procedures involving contact with normally sterile areas of the body or during procedures where sterility has been established and must be maintained. Use nonsterile examination gloves for procedures that do not require the use of sterile gloves.
   B. Wear gloves when processing blood specimens, reagents derived from blood products, and blood products. Disposable (single-use) gloves such as surgical or examination gloves must be replaced as soon as practical when contaminated or as soon as feasible if they are torn or punctured or when their ability to function as a barrier is compromised.
   C. Disposable (single-use) gloves must not be washed or decontaminated for reuse. Washing with detergents may cause increased penetration of liquids through undetected holes in the gloves.
   D. Rubber utility gloves may be decontaminated and reused if the integrity of the glove is not compromised. However, disinfectants may cause deterioration. Rubber gloves should be discarded if they are punctured, torn, cracked, or show other signs of deterioration such as peeling or discoloration. These conditions compromise the gloves' ability to function as a barrier.

   Gloves must be used for the collection of blood (phlebotomy) when it can be reasonably anticipated that the employee may have direct contact with blood or other potentially infectious substances. The exposure of mucous membrane or nonintact skin to blood or body fluids can be dangerous. Circumstances that could present this type of situation include the following:
   (1) A phlebotomist with cuts or skin abrasions on his or her hands
   (2) A phlebotomist performing a finger or heel puncture on a newborn or young child
   (3) A student receiving training in phlebotomy

   The use of gloves is optional and at the discretion of the phlebotomist in other circumstances, such as routine collection of blood from patients not believed to be at high risk of blood-borne diseases.

2. Frequent handwashing is an important safety precaution in the prevention of the spread of nosocomial infections. It should be performed after contact with patients and laboratory specimens. Hands should be washed with soap and water
   A. After completing lab work and before leaving the laboratory
   B. After removing gloves
   C. Before eating, drinking, applying makeup, changing contact lenses, or using the lavatory
   D. Before all activities that involve hand contact with mucous membranes or nonintact skin
   E. Immediately after accidental skin contact with blood, body fluids, or tissues

   When accidental skin contact occurs through breaks in gloves, the gloves should be removed immediately and the hands should be thoroughly washed. If accidental contamination occurs to an exposed area of the skin or because of a break in gloves, wash first with a liquid soap, rinse well with water, and apply a 1:10 dilution of bleach or 50% isopropyl or ethyl alcohol. Leave the bleach or alcohol on the skin for at least 1 minute before a final washing with liquid soap and water.

3. Used needles should be placed intact into specifically designated red, puncture-proof biohazard containers. Needles should *not* be bent, reinserted into their original plastic sheath, removed by hand from syringes, or otherwise manipulated by hand because this can produce an accidental needle wound. The most significant occupational hazard to laboratory personnel is exposure to HBV due to accidental needle sticks.

   The same criteria should be applied to used scalpel blades and any other sharp device that may be contaminated with blood. The container should be located as close as possible to the work area.

   Phlebotomists should carry red, puncture-resistant containers in their collection trays. Needles should not project from the top of the container. To discard the containers, close and place them into the biohazard waste receptacle. An accidental needle stick must be reported to the appropriate individual.

4. Immediately report all accidents such as needle punctures or glassware cuts to the supervisor. Allow this type of wound to bleed freely and then rinse with alcohol.

5. Wipe off the outside of containers that are visibly contaminated with blood or body fluids with a 1:10 dilution of household bleach (Table 1.2) before handling.

6. All work areas should be kept clean and well organized. Clean up spilled specimens or chemicals immediately. It is equally important to clean and disinfect work areas frequently during the workday as well as before and after the workday. Diluted household bleach prepared daily inactivates HBV in 10 minutes and HIV in 2 minutes.

   All work surfaces should be cleaned and sanitized at the beginning and end of the shift with a 1:10 dilution of household bleach. Instruments such as scissors or centrifuge carriages should be sanitized daily with a dilute solution of bleach. Decontaminate nondisposable equipment, such as counting chambers used for spinal fluid

TABLE 1.2 Preparation of Diluted Household Bleach

Volume of Bleach	Volume of H_2O	Ratio	% Sodium Hypochlorite	% Solution
1 mL	9 mL	1:10	0.5	10

Note: A 10% solution of bleach is stable for 1 week at room temperature when diluted with tap water.

cell counts, by soaking overnight in a dilute bleach solution and rinsing with methyl alcohol and water before reuse. Disposable glassware or supplies that have come in contact with blood should be autoclaved or incinerated.

All blood spills should be treated as *potentially* hazardous. In the event of a blood spill, the following procedure for cleaning up the spill should be used.
A. Wear gloves and a lab coat.
B. Absorb the blood with disposable towels. Bleach solutions are less effective in the presence of high concentrations of protein. Remove as much liquid blood or serum as possible before decontamination.
C. Using a diluted bleach solution, clean the spill site of all visible blood.
D. Wipe down the spill site with paper towels soaked with diluted bleach.
E. Place all disposable materials used for decontamination into a biohazard container.
7. Specimens needing centrifugation should be capped and placed into a centrifuge with a sealed dome. Slowly and carefully open rubber-stoppered test tubes with a 2-×-2-inch gauze square placed over the stopper in order to minimize aerosol production (the introduction of substances into the air). Tubes should be pointed away from the face as well as other workers.
8. Use autodilutors or safety bulbs for pipetting. Pipetting *by mouth* of any clinical material is strictly forbidden.
9. Use a sodium azide free diluent in cell-counting systems requiring an isotonic diluent. Several violent explosions have occurred because of the waste disposal hazard associated with sodium azide. These explosions occurred in plumbing containing brass, copper, lead, or alloy metals that react with sodium azide to form heavy metal azides that are unusually sensitive to mechanical shock, which can occur during maintenance procedures such as clearing a clogged drain.
10. Store xylene and other volatile chemicals in an adequately ventilated area or directly under a laboratory hood. Store alcohol in metal safety cans. Care must be taken to store and use acetone away from an open flame.
11. Food and drinks should not be consumed in work areas or stored in the same area as specimens. Containers, refrigerators, and freezers used for specimens should be marked as containing a biohazard.

Other Safety Issues

Each laboratory *must* have an up-to-date safety manual. This manual should contain a comprehensive listing of acceptable practices and precautions. Specific regulations that conform to current state and federal requirements such as OSHA regulations must be included in the manual. Other sources of mandatory and voluntary standards include the Joint Commission on Accreditation of Healthcare Organizations (JCAHO), the College of American Pathologists (CAP), and the CDC guidelines.

Personal Protective Equipment Standard

OSHA requires laboratories to have a Personal Protective Equipment (PPE) program. The components of this regulation include the following:

- A workplace hazard assessment with a written hazard certification
- Proper equipment selection
- Employee information and training, with written competency certification
- Regular reassessment of work hazards

Laboratory personnel should not rely solely on devices for PPE to protect themselves against hazards. However, they should apply protective equipment standards when using various forms of safety protection.

Hazardous Chemicals

In addition to the safety practices common to all laboratory situations, such as the proper storage of flammable materials, certain procedures are *mandatory* in a medical laboratory. Proper procedures for the handling and disposal of toxic, radioactive, and potentially carcinogenic materials must be included in the safety manual. Information regarding the hazards of particular substances must be included as a safety practice and to comply with the legal right of workers to know about the hazards associated with these substances. Some chemicals (e.g., benzidine) that were previously used in the laboratory are now known to be carcinogenic and have been replaced with safer chemicals.

Laboratory Policies

Laboratory policies should be included in a laboratory reference manual that is available to all hospital personnel. This manual should contain information regarding patient preparation for laboratory tests. Approved policies regarding the reporting of abnormal values should be clearly stated in this document.

Laboratory Procedures

The procedure manual should be a current and complete document of laboratory procedures, including safety rules and approved policies for the reporting of results. The laboratory procedure manual should detail each procedure performed in the hematology laboratory. This manual should comply with the National Committee for Clinical Laboratory Standards (NCCLS) format standards for a procedure manual. (The NCCLS is a nationally recognized group of laboratory professionals who lead quality assurance efforts in the United States.) Minimally, the manual should include the name of the test method; the principle of the test and its clinical applications; the protocol for specimen collection and storage; quality control information; names of special chemical reagents, equipment, or supplies; the procedural protocol; normal values; and technical sources of error. The procedural format found in Chapter 24 of this text follows these guidelines.

In order to support a quality contol program, methods for documenting laboratory results should be included in the procedure manual. Proper documentation ensures that control specimens have been properly monitored.

Quality Assurance in the Hematology Laboratory

Quality assurance is employed in the clinical hematology laboratory to ensure excellence in analytical performance. A systematic approach to quality assures that correct laboratory results are obtained in the shortest possible time and at a reasonable cost. A quality assurance system can be divided into two major components: nonanalytical factors and the analysis of quantitative data (quality control).

Nonanalytical Factors in Quality Assurance

In order to guarantee the highest quality patient care through laboratory testing, a variety of pre-analytical and post-analytical factors in addition to analytical data must be considered. In order for laboratories to comply with the Clinical Laboratory Improvement Act of 1988 (CLIA'88) and be certified to perform testing, they must meet minimum standards. In some cases, deficiencies are noted (Table 1.3) and must be corrected.

Nonanalytical factors that support quality testing include the following:

1. Qualified personnel
2. Established laboratory policies
3. The laboratory procedure manual
4. Proper procedures for specimen collection and storage
5. Preventive maintenance of equipment
6. Appropriate methodology
7. Established quality assurance techniques
8. Accuracy in reporting results

Qualified Personnel

The entry-level examination competencies of all certified persons in hematology should be validated. Validation should take the form of both external certification and new-employee orientation to the work environment. Continuing competency is equally important. Participation in continuing education activities is essential to the maintenance of competency.

Established Laboratory Policies

Laboratory policies should be included in a laboratory reference manual that is available to all hospital personnel. Refer to the previous section on laboratory documents in this chapter.

The Laboratory Procedure Manual

Refer to the previous section on laboratory documents in this chapter for a complete discussion of the contents of the manual.

TABLE 1.3 **Top Eight CLIA Deficiencies for First Cycle Inspections of Hospital and Independent Laboratories**

1. *Quality Control*
The lab must perform and document at least 2 levels of controls each day of testing

2. *Quality Assurance*
The lab must establish and follow a comprehensive, written quality assurance program to monitor its overall operation.

3. *Quality Control*
The lab must follow the manufacturer's instructions for instrument operation and test performance.

4. *Personnel*
The lab director must specify in writing the responsibilities and duties of all personnel.

5. *Quality Control*
The lab must have a procedure manual.

Quality Assurance
The lab must have a system for verifying accuracy and reliability twice each year for tests not covered under the lab's proficiency testing program.

6. *Patient Test Management*
The test report must have the name and address of lab, location where test was performed, test performed, result, and units of measurement.

7. *Patient Test Management*
The lab must record the identity of the personnel who performed the test(s).

8. *Proficiency Testing*
The lab must be enrolled in a proficiency testing program for each specialty and subspecialty of tests it performs.

Proficiency Testing
Laboratory must keep lab proficiency records a minimum amount of time.

Source: HCFA CLIA data base (July, 1997).

Proper Procedures for Specimen Collection and Storage

Strict adherence to correct procedures for specimen collection and storage is critical to the accuracy of any test. Preanalytical errors are the most common source of laboratory errors. For example, identification errors, either of the patient or of the specimen, are major potential sources of error. The use of computerized bar code identification of specimens is an asset to specimen identification.

Correct storage of specimens (also refer to Chapter 24, Manual Procedures) is critical to obtaining accurate results. Specimen integrity is an important issue when blood is collected at a site away from the testing facility. Samples may need to be drawn several hours before testing. In many cases, cooling of specimens on ice is critical. This is particularly true for coagulation testing, e.g., prothrombin time (PT) and activated partial thromboplastin time (aPTT).

According to NCCLS (Collection, Transport, and Processing of Blood Specimens for Coagulation Testing and Performance of Coagulation Assays, 2nd ed, Approved Guidelines, H21-A2, Dec., 1991), blood samples collected for PT and aPTT analysis in tubes with sodium citrate should be handled using this sample protocol when drawn off-site.

- The sample tube should remain unopened prior to testing.
- Centrifugation and testing of such samples can be delayed for up to 2 hours at 22° to 24°C (71.6° to 75.2°F) or for up to 4 hours at 2° to 4°C (35.6° to 39.2°F).
- Keep the sample in a well-chilled, properly insulated cooler or a refrigerated block. Either storage device should have a thermometer to monitor its temperature to prevent overheating or partial freezing of whole blood samples. Separation of the sample upon standing should not affect sample integrity.

In addition, this method of storage should be confirmed for compatibility by contacting both the manufacturer of the evacuated tube collection system and the technical supervisor of coagulation testing.

Preventive Maintenance of Equipment

Continual monitoring of the temperatures of water baths and refrigerators is important to the maintenance of reagent quality and test performance. Equipment such as microscopes, centrifuges, and spectrophotometers should be cleaned and checked for accuracy on a regular schedule. A preventive maintenance schedule should be followed (refer to the Instrument Protocol section in Chapter 25 for examples) for all pieces of automated equipment (e.g., cell-counting instruments). Failure to monitor equipment regularly can produce inaccurate test results and lead to expensive repairs.

Appropriate Methodology

When new methods are introduced, it is important to check the procedure for accuracy and variability. Replicate analyses using control specimens are recommended to check for accuracy and to eliminate factors such as day-to-day variability, reagent variability, and differences between technologists.

Established Quality Assurance Techniques

Each procedure should have an established protocol to assure the quality of the results. Usually, normal and abnormal control samples are analyzed at the same time patient specimens are analyzed. Established limits of acceptable performance must be determined for each type of test. If control results are not within acceptable limits, patient results cannot be guaranteed to be accurate. In these cases, the source of error must be identified and all of the tests repeated before a patient's result can be reported.

Participation in various external quality control programs, such as the CAP Survey Program, ensures the continuing accuracy of laboratory testing through proficiency testing.

Accuracy in Reporting Results

Many laboratories have established **critical values** or the **Delta check system** to monitor individual patient results. Highly abnormal individual test results in the case of panic values and significant differences from previous results in the Delta check system alert the technologist to a potential problem. Other control systems (discussed in the section on Statistical Analysis of Results in Quality Assurance) are also used to ensure the quality of test results.

When extremely abnormal results or differences from previous test values are found, the laboratory protocol should establish the method of rechecking and reporting such results to the attending physician.

Appropriate communication is critical to high-quality patient care. In most situations, laboratory reports should be recorded and sent to the appropriate patient area rather than conveyed by telephone. There is too much risk of error in depending on verbal reports alone. In emergency "stat" situations, verbal reports may be necessary but must be followed by written reports as soon as possible. It is equally important in reporting results to be on the alert for clerical errors, particularly transcription errors. The introduction of computer interfaced on-line reporting is useful in communicating information correctly and efficiently.

Analysis of Quantitative Data

It is important for a hematology technologist or technician to understand basic statistical concepts used in quality control. Knowledge of specific elements of statistics is important in hematology for two reasons:

1. Application of statistical analysis of results in quality assurance protocols
2. Instrumental applications of statistics to erythrocyte, leukocyte, and platelet reports

Terms Used in Clinical Quality Assurance

In the clinical hematology laboratory, several terms are used to describe different aspects of quality assurance:

1. **Accuracy** describes how close a test result is to the true value. This term implies freedom from error. Reference samples and standards with known values are needed to check accuracy.
2. **Calibration** is the comparison of an instrument measurement or reading to a known physical constant.
3. **Control** (noun) represents a specimen that is similar in composition to the patient's whole blood or plasma. The value of a control specimen is known. Control specimens are tested in exactly the same way as the patient specimen and are tested daily or in conjunction with the unknown (patient) specimen. Controls are the best measurements of precision and may represent normal or abnormal test values.
4. **Precision** describes how close the test results are to one another when repeated analyses of the same material are performed. Precision refers to the reproducibility of test results. It is important to make a distinction between precision and accuracy. The term accuracy implies freedom from error; the term precision implies freedom from variation.
5. **Standards** are highly purified substances of a known composition. A standard may differ from a control in its overall composition and in the way it is handled in the test. Standards are the best way to measure accuracy. Standards

are used to establish reference points in the construction of graphs (e.g., manual hemoglobin curve) or to calculate a test result.

6. **Quality control** is a process that monitors the accuracy and reproducibility of results through the use of control specimens.

The Functions of a Quantitative Quality Control Program

Assaying control specimens and standards along with patient specimens serves several major functions:

1. Providing a guide to the functioning of equipment, reagents, and individual technique
2. Confirming the accuracy of testing when compared with reference values
3. Detecting an increase in the frequency of both high and low minimally acceptable values (dispersion)
4. Detecting any progressive drift of values to one side of the average value for at least 3 days (trends)
5. Demonstrating an abrupt shift or change from the established average value for 3 days in a row (shift)

Basic Statistical Concepts

Before applying the results from controls to a systematic quantitative quality control program, or in order to understand the statistical reporting of instrumental results, the basic terms and concepts of statistics should be reviewed.

Terms and Definitions

Average equals the sum of the test results divided by the number of tests. The average is the arithmetic mean value.

Mean is the term used to express the average or arithmetic mean value. The mean value is 13.6 for the following series of values: 10, 11, 14, 16, and 17.

Median is the middle value of a set of numbers arranged according to their magnitude. If two middle values exist in an even number of mathematical observations, the median is the arithmetic mean of the two middle values. The median value is 14 if the following five test values are arranged in order of size: 10, 11, 14, 16, and 17.

Mode is the term used to indicate the number or value that occurs with the greatest frequency. The mode is 45 if the following values are obtained for a control blood: 45, 48, 35, 39, 51, 42, 45, 39, 45, 44, and 45.

Measurements of Variation

In the laboratory, measures of variation can include the range, the variance, the standard deviation, the coefficient of variation, and the z score.

Range is the term used to express the difference between the highest and lowest measurements in a series. The range is expressed in the same units as the raw data. Therefore, if the value of the raw data is expressed as a percentage (%), the range is also expressed as a percentage. If the following values are obtained, the range can be determined. The range is 0.5% to 2.0% for the following values (expressed as percentages): 1, 1.5, 1, 0.5, 2.0, 1.5, and 1.0.

Variance is an expression of the position of each observation or test result in relationship to the mean of the values.

The variance is determined by examining the deviation from the mean of each individual value. If the mean value for this series of assays is 8, the variance can be determined in this example. The following test results were obtained: 3, 4, 5, 6, 8, 9, 10, 12, and 15. The variance from the mean (deviance from the mean) of each individual result is -5, -4, -3, -2, 0, 1, 2, 4, and 7. To compute the variance, the squares of each deviation are used. The formula for computing a population variance is as follows:

$$\sigma^2 = \frac{\Sigma\,(X - \mu)^2}{N}$$

where σ^2 = the variance
X = the observation
μ = the mean
N = finite population size

Standard deviation expresses the degree to which the test data tend to vary about the average value (mean). To obtain a measure of variation expressed in the same units as the raw data, the square root of the variance or the standard deviation is used.

Standard deviation, as a measure of variability, has meaning only when two or more sets of data having the same units of measurement are compared. However, the principle of standard deviation can be used to describe the single-set measurement.

The traditional formula for calculating the standard deviation (SD) is the square root of the sum of all the differences from the mean squared and subsequently divided by the number of determinations (tests) minus one. The traditional formula is as follows:

$$SD = \sqrt{\frac{\Sigma\,(X - \overline{X})^2}{N - 1}}$$

where Σ = sum
X = individual value
$\overline{X}$ = mean individual value
N = number of individual values

To calculate the standard deviation of a laboratory test in the traditional manner, the following steps should be used:

1. A minimum of 20 results are needed. These results represent 20 consecutive days of testing of a control from the same pool sample.
2. Calculate the average (mean).
3. Determine the variance of each number from the mean.
4. Square each variance.
5. Add the squared variances.
6. Divide by the number of test results minus 1.
7. Find the square root of this number. The value obtained represents 1 standard deviation.

In many cases, the traditional formula is *not* appropriate because the mean does not lend itself to easy manipulation and the *sum of the differences* does not add up to a sum of zero. In these cases, the alternate formula, which is also the formula programmed into a scientific calculator, should be used. This formula is:

$$s^2 = \frac{n\Sigma x^2 - (\Sigma x)^2}{n(n - 1)}$$

The **coefficient of variation (CV),** or **related standard deviation,** is a statistical tool used to compare variability in nonidentical data sets. The CV of each data set allows comparison of two or more test methods, laboratories, or specimen sets. To do this, the variability in each data set must be expressed as a relative rather than an absolute measure. This is accomplished for each data set by expressing the standard deviation as a percentage of the mean. The formula for this calculation is as follows:

$$\text{Coefficient of variation (\%)} = \frac{\text{SD}}{\overline{X}} \times 100$$

where SD = standard deviation
$\overline{X}$ = mean

The **z score** measures how many standard deviations a particular number is from the right or left of the mean (Fig. 1.1A). A positive z score measures the number of standard deviations an observation is above the mean, and a negative z score gives the number of standard deviations an observation is below the mean. The z score is a unitless measure.

In order to compare the ranking of two observations from two different populations, the ranking is converted into standard units referred to as z scores or z values. The formula to compute the z score is:

$$z = \frac{x - \mu}{\sigma}$$

where x = an observation from a population
μ = the mean
σ = standard deviation

Statistical Analysis of Results in Quality Assurance

Statistical analysis of results has been used in the clinical laboratory since the original introduction of the Levey-Jennings chart. With the advent of computer technology and computerized instrumentation in hematology, many additional systems have been introduced to monitor test results numerically.

In this section the following methods will be presented:

1. The Levey-Jennings chart
2. The cumulative sum (Cusum) method
3. Trend line analysis
4. Power functions

The Levey-Jennings Chart

Quality control charts are used in the clinical laboratory to graphically display the assay values of controls versus time (e.g., day or specimen run). The **Levey-Jennings** chart is the traditional approach to monitoring quality control (e.g., instrument calibration or lot-to-lot reagent changes).

Confidence or control limits are calculated from the mean and the standard deviation. The confidence limits represent a set of mathematically established limits into which the majority of values (results) will fall. Within the confidence limits, the results are assumed to be accurate. It is common practice to use ±2 standard deviations as the limit of confidence.

In the Levey-Jennings control chart (Fig. 1.2), the control results are plotted on the y axis versus time on the x axis. This chart shows the expected mean value by the solid line in the center and indicates the control limits or range of acceptable values by the dotted points. If the control assay

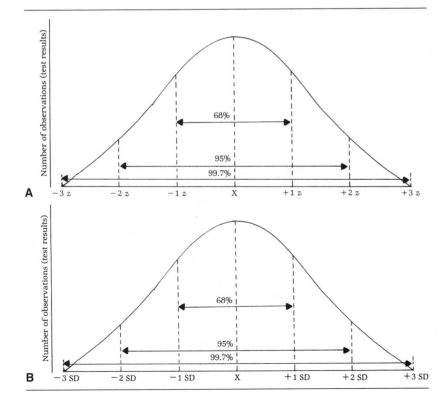

FIGURE 1.1 Frequency distribution. **A.** *Z* score. **B.** Gaussian distribution: normal frequency distribution curve.

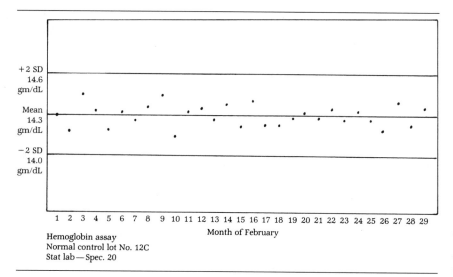

+2 SD
14.6
gm/dL

Mean
14.3
gm/dL

−2 SD
14.0
gm/dL

1 2 3 4 5 6 7 8 9 10 11 12 13 14 15 16 17 18 19 20 21 22 23 24 25 26 27 28 29

Month of February

Hemoglobin assay
Normal control lot No. 12C
Stat lab — Spec. 20

FIGURE 1.2 Levey-Jennings control chart. The normal or abnormal control value is plotted each day. This value must be within 2 standard deviations (SD) of the mean value.

value is outside the confidence limits, the control value and the patients' values are considered to be "out of control" and *cannot* be reported. If the control assay value falls within the confidence limits, the control value and patient specimens assayed at the same time are considered to be "in control," and the results can be reported.

Types of Change. The classification of changes in a quality control system is important because different kinds of changes suggest different sources. Three types of change are commonly observed in the Levey-Jennings quality control approach (Fig. 1.3):

1. Systematic drift
2. Increased dispersion of results
3. Shift or abrupt change in results

Systematic drift or **trend** is displayed when the control value direction moves progressively in one direction from the mean for at least 3 days. Systematic drift or a trend in control values suggests that a problem is progressively developing. This problem may be due to the deterioration of a reagent or control. Diluent contamination affects erythrocyte and leukocyte controls with an upward trend as bacterial growth increases.

Dispersion is observed when random errors or the lack of precision increase. This type of pattern indicates inconsistency in technique or a stability problem, for example, fluctuating electrical voltage or poor mixing of a cellular control specimen.

Shift or **abrupt change** is observed when a problem develops suddenly. This type of change can be associated with the malfunction of an instrument or an error in technique.

Computed-Based Control Systems

Cumulative Sum (Cusum) Method. This was an early supplementary control method. Decision limits can be manually calculated from the standard deviation with this method; however, computer systems are more efficient. This method allows for the rapid detection of trends and shifts from the mean. Its major disadvantages are that too many "out of

control" results are obtained, and it does not readily control for random error (precision). Cusum can be used as a supplement to the Levey-Jennings system.

Trend Line Analysis. Observed daily results of either the control value or the change in the standard deviation introduced by the control value are tracked. The tracking value at each point is plotted and compared against known error limits for the control of both the mean (accuracy) and the standard deviation (precision). If the value exceeds determined limits, a message is sent to the technologist.

Power Functions. These systems are a means of displaying the performance of a quality control rule by plotting the probability for rejection versus the size of the analytical error. This computerized method can be used to determine what control rule is most useful in detecting an error of given magnitude when a specific number of controls is evaluated.

USING STATISTICAL DATA IN THE HEMATOLOGY LABORATORY

Frequency Distribution

In any large series of measurements (test results) of a normal population, the results are evenly distributed about the average value. Grouping of data in classes and determining the number of observations that fall in each of the classes is a frequency distribution of grouped data (Table 1.4).

Histogram

Information regarding frequency distribution is easier to understand if presented graphically. A bar chart provides immediate information about a set of data in a condensed form; the related pictorial representation is a **histogram.**

Histograms can have almost any shape or form. The most frequently encountered type of distribution is the bell-shaped histogram, which is symmetrical. The bell shape may vary, with some curves being flatter and wider than others; however, most values cluster about the mean, with a few

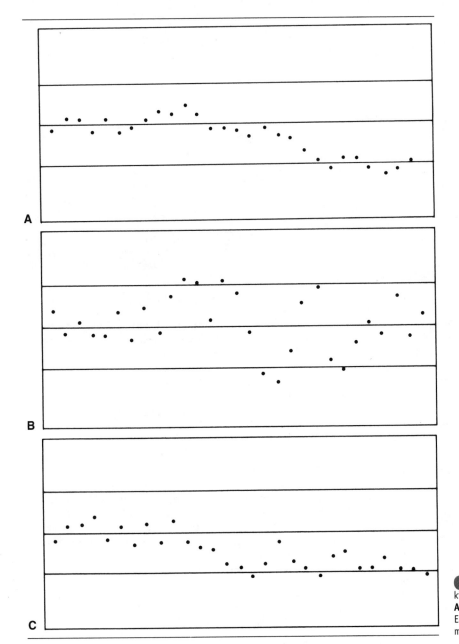

values falling in the extreme tails of the curve. This normal curve is referred to as a **Gaussian distribution** (see Fig. 1.1B).

In the bell-shaped normal curve, ±1 SD includes 68% of all of the values, ±2 SD includes 95% of the values, and ±3 SD includes 99.7% of the values. For biological studies, control confidence limits are usually established at ±2 SD. When values fall outside these limits, the procedure is considered out of control. In the establishment of reference values for a procedure, the reference range for a specific assay reflects the statistical processing of a large number of normal samples and represents the values found within 2 or 3 standard deviations.

In Chapter 25, Instrumentation in Hematology, histogram data generated by automated cell-counting systems are presented. The interpretation of patient histograms compared to histograms based on established normal values for erythrocytes, leukocytes, and platelets is presented in detail.

SUMMARY

An Overview of the Hematology Laboratory

The medical technologist (clinical laboratory scientist) and medical laboratory technician (clinical laboratory technican) play a major role in delivering quality patient care through the assay of blood and body fluids. The results reported by the laboratory can confirm clinical impressions, establish a diagnosis, exclude a diagnosis, screen for undetected disorders, or monitor the effects of therapy on a patient.

TABLE 1.4 An Example of a Frequency Distribution of Grouped Data

Class Boundaries	Frequency (f)
0.5–3.5	3
3.5–6.5	8
6.5–9.5	10
9.5–12.5	7
12.5–15.5	4

Safety in the laboratory should be detailed in a laboratory safety manual that complies with various agency regulations. The purpose of safety practices is to protect both patients and laboratory personnel. Certain procedures are *mandatory* in a medical laboratory.

The prevention of disease transmission is particularly important in the medical environment. In addition to specific practices dictated by particular situations, the most effective means of reducing **nosocomial infections** is frequent and thorough handwashing between patient contacts.

Laboratory policies must be clearly stated in a laboratory reference manual. The laboratory procedure manual should comply with the guidelines established by the NCCLS.

Quality Assurance in the Hematology Laboratory

Quality assurance or quality control ensures excellence in performance. A comprehensive program consists of nonanalytical and analytical components. Eight factors are important nonanalytical elements in quality assurance. These factors include the entry-level and continuing competence of laboratory personnel, established laboratory policies, the laboratory procedure manual, proper specimen collection and storage protocol, preventive maintenance of equipment, appropriate methodology, established quality assurance techniques, and accuracy in reporting results.

The analysis of quantitative data generated in the laboratory requires a basic knowledge of statistics. Quality control programs have five major functions, all important to observe. The basic statistical concepts of importance to quality assurance are the average (mean), median, mode, range, variance, standard deviation, coefficient of variation, and z score.

Statistical analysis of results includes the graphic display of control data. The traditional quality control system is the Levey-Jennings approach. Confidence limits are determined and the control results are plotted. This system allows for the visual observation of "in control" and "out of control" results. Changes such as systematic drift, increased dispersion, and an abrupt change in results can be observed through the use of this type of graphic display. Computer-based control systems are continually being introduced into the laboratory as clinical instrumentation becomes more sophisticated. These systems include the cumulative sum (Cusum) method, trend line analysis, and power functions.

Using Statistical Data in the Hematology Laboratory

Frequency distribution is an important method of grouping large quantities of data. Information regarding frequency distribution is easier to understand if presented graphically. A bar chart provides information about a set of data in a condensed form, and the related pictorial representation is a histogram.

Histograms can have almost any shape, but the most frequent is the bell shape. In a bell-shaped distribution, ±1 SD includes 68% of the values, ±2 SD includes 95% of the values, and ±3 SD includes 99.7% of the values. In biological studies, such as hematology, control confidence limits are usually established at ±2 SD.

The normal range values for a procedure are determined using the technique and knowledge of histograms and standard deviation. Histograms generated by modern instrumentation (discussed in Chapter 25) are used to study erythrocytes, leukocytes, and platelets.

BIBLIOGRAPHY

Alpert, L. I. "OSHA: New Player in the Battle Against AIDS." *Med. Lab. Observer*, Vol. 22, No. 4, April, 1990, pp. 49–52.

Arkin, C. F. "Quality Control in the New Environment: Statistics." *Med. Lab. Observer*, Vol. 18, No. 12, December, 1986, pp. 51–54.

Bachner, Paul and Stephen C. Kimber. "Quality Control in the New Environment: Automated Hematology." *Med. Lab. Observer*, Vol. 18, No. 11, November, 1986, pp. 49–54, 60–62.

Baer, D. M. "Bleach Stability." *Med. Lab. Observer*, Vol. 22, No. 4, April, 1990, p. 9.

Bender, James L. (Chairholder) *Clinical Laboratory Procedure Manual* (2nd edition). Villanova, PA: National Commission for Clinical Laboratory Standards, 1992.

"Bloodborne Pathogens." *Fed. Reg.*, Vol. 58, No. 235, December 6, 1991, pp. 63861–64186.

Brown, James W. "Biosafety in the Laboratory." *Testrends*, Vol. 5, No. 1, May, 1991, pp. 1–3.

Carlson, D. J. "Guidelines for Laboratory Safety for Medical Technologists: Policies and Procedures," in *Clinical Laboratory Improvement Seminar*. Chicago: Commission on Inspection and Accreditation, American Society of Clinical Pathologists, 1980.

Centers for Disease Control and Prevention. *HIV / AIDS Surveillance Report*. Vol. 9, No. 2, 1997, pp. 1–43.

"Ensuring Specimen Quality in Phlebotomy." *Lab. Med.*, Vol. 27, No. 1, January, 1996, p. 17.

Fahey, B. J. and D. K. Henderson. "Minimizing Risks for Occupational Blood-borne Infections." *JAMA*, Vol. 264, No. 9, September 5, 1990, pp. 1189–1190.

Hatfield, Scott. "CDC Updating On-Job HIV Post-Exposure Guidelines." *Advance for Medical Laboratory Professionals*, Vol. 28, Oct 6, 1997, p. 15.

Miller, L. E. "Recommended Concentrations of Bleach." *Lab. Med.*, Vol. 21, No. 2, February, 1990, p. 116.

Oman, D. S. "Calibration, Calibration Verification and Reportable Range." *Advance*, Vol. 27, No. 6, June, 1996, pp. 78–84.

Parks, D. G. "OSHA's Personal Protective Equipment Standard." *Lab. Med.*, Vol. 27, No. 2, February, 1996, pp. 86–87.

Perry, S., J. Ryan, and H. J. Polan. "Needlestick Injury Associated with Venipuncture." *JAMA*, Vol. 267, No. 1, January, 1992, p. 54.

Statland, Bernard E. and James O. Westgard. "Quality Management," in *Clinical Diagnosis and Management by Laboratory Methods*

(18th edition). John B. Henry (ed.). Philadelphia: Saunders, 1991, pp. 81–99.

U.S. Department of Health and Human Services. "Guidelines for Prevention of Transmission of Human Immunodeficiency Virus and Hepatitis B Virus to Health-Care and Public Safety Workers." *MMWR*, Vol. 38, No. S-6, June 23, 1989, pp. 4, 5, 9, 11.

Walpole, Ronald E. *Elementary Statistical Concepts.* New York: Macmillan, 1976, pp. 14–22, 27.

Wilson, C. N. and P. W. Cavnar. "The Economic Impact of OSHA's Proposed Rule on Occupational Exposure to Bloodborne Pathogens." *Lab. Med.*, Vol. 23, No. 1, January, 1992, pp. 29–32.

Winkel, Per and Bernard E. Statland. "Interpreting Laboratory Results: Reference Values and Decision Making," in *Clinical Diagnosis and Management by Laboratory Methods* (18th edition). John B. Henry (ed.). Philadelphia: Saunders, 1991, pp. 49–67.

Wong, E. S., et al. "Are Universal Precautions Effective in Reducing the Number of Occupational Exposures Among Health Care Workers?" *JAMA*, Vol. 265, No. 9, March 6, 1991, pp. 1123–1128.

Wood, A. J. J. "Management of Occupational Exposures to Blood-Borne Viruses." *N. Engl. J. Med.*, Vol. 332, No. 7, February 16, 1995, pp. 444–451.

REVIEW QUESTIONS

1. The function (or functions) of a hematology laboratory is (are):

   A. Confirm physician's impression of a possible hematological disorder.

   B. Establish or rule out a diagnosis.

   C. Screen for asymptomatic disorders.

   D. All of the above.

2. The major intended purpose of the laboratory safety manual is:

   A. To protect the patient and laboratory personnel.

   B. To protect laboratory and other hospital personnel.

   C. To comply with local health and state regulatory requirements.

   D. To comply with OSHA regulations.

3. Which of the following chemicals has been replaced in laboratory tests because of carcinogenic potential?

   A. Benzidine.   C. Ether.

   B. Chloroform.   D. Methanol.

4. Which of the following is *not* an appropriate safety practice?

   A. Disposing of needles in biohazard, puncture-proof containers.

   B. Frequent handwashing.

   C. Sterilizing lancets for reuse.

   D. Keeping food out of the same areas as specimens.

5. If a blood specimen is spilled on a laboratory bench or floor area, the first step in cleanup should be:

   A. Wear gloves and a lab coat.

   B. Absorb blood with disposable towels.

   C. Clean with freshly prepared 1% chlorine solution.

   D. Wash with water.

6. Which of the following procedures is the most basic and effective in preventing nosocomial infections?

   A. Washing hands between patient contacts.

   B. Wearing laboratory coats.

   C. Isolating infectious patients.

   D. Isolating infectious specimens.

7. The laboratory procedure manual does *not* need to include:

   A. Test method, principle of the test, and clinical applications.

   B. Specimen collection and storage procedures.

   C. The name of the supplier of common laboratory chemicals.

   D. Quality control techniques, procedures, normal values, and technical sources of error.

8. Which of the following statements is *not* a nonanalytical factor in a quality assurance system?

   A. Qualified personnel and established laboratory policies.

   B. Monitoring the standard deviation and reporting results of normal and abnormal controls.

   C. Maintenance of a procedure manual and the use of appropriate methodology.

   D. Preventive maintenance of equipment and correct specimen collection.

9. In which of the following laboratory situations is a verbal report *permissible*?

   A. When the patient is going directly to the physician's office and would like to have the report available.

   B. When the report cannot be found at the nurse's station.

   C. When preoperative test results are needed by the anesthesiologist.

   D. None of the above.

Questions 10 through 12: match the following terms with the best description.

10. _B_ Accuracy.   A. The value is known.

11. _D_ Calibration.   B. Closeness to the *true* value.

12. _A_ Control.   C. The process of monitoring accuracy.

                                D. Comparison to a known physical constant.

Questions 13 through 15: match the following terms with the best description.

13. _A_ Precision.   A. How close test results are when repeated.

14. _B_ Standards.   B. A purified substance of a known composition.

15. _C_ Quality control.   C. The process of monitoring accuracy and reproducibility of known control results.

                                D. The value is unknown.

16. Which of the following is *not* a function of a quantitative quality control program?

    A. Monitors the correct functioning of equipment, reagents, and individual technique.
    B. Confirms the correct identity of patient specimens.
    C. Compares the accuracy of controls to reference values.
    D. Detects shifts in control values.

Questions 17 through 20: match the following terms with the appropriate description.

17. ___ Mean.
18. ___ Range.
19. ___ Variance.
20. ___ Standard deviation.

A. The difference between the upper and lower measurements in a series of results.
B. The expression of the position of each test result to the average.
C. The arithmetic average.
D. The degree to which test data vary about the average.

21. The coefficient of variation is the:

    A. Sum of the squared differences from the mean.
    B. Square root of the variance from the mean.
    C. Standard deviation expressed as a percentage of the mean.
    D. The degree to which test data vary about the average.

22. The z score measures:

    A. How many standard deviations a particular number is from the right or left of the mean.
    B. Sum of the squared differences from the mean.
    C. Square root of the variance from the mean.
    D. The expression of the position of each test result to the average.

23. Acceptable limits of a control value must fall:

    A. Within ±1 standard deviation of the mean.
    B. Between 1 and 2 standard deviations of the mean.
    C. Within ±2 standard deviations of the mean.
    D. Within ±3 standard deviations of the mean.

24. A trend change in quality control data is:

    A. A progressive change all in one direction away from the mean for at least 3 days.
    B. An abrupt shift in the control values.
    C. Scattered variations from the mean.
    D. A progressive change in various directions away from the mean for at least a week.

25. A continuously increasing downward variation in a control sample in one direction from the mean can indicate:

    A. Deterioration of reagents used in the test.
    B. Deterioration of the control specimen.
    C. Deterioration of a component in an instrument.
    D. All of the above.

26. Which of the following statements is true of a Gaussian curve?

    A. It represents the standard deviation.
    B. It represents the coefficient of variation.
    C. It represents variance of a population.
    D. It represents a normal bell-shaped distribution.

27. Two standard deviations (2 SD) from the mean in a normal distribution curve would include:

    A. 99% of all values.
    B. 95% of all values.
    C. 75% of all values.
    D. 68% of all values.

Principles of Blood Collection

OBJECTIVES

Introduction
- Describe the importance of treating the patient with excellent interpersonal skills as well the collection of a blood specimen.

Blood collection supplies and equipment
- Name the major potential type of error in specimen collection.
- Name the three anticoagulants most commonly used in hematology and briefly explain their mode of action.
- Compare the color codes of evacuated tubes with the additive contained in the tube.
- Describe the equipment used for venous blood collection.
- Explain various considerations to meet specimen handling requirements.

Blood collection techniques
- Describe the proper technique for the collection of a venous blood specimen.
- Name and explain five specific venipuncture site selection situations.
- Name and describe the solutions to eight typical phlebotomy problems.
- Explain some techniques for obtaining blood from small or difficult veins.
- Describe special considerations for pediatric and geriatric patients in the collection of a blood specimen.

- Name the six categories of phlebotomy complications and describe the symptoms and treatment for each type of complication.
- Describe the proper technique for the collection of a capillary blood specimen.

Preparation of a blood smear
- Describe the procedure for preparing a push-wedge blood smear.
- List the characteristics of a good push-wedge smear.
- Explain the factors that influence the preparation of a high-quality push-wedge blood smear.
- Describe the coverslip method of blood film preparation.

Special collection procedures
- Describe the purpose and use of the Unopette system.
- Name the appropriate sites for bone marrow aspiration in adults and children.
- Explain the proper technique for preparing bone marrow specimens.

Routine staining of peripheral blood films
- Explain the principle of the Wright stain.
- Cite the reasons Romanowsky-type stains produce too red or too blue an appearance on microscopic examination of blood cells.
- Describe the manual procedure of the Wright stain, including sources of error in the technique.

INTRODUCTION

The role of the phlebotomist has never been more important. More than two thirds of laboratory errors are due to preanalytical mistakes. Most of these mistakes are related to specimen collection and handling. Phlebotomists can reduce these mistakes by being well trained and constantly alert to sources of error.

In addition, the phlebotomist is usually the only laboratory staff member that a patient sees. This means that the professional image of the laboratory is solely represented by the phlebotomist.

The phlebotomist is expected to deliver unexcelled customer satisfaction. It is important to understand and know the patient's expectations, manage unrealistic expectations through patient education, and be diplomatic with customer complaints. If a patient is unhappy, sincerely apologize and listen to find out about the details of the problem. Be sure to understand and confirm the problem, act on the complaint, keep your promises, and follow-up on resolution of the problem.

Pediatric Considerations. When working with children, it is important to be gentle and treat them with compassion, empathy, and kindness. Attempt to interact with the pediatric patient, realizing that both the patient and the parent (if present) may have anxiety about the procedure and be unfamiliar with the new settings. Acknowledge the parent as well as the child. Be friendly, courteous, and responsive. Allow enough time for the procedure.

Adolescent Patients. When obtaining a blood specimen from an adolescent, it is important to be relaxed and perceptive about any anxiety that he or she may have. General interaction techniques include allowing enough time for the procedure, establishing eye contact, and allowing the patient to maintain a sense of control.

Geriatric Patients. It is extremely important to treat geriatric patients with dignity and respect for their age. Do not demean the patient. It is best to address the patient with a more formal title such as Mrs., Ms., or Mr. rather than by his or her first name.

Senior patients may enjoy a short conversation. Keep a flexible agenda so that enough time is allowed for the patient. Speak slowly because elderly patients are frequently hearing-impaired. Allow enough time for questions. The elderly have the right of informed consent. Too many times this fact is lost in dealing with any patient, but it seems more prevalent in dealing with aging patients.

BLOOD COLLECTION SUPPLIES AND EQUIPMENT

In order to make the phlebotomy procedure easier for the technician, the following suggestions should be remembered:

- Have supplies prepared and at hand.
- Know the minimal acceptable amount of blood for an individual assay or a group of assays.
- Know the minimal acceptable amount of blood for each type of evacuated tube.
- Have a plan and an alternative plan in mind each time a phlebotomy procedure is preformed.

A properly collected blood specimen is essential to quality performance in the laboratory. Strict adherence to the rules of specimen collection is critical to the accuracy of any test. Preanalytical errors such as identification errors, either of the patient or of the specimen, are major potential sources of error.

For hematological studies, anticoagulated blood is the type of specimen most frequently used. When fresh whole blood is mixed with substances that prevent blood clotting, **anticoagulants,** the blood can be separated into **plasma,** a straw-colored fluid, and the cellular components: erythrocytes, leukocytes, and platelets (thrombocytes). Whole blood that is allowed to clot normally produces the straw-colored fluid **serum.**

Anticoagulants

Three types of anticoagulants are commonly used in the hematology laboratory: tripotassium ethylenediaminetetraacetate (EDTA), heparin, and sodium citrate. Each of the anticoagulant types prevents the coagulation of whole blood in a specific manner. The proper proportion of anticoagulant to whole blood is important in order to avoid the introduction of errors into test results. The specific type of anticoagulant needed for a procedure should be stated in the laboratory procedure manual.

Another anticoagulant, ammonium-potassium oxalate (double oxalate), is no longer in general use in the hematology laboratory. Among the disadvantages of ammonium-potassium oxalate is the fact it rapidly causes crenation of erythrocytes and vacuolization or distortion of leukocytes on blood smears.

EDTA (K3 EDTA) is tripotassium ethylenediaminetetraacetate. It may be referred to as Versene or Sequestrene. EDTA is used in concentrations of 1.5 mg per 1 mL of whole blood. The mode of action of this anticoagulant is that it removes ionized calcium (Ca^{2+}) through a process referred to as chelation. This process forms an insoluble calcium salt that prevents blood coagulation. EDTA is the most commonly used anticoagulant in hematology for tests such as the complete blood cell count (CBC) or any of its component tests (hemoglobin, packed cell volume-microhematocrit, total leukocyte count, and leukocyte differential count) and platelet count. The proper ratio of EDTA to whole blood is important because some test results will be altered if the ratio is incorrect. Excessive EDTA produces shrinkage of erythrocytes, thus affecting tests such as the manually performed packed cell volume-microhematocrit.

Heparin is used as an anticoagulant in a concentration of 0.2 mL of saturated heparin per 1 mL of whole blood. It acts as an antithrombin, or substance that inactivates the blood-clotting factor thrombin. This inactivation of thrombin is caused by the interaction of heparin with the antithrombin III molecule, which can inhibit the action of thrombin and the subsequent formation of blood clots. Heparin is the preferred anticoagulant for the osmotic fragility test and is used to coat micro (capillary blood) collection tubes. It is an inappropriate anticoagulant for many hematological tests, including Wright-stained blood smears, because the smear will stain too blue.

Sodium citrate in the concentration of a 3.2% solution has been adopted by the International Committee for Standardization in Hematology and the International Society for Thrombosis and Hemostasis as the appropriate concentration. Tubes containing 3.2% trisodium citrate replace those with 3.8% solution previously used for coagulation studies. Sodium citrate removes calcium from the coagulation system by precipitating it into an unusable form. This anticoagulant is used for many coagulation assays and for the Westergren erythrocyte sedimentation rate (ESR). The correct ratio of one part anticoagulant to nine parts of whole blood in blood collection tubes is critical. An excess of anticoagulant can alter the expected dilution of blood and produce errors in the results. Because of the dilution of anticoagulant to blood, sodium citrate is generally unacceptable for most other hematology tests.

Blood Collection Equipment

Needles

The standard needle for blood collection with a syringe or evacuated blood collection tubes is a 21G needle. Needles themselves haven't changed much yet regarding safety features. However, the Puncture-guard (Bio-Plexus, Tolland, CT, available through Baxter Scientific) blunts needles after venipuncture through passive use of a blunting member advanced through the needle bore. As more awareness is directed toward safety issues, look for use of this type of needle to increase.

Butterfly needles are being used more frequently as the acuity of patients increases. Newer designs of this equipment are reducing the incidence of postphlebotomy needle stick. The Safety-Lok (BD Vacutainer Systems) allows the needle to be retracted and locked into a protective shield when the venipuncture is completed. Another product, the Shamrock Safety Winged Set (Winfield Industries, San Diego, CA) features a retractable needle with an audible locking mechanism. A luer hub connects to the syringe or multiple tube collection device.

Evacuated Blood Collection Tubes

Evacuated tubes are the most widely used system for collecting venous blood samples. This system (Fig. 2.1) consists of a collection needle, a holder, and a glass tube containing enough vacuum to draw a specific amount of blood.

The collecting needle is a double-pointed needle. The longer end is for insertion into the patient's vein, and the shorter end pierces the rubber stopper of the collection tube. Sterile needles that fit a standard holder are used. Various needle sizes are available. In addition to length, needles are noted by gauge size. The higher the gauge number, the smaller the inner diameter, or bore. These double-pointed needles are either single-sample or multiple-sample types. The multiple-sample type has a short rubber sleeve on the short end of the needle, which punctures the rubber stopper. The rubber sleeve prevents blood from leaving the system when more than one evacuated tube is needed for testing.

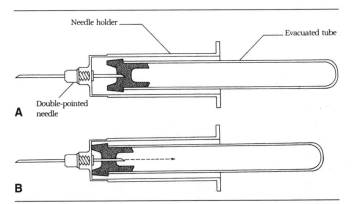

FIGURE 2.1 Evacuated tube system. **A.** The end of the double-pointed needle is partially inserted into the rubber stopper. This is the preferred position of the needle prior to entering the blood vessel. **B.** After the opposite end of the needle successfully enters the blood vessel, the evacuated tube is gently pushed until the partially inserted needle fully pierces the rubber stopper. This allows the blood to enter the evacuated tube.

The specially designed needle holder is used to secure the needle. This holder can be washed and reused. Phlebotomists should be aware of the fact that the highest accidental needle sticks occur with the use of needle holders. This may be due to their prevalence of use, design, or reusable nature. A number of needle holders, most of them disposable, have recently come on the market to protect users from postphlebotomy needle sticks. A one-handed technique (Needle Pro, Smith Industries, Keene, NH) allows a protective shield to be snapped securely over the needle after use. Another, the disposable Safety-Lok needle holder (BD Vacutainer Systems), permanently retracts the needle into a holder after use. The company also offers a reusable needle holder, the Safety Guard. It uses a one-handed needle shielding feature. In addition, the Saf-T Clik needle (Winfield Industries) is retracted and locked into a holder after use. It can be activated with one hand.

Evacuated tubes come in various (mL) sizes, including pediatric sizes, with color-coded stoppers. The stopper color denotes the type of anticoagulant or the presence of a gel separator (Table 2.1). The use of plastic tubes is becoming more widespread. Evacuated tubes are intended for one-time use. Use of the evacuated tubes with the double-pointed collection needles makes possible a closed sterile system for specimen collection. This preserves the quality of the specimen during transport prior to testing and protects the patient from infection.

TABLE 2.1 Color Codes for Evacuated Tubes and Anticoagulants

Color	Anticoagulant
Lavender	EDTA
Green	Heparin
Blue	Sodium citrate
Red	None

Syringe Technique

Disposable plastic syringes are used for special cases of venous blood collection. Such a syringe has a sterile disposable needle with a hub that attaches to the syringe. The syringe consists of a plunger and a barrel that is graduated into fractions of a milliliter. If a patient has particularly difficult veins, or if other special circumstances exist, the syringe technique may be used.

Capillary Blood Collection

Several types of micro collection tubes are available for use in capillary blood collection. Normally, the microhematocrit type of capillary tube is the most frequently used. This small tube may be heparinized or plain. For special tests, a 100 or 200 lambda micropipette may be used.

Laser Equipment

Laser technology is the first radical change in phlebotomy in more than 100 years. The risk of an accidental needle stick haunts every phlebotomist. But two new revolutionary devices (Fig. 2.2) received approval from the Food and Drug Administration (FDA) in 1997. The Laser Lancet™ (Transmedica International, Inc.) and Lasette™ (Cell Robotics) can draw blood without the use of sharp objects.

The Laser Lancet is intended for use by professional health care providers for the perforation of skin to draw capillary blood for screening purposes; the Lasette laser finger perforator is for all adults in a clinical setting, including diabetic patients.

Both devices emit a pulse of light energy that lasts a minuscule fraction of a second. The laser concentrates on a very small portion of skin, literally vaporizing the tissue about 1 to 2 mm to the capillary bed. Both devices can draw a 100-μL blood sample, a sufficient amount for certain tests.

The laser process is less painful and heals faster than when blood is drawn with traditional lancets. The patient feels a sensation similar to heat, as opposed to the prick of a sharp object.

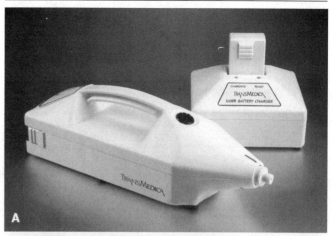

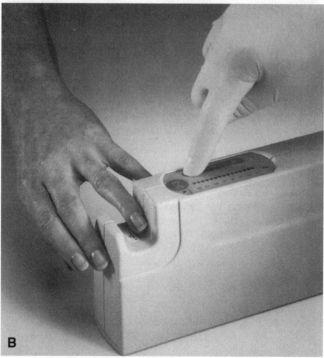

FIGURE 2.2 **A.** The Laser Lancet™ (TRANSMEDICA International, Inc.). **B.** The Lasette™ (Cell Robotics, Inc.).

Specimen Handling Requirements

The proper handling of blood and body fluids is critical to the accuracy of laboratory results. In addition, the safety of all individuals who come in contact with specimens must be guaranteed.

If a blood specimen is to be shipped by public transport, the shipping container must meet the requirements for shipping clinical specimens and infectious substances. If the specimen is less than 50 mL (five 10-mL containers), a product, SAFETEX Tube, is a newly FDA-approved Class I medical device with general controls for transporting medical materials and clinical and diagnostic specimens. This product is particularly useful because it eliminates the need for paperwork associated with shipping more than 50 mL of blood or body fluid specimens.

Greater quantities of specimen or other shipping containers must meet the packaging requirements of major couriers and Department of Transportation hazardous materials regulations. Approved reclosable plastic bags for handling biohazard specimens and amber bags for specimens for analysis of light-sensitive drugs are available. These bags must be approved to meet National Committee for Clinical Laboratory Standards (NCCLS) M29-T2 specimen handling guidelines—"Protection of Laboratory Workers from Infectious Disease Transmitted by Blood, Body Fluids and Tissue" (2nd edition) and OSHA Fed. Reg. 29 CAR 1910.1030 Blood borne Pathogens for containment and biohazard graphics. Approved bags such as LabGuard™ Reclosable Bags have bright orange and black graphics that clearly identify bags as holding hazardous materials.

Some products have an additional marking area that allows phlebotomists to identify contents that must be kept frozen, refrigerated, or at room temperature.

Maintaining specimens at the correct preanalytical temperature is extremely important. Products such as the Insul-Tote (Palco Labs) are convenient for specimen transport from the field to the clinical lab. This particular product has a reusable cold gel pack that keeps temperatures below 70°F for 8 hours even if the exterior temperature is above 100°F.

BLOOD COLLECTION TECHNIQUES

The two sources of blood for examination in the hematology laboratory are venous blood and capillary blood. Although arterial blood may be needed to perform procedures such as blood gas analysis, this procedure is not usually performed in the hematology laboratory. In order to obtain quality specimens for assay, strict adherence to proper specimen collection is necessary.

General Protocol

1. All medical personnel should pleasantly introduce themselves to the patient and briefly explain the procedure that is to be performed, in easy-to-understand terms.
2. Patient identification is the *critical* first step in blood collection. It is necessary both to ask the patient's name and to check the identification band that is physically attached to the patient. When the patient is unable to give his or her name, or when identification is attached to the bed or is missing, nursing personnel should be asked to physically identify the patient. Verbal identification of a patient should be noted on the test requisition.
3. Test requisitions should be checked and the appropriate equipment assembled. The type of evacuated tubes and proper transport of the specimen should be confirmed.
4. All specimens should be properly labeled *immediately after* the specimen is drawn. Prelabeling is unwise because an unsuccessful attempt to obtain blood results in a labeled tube or tubes in a collection tray that could inadvertently be used for another patient.

Capillary blood collection is performed with a sterile, disposable lancet. These lancets are individually wrapped and should be properly discarded in a puncture-proof container after a single use.

Venous Blood Collection (Phlebotomy)

Supplies and Equipment

1. Test requisition
2. Tourniquet and disposable gloves
3. Alcohol (70%) and gauze square or alcohol wipes
4. Sterile disposable needles (double-pointed or syringe type)
5. Evacuated blood tubes (appropriate to the test ordered) and a needle holder or a syringe (in special cases)
6. Any special equipment such as a stopwatch or warm water—refer to equipment required for special procedures
7. Spirits of ammonia breakable capsule (emergency use only)
8. Adhesive plastic strips or spots

Initiation of the Procedure

1. Identify the patient.
2. Assemble all necessary equipment at the patient's bedside.
3. Put on gloves.
4. If a needle and syringe are to be used, firmly secure the hub of the needle with its shield in place on the syringe. If an evacuated tube is to be used, screw the short end of the needle on the needle holder. The plastic shield is to remain on the needle until *immediately* prior to the venipuncture. The evacuated tube is placed into the holder and gently pushed until the top of the stopper reaches the guideline on the holder. *Note:* Do not push the tube all the way into the holder, or a loss of vacuum will result.

Selection of an Appropriate Site

Note: Venous blood should not be drawn near an intravenous (IV) infusion. It is preferable to draw the sample from the opposite arm, if possible, or from below the infusion site. If possible, the IV infusion should be shut off for 2 to 3 minutes before the sample is drawn. It should be noted on the test requisition whether the sample was drawn from below an IV site as well as the type of solution being administered. Obtaining a blood specimen from an IV line should be avoided because it increases the risk of mixing the fluid with the blood sample and producing incorrect test results.

1. Visually inspect both arms. Choose the arm that has not been repeatedly used for venipunctures and one that is free of bruises, abrasions, and sites of infection. In the arm, three veins are commonly used for venipuncture: the cephalic, basilic, and median cubital veins (Fig. 2.3).
2. Applying the tourniquet. Two general types of tourniquets are available. One type is a flat or rounded rubber tube, and the other has Velcro ends for simple adjustment to the arm.
   A. If a rubber tourniquet is used, slide the tourniquet under the arm a few inches above the expected venipuncture site. Evenly adjust both ends of the tourniquet (Fig. 2.4A).
   B. Grasp both ends of the tourniquet a few inches above the patient's arm. Pull up on the ends to create tension in the tourniquet. Cross the right side of the tourniquet over the left side. With the index finger of the right hand, create a small loop in the right side of the tourniquet while continuing to hold tension in the tourniquet (see Fig. 2.4B).
   C. Slip this small loop under the left side of the tourniquet. The resulting application will allow for easy removal of the tourniquet with one hand, after the needle has been inserted into the vein (see Fig. 2.4C). *Note:* Prolonged tourniquet application can elevate certain blood chemistry analytes. These are albumin, aspartate aminotransferase (AST), calcium, cholesterol, iron, lipids, total bilirubin, and total protein.

(continued)

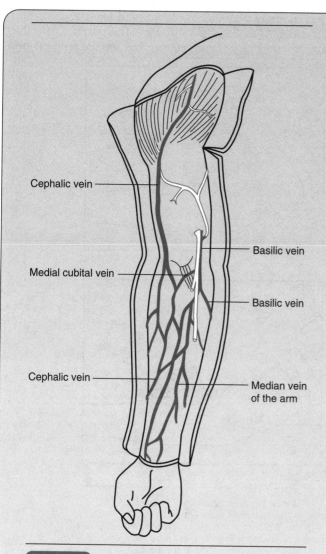

FIGURE 2.3 Anatomy of the veins of the arm. In the arm, three veins can be used for venipuncture: the cephalic, basilic, and median cubital veins.

Cephalic vein

Medial cubital vein

Cephalic vein

Basilic vein

Basilic vein

Median vein of the arm

3. Ask the patient to make a fist (sometimes a roll of gauze is placed in the patient's hand). This usually makes the veins more prominent. With the index finger, palpate (feel) for an appropriate vein (see Fig. 2.4D). Palpation is important for identifying the vein, which has a resilient feeling compared with the surrounding tissues. Large veins are not always a good choice because they have a tendency to roll as you attempt the venipuncture. Superficial and small veins should also be avoided. The ideal site is generally near or slightly below the bend in the arm. If no appropriate veins are found in one arm, examine the other arm by applying the tourniquet and palpating the arm. Do not leave the tourniquet on for more than 2 minutes. Veins in other areas such as the wrist, hands, and feet can be used as venipuncture sites; however, only experienced phlebotomists should use them.

Special Site Selection Situations

Five specific situations can create the potential for a difficult venipuncture or are potential sources of preanalytical error. These situations are:

1. Edema of the extremities
2. Intravenous lines
3. Scarring or burn patients
4. Dialysis patients
5. Postmastectomy patients

Edema

Edema is the abnormal accumulation of fluid in the intracellular spaces of the tissue. Venipuncture should not be performed in edematous areas because the extra fluid can make it difficult to palpate the veins and the specimen may be contaminated with the fluid and produce erroneous test results.

Intravenous Lines

Patients with fluid running in intravenous lines in their arms pose a common problem to phlebotomists. A limb with an IV running should not be used for venipuncture because of contamination to the specimen. The patient's other arm or an alternate site should be selected. If no alternate site can be found, the IV should be turned off by the physician and blood can be drawn from below the infusion site after a few minutes. The contents of the IV fluid should be documented on the requisition. After completing the venipuncture, the appropriate person should be notified to restart the infusion.

Scarring or Burn Patients

Veins are very difficult to palpate in areas where there is extensive scarring or burns. Burn areas also are more susceptible to infection because the protective barrier (the epidermis) has been disrupted. Venipunctures performed at these sites are unusually painful for the patient. Alternate sites or capillary blood collection should be used.

Dialysis Patients

Dialysis patients pose special problems when it comes to blood collection: frequency of testing and limited vein access. Blood should never be drawn from a vein in an arm with a cannula (temporary dialysis access device) or fistula (a permanent surgical fusion of a vein and an artery).

A trained staff member can draw blood from a cannula. Blood should never be drawn from a fistula or from a vein in an arm with a fistula. The preferred venipuncture site is a hand vein or a vein away from the fistula on the underside of the arm. In this case, a tourniquet may be used below the fistula but should be released as soon as the vein has been located.

In addition, special precautions should be taken to ensure that the dialysis patient does not bleed from the venipuncture site since most of these patients are medicated with heparin.

Mastectomy Patients

If a mastectomy patient has had lymph nodes adjacent to the breast removed, lymphostasis (a lack of flow of lymphatic fluids in the affected area) results. Specimens drawn from the affected side of the body may not be representative. In addition, the patient is much more susceptible to infections. Therefore, venipuncture should not be performed on the same side as the mastectomy.

Preparation of the Venipuncture Site

1. After an appropriate site has been chosen, release the tourniquet.

(continued)

BLOOD COLLECTION TECHNIQUES (continued)

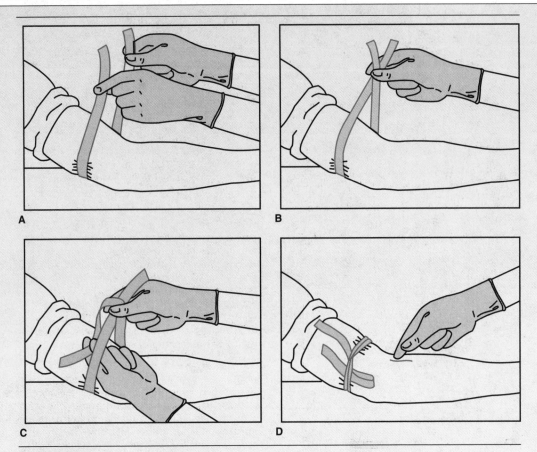

FIGURE 2.4 Selection of appropriate venipuncture site. **A.** Tourniquet adjustment: adjust both ends of the tourniquet evenly. **B** and **C.** Applying the tourniquet. Place tension on the tourniquet, cross one side over the other, and slip a small loop under one side of the tourniquet. A properly applied tourniquet can be removed with one hand by simply pulling on one end of it. **D.** Palpating the site. The index finger is used to feel for a suitable vein. This is the ideal site for venipuncture, usually near or slightly below the bend in the arm.

2. Using a cotton ball saturated with 70% alcohol or an alcohol pad saturated with 70% alcohol, cleanse the skin in the area of the venipuncture site. Using a circular motion, clean the area from the center and move outward. Do not go back over an area once it has been cleansed.
3. Allow the site to dry.

Performing the Venipuncture
Note: It is preferable to avoid touching the cleansed venipuncture site. In unusual situations, it may be allowable to touch the area with an alcohol-wiped finger to reestablish the location of the vein.

1. Use one hand to hold the evacuated tube assembly or syringe. Use one or more fingers of the other hand to secure the skin area of the forearm below the intended venipuncture site. This will tighten the skin and secure the vein. Position the patient's arm in a slightly downward position.
2. Hold the needle with attached syringe or evacuated tube about 1 to 2 inches below and in a straight line with the intended venipuncture site. Position the blood drawing unit at

an angle of about 20 degrees. The bevel of the needle should be upward.
3. Gently insert the needle through the skin and into the vein. This insertion motion should be smooth. If an evacuated tube is used, one hand should steady the needle holder unit while the other hand pushes the tube to the end of the plastic holder. It is important to hold the needle still during the collection process to avoid interrupting the flow of blood.

Multiple samples can be drawn by inserting each additional tube as soon as the tube attached to the needle holder has filled. The NCCLS standards for the order of drawing multiple evacuated tubes are:

1. Blood culture tubes (yellow top) or blood culture bottles
2. Nonadditive or serum tubes (red top)
3. Coagulation tubes (light blue top)
4. Additive tubes (green, lavender, gray, or gel separator tubes—mottled top)

To decrease the chance of bacterial contamination, blood cultures are always collected first.

(continued)

If a syringe is used, one hand should steady the barrel of the syringe while the other hand slowly pulls the plunger backwards.

Termination of the Procedure

1. The tourniquet may be released as soon as the blood begins to flow into the evacuated tube or syringe or immediately before the final amount of blood is drawn.
2. Ask the patient to open the hand.
3. After the desired amount of blood has been drawn, place a gauze pad over the venipuncture site.

4. Withdraw the blood collecting unit with one hand and *immediately* press down on the gauze pad with the other hand (Fig. 2.5).
5. If possible, have the patient elevate the entire arm and press on the gauze pad with the opposite hand. If the patient is unable to do this, apply pressure until bleeding ceases.
6. Place a nonallergenic adhesive spot or strip over the venipuncture site. *Note:* Failure to apply sufficient pressure to the venipuncture site could result in a **hematoma** (a collection of blood under the skin that produces a bruise).

(continued)

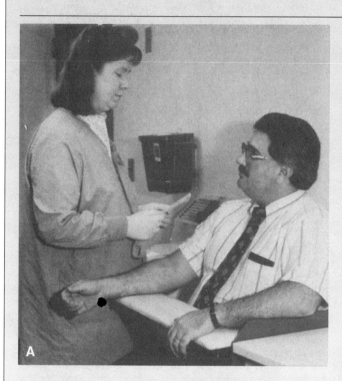

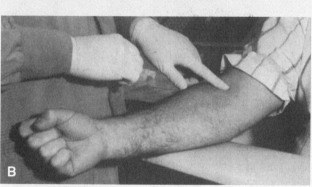

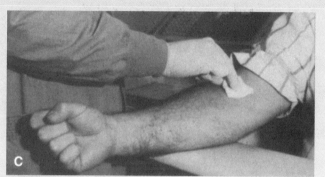

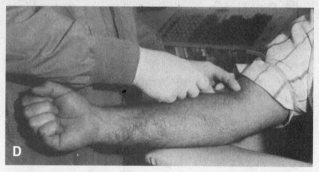

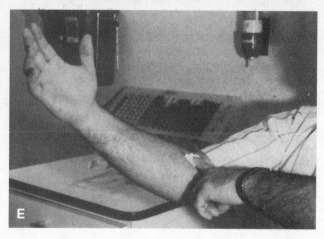

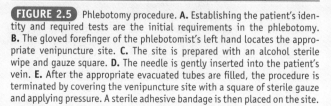

FIGURE 2.5 Phlebotomy procedure. **A.** Establishing the patient's identity and required tests are the initial requirements in the phlebotomy. **B.** The gloved forefinger of the phlebotomist's left hand locates the appropriate venipuncture site. **C.** The site is prepared with an alcohol sterile wipe and gauze square. **D.** The needle is gently inserted into the patient's vein. **E.** After the appropriate evacuated tubes are filled, the procedure is terminated by covering the venipuncture site with a square of sterile gauze and applying pressure. A sterile adhesive bandage is then placed on the site.

BLOOD COLLECTION TECHNIQUES (continued)

7. Mix tubes with anticoagulant by inverting the tubes several times. If a syringe was used, carefully remove the needle before dispensing the blood into a test tube. Blood should never be forced back through the needle, and the syringe plunger should be slowly depressed. Discard the used needle into an appropriate safety container.
8. Label all test tubes as required by the laboratory.
9. Clean up supplies from the work area, remove gloves, and wash hands. *Note:* If the patient is an outpatient, wait a few minutes after the venipuncture is complete, and check to be sure that the patient does not feel dizzy or nauseated before discharge. Discard all contaminated supplies in a biohazard disposal bag.

Phlebotomy Problems

Occasionally, a venipuncture is unsuccessful. Do not attempt to perform the venipuncture more than two times. If two attempts are unsuccessful, notify the hematology supervisor. Problems encountered in phlebotomy can include the following:

1. Refusal by the patient to have blood drawn. The response to this problem is to politely excuse yourself from the patient's room, note the refusal on the requisition, and notify the hematology supervisor.
2. Difficulty in obtaining a specimen because the bore of the needle is against the wall of the vein. Slightly pulling back on the needle may solve this problem.
3. Movement of the vein. To guard against this problem, always have firm pressure on the arm below the intended venipuncture site. The needle can be moved to reach the vein, but *excessive* probing in the tissues must be avoided. Care must be exercised in moving the needle because a *hematoma* can form if both sides of the vessel wall are pierced.
4. An inadequate amount of blood in an evacuated tube. A "short-draw," or lack of complete filling of an anticoagulated tube, can produce errors in test results. An excessive amount of EDTA will produce shrinkage of erythrocytes, and an insufficient amount of blood in a sodium citrate tube will introduce a dilutional problem if the specimen is tested for coagulation studies.
5. Improper anticoagulant. In most cases, anticoagulants cannot be substituted in a test. For example, blood smears cannot be prepared from a heparinized blood sample because with Wright stain the erythrocytes will stain too blue.
6. Sudden movement by the patient or phlebotomist that causes the needle to come out of the arm prematurely. Always anticipate this possibility. Quick action is needed! Immediately remove the tourniquet, place a gauze pad on the venipuncture site and apply pressure until bleeding has stopped to prevent the formation of a hematoma. It is a good practice to have easy access to gauze pads whenever a venipuncture is being performed.
7. Blood clot formation in anticoagulated tubes. In the phlebotomy procedure, red-top (plain) evacuated tubes should be drawn *first.* Promptly after termination of the venipuncture procedure, any tubes containing an anticoagulant should be gently inverted several times to mix the specimen.
8. Fainting or illness subsequent to venipuncture. The first aid procedures of the laboratory should be practiced in this event. It is very important to prevent injury to the patient because of fainting or dizziness.

Ten Tips for Locating and Drawing From Difficult or Small Veins

It is not uncommon to have difficulty drawing a venous blood specimen. Tips for locating or drawing blood from difficult or small veins are:

1. Adjust the position of the arm.
2. Use a smaller gauge needle.
3. Use a small syringe.
4. Use a butterfly needle and multiple small syringes.
5. Tighten the tourniquet.
6. Loosen the tourniquet.
7. Apply hot packs to the arm.
8. Use a second tourniquet below the site.
9. Use a hand or wrist vein or veins on underside of the arm.
10. Use a transilluminator device to identify the location of a vein.

Special Considerations for Pediatric and Geriatric Patients

Pediatric Patients

A phlebotomist should consider the limitations of their skills and self-confidence and consult with their immediate supervisor before attempting a difficult phlebotomy.

Table 2.2 lists some general tips in performing pediatric phlebotomy. Premature infants do not tolerate prolonged agitation or stimulation, so procedures should be done swiftly and efficiently. The amount of blood needed should be considered before selecting the site. It is also very important to examine all possible sites for venipuncture, if an obvious vein is not initially determined. Under no circumstances should a venipuncture be attempted on a child if the phlebotomist is uncertain of the vein or the feasibility of collecting all of the ordered tests in one needle stick.

Phlebotomists should always inspect the areas around a blood collection site for redness or bruising prior to collection of a sample. Also, excessive use of any area should be avoided and reported to the child's nurse. Warming a skin puncture site for a couple of minutes increases the blood flow up to eight times and will preclude excessive squeezing and subsequent injury. Phlebotomist should report any difference in the condition of a site if immediately noted after blood collection.

Specimens From Children Under Age 1

Guidelines should be developed and revised as needed to reflect common practice for children under 1 year of age. Competency checklists should separate when a heelstick rather than venous blood can be used for an assay.

(continued)

TABLE 2.2 **Pediatric Phlebotomy: General Tips**

- Work quickly on premature infants.
- Warm blood collection site to increase flow of blood.
- Check potential blood collection sites for redness or bruising.
- Do not attempt venipuncture unless obtaining enough blood for all of the ordered tests in one attempt is certain.
- Report any changes in the condition of the site immediately after venipuncture.

Some important points for phlebotomists who draw specimens from children under 1 year of age include:

1. Venipunctures should not be performed on children under 6 months of age unless there are specific testing requirements necessitating a venipuncture,
2. Venipunctures on infants between 6 and 12 months of age should be done if the child is of at least average weight for age and the quantity of blood and/or the assays require a venipuncture,
3. Paternity testing on newborns, infants, and children requires from 1 mL to 3 mL of whole blood. Limiting the number of staff who are trained to perform paternity testing will assure proper procedure for "chain of custody."
4. Lead levels can be drawn via capillary, but preferably are obtained by venipuncture because of the potential for contamination and the subsequent need for recollection and/or confirmation.
5. If an extensive number of tests are ordered on a small child, an experienced phlebotomist should perform the procedure.

Geriatric Patients

Aging produces physiological conditions that accentuate naturally occurring changes in the skin and subcutaneously, e.g., slower healing time and more chance of infection. Because of increased susceptibility, venipuncture site preparation becomes even more important in the elderly than in other patients.

In addition, arteries and veins change drastically with age. Blood vessels become less elastic and more fragile with aging and can be easily injured during a venipuncture attempt.

There are some important steps to consider when performing venipuncture on an elderly person. These include:

1. Carefully identify the patient. Elderly patients may be confused and disoriented.
2. Take your time locating the "perfect" spot for the venipuncture. Look at both arms, the wrists, hands, and complete forearms.
3. Never slap the arm to dilate the vein because this could cause the patient to bruise.
4. Warm up the skin if the patient's limb feels cold and clammy.
5. Be very cautious when using tourniquets or bandages because the skin is fragile. Try placing the tourniquet over clothing, which will be more comfortable for the patient.
6. Remove the tourniquet just before inserting the needle to reduce the risk of rupturing the vein and causing a hematoma.
7. Consider using a smaller gauge needle, e.g., butterfly needles to reduce trauma to the vein.
8. Use smaller pediatric vacuum tubes to reduce the vacuum draw back, if the vein is fragile and small.
9. Use one quick motion when inserting the needle—it is more effective and less painful.
10. Never probe for a vein.
11. Veins must be well anchored by holding the skin alongside the vein instead of directly over the vein before a venipuncture attempt is made. This will prevent obstructing the vein and causing it to collapse.
12. Ask for assistance from another person to prevent a hematoma, if you anticipate that the patient will not hold still during the venipuncture or will not be able to apply pressure to the site after the procedure.
13. Pay special attention to the fragility of the skin. Bandages or tape can cause the skin to become raw and develop seep-

ing areas. Elastic bandages will hold the gauze in place and not adhere to the skin.

Phlebotomy Complications

Patients can experience complications resulting from a phlebotomy procedure. These complications can be divided into six major categories: vascular (the most common), infection, cardiovascular, anemia, neurologic, and dermatologic.

Vascular Complications

Bleeding from the site of the venipuncture and hematoma formation are the most common vascular complications. The reasons for these mishaps include medications and existing medical conditions, e.g., coagulation disorders produced by a genetic defect or cancer. Bruises don't usually affect patient satisfaction. Uncommon vascular complications that are not usually related to technique include pseudoaneurysm, thrombosis, reflex arteriospasm, and arteriovenous fistula formation (Table 2.3).

Infections

The second most common complication of venipuncture is infection. The most common infectious complications are cellulitis (inflammation of tissue), and phlebitis (inflammation of vessel or infection of vessel). Other infectious complications include sepsis (infection of the blood), septic arthritis (infection of the joint space), and osteomyelitis (infection of the bone). Infection of the joint space usually occurs in children in the femoral joint after an arterial puncture. Osteomyelitis is usually associated with capillary puncture because most skin preparation regimens remove the majority of microorganisms but not all of them. Deep puncturing of the skin allows microorganisms to enter and infect the deep tissues and bone

Cardiovascular Complications

Cardiovascular complications include orthostatic hypotension, syncope, shock, and cardiac arrest.

Orthostatic hypotension results from changing from a sitting to a standing position or as the result of certain medications. The lack of a compensatory blood pressure response produces hypotension that in turn produces syncope.

(continued)

TABLE 2.3 Vascular Complications of Phlebotomy

Condition	Description
Pseudoaneurysm	A fibrous capsule around encapsulated blood due to a break in the blood vessel.
Thrombosis	Patient usually has a coagulation disorder. Thrombosis in a vein produces edema and swelling. If thrombosis is in an arterial blood vessel, a decreased oxygen supply due to impaired circulation can occur beyond the thrombus.
Reflex arteriospasm	Occurs when a needle sticks an artery. The condition prevents blood from moving through the vessel.
Arteriovenous fistula	This abnormal connection between a vein and an artery can occur after repeated venipunctures.

BLOOD COLLECTION TECHNIQUES (continued)

Syncope can be manifested as temporary loss of consciousness, fainting, lightheadedness, dizziness, sweating, or nausea. The causes of syncope include vasovagal response, arrhythmia, orthostatic hypotension, volume depletion, shock, and cardiac arrest. A vasovagal response is a neurologic response that can be triggered by emotion, stress, prolonged standing, warm temperature, fasting, pregnancy, or dehydration. The manifestations of this response are increased autonomic response, decreased heart rate and vasodilation, increased hypotension, and syncope. Treatment for syncope consists of having the patient lie down, loosening tight clothing, elevating the legs, ruling out chest pain and shortness of breath, and waiting for pressure and pulse to normalize.

Shock is manifested by the presence of cool, clammy, mottled skin; a weak and rapid pulse; and hypotension. The immediate treatment is to elevate the legs, use a warming blanket, and call a code.

Cardiac arrest manifests itself as chest pain, shortness of breath, arm or shoulder pain, nausea, and sweating. Treatment consists of *immediately* calling a code and beginning CPR efforts.

Anemia
Iatrogenic anemia is also known as nosocomial anemia, physician-induced anemia, or anemia resulting from blood loss for testing. Pediatric patients as well as adults in intensive care units and transplant patients are the most likely candidates to develop this iron deficiency anemia. The medical consequences of iatrogenic anemia are fatigue, shortness of breath, and impaired performance of physical work. In severe cases, the treatment is blood transfusion.

Neurologic Complications
Postphlebotomy patients can exhibit some neurologic complications. These include diaphoresis, seizure, pain, and nerve damage. A physician should be consulted immediately.

Dermatologic Complications
The most common dermatologic consequence of phlebotomy is an allergic reaction to iodine in the case of blood donors. Other dermatologic complications include necrosis, basal cell carcinoma (1 case described), and scarring.

....

Capillary Blood Collection

Supplies and Equipment
1. Alcohol (70%) and gauze squares or alcohol wipes
2. Disposable gloves and sterile small gauze squares
3. Sterile disposable blood lancets
4. Equipment specific to the test ordered, such as glass slides for blood smears, micropipette and diluent for CBCs, or microhematocrit tubes

Selection of an Appropriate Site
1. The fingertip (usually of the third or fourth finger), heel, and big toe are appropriate sites for the collection of small quantities of blood. The earlobe may be used as a site of last resort in adults. *Do not* puncture the skin through previous sites, which may be infected.

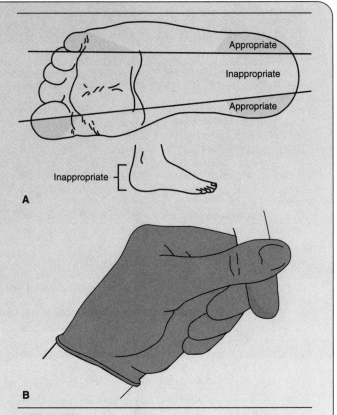

FIGURE 2.6 **A.** Heel puncture. The heel is the preferred site for drawing capillary blood from the newborn. The puncture should be in either the heel or the toe areas designated in the drawing. The posterior curvature of the heel should *never* be used. (Modified from T. A. Blumenfeld, B. K. Turi, and W. A. Blanc, "Recommended Sites and Depth of Newborn Heel Skin Punctures Based on Anatomic Measurements and Histopathology," *Lancet*, Vol. 1, 1979, p. 213.) **B.** Fingertip puncture. The shaded area is the preferred site for the collection of capillary blood from the finger.

The plantar surface (sole) of the heel or big toe is an appropriate site in infants (Fig. 2.6A) or in special cases such as burn victims. *Note:* The ideal site in infants is the medial or lateral plantar surface of the heel, with a puncture no deeper than 2.4 mm. NCCLS recommendations are not to use fingers of infants. The back of the heel should *never* be used because of the danger of injuring the heel bone. The arch should *never* be punctured because tendons, cartilage, and nerves may be injured in this area.

2. The site of blood collection must be warm to ensure the free flow of blood, otherwise the blood sample will not be truly representative of the blood in the vascular system. If necessary, massage the finger several times or place a warm cloth on the area for a few minutes to increase blood circulation to the site.

3. Osteomyelitis (infection of bone) is a potential complication in pediatric patients. This complication can be prevented by using good technique. It is important to avoid pushing too

(continued)

hard or too deeply with the lancet. Sites for the development of osteomyelitis are the heel, toes, or fingers. Treatment is long-term IV antibiotics.

Osteomyelitis can be prevented by warming an area to increase blood flow up to 5 times, selecting an appropriate site, cleansing the skin thoroughly, penetrating the skin no deeper than 2.4 mm, avoiding extra pressure, avoiding double cuts and previous puncture sites, and reducing the number of collections.

Preparation of the Site
1. Hold the area to be punctured with the thumb and index finger of a gloved hand.
2. Wipe the area with 70% alcohol and allow to air dry.
3. Wipe the area with a dry gauze square or cotton ball. If the area is not dry, the blood will not form a rounded drop and will be difficult to collect.

Puncturing the Skin
1. Use a disposable sterile lancet *once* and discard it properly in a puncture-proof container.
2. Securely hold the area and puncture once with a firm motion. The lancet should puncture across the creases of the fingerprint, not parallel with the grooves. If the finger is the chosen site, the area to be punctured should be in the portion of the finger that is rich in capillaries—not the fleshy part (see Fig. 2.6B).
3. Wipe away the first drop of blood, because it is not a true sample. The first drop of blood is mixed with lymphatic fluid and possibly alcohol.

4. Apply gentle pressure to the area to obtain subsequent drops. A good capillary puncture should require *no* forcing or hard squeezing of the site. If the site is squeezed too hard, lymphatic fluid will mix with the blood and produce inaccurate test results.

Collecting the Sample
1. If a blood smear is needed, follow the procedure in the next section of this chapter for the preparation of a push-wedge blood smear.
2. Allow micropipette or microhematocrit tubes to fill with free-flowing blood by capillary action. The tubes must be held horizontally to avoid introducing air bubbles or breaks in the column of blood.
3. If dilutions of the blood specimen are necessary, perform them promptly before the blood clots in the collecting tubes. Follow the specific methodology of the procedure to determine the quantities of diluent and whole blood that are needed.
4. Wipe the site frequently with a plain gauze square in order to prevent the accumulation of platelets, which will slow down or stop the blood flow.

Termination of the Procedure
1. Wipe the area with alcohol.
2. Place a clean gauze square on the site and apply pressure. If the patient is unable to apply pressure to the site, hold the gauze square until the bleeding has stopped.
3. Label all specimens.
4. Place the used lancet into a puncture-proof container, remove gloves, and wash hands.

PREPARATION OF A BLOOD SMEAR

The preparation of a blood smear may be conducted at the patient's bedside or in the laboratory, if EDTA-anticoagulated blood is used. Two of the most basic procedures conducted by the hematology technologist or technician are the preparation and staining of blood smears. In this section, the push-wedge and coverslip methods of blood smear preparation are presented.

The Push-Wedge Method

Specimen
Either EDTA-anticoagulated whole blood or free-flowing capillary blood can be used. If EDTA is used, smears must be prepared within *1 hour* of collection. Before preparing the smear, store the blood at 18° to 25°C. Adequate mixing is necessary before blood smear preparation.

Supplies and Equipment
Clean glass slides (plain or with one frosted end), a No. 2 lead pencil, and (optional) a specially designed pusher slide or a hemocytometer coverslip and pusher assembly.

Procedure
1. Place a small drop (0.05 mL) of well-mixed blood either directly from the freshly wiped fingertip puncture or with an applicator stick approximately 1/2 inch from one end of the slide. If frosted slides are used, place the blood near the frosted end of the slide.
2. Place the slide on a flat surface with the blood specimen to your right. Reverse this direction if left-handed.
3. Using a second pusher slide, place this slide slightly in front of the drop of blood. The angle of this pusher slide must be at approximately 45 degrees (Fig. 2.7A).
4. Draw the pusher slide back toward the drop of blood. Allow the drop of blood to spread about three-fourths of the way across the bevel of the pusher slide. Do not allow the blood to spread to the edges. Quickly push this slide forward (away from the drop). This forward movement must be smooth and continue to the end of the slide.
5. Allow the smear to air dry before staining. The slides ~~can~~ most be fanned in the air to rapidly dry them.
6. Label the slide using a No. 2 pencil. The labeling may be on the thick end (or frosted end) of the slide or on one edge of the slide.

(continued)

PREPARATION OF A BLOOD SMEAR (continued)

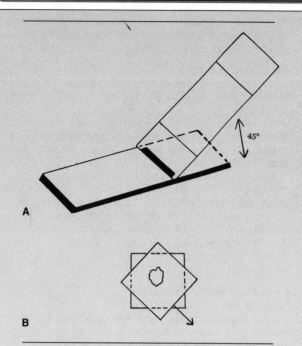

FIGURE 2.7 Push-wedge smear. **A.** Angle of slide. The proper angle of the pusher slide is approximately 45 degrees. **B.** Coverslip preparation. Once a small drop of blood has spread by capillary action between the coverslips, they should be *pulled* apart smoothly in a horizontal plane.

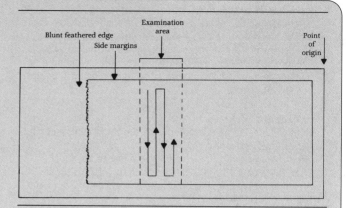

FIGURE 2.8 Ideal blood smear. An ideal peripheral blood smear should have side margins that do not touch the outer edges of the glass slide. The smear should become thinner from the point of origin to the termination in a blunt feathered edge. The area of examination and proper method of examining a blood smear are discussed in Chapter 17. (Modified from J. A. Koepke, "Standardization of the Manual Differential Leukocyte Count." *Lab. Med.*, Vol. 11, 1980, p. 371.)

Procedure Notes

1. A special pusher or spreader slide is commercially available to spread blood smears with margin-free edges. Some laboratories use a spreader device consisting of a straight artery clamp with the ends covered with rubber tubing. A rectangular (20 × 26 mm) hemocytometer coverslip is inserted between the ends of the clamp. The advantage of using a commercial spreader slide or the coverslip and pusher assembly is that the resulting smear has even slide margins that can be counted during the differential cell count.
2. The push-wedge method is recommended by NCCLS as the reference method for differential leukocyte counting.
3. Normally two smears are prepared. If free-flowing capillary blood is used, more than two smears may be desired.

Visual Evaluation of a Good Blood Smear

An ideal smear (Fig. 2.8) has the following characteristics.

1. It progresses from being thick at the point of origin to thin with a uniform edge at the termination point.
2. It does not touch the outer borders of the slide or run off the sides or ends of the slide.
3. It appears smooth, without waves or gaps.
4. It does not have any streaks, ridges, or troughs, which indicate an increased number of leukocytes carried to that area.
5. It is prepared with a proper amount of blood and spread to occupy about two-thirds of the length of the glass slide.

Causes of a Poor Blood Smear

1. Prolonged storage of anticoagulated whole-blood specimens. This can produce cellular distortion.

2. A delay in smear preparation. It is important to perform the blood smear *immediately* after placing the drop of blood on the slide. If this process is delayed, larger cells such as neutrophils and monocytes will be disproportionately located at the feathered edge when examined microscopically.
3. Dirty or poor-quality slides. Slides should be free of dust and grease spots.
4. Inappropriate size of blood droplet. Too large a drop of blood will produce a thick, long smear. Too small a drop of blood will produce a thin, short smear.
5. Improper angle of the pusher slide. The more the angle of the pusher slide is decreased, the longer the smear will be. The greater the angle, the thicker the smear will be.
6. Improper speed of the pushing movement. Slowly pushing the drop of blood will produce irregularities and affect the distribution of cells on the smear.
7. Improper pressure. The greater the pressure, the thinner the smear.
8. Humidity of the laboratory environment. High humidity can cause slides to dry too slowly. The prolonged drying of slides will produce erythrocyte distortion on microscopic examination.

Coverslip Method of Blood Film Preparation

Procedure

1. Hold two clean coverslips by their edges with the thumb and forefinger of each hand. Touch the center of one coverslip to a small drop of blood.
2. Immediately place the second coverslip on top of a very small drop of blood in a diagonal position.
3. Allow the blood to spread by capillary action. Just before the spreading action has almost stopped, evenly and smoothly

(continued)

pull the coverslips apart in the horizontal plane (see Fig. 2.7B).

4. Place the smears in an upright position and allow to air dry before staining.

Procedure Notes

1. The coverslip method produces a good distribution of leukocytes in all areas of the preparation.

2. Because of the smaller specimen amount, 50 leukocytes are counted per coverslip.

3. Owing to the small size of the coverslip, it is usually mounted (attached) to a conventional glass slide for staining.

SPECIAL COLLECTION PROCEDURES

In addition to the collection of venous or capillary blood specimens and the preparation of blood smears, some procedures are performed by the technologist or technician at the patient's bedside. Procedures such as the bleeding time are described in Chapter 24, Manual Procedures. In this section, basic procedures are described.

Capillary Blood Collection: The Unopette System

Principle

The Unopette system (Fig. 2.9) is a microsample collection system for use in certain manual or automated procedures. Different systems are available for hematological procedures such as total erythrocyte or leukocyte counts, hemoglobin assay, platelet counts, eosinophil counts, erythrocyte fragility studies, and reticulocyte counts, and for use with automated cell-counting systems.

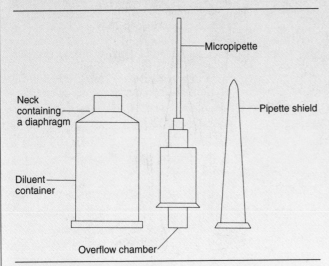

Micropipette

Pipette shield

Neck containing a diaphragm

Diluent container

Overflow chamber

FIGURE 2.9 Components of the Unopette system. The Unopette system consists of the reservoir, which contains diluent appropriate for a specific test, a microcapillary pipette, and a pipette shield. These components are manufactured of disposable plastic.

Supplies and Equipment

Although various diluents and sample sizes differ from test to test, the blood collection procedures are basically similar. Universal precautions should be practiced as required during specimen processing and the disposal of supplies. Each system consists of a capillary pipette and a reservoir containing a premeasured amount of specific diluent.

Collection and Dilution Procedure

1. Place the reservoir on a flat surface. Hold the reservoir with one hand. With the other hand, take the micropipette, covered with a pipette shield, and firmly push the tip of the pipette shield unit through the diaphragm into the neck of the reservoir.

2. Remove the pipette and shield from the neck of the reservoir. Remove the shield from the pipette.

3. Collect the free-flowing capillary blood into the pipette section using the technique described in the procedure for collection of capillary blood. When the pipette has filled up to the end of the capillary bore in the neck of the pipette, it will no longer draw any more blood.

4. Wipe any excess blood from the outside of the pipette, being careful not to touch the blood sample in the capillary tube.

5. While squeezing the reservoir slightly with one hand, cover the flagged end of the pipette with the index finger of the other hand and insert the capillary pipette into the reservoir.

6. Simultaneously, release the pressure on the reservoir and the index finger from the pipette. This action will draw the blood into the diluent.

7. Rinse the bore of the pipette by squeezing and releasing the reservoir (repeat steps 5 and 6) two or three times. This will thoroughly rinse the blood from the capillary pipette.

8. Place the index finger over the top of the inverted pipette, and gently tilt the entire unit up and down several times to mix.

9. To transport the specimen, remove the pipette from the reservoir and place the flagged end into the reservoir. Label the container with the patient's name and other appropriate identification.

10. To use this unit for testing, invert the specimen to mix it, and expel several drops of the dilution. The unit can then be used as a pipette to perform such procedures as loading a hemocytometer.

(continued)

SPECIAL COLLECTION PROCEDURES (continued)

Bone Marrow Preparation

Principle

Bone marrow examination is useful in the diagnosis of hematological disorders associated with cellular abnormalities. The diagnosis of disorders such as acute leukemia or multiple myeloma is usually confirmed by bone marrow examination. The management of patients undergoing treatment can also be monitored through the use of this procedure. Aspiration of bone marrow is performed only by a physician.

Sites of Aspiration

A specimen from a hematopoietically active area of the skeleton is needed (Fig. 2.10). Appropriate sites in an adult include the posterior iliac crest (preferred site), anterior iliac crest, and sternum. The tibia may be used in infants under 18 months of age.

Supplies and Equipment

Bone marrow aspiration/biopsy equipment packs are frequently assembled and autoclaved in the central supply section of many hospitals, or they may be purchased in kit form. If the laboratory is responsible for assembling the equipment, the following items are usually included:

1. Aspiration needles, biopsy needle, and various sizes of syringes and needles
2. Cotton balls and gauze, hemostat, 1% or 2% lidocaine, antiseptic solution, and surgical gloves
3. A bottle of Zenker solution or formalin fixative
4. A sterile container if microbiological cultures are requested
5. The laboratory may additionally supply liquid heparin, glass slides, a watch glass, and microbiological loop or capillary blood collection tubes with a small rubber bulb.

(continued)

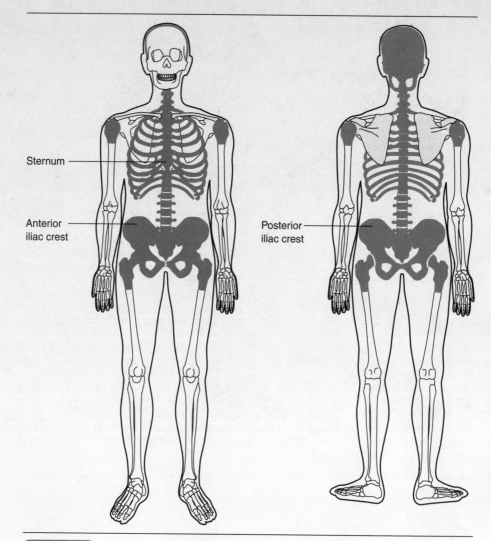

Sternum

Anterior iliac crest

Posterior iliac crest

FIGURE 2.10 Sites of bone marrow aspiration. The red-shaded areas indicate the sites in the skeletal system that contain productive marrow in adults.

Procedure

After the physician has aspirated the specimen, the technician or technologist may be asked to prepare bone marrow films at the patient's bedside. Universal precautions must be observed throughout the procedure and during the clean-up phase.

1. Peripheral blood is usually mixed with the bone marrow aspirate in the syringe. A simple way of removing most of the unwanted peripheral blood is to place the entire contents of the syringe onto a watch glass and remove the small pieces of marrow with a microbiological loop or capillary pipette with a rubber bulb.
2. Depending on the established procedure, three different types of smears may be made: conventional push-wedge, coverslip, and squash techniques.
3. The previously described procedures for the push-wedge and coverslip techniques are followed. Squash preparations are prepared by placing the specimen in the middle of one slide and covering the specimen with a second slide. The slides are pressed together and then pulled apart longitudinally (see Fig. 2.7B).
4. The specimen remaining in the watch glass, and any additional specimens (e.g., from bone biopsy), are usually placed in fixative solution for histological processing.
5. All specimens must be labeled before leaving the patient's room. Properly dispose of contaminated supplies.

ROUTINE STAINING OF PERIPHERAL BLOOD FILMS

In order to examine cells on a blood smear in detail, it is necessary to stain the smear. The beginning student in hematology should become familiar with the principles and practice of routine staining of a blood smear before investigating specific characteristics of cells or performing other staining procedures. The most commonly used stain in the hematology laboratory is a Romanowsky-type stain.

Staining Principles

In 1891, Romanowsky and Malachowski first described the use of a stain that combined a polychromed (oxidized) methylene blue solution with eosin as a blood stain. Ten years later, this stain was refined by Leishmann, who combined eosin with polychromed methylene blue, recovered the precipitate, and dissolved this precipitate in methyl alcohol. Today, Romanowsky-type stains are prepared by use of this modified technique.

A Romanowsky stain is defined as any stain containing methylene blue and/or its products of oxidation and a halogenated fluorescein dye, usually eosin B or Y. Romanowsky-based stains, such as Wright, Giemsa, or May-Grünwald stains, are alcoholic solutions with basic and acidic components. Stains of this type are referred to as polychrome stains because they can impart many colors and produce the Romanowsky effect. This effect imparts a typical color to certain cell components and reflects the combined action of the dyes contained in the stain at a pH of 6.4 to 7.0. The characteristic colors are purple in the cell nucleus, blue and pink in the cytoplasm, and various colors in specific granules.

Stain Preparation

The oxidation of methylene blue results in a solution containing primarily methylene blue; azures A, B, and C; methylene violet; and thionin symdimethylthionin. When eosin dye is added to this solution, the precipitate formed consists of eosinates of these products. Azure B eosinate appears to be the complex responsible for the characteristic Romanowsky effect. Stains with greater quantities of the azure B eosin will react rapidly and provide a better Romanowsky effect than those products containing a lesser amount of this salt. The content of azure B and eosin Y must be consistent and in correct proportions. Solutions of known composition and weights of azures can be prepared, for example, Giemsa stain. A stock solution of the stain is dissolved in a mixture of glycerol and absolute methyl alcohol. The stock stain is then diluted with phosphate buffer pH 6.8 to permit ionization of the stains.

Staining Reactions

The specific stains in a Romanowsky-type stain and their associated reactions are as follows.

Methylene blue is a basic stain, which stains the nucleus and some cytoplasmic structures a blue or purple color. These stained structures are thus **basophilic** (e.g., DNA or RNA).

Eosin is an acidic stain, which stains some cytoplasmic structures an orange-red color. The orange-red staining structures are **acidophilic** (e.g., proteins with amino groups).

When both the basic and the acidic components of the mixture stain a cytoplasmic structure, a pink or lilac color develops. This is referred to as a **neutrophilic** reaction.

Staining Procedure

Blood and other types of specimens can be stained using Romanowsky-based stains. These stains can be prepared in the laboratory or purchased in a ready-to-use form. Either manual or automated techniques can be used.

In some laboratories, blood smears are fixed separately in alcohol before the staining procedure is performed. This step enhances the retention of granules in blood cells. The usual fixative is methyl alcohol. Slides can be placed in anhydrous and acetone-free methanol for 1 minute or longer. Wright and other Romanowsky-based stains are dissolved in methyl alcohol; therefore, fixation normally takes place when the stain is applied to the blood smear.

(continued)

ROUTINE STAINING OF PERIPHERAL BLOOD FILMS (continued)

Reagents and Equipment

1. Stains may be purchased in a ready-to-use form or may be prepared by diluting preweighed vials in methyl alcohol according to the manufacturer's directions.
2. A staining rack or Coplin staining jars are needed.

Procedure

1. Place a thoroughly dried and labeled slide on a level staining rack with the smear side facing up.
2. Place freshly *filtered* stain slowly on the slide until the smear is completely covered. Do not add excess stain. Staining times will vary. Commonly, 3 to 10 minutes may be needed for an acceptably stained blood smear.
3. At the end of the staining time, gently add buffer (pH 6.4) to the slide without removing the stain. The buffer should form a large bubble (convex shape) on the slide. Do not add excess buffer. Some technologists prefer to use ordinary tap water in place of the buffer.
4. Mix the stain and buffer by gently blowing on the slide. A well-mixed slide will have a metallic green sheen rise to the surface of the slide. The timing for this stage ranges from 2 to 5 minutes. If a Coplin jar is preferred for staining, the slides are dipped into the stain and buffer solutions.
5. Wash the stain and buffer off the slide with a gentle flow of tap water. Pick the slide up by its edges and wipe the back of the slide to remove any stain.
6. Allow the slide to air dry.

Sources of Error in Staining

Poor-quality staining can result from several factors:

1. Failure to filter the stain daily, or prior to use, can produce sediment on blood films. If the precipitated sediment is very heavy, it will be impossible to view the blood cell microscopically. Small amounts of sediment can be mistaken for platelets on microscopic examination.
2. Inaccurate buffer pH can produce too bright or too dark a staining reaction. The buffer solution must control the acid-base balance of the stain to produce the proper colors in the various components of the blood cells. An overly acidic buffer produces a blood smear that is too red on microscopic examination. If the buffer is too basic (alkaline), the blood smear will be too blue on microscopic examination.
3. Improper timing of staining or buffering can produce faded staining or altered colors of the blood smears. Too short a staining time produces a blood smear that is too red on microscopic examination. If the staining time is too long, the blood smear will be too dark on microscopic examination.
4. Deteriorated reagents or improper ratios of stain and buffer in the staining process can produce washed-out cellular colors.

SUMMARY

Blood Collection Supplies and Equipment

A properly collected blood specimen is essential to quality results in the laboratory. The usual type of blood specimen used in the hematology laboratory is an anticoagulated sample. Three types of anticoagulants are used: EDTA, heparin, and sodium citrate. Each prevents the coagulation of blood by a specific mechanism. Although EDTA is the most frequently used anticoagulant, it is not appropriate for all tests. Each laboratory procedure should specify the type of anticoagulant needed for that technique.

An evacuated tube system consisting of a double-pointed collection needle, a holder, and a sterile evacuated test tube is the most widely used device for venous blood collection. In special cases, disposable plastic syringes can be used to collect venous blood.

Capillary blood from sites such as the fingertip can be collected in various types of microcollection tubes. The microhematocrit type of tube is the one most frequently used in hematology tests. These tubes may be plain or contain the anticoagulant heparin.

Venous and Capillary Blood Collection Techniques

Specific procedures must be followed in the collection of any type of blood sample. The proper identification of the patient is critical to the accuracy of laboratory testing.

In the collection of venous blood, several procedural phases must be followed: initiation of the procedure, selection of an appropriate site, preparation of the site, performance of the venipuncture, and termination of the procedure. Problems can be encountered in the phlebotomy procedure. The competent technologist should be familiar with the various types of problems and their solutions. Capillary blood collection consists of selection of an appropriate site, preparation of the site, puncture of the skin, collection of the sample, and termination of the procedure.

Preparation of a Blood Smear

The preparation of the push-wedge type of blood smear is a common laboratory procedure. This procedure may need to be conducted at the patient's bedside, although it is most frequently performed on EDTA-anticoagulated blood. The preparation of a high-quality blood smear is essential to the quality of the microscopic examination of erythrocytes, leukocytes, and thrombocytes (platelets). The hematology technologist/technician should know the characteristics of a good smear and be familiar with the causes of poor-quality smears. In addition to the push-wedge type of smear, a coverslip method of blood film preparation exists.

Special Collection Procedures

In addition to the collection of venous or capillary blood specimens and the preparation of blood smears, some procedures are performed by the technologist or technician at the patient's bedside. Basic procedures include capillary blood dilutions and bone marrow samples.

The Unopette system is a microsample collection system for use in certain manual or automated procedures. The hematology laboratory technologist/technician may also be asked to assist with the special technique of bone marrow aspiration. Although a physician collects the sample, bone marrow slides must be prepared immediately at the patient's bedside.

Routine Staining of Peripheral Blood Films

Romanowsky-type stains, such as the Wright, May-Grünwald, and Giemsa stains, are most commonly used to stain blood smears in the hematology laboratory. The Romanowsky effect imparts specific color to the various components of a cell. Staining characteristics serve as a guide to the morphological identification of cells. Poor-quality staining can result from several factors, such as inaccurate buffer pH. Because of the importance of well-stained preparations, these sources of error and corrective measures should be understood.

BIBLIOGRAPHY

Clark, Kathleen. "Phlebotomy: Beyond the Basics," *Advance for Medical Laboratory Professionals*, Vol. 28, No.9, Sept. 27, 1997, pp. 12–15.

Dale, Jane C. "Phlebotomy Complications," presented at Mayo Laboratory's Phlebotomy Conference, August, 1996, Boston, MA.

Faber, Virginia. "Phlebotomy and the Aging Patient," *Advance for Medical Laboratory Professionals*, Vol. 29, No. 1, Jan. 5, 1998, pp. 24–25.

Haraden, Leah. "Pediatric Phlebotomy: Great Expectations," Vol. 28, No. 11, Nov. 3, 1997, pp. 12–13.

Hurley, Theresa R. "Considerations for the Pediatric and Geriatric Patient," presented at Mayo Laboratory's Phlebotomy Conference, August, 1996, Boston, MA.

Iverson, Linda K. "Changing Roles of Phlebotomist/Customer Satisfaction," presented at Mayo Laboratory's Phlebotomy Conference, August, 1996, Boston, MA.

Jacoby, H. (ed.). *Standard for Evacuated Tubes for Blood Specimen Collection*, 3 ed. NCCLS Approved Standard: H1-A3. Villanova, PA: National Committee for Clinical Laboratory Standards, 1991.

Koepke, John A. (Chairholder). *Leukocyte Differential Counting*. Tentative Standard, Vol. 4, No. 11. Villanova, PA: National Committee for Clinical Laboratory Standards, 1984, pp. 257–268, 277.

Latshaw, Jamie. "Laser Takes Sting Out of Phlebotomy," *Advance for Medical Laboratory Professionals*, Vol. 28, No. 12, Dec. 1, 1997, pp. 40–41.

Linke, E. George and John B. Henry. "Clinical Pathology/Laboratory Medicine Purposes and Practice," in *Clinical Diagnosis and Management by Laboratory Methods*, 18th ed. John B. Henry (ed.). Philadelphia: Saunders, 1991.

Loschen, D. J. et al. *Physician's Office Laboratory Procedure Manual*, Vol. 12, No. 7, Villanova, PA: National Committee for Clinical Laboratory Standards, 1992, pp. b-1–b-16.

Pendergraph, Garland E. *Handbook of Phlebotomy*. Philadelphia: Lea & Febiger, 1984, pp. 56–70.

Sigma Diagnostics Summary Technical News and Notes, Vol. 1 and Vol. 2. St. Louis, MO: Sigma Diagnostics, 1985.

Stockblower, Jean M. (Chairholder). *Standard Procedures for the Collection of Diagnostic Blood Specimens by Venipuncture*, 3rd ed. (H3-A3) Villanova, PA: National Committee for Clinical Laboratory Standards, 1991.

Stockblower, Jean M. and Thomas A. Blumenfeld. *Collection and Handling of Laboratory Specimens*. Philadelphia: Lippincott, 1983, pp. 3–54.

Thomas, Clayton L. *Taber's Cyclopedic Medical Dictionary*, 13th ed. Philadelphia: Davis, 1977.

INTERNET SITES

Phlebotomy: Blood Collection: Routine Venipuncture and Specimen Handling
http://telpath2.med.utah.edu/WebPath/TUTORIAL/PHLEB/PHLEB.html.

Phlebotomy Competence Log
http:www.human.cornell.edu/youthwork/ptolls/notebook/hc/laborat/phleb.htm.

REVIEW QUESTIONS

1. When the coagulation of fresh whole blood is prevented through the use of an anticoagulant, the straw-colored fluid that can be separated from the cellular elements is:

   A. Serum. C. Whole Blood.
   B. Plasma. D. Platelets.

2. Which characteristic is inaccurate with respect to the anticoagulant tripotassium ethylenediaminetetraacetate (K3 EDTA)?

   A. Removes ionized calcium (Ca^{2+}) from fresh whole blood by the process of chelation.
   B. Is used for most routine coagulation studies.
   C. Is the most commonly used anticoagulant in hematology.
   D. Is conventionally placed in lavender stoppered evacuated tubes.

3. Heparin inhibits the clotting of fresh whole blood by neutralizing the effect of:

   A. Platelets. C. Fibrinogen.
   B. Ionized calcium (Ca^{2+}). D. Thrombin.

Questions 4 through 7: match the conventional color-coded stopper with the appropriate anticoagulant.

   4. ___ EDTA. A. Red
   5. ___ Heparin. B. Lavender.
   6. ___ Sodium citrate. C. Blue.
   7. ___ No anticoagulant. D. Green.

Questions 8 through 12: the following five procedural steps are significant activities in the performance of a venipuncture. Place these steps in the correct sequence.

A. Select an appropriate site and prepare the site.
B. Identify the patient, check test requisitions, assemble equipment, wash hands, and put on latex gloves.
C. Remove tourniquet, remove needle, apply pressure to site, and label all tubes.
D. Reapply the tourniquet and perform the venipuncture.
E. Introduce yourself and briefly explain the procedure to the patient.

8. ___ .

9. ___ .

10. ___ .

11. ___ .

12. ___ .

13. The appropriate veins for performing a routine venipuncture are the:

A. Cephalic, basilic, and median cubital.
B. Subclavian, iliac, and femoral.
C. Brachiocephalic, jugular, and popliteal.
D. Saphenous, suprarenal, and tibial.

14. A blood sample is needed from a patient with intravenous (IV) fluids running in both arms. Which of the following is an acceptable procedure?

A. Any obtainable vein is satisfactory.
B. Obtain sample from above the IV site.
C. Obtain sample from below IV site with precautions.
D. Disconnect the IV line.
E. Do not draw a blood specimen.

15. The bevel of the needle should be held ___ in the performance of a venipuncture.

A. Sideways.   C. Downward.
B. Upward.   D. In any direction.

16. A hematoma can form if:

A. Improper pressure is applied to a site after the venipuncture.
B. The patient suddenly moves and the needle comes out of the vein.
C. The needle punctures both walls of the vein.
D. All of the above.

17. Phlebotomy problems can include:

A. The use of improper anticoagulants.
B. Misidentification of patients.
C. Improper angle of the needle or having the needle up against the side of the vessel wall.
D. All of the above.

18. Which of the following area(s) is (are) acceptable for the collection of capillary blood from an infant?

A. Previous puncture site.
B. Posterior curve of the heel.
C. The arch.
D. Medial or lateral plantar surface.

19. The proper collection of capillary blood includes:

A. Wiping away the first drop of blood.
B. Occasionally wiping the site with a plain gauze pad to avoid the buildup of platelets.
C. Avoiding the introduction of air bubbles into the column of blood in a capillary collection tube.
D. All of the above.

20. A peripheral blood smear can be prepared from:

A. EDTA-anticoagulated blood within 1 hour of collection.
B. Free-flowing capillary blood.
C. Heparinized whole blood.
D. All of the above.

21. Identify the characteristic(s) of a good peripheral blood smear.

A. It progresses from thick at the point of origin to thin.
B. It has a blunt feathered termination.
C. The outer margins do not touch the edges of the slide.
D. All of the above

22. Poor blood smears can be caused by:

A. Delay in preparing the smear once the drop of blood has been placed on the slide.
B. A drop of blood that is too large or too small.
C. Holding the pusher slide at the wrong angle and poor drying conditions.
D. All of the above.

23. If a blood smear is too long, the problem can be resolved by:

A. Decreasing the angle of the pusher slide.
B. Increasing the angle of the pusher slide.
C. Using a larger drop of blood.
D. Pushing the slide slower in smearing out the blood.

24. The examination of bone marrow is useful in:

A. Diagnosing a bleeding disorder.
B. Diagnosing disorders associated with erythrocytes and leukocytes.
C. Diagnosing acute leukemias.
D. Both B and C.

25. Appropriate bone marrow aspiration sites in an adult are:

A. The anterior and posterior iliac crest.
B. The sternum and posterior iliac crest.
C. The tibia and sternum.
D. Both A and B.

Questions 26 through 28: match the following type of staining effect with the color it imparts to blood cells.

26. ___ Basic stain.   A. Orange-red color.

27. ___ Acidic stain.   B. Pink-lilac color.

28. ___ Neutrophilic.   C. Blue-purple color.

Questions 29 through 32: identify the following as Romanowsky-type or non–Romanowsky-type stains.

29. ___ Wright.

30. ___ May-Grünwald.

31. ___ Giemsa.

32. ___ Methylene blue.

A. Romanowsky-type.

B. Non–Romanowsky-type.

33. If a blood smear stains too red on microscopic examination of a Wright-stained preparation, possible causes include:

A. The staining time was too long.

B. The stain was too basic.

C. The buffer was too acidic and the exposure time was too short.

D. The buffer was too basic and the exposure time was too long.

Molecular Genetics and Cellular Morphology

OBJECTIVES

Cellular ultrastructure and organization

- Describe the chemical composition and general function of cellular membranes.
- Explain the general membrane activities of passive and facilitated diffusion, active transport, osmosis, and endocytosis.
- Name and describe the structure and function of each of the cytoplasmic organelles found in a typical mammalian cell.
- Describe two cellular metabolites that are of importance to hematologists.
- Draw and describe the features of the nucleus.

- Define the terms **heterochromatin** and **euchromatin.**
- Relate the nuclear structures to the cellular activities that are associated with the nucleus.
- Describe the processes of mitosis and meiosis.

Molecular genetics in hematology

- Name at least three hematologic abnormalities that can be detected by molecular methods.
- Describe the use of the following molecular techniques: restriction endonucleases, Southern blotting, hybridization, polymerase chain reaction (PCR), and Northern blotting.

CELLULAR ULTRASTRUCTURE AND ORGANIZATION

Cells, as the smallest organized units of living tissues, have the ability to individually perform all the functions essential for life processes. Although the range of morphological features varies widely, all cells conform to a basic model (Fig. 3.1A). Large cellular structures are observable on stained preparations with the light microscope. Smaller ultrastructures or organelles must be viewed with an electron microscope.

Cellular Membranes

Structure

Cellular membranes provide a semipermeable separation between the various cellular components, the organelles, and the surrounding environment. The cytoplasmic membrane, or outer membrane, defines the boundaries of the cell, while being resilient and elastic. Differences in membrane thickness reflect the various functional properties of specific cell types or organelles within the cell.

Chemically, membranes consist of proteins, phospholipids, cholesterol, and traces of polysaccharide. The most popular hypothesis to explain the arrangement of these molecular components is the **fluid mosaic model** (see Fig. 3.1B). According to this model, the cell membrane is a dynamic fluid structure with globular proteins floating in lipids. The lipids, as phospholipids, are arranged in two layers. The polar (charged) phosphate ends of the phospholipids are oriented toward the inner and outer surfaces, while the nonpolar (fatty acid) ends point toward each other in the interior of the membrane. Protein molecules may be either integral (incorporated into the lipid bilayer) or peripheral (associated with either the outer or the inner surface of the membrane). Polysaccharides in the form of either glycoproteins or glycolipids can be found attached to the lipid and protein molecules of the membrane.

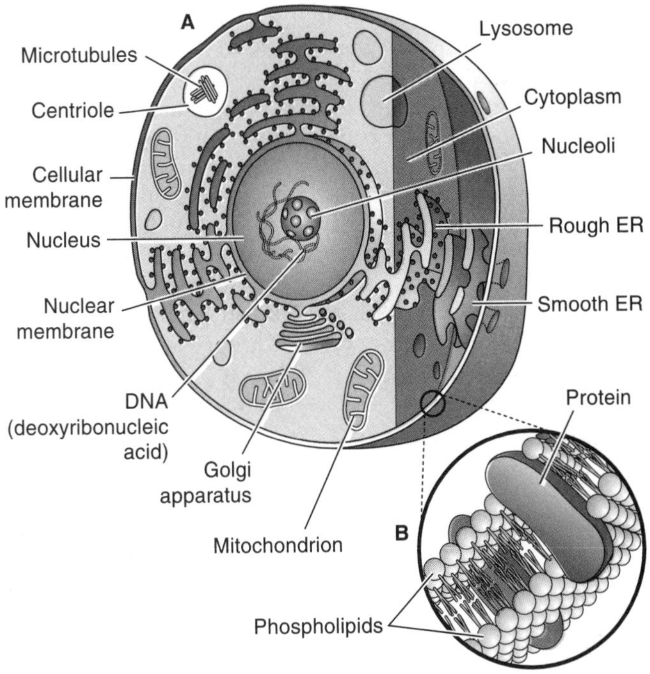

Membrane Functions

The lipid bilayer is directly responsible for the impermeability of the membrane to most water-soluble molecules. Proteins within the membrane act as transport molecules for the rapid penetration of polar and non–lipid-soluble substances. Additionally, protein molecules determine and protect the shape and structure of the membrane, often through attachment to underlying microtubules and microfilaments. In human red blood cells, the extrinsic protein, spectrin, in conjunction with the protein actin, forms a contractile network just under the cell membrane and provides the cell with the resistance necessary to withstand distorting forces during movement through the blood circulation. Membrane-bound carbohydrates act as surface **antigens,** which function in the process of cellular recognition and interaction between cells.

As a unit, the cytoplasmic membrane maintains cellular integrity of the interior of the cell by controlling and influencing the passage of materials in and out of the cell. This function is accomplished through the major membrane processes of osmosis, diffusion, active transport, and endocytosis.

The term **osmosis** is used to describe the net movement of water molecules through a semipermeable membrane (Fig. 3.2). Normally, water molecules move in and out of the cell membrane at an equal rate, producing no net movement. If a concentration gradient exists, the movement of water molecules will be greater from areas of low solute (e.g., sodium and chloride ions) concentration to areas of higher solute concentration. Osmosis is the basic principle underlying the erythrocyte, or red blood cell, fragility test (described in Chapter 24), which demonstrates changes in the erythrocytic membrane. Alterations in the erythrocytic

FIGURE 3.1 Cellular organization. Most of the organelles depicted in **A** are visible only with electron microscope examination. **A.** Cellular ultrastructures. **B.** Fluid mosaic model. The unique positioning of the phospholipids and free-floating proteins is characterized by the fluid mosaic model of the cellular membrane. ER = endoplasmic reticulum.

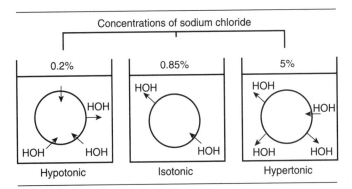

FIGURE 3.2 Osmosis. A schematic comparison of erythrocytes in three concentrations of sodium chloride solution demonstrates the net movement of water molecules into and out of the cell. If the net movement of water into the cell is in excess, the cell will lyse. If the net movement of water out of the cell is in excess, the cell will crenate. HOH = water.

membrane, such as the loss of flexibility, can be observed by placing erythrocytes in solutions with varying solute concentrations.

Diffusion is an important process in overall cellular physiology, such as the physiological activities of the erythrocyte. This passive process through a semipermeable membrane may also be referred to as **dialysis.** Substances passively diffuse, or move down a concentration gradient from areas of high solute concentration to areas of low solute concentration, by dissolving in the lipid portion of the cellular membrane. Diffusion through the membrane is influenced by the solubility of molecules in lipids, temperature, and the concentration gradient. Lipid-soluble substances diffuse through the lipid layer at rates greater than through the protein portions of the membrane.

Small molecules, such as those of water or inorganic ions, are able to pass down the concentration gradient via **hydrophilic** regions. These hydrophilic regions are associated with the points where some of the membrane's protein molecules create a polar area, resulting in pore-like openings. However, movement of molecules through these regions is affected by electrical charges along the surface of the region, the size of the region, and the specific nature of the protein. Calcium ions affect the permeability of membranes. An increase in the concentration of calcium ions in the fluid surrounding the cell, or accumulation of calcium ions in the cytoplasm, can decrease the permeability of the membrane and has been demonstrated as a factor in the aging process of erythrocytes.

Active transport is another essential membrane function. Because the cellular membrane also functions as a metabolic regulator, enzyme molecules are incorporated into the membrane. One such enzyme, particularly important as a metabolic regulator, is sodium-potassium-adenosine triphosphatase (Na-K-ATPase). This enzyme provides the necessary energy to drive the sodium-potassium pump, a fundamental ion transport system. Sodium ions are pumped out of the cells into extracellular fluids, where the concentration of sodium is higher than it is inside the cell. This movement of molecules is referred to as moving against the concentration gradient. The energy-producing activities of the mitochondria are heavily dependent on this process (refer to the function of mitochondria in this chapter).

Endocytosis is the process of engulfing particles or molecules, with the subsequent formation of membrane-bound vacuoles in the cytoplasm. Two processes, **pinocytosis** (the engulfment of fluids) and **phagocytosis** (the engulfment and destruction of particles), are forms of endocytosis. The vesicles formed by endocytosis either discharge their contents into the cellular cytoplasm or fuse with the organelles and the lysosomes. Phagocytosis is an important body defense mechanism and is discussed in more detail in Chapter 14.

Cell Volume Homeostasis

Maintenance of a constant volume despite extracellular and intracellular osmotic challenges is critical to the integrity of a cell. In most cases, cells respond by swelling or shrinking by activating specific metabolic or membrane-transport processes that return cell volume to its normal resting state. These processes are essential for the normal function and survival of cells.

Cells respond to volume changes by activating mechanisms that regulate their volume. The processes by which swollen and shrunken cells return to a normal volume are called regulatory volume decrease and regulatory volume increase, respectively. Cell volume can only be regulated by the gain or loss of osmotically active solutes, primarily inorganic ions such as sodium, potassium, and chloride or small organic molecules called organic osmolytes.

Regulatory loss and gain of electrolytes are mediated by membrane transport processes. In most animal cells, regulatory decreases in volume are accomplished by the loss of potassium chloride as a result of the activation of separate potassium and chloride channels or of the K^+/Cl^- cotransporter. Regulatory increases in volume occur through the uptake of both potassium chloride and sodium chloride. Certain ion transport systems have multiple roles, participating in volume regulation, intracellular pH control, and transepithelial movement of salt and water.

Organic osmolytes are found in high concentrations in the cytosol of all organisms, from bacteria to humans. These solutes have key roles in cell volume homeostasis and may also function as general cytoprotectants. The accumulation of organic osmolytes is mediated either by energy-dependent transport from the external medium or by changes in the rates of osmolyte synthesis and degradation.

Volume accumulation induces a very rapid increase in the passive efflux of organic osmolytes. Generally, this process is slow. Cell swelling inhibits transportation of the genes coding for organic-osmolyte transporters and the enzymes involved in osmolyte synthesis. As transcription decreases, levels of messenger RNA (mRNA) drop and the number of functional proteins declines over a period of many hours to days.

The sensing mechanism for cell size is not yet understood. A number of volume signals have been postulated, including swelling- and shrinkage-induced changes in membrane tension, cytoskeletal architecture, cellular ion concentrations, and the concentration of cytoplasmic macromolecules. No one signaling mechanism can account for the volume sensitivity of the various genes and membrane transport pathways that reactivate or are inactivated in response to perturbations in cell volume. Recent evidence suggests that cells can detect more than simple swelling or shrinkage. Disruption of cellular osmoregulatory mechanisms can give rise to a diverse group of disease states and their complications.

Reactive and Neoplastic Growth Processes

The size and shape of particular cell types are constant. Individual cell features can vary because of infectious disease or malignancy and groups of cells (tissues) can manifest a variety of changes as well. Terms that may be encountered in the study of hematological diseases include:

Anaplasia—highly pleomorphic and bizarre cytologic features associated with malignant tumors that are poorly differentiated

Atrophy—decrease in the number or size of cells that can lead to a decrease in organ size or tissue mass

Dysplasia—abnormal cytologic features and tissue organization, often is a premalignant change

Hyperplasia—increase in the number of cells in a tissue

Hypertrophy—increase in the size of cells that can lead to an increase in organ size

Metaplasia—change from one adult cell type to another, e.g., glandular to squamous metaplasia

Cytoplasmic Organelles and Metabolites

Organelles (see Fig. 3.1A) are functional units of a cell. Most of the smaller organelles must be viewed with an electron microscope. Staining techniques are of value in the identification of larger organelles and soluble substances in the cytoplasm.

Stains such as Wright stain (discussed in Chapter 2) aid in differentiating the features of cells found in the blood and bone marrow. The staining and morphological characteristics of blood cells are presented in the last section of this chapter. Specialized stains (discussed in Chapter 24) can be used to identify constituents such as lipids, glycogen, iron, enzymes, and nucleic acids in cells. In abnormal cells, the soluble substances in the cytoplasm can provide important clues to the cell's identity. A detailed discussion of cytochemical staining is included in Chapters 19, 21, and 24. The organelles and their respective functions are listed here.

Centrioles are two central spots inside of the centrosomes. These paired structures are cylindrical and the long axes are always oriented at right angles to each other. Internally, each structure consists of nine (triplet) groups of microtubules. The centrioles divide and move to the opposite ends of the cell during cell division. They serve as points of insertion of the spindle fibers during cell division.

The **endoplasmic reticulum** (ER), an extensive lacelike network, is composed of membranes enclosing interconnecting cavities or cisterns. It is classified as either rough (granular) or smooth (agranular). The rough sections contain **ribosomes.** Rough ER is associated with protein production; smooth ER is thought to be the site of the synthesis of lipids such as cholesterol and also the site of the breakdown of fats into smaller molecules that can be used for energy.

The **Golgi apparatus** appears as a horseshoe-shaped or hook-shaped organelle with an associated stack of vesicles or sacs. In stained blood smears, the Golgi apparatus appears as the unstained area next to the nucleus. Functionally, the Golgi apparatus is the site for concentrating secretions of granules, packing, and segregating the carbohydrate components of certain secretions. Part of the Golgi apparatus and adjacent portions of the ER appear to form lysosomes. The Golgi-associated endoplasmic reticulum lysosome (GERL) concept focuses on the coordination of these cellular components. Products of the Golgi apparatus are usually exported from the cell when a vesicle of the Golgi apparatus fuses with the plasma membrane.

Lysosomes contain hydrolytic enzymes. Three types of lysosomes have been identified: primary, secondary, and tertiary lysosomes. Lysosomes are responsible for the intracellular digestion of the products of **phagocytosis** or the disposal of worn-out or damaged cell components. In some instances, lysosomes fuse with vacuoles containing foreign substances engulfed by the cell. In this process, the lysosomes may rupture and these internal enzymes actually autolyse the entire cell.

Microbodies are small, intracytoplasmic organelles, limited by a single membrane that is thinner than the lysosome. Microbodies contain enzymes. These organelles are especially likely to contain oxidase enzymes that produce hydrogen peroxide. Their function, related to oxidative activity, is an important aspect of phagocytosis.

Microfilaments are solid structures, consisting of the protein **actin** and the larger **myosin** filaments. Microfilaments are the smallest components of the cytoskeleton. These structures are responsible for the amoeboid movement of cells, such as the phagocytic cells. In **cytokinesis,** the plasma membrane pinches in because of the contraction of a ring of microfilaments.

Microtubules are small, hollow fibers composed of polymerized, macromolecular protein subunits, **tubulin.** They are narrow and have an indefinite length. The formation of tubules occurs through rapid, reversible self-assembly of filaments. Microtubules may be concerned with cell shape (the cytoskeleton) and the intracellular movement of organelles, and may have a passive role in intracellular diffusion. The mitotic spindle is composed of microtubules.

Mitochondria are composed of an outer smooth membrane and an inner folded membrane. Cells contain from hundreds to thousands of these rod-shaped organelles; however, mature erythrocytes lack mitochondria. The inner membrane functions as a permeable barrier. Each of the membranes has distinct functional differences. The cristae contain the enzymes and other molecules that carry out the energy-producing reactions of the cell. The granules of the matrix function as binding sites for calcium and contain some **deoxyribonucleic acid (DNA)** and some ribosomes that are similar to those found in microorganisms. The reaction located on the inner membrane of the mitochondria is enzyme-controlled, energy-producing, and electron transfer-oxidative.

Ribosomes, small dense granules, show a lack of membranes and are found both on the surface of the rough ER and free in the cytoplasm. They contain a significant proportion of **ribonucleic acid (RNA)** and are composed of unequally sized subunits. Ribosomes may exist singly, in groups, or in clusters. The presence of many ribosomes produces cytoplasmic basophilia (blue color) when a cell is stained with Wright stain. The complex of messenger RNA (mRNA) and a ribosome serves as the site of protein synthesis. Numerous cytoplasmic ribosomes with few associated membranes suggest significant protein synthesis activity for internal use, such as in growing and dividing cells or in erythrocytic precursors in which hemoglobin is retained as it is synthesized. Cells, such as the plasma cell, that synthesize proteins for use outside of the cell tend to have greater amounts of rough ER except in the Golgi area.

Cellular Inclusions and Metabolites

Cells contain a variety of inclusions. Some of these structures are vacuoles with ingested fluids or particles, stored fats, and granules of glycogen and other substances. Numerous soluble cellular metabolites are present in the cytoplasm, but few have a clearly defined ultrastructural identity. Two metabolites of importance to hematologists are glycogen and ferritin.

Glycogen is a long-chain polysaccharide, a storage form of carbohydrate that is detectable with a special stain, the periodic acid-Schiff (PAS) stain (refer to Chapter 24). The size of these particles is about twice that of a ribosome. The beta form of glycogen is found in single particles in the neutrophilic leukocytes. Undoubtedly, increased glycogen concentrations in cells such as the neutrophilic leukocyte are related to the needs of the cells for a high energy reserve in order to carry out their body defense functions.

Ferritin is a common storage form of iron. Ferritin measures approximately 9 nm in diameter, which makes it substantially smaller than a ribosome. It is often found in iron-rich dense bodies referred to as **telolysosomes.** The term **siderosome** is used to refer to iron-saturated telolysosomes. Histologists refer to granular, iron-rich brown pigment as **hemosiderin.** Ferritin can be found in the macrophages of the spleen and bone marrow. The presence of ferritin in macrophages is indicative of the role these cells play in the recycling and storage of iron for hemoglobin synthesis (discussed in Chapter 5).

Nuclear Characteristics

Structure and Function

The overall average size of the nucleus is 10 to 15 μm. This structure, which is the largest organelle, functions as the control center of the cell and is essential for its long-term survival. The nucleus is surrounded by a nuclear envelope, which consists of an inner and an outer membrane with a gap between them of approximately 50 nm. The outer membrane is probably continuous at scattered points with the ER. Many large pores extend through this membrane envelope. The nuclear pores are usually bridged by a diaphragm that is more diffuse than a membrane and prevents materials from passing in and out freely.

Inside the nucleus, within the inner nucleoplasm, are the **nucleoli** (singular, nucleolus) and **chromatin.** Normally, the nucleus contains one or more small nucleoli that are not separated from the nucleoplasm by a specialized membrane. Morphologically, the nucleoli are irregularly shaped. Chemically, the nucleoli are composed mainly of RNA. Functionally, the nucleoli are the site of synthesis and processing of various species of ribosomal RNA. As the cell goes through various stages of growth and cellular division, the appearance of the nucleoli changes. These changes in the appearance are related to the rate of synthesis of ribosomal RNA.

Chromatin Characteristics

Genetic material is composed of nucleic acids and protein (nucleoprotein) which is referred to as **chromatin.** Despite the presence of protein in the chromatin, the DNA component stores genetic information. DNA has two functions:

1. To dictate the nature of proteins that can be synthesized, thereby controlling the function of the cell
2. To transmit information for cellular control from one generation to the next

Proteins associated with the nucleic acids are divided into basic, positively charged **histones** and less positively charged **nonhistones.** The histones are believed to be essential to the structural integrity of chromatin. Histones may be important in facilitating the conversion of the thin chromatin fibers seen during interphase into the highly condensed chromosomes seen in mitosis. The nonhistone proteins are thought to play other roles, including genetic regulation. A general model of the organization of DNA and histones (Fig. 3.3) depicts a regular spacing arrangement. The complete unit, the **nucleosome,** consists of a string of DNA wrapped around a histone core.

The chromatin arrangement within the nucleus demonstrates characteristic patterns when stained and viewed with a light microscope. These patterns are the most distinctive feature of a cell in terms of recognition of cell types and cell maturity. Chromatin can be divided into two types: **heterochromatin** (previously called chromatin), the condensed, dark-staining areas, and **euchromatin** (previously called parachromatin), the uncoiled, pale-staining areas. Heterochromatin may be in patches or clumped toward the nuclear envelope in a thin rim. Small patches of heterochromatin may be associated with the nucleolus. In general, the more restricted the function of a cell, the more predominant the heterochromatin. In the maturation of an erythrocyte, the chromatin distribution is very diffuse in the young cells with abundant euchromatin. As the erythrocyte matures, dense aggregates of heterochromatin predominate before the nucleus is lost in the mature cell.

Several functional characteristics distinguish heterochromatin from euchromatin. Heterochromatin areas are genetically inactive because they either lack genes or contain genes that are repressed. Heterochromatin replicates later during the S phase (described in the next section) of the cell cycle than does euchromatin. Labeled RNA shows that active transcription occurs within the euchromatin areas.

Chromosomes

Genetic material exists as diffuse elongated chromatin fibers during cellular interphase. However, during cellular division (mitosis), the individual strands condense into short

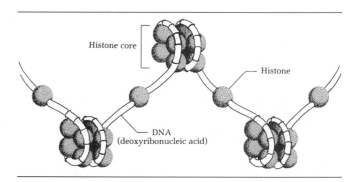

FIGURE 3.3 A general model of the organization of DNA and histones.

visible structures, the **chromosomes.** The number of chromosomes in each cell is constant within each species. Humans have a complement of 46 chromosomes arranged into 23 pairs; one member of each pair is inherited from the father and the other from the mother. Each of the members of one chromosome pair is referred to as a chromosome homologue. Of the pairs, 22 are called autosomes; the remaining pair represents the sex chromosomes of which males have an X and a Y and females have two Xs.

The technique of staining cells to bring out the different parts more clearly was discovered about 1873. Basic dyes were used to stain the cells. The name "chromosome" was chosen because these structures showed the bright colors of the basic stain.

Chromosomes were first seen in human cells by Flemming in 1882; however, there were so many and they were so small that he could not accurately estimate the actual number. As a result of the squash technique developed in 1956, the entire chromosome complement of a cell can be spread out and flattened so that each chromosome can be seen clearly. Cells for chromosome studies can be taken from any area of the body including the bone marrow, circulating blood, and amniotic fluid. Most studies use leukocytes (white blood cells). Tissue culture technique allows these cells to be placed in a nutrient medium and stimulated to grow and divide very rapidly. Normally, mature blood cells do not divide, but the addition of a **mitogen,** such as colchicine, stimulates cell division in white blood cells of the lymphocyte type. Other cells such as red blood cells cannot divide. The cell selected for chromosome analysis is usually in the metaphase stage of cellular division.

In 1961, the Denver system of identifying human chromosomes was established (Fig. 3.4). Chromosome pairs were numbered according to relative size and the position of their centromeres (the constricted area of a chromosome) and placed in groups according to letters. This arrangement of chromosome constitutes a **karyotype.** Differential staining of chromosomes using newer cytological techniques was introduced in the early 1970s. These methods, **chromosome banding techniques,** provide more information about the individual identity of chromosomes than previous methods. If chromosome preparations are denatured with heat and treated with Giemsa stain, a unique staining pattern emerges. The staining pattern with this technique is referred to as **C-banding.** Other banding techniques include fluorescent dyes that bind to nucleoprotein complexes. When chromosomes are treated with fluorochrome quinacrine mustard and viewed with a fluorescent microscope, precise patterns of differential brightness are seen. Each of the 23 human chromosome pairs can be distinguished by this technique; the bands produced are called **Q-bands.** Another technique that produces patterns similar to Q-bands involves the digestion of chromosomes with the enzyme trypsin, followed by Giemsa staining, that produces **G-bands** (Fig. 3.5). Chromosome analysis is being performed today by use of a laser technology (discussed in Chapter 25) that generates chromosome histograms.

The study of individual karyotypes and chromosome banding patterns is important to hematologists as well as geneticists. Supplementary information on hematological disorders, such as the leukemias (discussed in Chapters 19 and 21), can aid in establishing a diagnosis and can provide information about the probable outcome (**prognosis**) in some cases.

Chromosomal Alterations

Chromosomes sometimes break, and a portion may be lost or attached to another chromosome. Deletion and translocation are the terms used to describe these conditions. **Deletion** is defined as the loss of a segment of chromosome. **Translocation** is the process in which a segment of one chromosome breaks away (is deleted) from its normal location. Translocation can happen frequently between homologous chromosomes while they are paired in meiosis (discussed in the next section). An abnormality or aberration can result when the detached portion is lost or reattached. The Philadelphia chromosome, the first chromosomal abnormality discovered in a malignant disorder, is an example of a translocation from chromosome 22 to chromosome 9. Additional examples of chromosomal

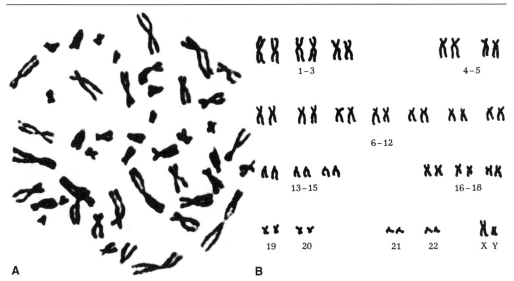

FIGURE 3.4 Denver system of chromosome grouping. **A.** A single cell is squashed in the study of human chromosomes. **B.** The Denver system of grouping chromosomes is by overall length and centromere position.

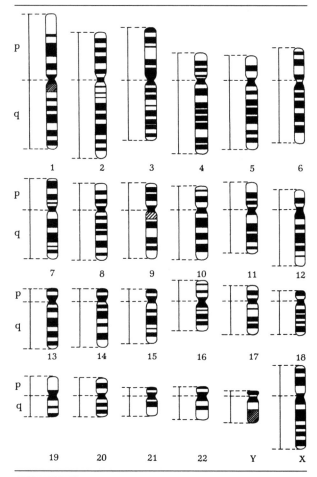

FIGURE 3.5 Chromosome banding. After the chromosomes are stained with Giemsa stain, the areas of the chromosomes referred to as G-bands can be seen. The p (*upper portion*) and q (*lower portion*) are easily visible.

translocations associated with malignant conditions are discussed in detail in Chapter 21.

Trisomy is another abnormality of chromosomes that is of interest to hematologists. In trisomy, one of the homologous chromosomes fails to separate from its sister chromatid. This failure to separate leads to a set of three chromosomes in place of the normal pair. Trisomy is encountered in a variety of hematological malignancies.

Clinical Use of Cytogenetics

Clinical cytogenetics contributes to understanding inborn or acquired genetic problems by providing a low-power screening method for detecting isolated or missing chunks of chromosomes. The human genome consists of 3×10^9 bp of DNA distributed among 46 chromosomes. This genome contains at least 100,000 (and possibly as many as 1 million) genes with gene sizes ranging from a few thousand to several hundred thousand base pairs. The resolution limit precludes microscopic recognition of genome regions smaller than 2 to 3 million bp, chromosome stretches sufficient to accommodate about 50 to 100 genes. In contrast, gene probing procedures are capable of discerning differences as small as 10 to 50 bp in fragments of individual cloned genes. The strength of cytogenetics is not in characterizing gene structure but in its utility in locating major rearrangements, which can then be characterized at the gene level by methods for DNA analysis.

Activities of the Nucleus

Mitosis

Mitosis (Fig. 3.6) is the process of replication in nucleated body cells (except ova and sperm cells). Cellular replication, or mitotic division, results in the formation of two identical daughter cells because the genes are duplicated and exactly segregated before each cell division. Originally, only two phases were recognized in mitosis: a resting or **interphase** phase (the period of time between mitoses) and the phase of actual cell division (**M phase**).

Mitosis, particularly the interphase period in bone marrow cells, is important to hematologists because special staining and flow cytometry techniques (discussed in Chapter 25) now make it possible to perform DNA cell cycle analysis in these cells. This type of analysis is useful in the treatment of various hematological disorders because the optimum

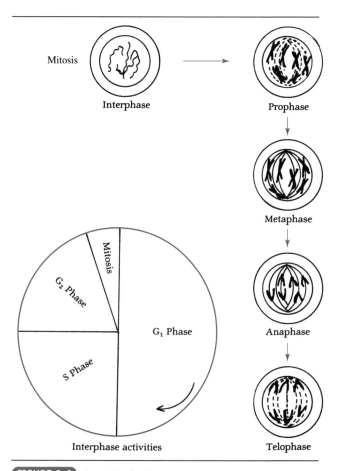

FIGURE 3.6 The cycle of cell growth (mitosis). The cell cycle begins with interphase. During this phase, the normal cell progresses through the G_1, S, and G_2 phases. Actual cell division, **mitosis,** follows the G_2 phase in a metabolically active cell.

time for the administration of chemotherapeutic drugs can be determined.

Interphase

Since the introduction of isotope techniques, it has been documented that in cells capable of reproduction, DNA is replicated or doubled during the interphase. Interphase is now divided into three subphases (see Fig. 3.6): G_1, first gap; S phase; and G_2, second gap. Under normal conditions, the amount of time that a cell spends in interphase is relatively constant for specific cell types.

1. The G_1 subphase lasts for approximately 6 to 8 hours. During this period, the nucleolus (nucleoli) becomes visible, and the chromosomes are extended and active metabolically. The cell synthesizes RNA and protein in preparation for cell division. As the G_1 period ends, cellular metabolic activity slows down.
2. The S subphase lasts for approximately 6 hours. This is the time of DNA replication, during which both growth and metabolic activities are minimal. However, all metabolic activities do not stop because not all the DNA is replicated at the same time. The shorter chromosomes are replicated first, and the others follow according to their length. Some DNA strands complete replication and resume the output of their messages while others are still replicating. The protein portion of the chromosome is also duplicated, so that at the end of the S stage, each chromosome homologue has doubled but is held together by a single centromere (Table 3.1).
3. The G_2 phase is relatively short, lasting approximately 4 to 5 hours. This is the second period of growth, when the

DNA can again function to its maximum in the synthesis of RNA and proteins in preparation for mitotic division. By the time a cell is ready to enter into mitotic division, proteins have been constructed in preparation for cell division, and both the DNA and the RNA are doubled. The centrioles have divided, forming a pair of new centrioles at right angles to each other.

The Four Phases of Mitotic Division

The **M phase** is the period of actual cell division, which lasts from 30 to 60 minutes; however, not all human body cells duplicate at this rate. The rate is most rapid in the early embryo, with a progressive slowing down throughout the rest of fetal life and childhood. In adults, most cells undergo mitotic division only fast enough to replace cells, with the eventual loss in old age of many types of cells. Abnormal conditions (malignancies) can alter the rate of mitosis of particular cell lines during any stage of growth and development.

During mitosis, the replicated DNA and other cellular contents are equally distributed between the daughter cells. The four mitotic periods are prophase, metaphase, anaphase, and telophase (Table 3.2). Each state is visible in stained preparations by use of a conventional light microscope.

Prophase. In this stage of mitosis, the replicated strands of chromatin become tightly coiled, distinctive structures. The identical halves, referred to as **chromatids,** are joined at the centromere. The nucleolus and nuclear envelope disintegrate, with the fragments scattering in the cytoplasm. The centrioles, composed of microtubules, separate and migrate to the opposite poles of the cell. The microtubules aggregate to form the mitotic spindle that is attached to the centrioles.

Metaphase. During metaphase, the identical sister chromatids move to the center of the spindle (the equatorial plate). Each of the chromatid pairs is attached to a spindle fiber and aligned along the equator of the cell. The point of attachment is the centromere, a constriction that divides the chromatid into an upper and a lower portion.

TABLE 3.1   Summary of DNA Structure and Activities

- A single strand of DNA is composed of a chain of phosphorylated deoxyribose sugars, each attached to a purine (adenine or guanine) or pyrimidine (cytosine or thymine) base to form nucleotides. The sugars are bonded together between the OH (hydroxyl) group of the 3′ carbon at one end and the PO_4 group on the 5′ carbon of the next group. Every strand has a free 5′ phosphate on one end and a free 3′ hydroxyl on the other. This configuration results in a structural direction or polarity on each strand.
- Each strand of DNA is arranged in a linear sequence consisting of any of the four nucleotide bases (adenine, thymine, cytosine, and guanine). These nucleotide bases come in close contact with the complimentary nucleotide bases on the opposite strand of the two DNA strands, the double helix.
- Hydrogen bonding produces interstrand pairing of complimentary bases (adenine with thymine; cytosine with guanine). Two hydrogen bonds exist between adenine and thymine; three hydrogen bonds exist between cytosine and guanine).
- The two strands of a DNA double helix run in opposite directions with the beginning 3′ carbon on one strand across from a free 5′ carbon on the opposing strand. This configuration is referred to as antiparallel.
- DNA synthesis in vivo and in vitro is unidirectional, proceeding from 5′ to 3′ end with growth of the new strand only at the 3′ end.

TABLE 3.2   Characteristics of the Four Mitotic Periods

Prophase
Chromatin becomes tightly coiled
Nucleolus and nuclear envelope disintegrate
Centrioles move to opposite poles of the cell

Metaphase
Sister chromatids move to the equatorial plate

Anaphase
Sister chromatids separate and move to opposite poles

Telophase
Chromosomes arrive at opposite poles
Nucleolus and nuclear membrane reappear
Chromatin pattern reappears

Anaphase. This phase begins as soon as the chromatids are pulled apart and lasts until the newly formed chromosomes reach the opposite poles of the spindle. In this phase, the chromatid pairs are separated, with one-half of each pair being pulled at their centromere by the spindle fibers toward each pole. Which half goes to which pole is random. Chromatids become chromosomes only after they have separated at the beginning of anaphase.

Telophase. The chromosomes arrive at opposite poles of the cell in early telophase. One of each kind of chromosome arrives at each of the poles of the cell. The nucleolus and nuclear membrane reappear and the spindle fibers disappear during this phase. Because the chromosomes uncoil and become longer and thinner, the chromosome structural formations disappear. The DNA and proteins (nucleoproteins) now assume their distinctive chromatin arrangement.

Following the stages that constitute nuclear division (**karyokinesis**), the cell undergoes cytokinesis. **Cytokinesis** is the division of cytoplasm. The cytoplasm around the two new nuclei becomes furrowed, and the cytoplasmic membrane pinches in. This pinching in is accomplished by the contraction of a ring of microfilaments that forms at the furrow. At the completion of cytokinesis, two new and identical daughter cells have been formed.

G_0 Phase

Following the M phase, some cells continue through the mitotic cycle repeatedly but others lose their mitotic ability and enter a protracted state of mitotic inactivity, the G_0 phase. In some cases, cells will be stimulated by factors such as hormones (refer to Chapter 5 for a discussion of the hormone erythropoietin in the production of erythrocytes) to reenter the mitotic cycle. Abnormal proliferation of cells may result from overstimulation by extrinsic or intrinsic factors. Other nucleated cells such as nerve cells lose their ability to undergo mitosis and remain in the G_0 (zero growth) phase permanently.

Meiosis

Meiosis (Fig. 3.7) is the process of cell division unique to **gametes** (ova and sperm). In contrast to mitosis, the process of meiosis produces four gametes with genetic variability. Gametes have *only* one of the homologues of each of the 23 pairs of chromosomes (the haploid [$1n$] number). Other nucleated human body cells contain 23 homologous pairs of chromosomes (the diploid [$2n$] number).

The phases of meiosis differ from mitosis in several important ways. During phase I of meiosis, the homologous sister chromatids in a tetrad formation undergo the process of **synapsis**, lining up end-to-end. Synapsis allows for the easy exchange of genetic material through **crossing over.** In phase II of meiosis, reduction division occurs, producing the haploid number in the resulting gametes.

The Foundations of Genetic Interactions

Genetics, the study of the transmission of inherited characteristics, is related to meiosis and is important in the study of inherited hematological disorders. During the last 30

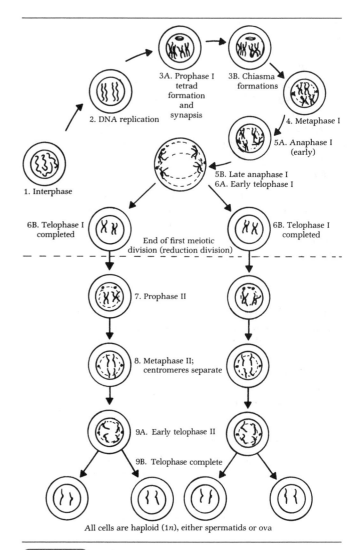

FIGURE 3.7 Meiotic division. The major events in the process of division of ova and spermatids are depicted. Meiosis, unlike mitosis, has two stages *without* the duplication of genetic material between the two stages.

years, a revolution has occurred in our understanding of genetic diseases. The identification of single-gene disorders is proceeding at an exponential rate. More than 200 human genes have been cloned and the chromosomal map location is known for more than 140 of these genes. More than 100 genes are known to be associated with one or more diseases. The hemoglobinopathies and thalassemias (discussed in Chapter 13) have been most extensively studied at the DNA level. Information is also rapidly emerging about alterations in genes for factors VIII:C and IX of the coagulation system.

In 1953 Watson and Crick described the double-helix model of DNA in which genetic information is encoded into linear arrays in the form of the deoxyribonucleotide bases adenine (A), thymine (T), cytosine (C), and guanine (G). The two strands of DNA have antiparallel complementary sequences that pair by hydrogen bonding between the bases; thymine pairs with adenine and cytosine with guanine. The genetic code, which stores hereditary information, is stored as triplets of nucleotides that encode for various amino acids. Genomes of different organisms are unique and distinguishable from one another. The human genome consists of double-stranded DNA molecules organized into chromosomes with cell nuclei. Most human DNA is in the right-handed beta configuration having 10.5 bp per helical turn.

A **gene** is a segment of DNA that is arranged along the chromosome at a specific position called a **locus.** Genes at a specific locus that differ in their nucleotide sequence are called **alleles.** Thus, in each somatic cell, one of the members of a set of alleles is maternally derived and the other paternally derived. Genes that lie close to each other in the linear array along the chromosomes have less opportunity for crossing over; genes that recombine once in every 100 meiotic opportunities are said to be 1 centimorgan (cM) apart. The relationship between the linear proximity of genetic loci and the recombinational frequency between them provides the basis for linkage mapping. However, this relationship is not always a linear one. Particular segments of DNA seem to be recombination hotspots and are predisposed to crossing over much more often than would be predicted from their DNA lengths.

Each gene has a unique sequence of nucleotides that is transcribed into mRNA. It is the sequence of nucleotides that determines gene function. In most cases the coding sequences, or **exons,** are interrupted by intervening sequences, or **introns.** The entire gene, including both exons and introns, is transcribed in a pre-mRNA; however, the exon sequences are ultimately translated on the ribosomes into protein but the intron sequences are spliced out as the pre-mRNA is processed into mature RNA. The sequences at the intron-exon junctions, called splices, are critical for mRNA processing and important potential sites of mutation.

Genetic Alterations

A gene, as the functional unit of a chromosome, is responsible for determining the structure of a single protein or polypeptide. Normally a gene is a very stable unit that undergoes thousands of replications, with perfect copies resulting each time. On rare occasions, a copy may be produced that varies slightly and leads to an alteration in transcription from the long DNA molecule, with far-reaching consequences. A change in the gene is caused by **mutation** producing a change in the actual structure of DNA. A single-nucleotide change among the thousands of base pairs in a gene may have crucial consequences to the gene product. An example of such a gene alteration has been traced to Queen Victoria or one of her immediate ancestors; the alteration led to classic hemophilia (discussed in Chapters 26 and 27) that spread throughout the royal families of Europe.

Mutations usually affect a single base in the DNA. The sequence of nucleotide bases in the DNA is altered by the substitution of a single different base at one point along the DNA molecule. These mutations may act by affecting transcription of the gene, RNA processing to produce the mature mRNA, or translation of the mRNA into protein; or they may act by altering an important amino acid in the protein products.

The sickle cell mutation (Fig. 3.8) is the best known example of a single-nucleotide alteration. Human hemoglobin was

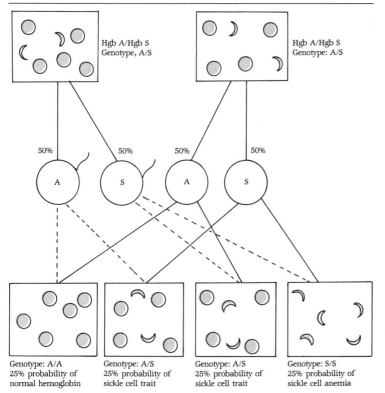

FIGURE 3.8 Sickle cell trait and anemia. When two persons with sickle cell trait (genotype: A/S) produce offspring, the expected genotypic ratio is 1:2:1, or a 25% chance of offspring with a normal hemoglobin (A/A), a 50% chance of offspring with sickle cell trait (A/S), and a 25% chance of offspring with sickle cell anemia (S/S). Hgb = hemoglobin.

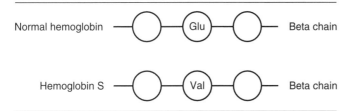

FIGURE 3.9 Hemoglobin S amino acid sequence. Hemoglobin S differs from hemoglobin A in one amino acid residue on the beta chain of the hemoglobin molecule. On this chain, valine (Val) is substituted for glutamic acid (Glu) at the sixth position of the chain.

one of the first proteins for which the genetic code was worked out and is a good example of the relationship between genes and proteins. The normal adult hemoglobin molecule (discussed in Chapter 5) consists in part of the protein globin. Globin is arranged into four chains in the form of two identical pairs. In each pair, the alpha chain consists of 141 amino acids and the beta chain contains 146 amino acids. The laboratory procedures of electrophoresis and chromatography allow determination of the exact sequence of amino acids on each of these two chains. In the case of sickle cell disease, hemoglobin S has a difference in one amino acid on the beta chain (Fig. 3.9). On this chain, valine is substituted for glutamic acid at the sixth position on the chain because an A in the sixth codon is changed to a T; this changes the codon GAG (glutamic acid) to GTG (valine). In hemoglobin C disorder, a substitution of lysine for glutamic acid at the same position in the beta chain occurs.

Through meiosis, a parent with the trait may pass the mutation to another generation. In the case of sickle cell disease (anemia), an individual is *homozygous* for the trait. Because in the genetic expression of this disorder a lack of dominance exists, both genes of an allelic pair are partially and about equally expressed. Those individuals who are heterozygous for the trait are designated as suffering from sickle cell trait. The mode of inheritance of hemoglobin S is depicted in Figure 3.10. A further discussion of abnormal hemoglobins is presented in Chapter 13.

Linkage studies can be used for those families where the precise mutation is unknown but the locus of the mutation is known, such as in the hemoglobinopathies. Linkage analysis has proved highly useful as an indirect method of distinguishing between chromosomes carrying normal and mutant alleles. These polymorphisms represent so-called neutral mutations. Indirect analysis of this type has been used in the prenatal diagnosis of beta-thalassemia (see Chapter 13) and is available for hemophilia A. At the present time, prenatal diagnosis by DNA analysis is available for several hematological disorders including hemophilia A, hemophilia B, sickle cell disease, alpha-thalassemia, and beta-thalassemia.

MOLECULAR GENETICS IN HEMATOLOGY

The techniques of molecular biology are now being applied to hematology. Molecular methods can be used in hematology to identify changes ranging from a single chromosome disorder to alterations involving the interchange of DNA between chromosomes. Abnormalities of erythrocytes (sickle cell anemia and alpha and beta thalassemias), leukocytes (acute myeloblastic leukemia, acute lymphoblastic leukemia, chronic myeloid leukemia, and lymphoma), and coagulation factors (hemophilia A, hemophilia B, and factor V defect) can be detected in this manner.

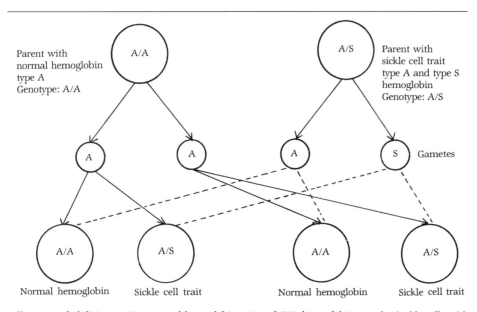

Offspring probabilities are 50% normal hemoglobin A/A and 50% hemoglobin A and S (sickle cell trait)

FIGURE 3.10 Inheritance of hemoglobin S.

Molecular Testing Techniques

Three basic techniques used for analyzing gene structure are restriction endonuclease mapping, molecular cloning, and DNA sequencing. The most versatile technique and the one most responsible for the explosive progress of molecular biology is DNA analysis by use of unique prokaryotic enzymes known as restriction endonucleases, because they can cut within strands of duplex DNA.

Restriction endonucleases are bacterial enzymes that protect their host from viral invasion through their ability to cut into double-stranded DNA at specific sites determined by the base sequence of individual strands. Each of the several hundred known restriction enzymes recognizes specific short oligonucleotides in foreign DNA.

Southern blotting (Fig. 3.11) is a technology for identifying small DNA fragments. Because certain restriction enzymes can divide DNA reproducibly into small pieces, this allows restriction sites around a particular sequence of interest to be mapped. After digestion of a DNA preparation with one or several restriction enzymes, the resulting frag-

ments are separated according to size by gel electrophoresis. Their distribution in the gel is preserved as they are denatured and transferred by blotting to a nitrocellulose or nylon membrane having a charged surface. After blotted DNA fragments complementary to the probe have completed hybridization, radiographic film is exposed to the membrane filter, resulting in an autoradiographic copy. The position and number of radioactive bands on multiple autoradiographs thus generated can be used to detect the presence and molecular size of fragments containing a specific gene.

Hybridization

Almost every molecular assay depends on the principle of hybridization or the interaction between two complementary nucleotide sequences of DNA or RNA molecules. Hybridization reactions involve a small piece of nucleotide base sequence which is used to search for its complementary sequence among the nucleotide base sequences present among the three billion base pairs comprising human genomic DNA. This results in a very specific reaction.

Short detector sequences of nucleotides are referred to as **probes** or primers, depending on the procedure in which they are used. Hybridization reactions depend on unwinding and separating the two strands of the DNA helix, a process called denaturation. Denaturation of DNA can be accomplished in a variety of ways, e.g., heating or treatment with alcohol. In the presence of complementary base sequences, hydrogen bonds can reform or hybridize.

After DNA is digested by restriction enzymes and the fragments are separated and fixed in the course of Southern blotting, the fragment containing a gene of interest can be located by use of nuclei acid probes. If attempting to detect a target sequence in solution, probes also can be immobilized on a solid support and used to capture target sequences from solution.

Discovery in 1985 of the **polymerase chain reaction** (PCR) (Fig. 3.12) has transformed the power of molecular genetics and provided a simple procedure for massively amplifying the DNA of cloned genes. The importance of PCR lies in its unlimited capacity to amplify DNA, fragmented or intact, by biochemical rather than biologic proliferation. The method makes it possible to amplify known DNA sequences ranging from 50 to over 2000 bp in length by more than a millionfold in only a few hours, and by a billionfold with a day or two.

PCR is unrivaled as a means for direct cloning and gene sequence analysis, for identifying point mutations, and for rapid sequencing of mitochondrial and viral DNA and RNA.

The first diagnostic application of PCR technology was in prenatal diagnosis of sickle cell anemia through amplification of beta globin sequences. Hybridization of labeled oligonucleotide probes allowed the distinction of mutant from normal alleles. PCR has become increasingly popular for detecting chromosomal breakpoints, fusion genes, and minimal residual disease after chemotherapy for leukemia and lymphoma. Its very sensitivity is its only limitation.

Northern blotting is used for analysis of the proximal product of gene expression, mRNA. Cloned DNA probes can be used to determine whether a given gene is being expressed, and if so, how vigorously.

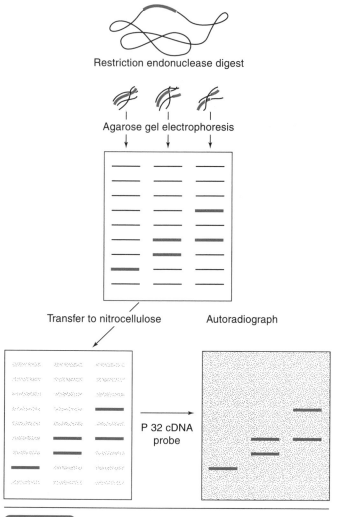

Restriction endonuclease digest

Agarose gel electrophoresis

Transfer to nitrocellulose

Autoradiograph

P 32 cDNA probe

FIGURE 3.11 The technique of Southern blotting identifies variable-length fragments of DNA with a P 32–labeled probe.

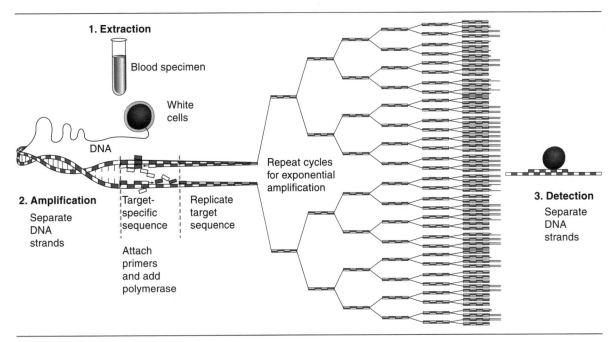

FIGURE 3.12 An example of polymerase chain reaction.

Recombinant DNA methodology, which relies on molecular hybridization, restriction endonuclease mapping, cloning, sequencing, and PCR technology, is only beginning to expedite advances against disease. To date, its greatest practical accomplishments have been in mass production of recombinant erythropoietin, in diagnosis and understanding of many disease states at a molecular level, and in antenatal prediction and family counseling for genetic disorders.

SUMMARY

Cells are the smallest organized units of a living organism. Cellular metabolism is responsible for the basic life processes within the human body.

Cellular Ultrastructure and Organization

The cellular membrane provides a semipermeable separation between cellular components and the surrounding environment. Chemically, membranes consist of proteins, phospholipids, cholesterol, and traces of polysaccharide. These components in the membrane are arranged according to the **fluid mosaic model.**

The cellular membrane has a variety of functions. These functions include cellular recognition and interaction between cells, osmosis, diffusion, active transport, and endocytosis. Endocytosis is important in defending the body against disease.

Organelles are functional units of the cell. Cellular organelles include the centrioles, ER (rough and smooth), the Golgi apparatus, lysosomes, microbodies, microfilaments, microtubules, mitochondria, and ribosomes. The cytoplasm may additionally contain vacuoles and metabolites, such as glycogen and ferritin.

The nucleus is a double-layered organelle containing both DNA in the form of chromatin and RNA in the nucleolus. The nucleus functions as the control center of the cell and is essential for its long-term survival. The RNA-containing nucleoli are contained within the nucleus. Nucleic acid (DNA) and protein within the nucleus are referred to as chromatin, which has characteristic patterns for different cell types. Chromatin can be classified as heterochromatin, an inactive form, and euchromatin, the site of active transcription. During mitosis, chromatin condenses into microscopically visible structures, the chromosomes. Chromosome analysis provides important supplementary information in various blood dyscrasias, such as the leukemias.

Nucleated body cells reproduce by the process of mitosis. Germ cells, ova and sperm, reproduce by the process of meiosis. Both processes are important for the hematologist to understand because genetic errors can produce defective proteins such as sickle cell hemoglobin.

Molecular Genetics in Hematology

Techniques in molecular genetics are beginning to be extensively used in hematology. A wide range of abnormalities can be detected with these techniques. Molecular testing techniques include three basic techniques for analyzing gene structure—restriction endonuclease mapping, molecular cloning, and DNA sequencing. Southern blotting is a technology for identifying small DNA fragments.

Almost every molecular assay depends on the principle of hybridization or the interaction between two complementary nucleotide sequences of DNA or RNA molecules. Techniques of importance include the polymerase chain reaction (PCR) and Northern blotting.

BIBLIOGRAPHY

Carr, Katharine E. and P. G. Toner. *Cell Structure: An Introduction to Biomedical Electron Microscopy.* New York: Churchill-Livingstone, 1982, pp. 6–43.

Creager, Joan G. *Human Anatomy and Physiology.* Belmont, CA: Wadsworth, 1983, pp. 47–61.

Jandl, James H. *Blood* (2nd ed.). Boston: Little, Brown & Co., 1996, pp. 71–134.

Klug, William S. and Michael R. Cummings. *Concepts of Genetics* (2nd ed.). Columbus, OH: Merrill, 1986, pp. 243–256.

Pansky, Ben. *Dynamic Anatomy and Physiology.* New York: Macmillan, 1975, pp. 36–53.

Strand, Fleur L. *Physiology* (2nd ed.). New York: Macmillan, 1986, pp. 8–25, 57–67.

Wheater, Paul R. et al. *Functional Histology.* London: Churchill-Livingstone, 1979, pp. 2–23.

Winchester, A. M. *Human Genetics* (2nd ed.). Columbus, OH: Merrill, 1975.

REVIEW QUESTIONS

1. The smallest organized unit of living tissue is the:
   - A. Nucleus.
   - B. Cell.
   - C. Organelle.
   - D. Cytoplasm.

2. The cell membrane's *major* components are:
   - A. Carbohydrates and proteins.
   - B. Proteins and lipids.
   - C. Lipids and glycoproteins.
   - D. Polysaccharides and lipids.

3. Which of the following is a characteristic of osmosis?
   - A. Requires energy (ATP).
   - B. Movement of water molecules.
   - C. An unusual cellular activity.
   - D. Requires a carrier molecule.

4. Which of the following is a characteristic of active transport?
   - A. Requires energy (ATP).
   - B. Movement of molecules up the concentration gradient.
   - C. Requires a carrier molecule.
   - D. All of the above.

5. Phagocytosis is:
   - A. A type of endocytosis.
   - B. The engulfment of fluid molecules.
   - C. The engulfment of particulate matter.
   - D. Both A and C.

Questions 6 through 9: match the following organelles with their appropriate function.

6. ___ Centrioles.
7. ___ Rough endoplasmic reticulum.
8. ___ Smooth endoplasmic reticulum.
9. ___ Golgi apparatus.

   - A. Protein production.
   - B. Concentration of secretory granules.
   - C. Lipid synthesis.
   - D. DNA synthesis.
   - E. Points of attachment of the spindle fibers.

Questions 10 through 13: match the following organelles with their appropriate function.

10. ___ Lysosomes.
11. ___ Microtubules.
12. ___ Mitochondria.
13. ___ Ribosomes.

   - A. Energy production and heme synthesis.
   - B. Protein synthesis.
   - C. Cytoskeleton.
   - D. Intracellular digestion.
   - E. Carbohydrate synthesis.

14. Glycogen is a:
   - A. Protein.
   - B. Lipid.
   - C. Carbohydrate.
   - D. Hormone.

15. A cellular inclusion that represents a common storage form of iron is:
   - A. Glycogen.
   - B. Vacuoles.
   - C. Auer body.
   - D. Ferritin.

16. The nucleus of the cell contains:
   - A. Chromatin, nucleoli, and nucleoplasm.
   - B. Chromatin, nucleoli, and ribosomes.
   - C. DNA, RNA, and ribosomes.
   - D. DNA, RNA, and mitochondria.

17. The overall function of DNA is:
   - A. Protein and enzyme production.
   - B. Control of cellular function and transmission of genetic information.
   - C. Control of heterochromatin and euchromatin synthesis.
   - D. Production of cellular energy and transmission of genetic information.

18. Heterochromatin is:
   - A. Genetically inactive.
   - B. Found in patches or clumps.
   - C. Genetically inactive and pale staining.
   - D. Both A and B.

19. Chromosomal translocation is:
   - A. A frequent activity of homologous chromosomes in meiosis.
   - B. A rearrangement of genetic material.
   - C. Attachment of a piece of chromosome to another nonhomologous chromosome.
   - D. All of the above.

20. A chromosomal deletion is:
   - A. Loss of a pair of chromosomes.
   - B. Loss of a segment of chromosome.
   - C. Attachment of a piece of a chromosome.
   - D. An exchange of genetic material.

Questions 21 through 24: match the following activities with the appropriate period of time. Use an answer only once.

21. ___ G_1.
22. ___ S.
23. ___ G_2.
24. ___ G_0.

A. DNA replication.

B. Protracted state of mitotic inactivity.

C. Immediately precedes actual mitotic division.

D. Actual mitotic division.

E. An active period of protein synthesis and cellular metabolism.

Questions 25 through 29: match the following mitotic activities with the appropriate cellular activity. Use an answer only once.

25. ___ Prophase.
26. ___ Metaphase.
27. ___ Anaphase.
28. ___ Telophase.
29. ___ Cytokinesis.

A. Chromosomes line up at the cell's equator.

B. Two identical daughter cells form.

C. Division of the cellular cytoplasm.

D. Chromatids separate and move to opposite ends of the mitotic spindle.

E. Chromosomes tightly coil and condense.

30. In meiosis, the cells produced contain:

A. A $2n$ number of chromosomes.
B. 22 pairs of chromosomes.
C. 23 pairs of chromosomes.
D. 23 chromosomes.

31. Hematologists are interested in inherited disorders. Which of the following are inherited disorders.

A. Sickle cell trait.
B. Sickle cell anemia.
C. Hemophilia.
D. All of the above

32. Molecular techniques are being used to detect abnormalities of:

A. Erythrocytes.
B. Leukocytes.
C. Some coagulation factors.
D. All of the above.

33. The molecular technique that is the most versatile and the one most responsible for the explosive progress of molecular biology is:

A. Hybridization.
B. Restriction endonucleases.
C. Southern blotting.
D. Northern blotting.

Questions 34 through 37: match the following.

34. ___ Polymerase chain reaction.
35. ___ Southern blotting.
36. ___ Restriction endonucleases.
37. ___ Northern blotting.

A. Used for analysis of mRNA.

B. Massive amplification of DNA of cloned genes.

C. Cut into DNA.

D. Identification of small DNA fragments.

Hematopoiesis

Hematopoiesis
Origin of blood cells
Blood cell development
Hematopoietic growth factors
Bone marrow sites and
    function

Maturational
    characteristics of
    hematopoietic cells
Summary
Bibliography
Review questions

OBJECTIVES

Hematopoiesis

- Explain the origin of blood cells and trace the sequential sites of cellular proliferation and development.
- Describe the development of cells from the stem cell level to the blast form of a cell.
- State the function of hematopoietic growth factors.
- Name at least three growth factors.
- Name the cells in developmental order that will mature into erythrocytes, thrombocytes, plasma cells, and the five leukocyte types.

- Name and describe in detail the two overall features of a cell that are important in the identification of a cell and that may vary as a cell matures.
- Compare the nuclear characteristics of shape, chromatin pattern, and nucleoli in specific cell types and according to the age of the cell.
- Compare the cytoplasmic features of color, granulation, shape, quantity, vacuolization, and inclusions to cell maturity.
- Name and describe the average percentage and cellular characteristics of the six mature leukocytes found in normal peripheral blood.

The microscopic examination of blood cells is an important aspect of the practice of hematology. Cell structure and function, hematopoiesis, and the morphological characteristics of blood cells are presented in this chapter. A basic understanding of these fundamental topics is required for a comprehensive understanding of hematological processes, and provides a foundation for the identification of specific peripheral blood cells.

HEMATOPOIESIS

Hematopoiesis is the process of blood cell production, differentiation, and development. The hematopoietic system consists of the bone marrow, liver, spleen, lymph nodes, and thymus. Before investigating the general maturational characteristics of cells, a knowledge of blood cell development is useful.

Origin of Blood Cells

Embryonic blood cells, excluding the lymphocyte type of white blood cell, originate from the mesenchymal tissue that arises from the embryonic germ layer, the mesoderm (Fig. 4.1). The sites of blood cell development follow a definite sequence in the embryo and fetus (see Fig. 4.1):

1. The first blood cells are primitive red blood cells (erythroblasts) formed in the islets of the yolk sac during the first 2 to 8 weeks of life.
2. Gradually, the **liver** and **spleen** replace the yolk sac as the sites of blood cell development. By the second month of gestation, the liver becomes the major site of hematopoiesis, and granular types of leukocytes have made their

initial appearance. The liver and spleen predominate from about the second to fifth months of fetal life.
3. In the fourth month of gestation, the **bone marrow** begins to function in the production of blood cells. After the fifth fetal month, the bone marrow begins to assume its ultimate role as the primary site of hematopoiesis (medullary hematopoiesis).

Blood Cell Development

The pluripotent stem cell is the first in a sequence of steps of hematopoietic cell generation and maturation (Plate 1). The progenitor of all blood cells is called the **multipotential hematopoietic stem cell.** These cells have the capacity for self-renewal as well as proliferation and differentiation into progenitor cells committed to one specific cell line.

Hematopoietic cells can be divided into three phases according to cell maturity. The most immature group consists of primitive multipotential cells capable of self-renewal and differentiation into all blood cell lines; the intermediate group consists of committed progenitor cells destined to develop into distinct cell lines; and the most developed group consists of mature cells with specific functions.

The multipotential stem cell is the progenitor of two major ancestral cell lines: lymphocytic and nonlymphocytic cells. The lymphoid stem cell is the precursor of either mature T cells or B cells/plasma cells. The nonlymphocytic (myeloid) stem cell progresses to the progenitor CFU-GEMM (colony-forming unit, granulocyte-erythrocyte-monocyte-megakaryocyte). The acronym CFU is used as a prefix to record the number of colony forming units of different progenitor cells that are identified through in vitro clonal assays. The unit colony of CFU-GEMM leads to the development of distinct subsets of committed progenitor cells. The CFU-GEMM can lead to the formation of CFU-GM (CFU-granulocyte macrophage/monocyte), CFU-Eo (CFU-eosinophil), CFU-Bs (CFU-basophil), and CFU-Meg (CFU-megakaryocyte). In erythropoiesis, the CFU-GEMM differentiates into the BFU-E (burst-forming unit-erythroid). Each of the CFUs in turn can produce a colony of one hematopoietic lineage under appropriate growth conditions.

The formation and development of mature blood cells from the bone marrow multipotential stem cell is controlled by growth factors and inhibitors and the microenvironment. The microenvironment or locale influences behavior and controls proliferation of multipotential cells. Bone seems to provide the microenvironment most appropriate for proliferation and maturation of cells.

Hematopoietic Growth Factors

The hematopoietic growth factors are glycoprotein hormones that regulate the proliferation and differentiation of hematopoietic progenitor cells and the function of mature blood cells. Semisolid culture systems that were developed in the late 1960s supported the growth of bone marrow progenitor cells in vitro and the subsequent identification of hematopoietic growth factors. These factors were referred to as **colony-stimulating factors (CSFs)** because they stimulated the formation of colonies of cells derived from individual bone marrow progenitors.

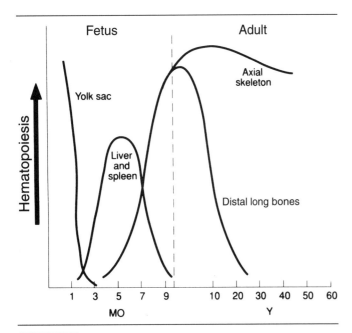

FIGURE 4.1 Sites of active hematopoiesis in the fetus and adult. During fetal development, hematopoiesis is established in the yolk sac and it progresses to the liver and spleen. Hematopoiesis is limited to the skeleton in adults, under normal circumstances. (From R. S. Hillman and C. A. Finch. *Red Cell Manual* [6th ed.], Philadelphia: Davis, 1992.)

Erythropoietin, granulocyte-macrophage colony-stimulating factor (GM-CSF), granulocyte colony-stimulating factor (G-CSF), macrophage colony-stimulating factor (M-CSF), and interleukin-3 are representative factors that have been identified, cloned, and produced through recombinant DNA technology. The hematopoietic growth factors interact with blood cells at different levels in the cascade of cell differentiation from the multipotential progenitor to the circulating mature cell.

Each growth factor is encoded by a single gene. The gene for erythropoietin is located on chromosome 7. The genes for GM-CSF, interleukin-3, and M-CSF are clustered on the long arm of chromosome 5. Chromosome 17 is the location of the G-CSF gene. The cellular sources and other characteristics of growth factors are presented in Table 4.1.

Protein molecules that work in conjunction with hematopoietic growth factors to stimulate proliferation and differentiation of specific cell lines are the interleukins: interleukin-1 (IL-1) to interleukin-7 (IL-7). Interleukins are cytokines that act independently or in conjunction with other interleukins to encourage hematopoietic growth. The interleukins are described in Table 4.2. This interacting network of inflammatory stimuli and cytokines suggests that these growth factors may have a limited role in hematopoietic homeostasis, but a major role in host responses to infection or antigenic challenge. The major role of the hematopoietic growth factors appears to be regulating the proliferation and differentiation of hematopoietic progenitor cells as well as regulating the survival and function of mature blood cells.

The biological effects of hematopoietic growth factors are mediated through specific binding to receptors on the surface of target cells. Hematopoietic growth factors are being used and tested in clinical trials for the treatment of a variety of hematological disorders. Specific factors are being used as adjunct therapy in a wide variety of diseases (e.g., to stimulate the production of granulocytes or lymphocytes).

Bone Marrow Sites and Function

Bone marrow is found within the cavities of all bones and may be present in two forms: yellow marrow, which is normally inactive and composed mostly of fat (adipose) tissue, and red marrow, which is normally active in the production of most types of leukocytes, erythrocytes, and thrombocytes. During the first few years of life, the marrow of all bones is red and cellular. The red bone marrow is initially found in both the appendicular and the axial skeleton (Fig. 4.2A) in young persons but progressively becomes confined to the axial skeleton and proximal ends of the long bones in adults (see Fig. 4.2B). By age 18, red marrow is found only in the vertebrae, ribs, sternum, skull bones, pelvis, and to some extent the proximal epiphyses of the femur and humerus.

In certain abnormal circumstances, the spleen, liver, and lymph nodes revert back to producing immature blood cells (**extramedullary hematopoiesis**). In these cases, enlargement of the spleen and liver is frequently noted on physical examination of the patient. This situation suggests that undifferentiated primitive blood cells are present in these areas and are able to proliferate if an appropriate stimulus is present. This situation occurs under the following conditions:

1. When the bone marrow becomes dysfunctional in cases such as aplastic anemia, infiltration by malignant cells, or overproliferation of a cell line, for example, leukemia
2. When the bone marrow is unable to meet the demands placed on it, as in the hemolytic anemias (a full discussion of the anemias is presented in Part 2, Chapters 8–13)

Maturational Characteristics of Hematopoietic Cells

The examination of a stained peripheral blood smear is an important component of the **complete blood cell count (CBC)** procedure, which is routinely performed in the hematology laboratory. In this procedure (refer to the leukocyte

---

TABLE 4.1 Characteristics of Human Hematopoietic Growth Factors

Growth Factor	Cellular Source	Progenitor Cell Target	Mature Cell Target
Erythropoietin	Peritubular cells of the kidney, Kupffer cells	CFU-E, late BFU-E, CFU-Meg	None
Interleukin-3	Activated T lymphocytes	CFU-blast, CFU-GEMM, CFU-GM, CFU-G, CFU-M, CFU-Eo, CFU-Meg, CFU-Baso, BFU-E	Eosinophils, monocytes
G-CSF	Monocytes, fibroblasts, endothelial cells	CFU-G	Granulocytes
M-CSF	Monocytes, fibroblasts, endothelial cells	CFU-M	Monocytes
GM-CSF	T lymphocytes, monocytes, fibroblasts, endothelial cells	CFU-blast, CFU-GEMM, CFU-GM, CFU-G, CFU-M, CFU-Eo, CFU-Meg, BFU-E	Eosinophils, monocytes, granulocytes

G-CSF = granulocyte colony-stimulating factor; M-CSF = macrophage colony-stimulating factor; GM-CSF = granulocyte-macrophage colony-stimulating factor; CFU-blast = colony-forming unit-blast; CFU-GEMM = colony-forming unit-granulocyte, erythrocyte, monocyte, and megakaryocyte; CFU-GM = colony-forming unit-granulocyte and macrophage; CFU-Eo = colony-forming unit-eosinophil; CFU-Meg = colony-forming unit—megakaryocyte; BFU-E = burst-forming unit-erythroid; CFU-G = colony-forming unit-granulocyte; CFU-M = colony-forming unit-macrophage; CFU-E = colony-forming unit-erythroid; and CFU-Baso = colony-forming unit-basophil.

TABLE 4.2 A Summary of Interleukin Functions

Interleukin-1 (IL-1)	A response modulator molecule that appears to influence different progenitor cells indirectly in hematopoiesis. It may act in synergy with IL-3, M-CSF, G-CSF, and GM-CSF to stimulate cells. IL-1 stimulates the lymphoid stem cell. It enhances the B cell response and proliferation of T cells.
Interleukin-2 (IL-2)	Influences the proliferation and regulation of T cells, B cells, natural killer (NK) cells, and monocytes. It acts on activated B cells as a growth and differentiation factor.
Interleukin-3 (IL-3)	Supports the proliferation of CFU-GEMM, CFU-M, CFU-Meg, CFU-Eo, and CFU-Bs colonies from bone marrow. IL-3 acts with M-CSF to stimulate proliferation of monocytes and macrophages. It also stimulates granulocyte, monocyte, eosinophil, and mast cell production and induces basophil histamine release.
Interleukin-4 (IL-4)	Influences T and B lymphocyte pathways and mast cells. IL-4 assists B cell maturation and stimulates growth of helper T lymphocytes. It enhances growth of mast cells in response to IL-3, and interacts with G-CSF to proliferate myeloid progenitor cells.
Interleukin-5 (IL-5)	Promotes differentiation of B cells and immunoglobulin M (IgM) secretion and proliferation by B cells. Also stimulates eosinophil colony production and differentiation and interacts with GM-CSF and IL-3 in eosinophil induction.
Interleukin-6 (IL-6)	Induces differentiation of B cells and enhances immunoglobulin secretion by B lymphocytes. IL-6 is active in the development of immature B cells and stimulates T lymphocytes.
Interleukin-7 (IL-7)	Is active in the development of immature B cells and stimulates T lymphocytes.
Interleukin-8 (IL-8)	Originally described as a monocyte-derived neutrophil chemotactic factor. IL-8 appears to be an inflammatory cytokine that is chemotactic for both neutrophils and T cells. It is a potent stimulator of neutrophils, and it activates the respiratory burst and the release of both specific and azurophilic granular contents.
Interleukin-9 (IL-9)	IL-9 is a potent CD4+ T lymphocyte growth factor. It stimulates the proliferation of activated CD4+ T cells and proliferation of mast cells. In addition, it has been demonstrated to support growth of erythroid blast-forming units (BFU-E). IL-9 may play a role in autocrine growth of tumors in large cell anaplastic lymphomas and Hodgkin's disease. Hodgkin and Reed-Sternberg cells produce IL-9 transcripts and protein and express surface-binding sites for IL-9.
Interleukin-10 (IL-10)	IL-10 is secreted by macrophage/monocytes and T lymphocytes. The cell targets are macrophage/monocyte inhibition and B lymphocyte activation. The ability of IL-10 to turn down cytokine synthesis provides negative feedback. In patients with intermediate or high-grade non-Hodgkin's lymphoma, the presence of detectable serum IL-10 at diagnosis has been correlated to a significantly shorter overall and progression-free survival. Patients with stage IV disease and detectable serum IL-10 have a particularly poor prognosis (less than 4 years of survival).
Interleukin-11 (IL-11)	IL-11 is a bone marrow, stromal-derived cytokine that appears to be a multifunctional regulator of hematopoiesis. IL-11 has been shown to synergize with IL-3 to stimulate the production of megakaryocyte and myeloid progenitors and to increase the number of Ig-secreting B lymphocytes both in vivo and in vitro. IL-11 acts in a manner similar to IL-6 on hematopoietic progenitor cells. It is known to promote differentiation of normal human B cells. IL-11 does not result in significantly increased DNA synthesis or Ig secretion of B cell alone. IL-11 promotes differentiation of human B lymphocytes only in the presence of accessory T cells and monocytes. A minor component of this effect may be through stimulation of IL-6 production by CD4+ T cells and monocytes. IL-11 might regulate malignant cells of the megakaryocytic line.
Interleukin-12 (IL-12)	This cytokine is secreted by macrophage/monocytes and dendritic cells. The primary targets are NK cells and T lymphocytes. The primary effects on each target are IFN-gamma synthesis, cytolytic function, and CD4+ T cell differentiation. In fact, it was originally identified as a macrophage/derived activator of NK cell cytologic function but is now appreciated to be a potent inducer of IFN-gamma production by T cells as well as NK cells. IL-12, also known as NK cell stimulatory factor (NKSF) or cytotoxic lymphocytic maturation factor (CLMF), can enhance the activity of cytotoxic effector cells. This cytokine was first identified by its ability to synergize with IL-2 in augmenting cytotoxic lymphocyte responses. Although IL-12 shares the functional properties of enhancing the cytotoxic function of NK cells and activated T cells with IL-2, it appears to act via a distinct mechanism independent of IL-2. In addition, IL-12 is a growth factor for activated NK/lymphokine-activated killer cells and for activated T cells of both the CD4+ and CD8+ subsets.
Interleukin-13 (IL-13)	The source of IL-13 is T cells. Inhibition of the release of inflammatory cytokines is its principal action.
Interleukin-14 (IL-14)	IL-14 is synthesized and secreted by T cells. The action of this cytokine is to induce proliferation of activated B cells.
Interleukin-15 (IL-15)	IL-15 is produced by macrophage/monocytes and other cells. The target cells are NK cells and T cell. Proliferation of these cells is the primary effect.

M-CSF = macrophage colony-stimulating factor; G-CSF = granulocyte colony-stimulating factor; GM-CSF = granulocyte-macrophage colony-stimulating factor; CFU-GEMM = colony-forming unit-granulocyte, erythrocyte, monocyte, and megakaryocyte; CFU-M = colony-forming unit-macrophage; CFU-Meg = colony-forming unit-megakaryocyte; CFU-Eo = colony-forming unit-eosinophil; CFU-Bs = colony-forming unit-basophil.

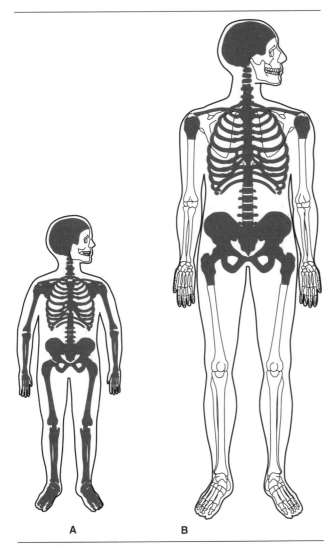

FIGURE 4.2 Sites of red bone marrow activity. **A.** Child. Red bone marrow (*red-shaded areas*) is located throughout the skeletal system in children. **B.** Adult. Yellow marrow replaces red marrow (*dark-shaded areas*) in the adult skeletal system. Red marrow activity occurs in the central portion of the skeleton.

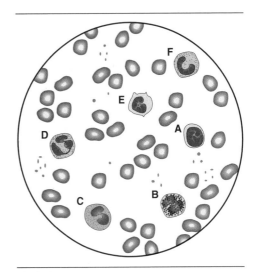

FIGURE 4.3 Normal peripheral blood cells. **A.** Lymphocytes. **B.** Basophils. **C.** Eosinophils. **D.** Segmented neutrophils. **E.** Monocytes. **F.** Band form neutrophil.

differential count in Chapter 24), white blood cells are examined, identified, and counted. Red blood cells and platelets are also carefully examined during this procedure.

In order to identify the normal cells (Fig. 4.3) that appear on a blood smear as well as recognize immature cells that may appear in various disorders or in the bone marrow (refer to bone marrow examination in Chapter 24), it is important to know the sequences of cellular development by name (Table 4.3) as well as the general maturational characteristics of blood cells. Specific cell-line maturational details and abnormalities that may be encountered in various types of cells are presented in relevant chapters in Parts 1, 2, and 3.

General Cellular Characteristics

The identification and stage of maturation of stained blood cells can be guided by a variety of systematic features (Table 4.4). Two important characteristics to observe initially in cell identification are:

1. Overall cell size
2. Nuclear-cytoplasmic ratio

Overall Cell Size

The overall size of a blood cell is usually compared with the size of a mature erythrocyte. Except for the megakaryocytic maturational series, erythrocytes and leukocytes *decrease* in overall size as maturation progresses.

Nuclear-Cytoplasmic Ratio

The amount of space occupied by the nucleus in relationship to the space occupied by the cytoplasm is the nuclear-cytoplasmic (**N:C**) ratio. The size of the nucleus generally *decreases* as a cell matures. Consequently, the N:C ratio *decreases* in many cell types with maturation. Blast forms of erythrocytes, leukocytes, and megakaryocytes have a high (4:1) N:C ratio. As these cells mature, the ratio is reduced to 2:1 or 1:1 in most cells, except in thrombocytes, mature erythrocytes, and the lymphocyte type of leukocyte. Thrombocytes and erythrocytes lack a nucleus (**anuclear**), and mature lymphocytes frequently retain the original 4:1 to 3:1 N:C ratio.

Nuclear Characteristics

Nuclear characteristics play an important role in cell identification. Important features of the nucleus include:

1. Chromatin pattern
2. Nuclear shape
3. The presence of nucleoli

Chromatin Patterns

The chromatin arrangement demonstrates characteristic patterns. These patterns are the most *distinctive* nuclear feature of a cell in terms of maturity and cell type recognition. In general, the overall pattern progresses from a loose-looking

TABLE 4.3   **Blood Cell Development Nomenclature of Normal Committed Cell Lines**

	Erythrocyte[a]		Megakaryocyte	Granulocyte	Monocyte	Lymphocyte
Immature	Rubriblast	Pronormoblast	Megakaryoblast	Myeloblast	Monoblast	Lymphoblast
	↓ Prorubricyte	↓ Basophilic normoblast	↓ Promegakaryocyte	↓ Promyelocyte	↓ Promonocyte	↓ Prolymphocyte
Bone marrow	↓ Rubricyte	↓ Polychromato-philic nor-moblast	↓ Megakaryocyte	↓ Myelocyte[b]		
	↓ Metarubricyte	↓ Orthochromatic normoblast or nucleated red blood cell		↓ Metamyelocyte[b]		
Circulating blood	↓ Reticulocyte or polychromato-philic erythrocyte (diffusely basophilic)			↓ Band or stab[b]		
Mature		↓ Erythrocyte	↓ Thrombocyte or platelet	↓ Segmented neutrophil[b]	↓ Monocyte	↓ Lymphocyte
					↓ Macrophage (tissues)	↓ B cell ↘ T cell
						↓ Plasma cell (bone marrow)

[a]Comparable terms.

[b]These cell types may be either neutrophilic, eosinophilic, or basophilic.

arrangement to a more clumped pattern as a cell matures. The terms used to describe various patterns include the following: smooth or homogeneous, fine, delicate, lacy or thready, smudged, clumped, or pyknotic (dense or compact). Examples of common chromatin features for each cell type are given here.

TABLE 4.4   **Summary of General Maturational Characteristics***

Morphological Feature	Usual Development
General cell size	Decreases with maturity
Nuclear-cytoplasmic ratio	Decreases with maturity
Nucleus	
Chromatin pattern	Becomes more condensed
Presence of nucleoli	Not visible in mature cells
Cytoplasmic Characteristics	
Color	Progresses from darker blue to lighter blue, blue-gray, or pink
Granulation	Progresses from no granules to non-specific to specific granules
Vacuoles	Increase with age

*The characteristics of specific cells vary.

Lymphocytes exhibit a smooth or homogeneous pattern of chromatin throughout development until the mature stage, when clumped heterochromatin is more obvious.
Granulocytes progress from having a fine to a highly clumped pattern.
Monocytes have a lacy pattern, which becomes finer as the cell matures.
Erythrocytes continue to develop a more clumped pattern as maturation progresses until the extremely dense (pyknotic) nucleus is lost (extruded) from the mature cell.

Nuclear Shape

The shape of the nucleus in young cells is either round or oval; however, monocytes may have a slightly folded nuclear shape. In the cells that retain their nucleus as they mature, nuclear shapes become very distinctive for particular cell types.

Lymphocytes usually continue to have a round or oval nucleus. Some cells may have a small cleft in the nucleus.
Monocytes have a kidney bean–shaped nucleus, but folded or horseshoe shapes are common.
Mature neutrophils, eosinophils, and **basophils** have segmented nuclei attached to one another by fine filaments. The number of distinctive lobes ranges from two to five depending on the cell type.

Presence of Nucleoli

The presence or absence of nucleoli is important in the identification of cells. The three cell lines of erythrocytes, leukocytes, and megakaryocytes all have nucleoli in the earliest cell stages. As cells mature, nucleoli are usually not visible. These changes in the appearance of the nucleoli are related to the rate of synthesis of ribosomal RNA.

The number of nucleoli varies depending on the cell type, as is shown in the following examples:

Lymphoblasts have one or two nucleoli.
Myeloblasts have one to five nucleoli.
Monoblasts usually have one or two nucleoli but occasionally may have three or four.
Erythroblasts may not have any nucleoli or may have up to two nucleoli that may stain darker than in other types of blast cells.
Megakaryoblasts typically have one to five nucleoli.

Cytoplasmic Characteristics

A variety of cytoplasmic features aid in the microscopic identification of cell maturity and type. These features include:

1. Staining color and intensity
2. Granulation
3. Shape
4. Quantity of cytoplasm
5. Vacuolization
6. Inclusion bodies

Staining Color and Intensity

The overall color and intensity of staining in a Wright-stained blood smear vary with cell maturity and type. In general, cytoplasmic color progresses from darker blue (indicating active protein synthesis) in younger cells to lighter blue or pink in mature cells. Most early cells have a medium-blue cytoplasm. Immature **erythrocytes** have a very distinctive dark-blue cytoplasm that becomes paler and gray-looking as the cell synthesizes hemoglobin. As mature cells, **lymphocytes** are usually noted for their pale sky-blue cytoplasmic color. Variations in cytoplasmic color develop in many cells because of abnormalities or the presence of granules.

Granulation

The presence, size, and color of granules are important in cellular identification. In general, granulation progresses from *no* granules to *nonspecific* granulation to *specific* granulation.

The earliest, blast forms of leukocytes and megakaryocytes do not have granules, and erythrocytes never exhibit granulation throughout their life cycle. The granulocytic cell line of leukocytes is noted for distinctive granulation. The complete development of granules in leukocytes is discussed in Chapters 14 and 16.

Granules vary in several ways:

1. In size, ranging from very fine to coarse
2. In color, including red (**azurophilic**), blue (**basophilic**), and orange (**eosinophilic**)
3. In the amount of granulation per cell

Cytoplasmic Shape

The cytoplasmic outline or shape is useful in cellular identification. The most distinctive variation in cytoplasmic shape occurs in some **blast forms, monocytes,** and **megakaryocytes. Pseudopods** may be observed in mature monocytes and in some leukocyte blast forms. The megakaryocyte develops a more irregular outline as the cell matures.

Quantity of Cytoplasm

In some cell types, the actual quantity of cytoplasm increases with age. The megakaryocyte, in particular, develops extensive quantities of cytoplasm. Abnormalities of lymphocytes frequently demonstrate increased amounts of cytoplasm.

Vacuolization

Monocytes are frequently noted for having vacuoles throughout their life cycle and under normal conditions. Except for the monocyte, vacuolization of the cytoplasm is commonly seen in older cells as well as in abnormal conditions. Anticoagulants can also produce vacuoles as **artifacts**

TABLE 4.5 Normal Adult Values and Selected Characteristics of Mature Leukocytes in Peripheral Blood

Type	Nuclear Shape	Chromatin	Cytoplasmic Color	Granules	Color of Granules	Average Percentage
Segmented neutrophil	Lobulated	Very clumped	Pink	Many	Pink, a few blue	56
Band form neutrophil	Curved	Moderately clumped	Blue/pink	Many	Pink	3
Lymphocyte	Round	Smooth	Light blue	Few or absent	Red	34
Monocyte	Indented or twisted	Lacy	Gray-blue	Many	Dusty blue	4
Eosinophil	Lobulated	Very clumped	Granulated	Many	Orange	2.7
Basophil	Lobulated	Very clumped	Granulated	Many	Dark blue	0.3

if the blood is stored for a longer-than-acceptable period of time. Severe bacterial infections, viral infections (e.g., infectious mononucleosis), and malignancies may produce a remarkable number of vacuoles in various leukocyte types.

Inclusion Bodies

Cytoplasmic inclusions such as **Auer bodies** or **Auer rods** (discussed in Chapter 14) in **myelocytic** or **monocytic blast** forms or ingested particles are important to observe because they aid in the identification of cell types. Various **erythrocytic inclusions** (refer to Chapter 5) and **leukocytic inclusions** (refer to Chapters 14 and 16) are indicative of specific diseases. Some types of inclusions may be seen on a Wright-stained blood smear, but other inclusions, such as iron particles, require special staining techniques.

Mature Leukocyte Forms in Peripheral Blood

Identification of blood cells by microscopic examination of a peripheral smear can be performed more systematically, if the morphologist assesses the various maturational features as outlined in the preceding section. This process will simplify the identification of cells, particularly those that do not have all of the classic features.

The normal average percentage of leukocytes in adults and selected characteristics of these cells found on a normal Wright-stained blood smear are presented in Table 4.5.

SUMMARY

Blood cells originate from the mesenchymal tissue that arises from the embryonic germ layer, the mesoderm. The sites of blood cell development, hematopoiesis, follow a definite sequence from embryonic life, to fetal life, to childhood, to adult life. In abnormal situations, blood production may revert to a more primitive state, referred to as extramedullary hematopoiesis.

The stem cell is the first in a sequence of steps of hematopoietic cell generation and maturation. Hematopoietic cells can be divided into three phases according to cell maturity. The multipotential stem cell is the progenitor of the two major cell lines: lymphoid and nonlymphoid. Colony-forming units (CFUs) precede the blast stage of cell development.

Hematopoietic growth factors regulate the proliferation and differentiation of progenitor cells and the function of mature blood cells. These factors are being used to treat a variety of diseases and disorders.

Each cellular element has a definite name and associated characteristics for each stage of development. Certain maturational characteristics are shared by most hematopoietic cells. Characteristics such as overall size and N:C ratio are important in determining the stages of development. Nuclear characteristics, such as the presence of nucleoli and chromatin patterns, vary with cell type and cell maturity. Cytoplasmic features, such as color and the presence of granules, must be carefully observed in a peripheral blood examination. The presence of granules is indicative of specific cell types and is a feature of cellular age. Identification of blood cells can be performed more systematically if the morphologist assesses the various maturational features. This process simplifies the identification of many cells that do not have all the classic features associated with a particular cell line, and is useful in determining the age of a cell.

BIBLIOGRAPHY

Crawford, J. et al. "Reduction by Granulocyte Colony-Stimulating Factor of Fever and Neutropenia Induced by Chemotherapy in Patients with Small-Cell Lung Cancer." *N. Engl. J. Med.*, Vol. 325, No. 3, July 18, 1991, pp. 164–170.

Delmonte, L. "Demystifying Blood Growth Factors." *Oncol. Times*, Vol. 12, No. 4, April, 1990, pp. 5–8.

Francomano, C. A. "DNA Analysis in Genetic Disorders." *Annu. Rev. Med.*, Vol. 37, 1986, pp. 377–395.

Golde, D. W. "Hematopoietic Growth Factors." *Hematol. Oncol. Clin. North Am.*, Vol. 3, No. 3, September, 1989.

Groopman, J. E., J. Molina, and D. T. Scadden. "Hematopoietic Growth Factors." *N. Engl. J. Med.*, Vol. 321, No. 21, November 23, 1989, pp. 1449–1459.

Hoelzer, D. "Hematopoietic Growth Factors." *N. Engl. J. Med.*, Vol. 336, No. 25, June 19, 1997, pp. 1822–1824.

Jaiyesimi, I., S. S. Giralt, and J. Wood. "Subcutaneous Granulocyte Colony-Stimulating Factor and Acute Anaphylaxis." *N. Engl. J. Med.*, Vol. 325, No. 8, August 22, 1991, p. 587.

Nemunaitis, J. et al. "Recombinant Granulocyte-Macrophage Colony-Stimulating Factor After Autologous Bone Marrow Transplantation for Lymphoid Cancer." *N. Engl. J. Med.*, Vol. 224, No. 25, June 20, 1991, pp. 1773–1778.

Nightingale, S. L. "Hematopoietic Growth Factors Workshop." *JAMA*, Vol. 262, No. 10, September 8, 1989, p. 1296.

O'Connor, Barbara H. *A Color Atlas and Instructional Manual of Peripheral Blood Cell Morphology*. Baltimore, MD: Williams & Wilkins, 1992.

Turgeon, Mary Louise. *Immunology and Serology in Laboratory Medicine* (2nd ed.). St. Louis: Mosby–Yearbook, Inc., 1996.

REVIEW QUESTIONS

1. The normal sequence of blood cell development is:

   A. Yolk sac—red bone marrow—liver and spleen.
   B. Yolk sac—thymus—liver and spleen—red bone marrow.
   C. Yolk sac—liver and spleen—red bone marrow.
   D. Liver and spleen—yolk sac—red bone marrow.

2. The maturational sequence of the thrombocyte (platelet) is:

   A. Megakaryoblast—promegakaryocyte—megakaryocyte—metamegakaryocyte—thrombocyte.
   B. Promegakaryocyte—megakaryocyte—metamegakaryocyte—thrombocyte.
   C. Megakaryoblast—promegakaryocyte—megakaryocyte—thrombocyte.
   D. Megakaryoblast—promegakaryocyte—metamegakaryocyte—thrombocyte.

3. The maturational sequences of the erythrocyte are:

   A. Rubriblast—prorubricyte—rubricyte—metarubricyte—reticulocyte—mature erythrocyte.

   B. Prorubricyte—rubricyte—metarubricyte—reticulocyte—mature erythrocyte.

   C. Pronormoblast—basophilic normoblast—polychromatophilic normoblast—orthochromic normoblast—reticulocyte—mature erythrocyte.

   D. Both A and C.

4. The cell maturation sequence of the segmented neutrophil is:

   A. Promyelocyte—myeloblast—myelocyte—metamyelocyte—band or stab—segmented neutrophil (PMN).

   B. Myeloblast—promyelocyte—myelocyte—metamyelocyte—band or stab—segmented neutrophil (PMN).

   C. Monoblast—promyelocyte—myelocyte—metamyelocyte—band or stab—segmented neutrophil (PMN).

   D. Promyelocyte—myelocyte—metamyelocyte—band or stab—segmented neutrophil (PMN).

5. As a blood cell matures, the overall cell diameter in most cases:

   A. Increases.   C. Remains the same.
   B. Decreases.

6. As a blood cell matures, the ratio of nucleus to cytoplasm (N:C) in most cases:

   A. Increases.   C. Remains the same.
   B. Decreases.

7. The chromatin pattern in most cells ___ as the cell matures:

   A. Becomes more clumped.   C. Remains the same.
   B. Becomes less clumped.

8. The presence of nucleoli is associated with:

   A. Immature cells.
   B. All young cells, except myeloblasts.
   C. Only erythroblasts.
   D. Disintegrating cells.

9. In the blast stage of development of leukocytes, the cytoplasm of the cell is:

   A. Dark blue and lacks vacuoles.
   B. Light blue and lacks granules.
   C. Light blue and has specific granules.
   D. Gray with many dark-blue granules.

Questions 10 through 14: match the cellular characteristics with the name of the appropriate mature leukocyte. Use an answer only once.

10. ___ Segmented neutrophil.
11. ___ Monocyte.
12. ___ Lymphocyte.
13. ___ Band form neutrophil
14. ___ Eosinophil.

A. Large orange granules.

B. An elongated and curved nucleus.

C. Light, sky-blue cytoplasm.

D. Kidney bean–shaped nucleus.

E. Averages about 56% of normal adult leukocytes in the peripheral blood.

CHAPTER

5

Normal Erythrocyte Lifecycle and Physiology

Erythropoiesis
Erythropoietin
Disorders of erythropoietin
Red cell increases
Development and maturation of erythrocytes
General characteristics
Developmental stages
Defective nuclear maturation
Reticulocytes
Characteristics and properties of hemoglobin
Chemical composition and configuration of hemoglobin

The role of 2,3-diphosphoglycerate (2,3-DPG)
Oxygen dissociation
Alterations in oxygen dissociation
Carbon dioxide transport
Synthesis of hemoglobin
Normal hemoglobin types
Variant forms of normal hemoglobin
Genetic inheritance of hemoglobin
Analysis of hemoglobin
Membrane characteristics and metabolic activities of erythrocytes

Membrane characteristics
Cytoplasmic characteristics
Metabolic activities
Catabolism of erythrocytes
Measurement of erythrocytes
Mean corpuscular volume (MCV)
Mean corpuscular hemoglobin (MCH)
Mean corpuscular hemoglobin concentration (MCHC)
Summary
Case studies
Bibliography
Review questions

OBJECTIVES

Erythropoiesis

- Name the sites of erythropoiesis from the early embryonic stage of development until fully established in adults.
- Name the substances necessary for proper erythropoiesis and cite examples of deficient substances that can produce various types of anemias.
- Describe the biochemical properties and sites of production of erythropoietin.
- Explain the normal condition that stimulates the production of erythropoietin and how it influences the production of erythrocytes.
- Compare the terms **secondary polycythemia** and **relative polycythemia.**
- Describe the various types of conditions that can produce disorders of erythropoietin production.

Development and maturation of erythrocytes

- List the maturational times for the various erythrocyte developmental phases.
- Describe the major morphological features of each of the erythrocyte maturational stages.
- Compare the morphological characteristics of defective erythrocyte maturation and **megaloblastic maturation** with normal developmental features.

- Explain the events that occur during reticulocyte maturation.
- Describe the normal distribution and replacement pattern of reticulocytes in the circulation.
- Define the terms **shift** or **stress** reticulocytes.
- Compare the morphological appearances of reticulocytes stained with Wright stain and a supravital stain, such as new methylene blue.
- Give the normal value of the uncorrected reticulocyte count.
- When given the necessary laboratory results, calculate the **corrected reticulocyte count** and the **reticulocyte production index** (RPI).

Characteristics and properties of hemoglobin

- Describe the chemical configuration of normal adult hemoglobin.
- Explain the physiological role of 2,3-diphosphoglycerate in the oxygenation of the hemoglobin molecule.
- Relate the oxygen dissociation curve to the oxygen-binding activities of the hemoglobin molecule.
- Cite at least two examples of clinical conditions that can alter oxygen dissociation and explain what effect these conditions have on the oxygen dissociation curve.

- Describe the **Bohr effect** and other physical or chemical factors that affect the oxygen dissociation curve.
- Explain the elimination and transport of carbon dioxide.
- Briefly describe the overall synthesis of heme.
- Name one congenital and two acquired disorders that are related to defects in heme (porphyrin) synthesis.
- Describe the sites and mechanism of transport and insertion of iron in the production of hemoglobin.
- Explain the factors that regulate the synthesis of globin in hemoglobin production.
- Specifically describe the outcomes of a deficiency in the production of globin.
- Name the embryonic hemoglobins and describe their chemical composition and site of formation.
- Explain the types of chains, developmental formation, and quantities of fetal hemoglobin.
- Identify the types of chains, site of formation, and quantities of adult hemoglobin A and A_2.
- Describe the formation and concentration of glycosylated hemoglobin in normal and hyperglycemic environments.
- Diagram and explain the inheritance patterns of normal hemoglobin and abnormal hemoglobin genotypes and phenotypes.
- Name at least four hemoglobin analysis methods and explain the purpose of each procedure.

Membrane characteristics and metabolic activities of erythrocytes

- Describe the general characteristics, including the physical properties, of the erythrocyte membrane.
- Explain the importance of enzymes in energy-yielding cellular reactions.
- Describe the importance and physiology of the **Embden-Meyerhof** glycolytic pathway.
- Explain the physiology of the **oxidative pathway** and the effects of a defect in this pathway.
- Explain the importance of the **methemoglobin reductase** pathway to heme iron.

- Describe the function of the **Luebering-Rapaport** pathway.
- Detail the changes that take place at the end of the erythrocytic life span and describe the removal of cells from the circulation.
- Explain the events of extravascular destruction of the erythrocyte.
- Describe the details of intravascular destruction of the erythrocyte.

Measurement of erythrocytes

- Name the procedures that assess the quantities of either erythrocytes or hemoglobin.
- Cite the normal values of the erythrocyte count, hemoglobin, and packed cell volumes for various age groups.
- Define each of the erythrocyte indices: mean corpuscular volume (MCV), mean corpuscular hemoglobin (MCH), mean corpuscular hemoglobin concentration (MCHC).
- Apply the appropriate formulas and calculate the MCV, MCH, and MCHC when given the erythrocyte values.

Case studies

- Apply the laboratory data to the stated case studies and discuss the implications of these cases to the study of hematology.
- The mature erythrocyte is a biconcave disc with a central pallor that occupies the middle one third of the cell. About 33% of the volume of the mature cell consists mainly of the respiratory protein hemoglobin, which performs the function of oxygen-carbon dioxide transport. Throughout the life span of the mature cell, an average of 120 days, this soft and pliable cell moves with ease through the tissue capillaries and splenic circulation. As the cell ages, cytoplasmic enzymes are catabolized, leading to increased membrane rigidity, phagocytosis by macrophages, and destruction.

ERYTHROPOIESIS

The term used to describe the process of erythrocyte production is **erythropoiesis.** This process (refer to **hematopoiesis** in Chapter 4 for a complete discussion) begins with the development of primitive erythrocytes in the embryonic yolk sac, continues in extramedullary organs such as the liver in the developing fetus, and is ultimately located in the red bone marrow during late fetal development, childhood, and adult life.

Transport of oxygen to the tissues and carbon dioxide from the tissues is accomplished by the **heme** pigment in hemoglobin, which is synthesized as the erythrocyte matures. The basic substances needed for normal erythrocyte and hemoglobin production are amino acids (proteins), iron, vitamin B_{12}, vitamin B_6, folic acid (a member of the vitamin B_2 complex), and the trace minerals cobalt and nickel. Abnormal erythropoiesis can result from deficiencies of any of these necessary substances. Defective erythropoiesis is frequently seen in underdeveloped countries where protein deficiencies are common. Other types of anemias (discussed in Chapters 10 and 11) can be due to deficiencies in vitamin B_{12}, folic acid, or iron.

Erythropoietin

The substance **erythropoietin** is produced primarily by the kidneys. Peritubular cells are the probable site of synthesis in the kidneys. Extrarenal organs such as the liver also secrete this substance. Ten to 15% of erythropoietin production occurs in the liver, which is the primary source of erythropoietin in the unborn. This glycoprotein hormone, with a molecular weight of 46,000, stimulates erythropoiesis and can cross the placental barrier between mother and fetus. Erythropoietin was the first human hematopoietic growth factor to be identified. The gene for erythropoietin is located on chromosome 7.

Erythropoietin is detectable in the plasma (average concentration, 25 mU per mL). The red cell mass of the body is continuously adjusted to the optimal size for its function as an oxygen carrier, by messages transmitted to the bone marrow from the oxygen sensor in the kidney. Tissue hypoxia, a decrease in the oxygen content within the tissues, produces a dramatic increase in the production of erythropoietin. A heme protein is thought to be involved in the oxygen-sensing mechanism. The messages from the sensing mechanisms are mediated by erythropoietin, are modulated by cardiovascular and renal factors, and form a key link in the feedback loop that controls red cell production. Through the action of erythropoietin, the number of hemoglobin-containing erythrocytes increases, the oxygen-carrying capacity of the blood increases, and the normal level of oxygen in the tissues can be restored.

Erythropoietin has its predominant effect on the committed erythroid cells, colony-forming unit-erythroid (CFU-E), promoting their proliferation and differentiation into pro-erythroblasts. It may also stimulate the differentiation of a more primitive erythroid progenitor, the burst-forming unit-erythroid, in association with so-called burst-promoting activity. In biochemical studies of the action of erythropoietin, it has been demonstrated that initially an increase in the production of several types of ribonucleic acid (RNA) takes place. This activity is followed by an increase in deoxyribonucleic acid (DNA) activity and protein synthesis. Increased erythrocyte production and hemoglobin synthesis are ultimately the result. Questions remain as to how many of the effects attributed to erythropoietin are direct. The androgen hormones and thyroid hormones can also stimulate erythropoiesis.

Erythropoietin also interacts with interleukin-3, granulocyte-macrophage colony-stimulating factor (GM-CSF), interleukin-1, and thrombocytopoiesis-stimulating factor to promote the production of megakaryocytes.

Recombinant human erythropoietin is produced from mammalian cells and was originally used in patients being treated with dialysis who had anemia due to chronic renal failure. In addition to possible uses in the treatment of various types of anemia, recombinant human erythropoietin is likely to be useful in a broad range of clinical applications.

Disorders of Erythropoietin

Polycythemia is the term used to refer to an increased concentration of erythrocytes (**erythrocytosis**) in the circulating blood that is above normal for sex and age. **Secondary,** or **absolute,** polycythemias reflect an increase in erythropoietin production and should *not* be confused with polycythemia vera (see Chapter 21) or relative polycythemias.

Secondary polycythemia due to increased erythropoietin production results from either tissue **hypoxia** caused by such diverse factors as defective high oxygen affinity type of hemoglobin, certain types of anemia, chronic lung disease, and inappropriate erythropoietin production. Smoking is a common cause of secondary erythrocytosis. Conditions of inappropriate erythropoietin production may result from **neoplasms,** usually renal, or renal disorders that produce local hypoxia within the kidney. A more unusual cause of inappropriate erythropoiesis is **familial polycythemia,** an autosomal dominant trait that produces a defect in the regulation of erythropoietin. A reduction in erythropoietin production may also exist. In situations such as hypertransfusion, the quantity of erythropoietin is reduced.

Red Cell Increases

Increases in erythrocytes can result from conditions that are not related to increased erythropoietin. These conditions include the **relative polycythemias.**

A relative polycythemia exists when an increase in the packed cell volume (hematocrit) or the total erythrocyte count is caused by decreased plasma volume. The total erythrocyte mass is not increased. Increases in the packed red blood cell volume or erythrocyte count reflect an increase in the volume or erythrocytes in proportion to the total blood volume. Loss of body fluids and plasma volume due to conditions producing dehydration, such as diarrhea or burns, can produce these increased results.

DEVELOPMENT AND MATURATION OF ERYTHROCYTES

General Characteristics

Erythrocytes are rapidly maturing cells. Once the stem cell differentiates into the erythroid cell line, a cell matures through the nucleated cell stages in 4 or 5 days. Bone marrow reticulocytes have an average maturation period of 2.5 days. Once young reticulocytes enter the circulating blood, they remain in the reticulocyte stage for an average of 1 day and represent approximately 0.5% to 1.5% of the circulating erythrocytes.

Developmental Stages

Early Cells

All hematopoietic cell lines are derived from an original, common pool of ancestral pluripotent stem cells. When the pluripotent stem cell, the first in a sequence of steps of cell generation and maturation, differentiates into a non-lymphoid multipotential stem cell, it can become a CFU-GEMM (colony-forming unit granulocyte-erythrocyte-monocyte-megakaryocyte) depending on the presence of specific growth factors (see Plate 1). In erythropoiesis, the CFU-GEMM differentiates into a burst-forming unit-erythroid (BFU-E).

The earliest cell in the erythrocyte series is the BFU-E. The next step in differentiation is the formation of colony-forming units (CFU-E). CFU-E produce erythroid colonies of up to 100 cells. Under the influence of erythropoietin, the CFU-E undergo a programmed series of cell divisions and cell maturation, culminating in the mature erythrocyte. Although BFU-E and CFU-E cannot be distinguished by light microscopic examination of aspirated bone marrow smears, the progeny of CFU-E are easily identified.

When cells differentiate into the erythroid line (Fig. 5.1), the maturational changes are consistent with the overall nuclear and cytoplasmic changes seen in other cell lines (see Chapter 4). However, the erythrocyte becomes an **anuclear** mature cell (Table 5.1).

Rubriblast (Pronormoblast)

The **rubriblast** (Plate 2) or **pronormoblast** (see Table 5.1) has an overall diameter of approximately 12 to 19 μm. The nuclear-to-cytoplasmic (N:C) ratio is 4:1. The large, round nucleus contains from zero to two nucleoli, is usually dark-appearing, and has a fine chromatin pattern.

The cytoplasm stains a distinctive blue (**basophilic**) color with Wright stain and lacks granules. The distinctive blue color reflects the RNA activity needed to produce the protein needed for hemoglobin synthesis. Studies with radioactive iron have demonstrated that most of the iron destined for hemoglobin synthesis is taken into the cell at this stage.

Prorubricyte (Basophilic Normoblast)

The second stage, the **prorubricyte** (Plate 3), or basophilic normoblast, has an overall cell diameter of 12 to 17 μm and is only slightly smaller than the rubriblast. The N:C ratio remains high (4:1); however, this stage demonstrates morphological evidence of increasing maturity.

The nuclear chromatin becomes more clumped. Nucleoli are usually no longer apparent. The cytoplasm continues to appear basophilic with a Wright stain. This cell contains no evidence of the pink color that indicates hemoglobin development.

Rubriblast
(pronormoblast)

Prorubricyte
(basophilic normoblast)

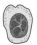

Rubricyte
(polychromatic normoblast)

Metarubricyte
(orthochromic normoblast)

Reticulocyte

Mature erythrocyte

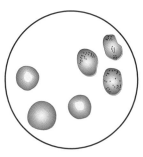

Reticulocyte appearance
with a supravital stain

FIGURE 5.1 Erythrocyte morphology. The morphological development of the erythrocyte is typical of blood cell maturation. The unique difference is that the erythrocyte loses its nucleus. If the erythrocyte is stained with a supravital stain, such as new methylene blue, reticulocytes, as depicted on the right, will be visible.

Rubricyte (Polychromatic Normoblast)

Hemoglobin appears for the first time in the third maturational stage, the **rubricyte** (Plate 4), or **polychromatic normoblast.** At this stage, the overall cell size of 11 to 15 μm is slightly decreased from that of the prorubricyte stage. Further maturation is also demonstrated by the decreased N:C ratio of 1:1.

The chromatin continues to become increasingly clumped. The cytoplasm of cells in this stage show variable amounts of pink coloration mixed with basophilia; this can give the cell a muddy, light gray appearance.

Metarubricyte (Orthochromic Normoblast)

The rubricyte matures into the **metarubricyte** (Plate 5) or **orthochromic normoblast.** The overall cell is smaller (8 to 12 μm). The chromatin pattern is tightly condensed in this maturational stage and can be described as **pyknotic** (dense or compact). In the later period of this stage, the nucleus will be extruded from the cell. The metarubricyte is characterized by an **acidophilic** (reddish-pink) cytoplasm. This coloration indicates the presence of large quantities of hemoglobin.

TABLE 5.1 Dual Nomenclature and Developmental Characteristics of Red Blood Cells

Name	Cellular Features
Rubriblast or pronormoblast	Size: 12–19 μm in diameter N:C ratio 4:1 *Nucleus* Large, round nucleus Chromatin has a fine pattern 0–2 nucleoli *Cytoplasm* Distinctive basophilic color Without granules
Prorubricyte or basophilic normoblast	Size: 12–17 μm in diameter N:C ratio 4:1 *Nucleus* Nuclear chromatin more clumped Nucleoli usually not apparent *Cytoplasm* Distinctive basophilic color
Rubricyte or polychromatic normoblast	Size: 11–15 μm in diameter N:C ratio 1:1 *Nucleus* Increased clumping of the chromatin *Cytoplasm* Color: variable, with pink staining mixed with basophilia
Metarubricyte or orthochromic normoblast or nucleated RBC (NRBC)	Size: 8–12 μm *Nucleus* Chromatin pattern is tightly condensed *Cytoplasm* Color: reddish-pink (acidophilic)
Reticulocyte (supravital stain) or polychromatic erythrocyte (Wright stain)	Size: 7–10 μm Cell is anuclear Diffuse reticulum *Cytoplasm* Overall blue appearance
Erythrocyte	Average diameter: 6–8 μm

Three mitoses are believed to occur in the 2- to 3-day interval between the rubriblast and the end of the metarubricyte stage. Two thirds of these mitoses have been shown to occur in the rubricyte stage. After this stage, the cell is no longer able to undergo mitosis.

Reticulocyte

The **reticulocyte** (Plate 6) stage is the next maturational stage. Part of this phase occurs in the bone marrow, and the later part of the stage takes place in the circulating blood. Reticulocytes are discussed in greater detail in the following section.

This cell demonstrates a characteristic reticular appearance due to remaining RNA if stained with a supravital stain, such as new methylene blue. In a Wright-stained blood smear young reticulocytes with a high amount of RNA residual have a blue appearance, which is referred to as **polychromatophilia** (Plate 7). The overall cellular diameter ranges from 7 to 10 μm. This cell is anuclear.

Mature Erythrocyte

After the reticulocyte stage, the **mature erythrocyte** is formed. This cell has an average diameter of 6 to 8 μm. The survivability of erythrocytes can be determined by using radioactive chromium (^{51}Cr). A shortened life span can be observed in the hemolytic anemias (see Chapter 12).

Defective Nuclear Maturation

A defect in maturation known as **megaloblastic maturation** can be seen in certain anemias, such as vitamin B_{12} or folate deficiencies (see Chapter 11). The most noticeable characteristic of this type of defect is that nuclear maturation lags behind cytoplasmic maturation. Because of an impaired ability of the cells to synthesize DNA, both the interphase and the phases of mitotic division are prolonged. This asynchronous pattern of maturation can be confusing because the nuclear development of the cell is much younger-looking than the actual developmental age, which is expressed by the cytoplasmic development. Other important features of megaloblastic maturation include an increased amount of erythrocytic cellular cytoplasm and increased overall erythrocyte size. The megaloblastic dysfunction also expresses itself in the maturation of leukocytes. Giant band-type leukocyte forms are frequently observed on blood smears.

Reticulocytes

As the erythrocyte develops, the nucleus becomes more and more condensed and is eventually lost. After the loss of the nucleus, an immature erythrocyte remains in the bone marrow for 2 to 3 days before entering the circulating blood. During this period in the bone marrow and during the first day in the circulation, this immature erythrocyte is referred to as a **reticulocyte.**

Although the reticulocyte lacks a nucleus, it contains various organelles, such as mitochondria, and an extensive number of ribosomes. The formation of new ribosomes ceases with the loss of the nucleus in the late metarubricyte; however, while RNA is present, protein and heme synthesis continues. During reticulocyte maturation, the RNA is catabolized, and the ribosomes disintegrate. The loss of ribosomes and mitochondria, along with full hemoglobinization of the cell, marks the transition from the reticulocyte stage to full maturation of the erythrocyte.

Under normal conditions, the quantity of reticulocytes in the bone marrow is equal to that of the reticulocytes in the circulating blood. In order to maintain a stable reticulocyte pool in the circulation, the bone marrow replaces the number of erythrocytes that have reached their full life span. Because the normal life span or survival time is 120 days, 1/120th of the total number of erythrocytes is lost each day, and an equal number of reticulocytes is released into the circulation.

If, under the stimulus of erythropoietin, increased numbers of young reticulocytes are prematurely released from the bone marrow because of such conditions as acute bleeding, these reticulocytes are referred to as **stress** or **shift** reticulocytes. This situation is analogous to the appearance of immature leukocytes in the peripheral blood during the stress of infection.

The Reticulocyte Count

Peripheral smears of normal blood stained with Wright stain may demonstrate a slight blue tint in some erythrocytes. This morphological condition of erythrocytes, which is described in more detail in the next chapter, is referred to as **polychromatophilia** or **polychromasia.** However, a supravital stain, such as new methylene blue, precipitates the ribosomal RNA in these cells to form a deep-blue, meshlike network. Stress reticulocytes are recognizable on Wright-stained blood smears by their larger size and increased blue tint, and may be accompanied by even younger erythrocytes, such as metarubricytes. When stained with a supravital stain, stress reticulocytes exhibit a much denser meshlike network.

The **reticulocyte count** procedure (see Chapter 24) is frequently performed in the clinical laboratory as an indicator of the rate of erythrocyte production. Usually, the count is expressed as a percentage of total erythrocytes. The normal range is 0.5% to 1.5% in adults. In newborn infants, the range is 2.5% to 6.5%, but this value falls to the adult range by the end of the second week of life.

The reticulocyte count is of value as an indication of a shorter-than-normal erythrocyte survival, which is based on the deduction that the total red blood cell mass in a steady state is equal to the number of new red blood cells produced, multiplied by the 120-day life span of individual cells. When the red blood cell mass falls, it is the result of decreased red blood cell production or a shortened life span. Normal erythropoiesis corrects for a shorter life span by increasing the production rate, which the reticulocyte count measures. Therefore, an elevated reticulocyte count accompanies a shortened red blood cell survival. **Reticulocytosis** indicates that the body is trying to maintain homeostasis.

Calculating and Expressing Reticulocyte Values

Traditionally, the reticulocyte count has been expressed as a percentage of the total number of circulating erythrocytes (e.g., 1%). However, this value may be erroneous because fluctuation in the percentage may be due to a change in the total number of circulating erythrocytes rather than a true change in the number of circulating reticulocytes. In order to account for variations due to erythrocyte quantity, expression of reticulocytes in absolute rather than proportional terms is becoming the preferred method of reporting. The correction for anemia is helpful for clinical interpretation, and several different methods are used. The National Committee for Clinical Laboratory Standards proposes that the correction for anemia, the **corrected reticulocyte count,** be made mathematically by correcting the observed reticulocyte count to a normal packed red blood cell volume (hematocrit; see Chapter 24).

Corrected Reticulocyte Count

$$\text{Corrected reticulocyte count} = \text{reticulocyte count (\%)}$$
$$\times \frac{\text{patient's packed cell volume (hematocrit)}}{\text{normal hematocrit based on age and sex}} = \%$$

Example: If an adult male has a hematocrit of 30% (0.30

L/L) and a reticulocyte count of 3%, the corrected reticulocyte count would be:

$$\text{corrected reticulocyte count}$$
$$= 3\% + \frac{0.30\,\text{L/L}}{0.45\,\text{L/L}}\ (\text{adult male normal value})$$
$$= 0.03 \times \frac{0.30\,\text{L/L}}{0.45\,\text{L/L}} = 0.03 = 3.0\%$$

The normal value based on correction for anemia is the same as the previously stated normal reticulocyte values of 0.5% to 1.5%.

Reticulocyte Production Index

A simple percentage calculation of reticulocytes does not account for the fact that prematurely released reticulocytes require from 1/2 to 1-1/2 days longer in the circulating blood to mature and lose their netlike reticulum. Therefore, the reticuloctye count, even if "corrected," will be elevated out of proportion to the actual increase in erythrocyte production because of the accumulation of these younger reticulocytes in the circulating blood. To correct for this situation, the use of the **reticulocyte production index (RPI)** was proposed.

The RPI measures erythropoietic activity when "stress" reticulocytes are present. The rationale for obtaining this value is that the life span of the circulating "stress" reticulocytes is 2 days instead of the normal 1 day. In order to compensate for the increased maturation time and consequent retention of residual RNA of the prematurely released reticulocytes, the corrected reticulocyte count is divided by a correction factor derived from the maturation time table (Table 5.2).

Calculation of the Reticulocyte Production Index

$$\text{RPI} = \frac{\text{corrected reticulocyte count in \%}}{\text{maturation time in days}}$$

If the corrected reticulocyte count is 2.0% and the patient's hematocrit is 0.30 L/L, the RPI is:

$$\text{RPI} = \frac{2.0}{1.75} = 1.14$$

Normal bone marrow activity produces an RPI index of 1. In hemolytic anemias, where there is increased destruction of erythrocytes in the peripheral blood and a functionally normal marrow, this index may be from three to seven times higher than normal. In cases of bone marrow damage, erythropoietin suppression, or a deficiency of vitamin B_{12},

TABLE 5.2 Maturation Time Correction Factor

Hematocrit (L/L)	Maturation Time (Days)
0.45	1.0
0.35	1.5
0.25	2.0
0.15	2.5

folic acid, or iron (hypoproliferative states), the index is 2 or less.

CHARACTERISTICS AND PROPERTIES OF HEMOGLOBIN

In 1862, Felix Seyler identified the respiratory protein **hemoglobin.** He discovered the characteristic color spectrum of hemoglobin and proved that this was the true coloring matter of the blood. Following this discovery, research began on the reaction of hemoglobin with oxygen. Today, the activities of hemoglobin and oxygen are well known and can be demonstrated by an oxygen dissociation curve.

Chemical Composition and Configuration of Hemoglobin

Normal adult hemoglobin (hemoglobin A) consists of four heme groups and four polypeptide chains with a total of 574 amino acids. The polypeptide chains are organized into two alpha chains and two beta chains. Each of the chains has an attached heme group (Fig. 5.2). Normal adult hemoglobin has 141 amino acids in each of the alpha chains and 146 amino acids in each of the beta chains. The specific sequence of these amino acids is known and is important in the identification of abnormal hemoglobins involving substitutions of specific amino acids.

In the native configuration of the hemoglobin molecule, the four hemes and four polypeptide chains are assembled in a very specific spatial configuration. Each of the four chains in the molecule coils into eight helices, forming an egg-shaped molecule with a central cavity. In the process of the binding of the first heme group to a molecule of oxygen, a change in the overall configuration of the hemoglobin molecule occurs. This altered configuration of the molecule favors the additional binding of oxygen to the remaining heme groups, if sufficient oxygen pressure is present. Meta-

bolic processes within the erythrocyte ensure a suitable intracellular environment for hemoglobin that protects it from chemical changes that might result in the loss of its native structure or denaturation. If hemoglobin is denatured, it loses its ability to carry oxygen.

The Role of 2,3-Diphosphoglycerate

The major function of the hemoglobin molecule is the transport of oxygen to the tissues. The oxygen affinity of the hemoglobin molecule is associated with the spatial rearrangement of the molecule and is regulated by the concentration of phosphates, particularly 2,3-diphosphoglycerate (2,3-DPG) in the erythrocyte. The manner in which 2,3-DPG binding to reduced hemoglobin (deoxyhemoglobin) affects oxygen affinity is complex. Basically, 2,3-DPG combines with the beta chains of deoxyhemoglobin and diminishes the molecule's affinity for oxygen (Fig. 5.3).

When the individual heme groups unload oxygen in the tissues, the beta chains are pulled apart. This permits the entrance of 2,3-DPG and the establishment of salt bridges between the individual chains. These activities result in a progressively lower affinity of the molecule for oxygen. With oxygen uptake in the lungs, the salt bonds are sequentially broken; the beta chains are pulled together, expelling 2,3-DPG; and the affinity of the hemoglobin molecule for oxygen progressively increases.

In cases of tissue hypoxia, oxygen moves from hemoglobin into the tissues, and the amount of deoxyhemoglobin in the erythrocytes increases. This produces the binding of more 2,3-DPG, which further reduces the oxygen affinity of the hemoglobin molecule. If hypoxia persists, depletion of free 2,3-DPG leads to increased production of more 2,3-DPG and a persistently lowered affinity of the hemoglobin molecule for oxygen.

Oxygen Dissociation

The structure of the hemoglobin molecule makes it capable of considerable molecular changes as it loads and unloads oxygen. Changes in oxygen affinity of the molecule are responsible for the ease with which hemoglobin can be loaded with oxygen in the lungs and unloaded in the tissues.

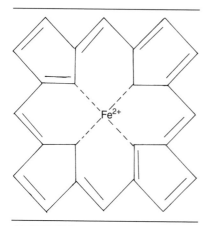

FIGURE 5.2 The heme portion of the hemoglobin molecule consists of one iron (Fe^{2+}) atom and four pyrrole rings that are joined to each other. A complete hemoglobin molecule consists of four heme molecules, each of which is attached to one molecule of the protein globin.

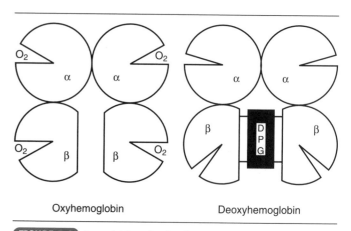

FIGURE 5.3 Hemoglobin molecular changes.

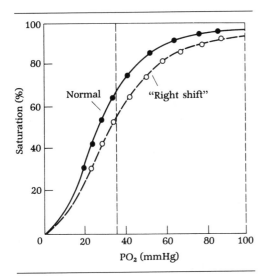

FIGURE 5.4 Oxygen dissociation curve. (From S. H. Robinson and P. R. Reich, *Hematology: Pathophysiologic Basis for Clinical Practice* [3rd ed.]. Boston: Little, Brown & Co. 1993.)

The shape and position of the oxyhemoglobin dissociation curve (Fig. 5.4) graphically describe the relationship between oxygen content (percentage of saturation) and partial pressure of oxygen (PO_2). For comparative purposes, the position of the curve is usually explained by the P_{50} value. The P_{50} value is defined as the partial pressure of oxygen required to produce half saturation of hemoglobin, when the deoxyhemoglobin (reduced hemoglobin) concentration equals the oxyhemoglobin (oxygenated hemoglobin) concentration at a constant pH and temperature. In humans, the P_{50} value is 26.52 mm Hg for whole blood under accepted standard conditions of pH 7.4 and temperature of 37.5°C. An increase in oxygen affinity is demonstrated by a shift to the left in the curve, whereas a decrease in oxygen affinity is represented by a shift to the right.

In addition to the effect of 2,3-DPG, the oxygen-binding sites are also affected by their state of oxygenation. Oxygenation of one site on a hemoglobin molecule enhances affinity for oxygen at a different but chemically identical site. The sequence of molecular changes during oxygenation of hemoglobin probably occurs as follows: the first oxygen molecule binds to an alpha chain, causing a change in the three-dimensional structure of that chain. The addition of a second oxygen to the other alpha chain produces a change in the molecular structure, and the alignment of the chains to each other rapidly changes. The 2,3-DPG is expelled from the molecule, resulting in increased oxygen affinity, and oxygen is added to the remaining beta chain. These changes in molecular configuration are demonstrated by the sigmoid form of the hemoglobin oxygen dissociation curve.

Alterations in Oxygen Dissociation

Fetal hemoglobin (hemoglobin F) has an increased affinity for oxygen. This increased affinity for oxygen is advantageous to the fetus because it results in increased placental oxygen transfer at low oxygen tension levels. The oxygen dissociation curve in the newborn is shifted to the left, owing to decreased levels of 2,3-DPG and the higher oxygen affinity of hemoglobin F. Hemoglobin variations due to an amino acid substitution can alter the oxygen dissociation curve. These alterations in amino acids within the hemoglobin molecule are important in modifying oxygen transport. A variety of genetic hemoglobin abnormalities may distort the molecular structure or restrict the oxygenation. Other genetic abnormalities in the amino acid sequence of the hemoglobin molecule may affect oxygen transport by causing the oxidation of heme iron to methemoglobin.

Oxygen dissociation as represented by the sigmoid curve can be shifted to the right (decreased oxygen affinity) by a decrease in pH (Bohr effect), an increase in temperature, or hypoxic conditions such as altitude adaptation or anemia. An alteration in blood pH is responsible for the fact that the oxygen dissociation curve is shifted to the right in the acid microenvironment of hypoxic tissues. This causes an enhanced capacity to release oxygen where it is most needed. The reason for this shift in the oxygen affinity of hemoglobin is related to the acidity of the hemoglobin molecule. Oxyhemoglobin is a stronger acid than deoxyhemoglobin. Because deoxygenated hemoglobin is more alkaline than is oxygenated hemoglobin, and an alkaline pH stimulates glycolysis, 2,3-DPG production is thereby increased. This, in turn, decreases molecular affinity for oxygen. In summary, increased amounts of deoxyhemoglobin and increased amounts of 2,3-DPG produce decreased affinity for oxygen.

Carbon Dioxide Transport

The transport function of hemoglobin also includes support for carbon dioxide transport from the tissues to the lungs. Carbon dioxide can be carried to the lungs by three different mechanisms. These mechanisms are indirect and direct transport by erythrocytes, and transport in solution in plasma.

In the predominant indirect erythrocyte mechanism, which accounts for about three fourths of the activity for removing carbon dioxide, carbon dioxide diffuses into the erythrocytes, is catalyzed by the enzyme carbonic anhydrase, and is transformed into carbonic acid.

$$H_2O + CO_2 \rightarrow H_2CO_3$$

The hydrogen ion of carbonic acid is accepted by the alkaline deoxyhemoglobin, and the bicarbonate ion diffuses back into the plasma.

$$H_2CO_3 \rightarrow H^+ + HCO_3^-$$

Free bicarbonate diffuses out of erythrocytes into the plasma in exchange for plasma chloride (Cl^-) that diffuses into the cell. This process is called the **chloride shift**. Bicarbonate is carried back to the lungs by the plasma. In the pulmonary capillaries, bicarbonate is converted back into carbon dioxide and water and eliminated through respiration.

About one fourth of the total carbon dioxide exchanged by erythrocytes in respiration is by a direct transport mechanism. In this mechanism, deoxyhemoglobin directly binds with carbon dioxide. This carbon dioxide reacts with uncharged amino groups of the four globin chains to form negatively charged carbamino hemoglobin. The carbamate groups form salt bridges with the positively charged deoxyhemoglobin molecule. This stabilizes the deoxy form and decreases oxygen affinity.

Approximately 5% of carbon dioxide is carried in solution in plasma to the lungs.

Synthesis of Hemoglobin

Hemoglobin is synthesized during most of the erythrocytic maturation process. About 65% of cytoplasmic hemoglobin is synthesized before the nucleus is extruded, and the remaining 35% is synthesized in the early reticulocyte. The major components of hemoglobin are heme and globin. Discussion of the synthesis of each of these components follows.

Formation of Heme from Porphyrin

Heme synthesis (Fig. 5.5) occurs in most body cells except for mature erythrocytes. Of all the body tissues, the red bone marrow and the liver are the most predominant heme (porphyrin) producers. Heme produced in the erythroid precursors is chemically identical with that in the cytochromes and myoglobin.

The preliminary activities in the synthesis of porphyrin, which precedes heme formation, begins when succinyl-coenzyme A (Co A) condenses with glycine. An unstable intermediate, adipic acid, is formed from this condensation and is readily decarboxylated to delta-aminolevulinic acid (ALA). This initial condensation reaction occurs in the mitochondria and requires vitamin B_6. The most important limiting step in this reaction is the rate of conversion to delta-ALA, which is catalyzed by the enzyme ALA synthetase. The activity of this enzyme is influenced by both erythropoietin and by the presence of the cofactor pyridoxal phosphate (vitamin B_6).

Following the formation of delta-ALA in the mitochondria, the synthesis reaction continues in the cytoplasm. Two molecules of ALA condense to form the monopyrrole porphobilinogen (PBG). This reaction is catalyzed by the enzyme ALA dehydrase. Four molecules of PBG condense into a cyclic tetrapyrrole to form uroporphyrinogen I or III. The type III isomer is converted, by way of coproporphyrinogen III and protoporphyrinogen, to protoporphyrin.

The final steps, carried out in the mitochondria, involve the formation of protoporphyrin and the incorporation of iron to form heme. Four of the six ordinate positions of ferrous (Fe^{2+}) iron are chelated to protoporphyrin by the enzyme heme synthetase ferrochelatase. This step completes the formation of heme (Fig. 5.6), a colored compound consisting of four pyrrole rings connected by methene bridges into a larger tetrapyrrole structure.

Disorders of Heme (Porphyrin) Synthesis

Disorders in the synthesis of porphyrin or the heme moiety may be either inherited or acquired. Inherited defects include a rare autosomal recessive condition, congenital erythropoietic porphyria.

Acquired defects include lead poisoning, which inhibits heme synthesis at several points. In this defect, inhibition of several enzymes, including heme synthetase, impairs synthesis reactions at several points, including ALA to PBG and protoporphyrin to heme. Not only are there morphological abnormalities of the erythrocytes (discussed in Chapter 6), but the quantity of ALA that is normally excreted in small amounts in the urine is also increased in lead poisoning.

Porphyrias of various types demonstrate alteration in the amount of PBG excreted in the urine. PBG is normally excreted in small amounts in urine; however, it appears in markedly elevated amounts in acute intermittent porphyria,

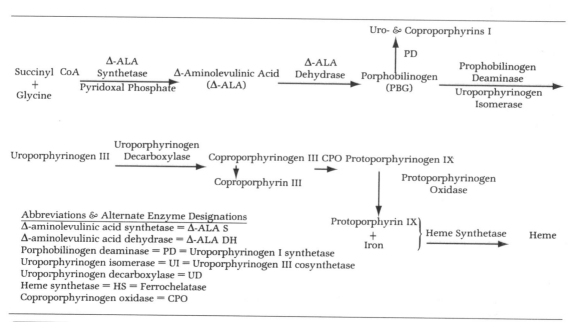

FIGURE 5.5 Heme synthesis flow chart. (From S. H. Robinson and P. R. Reich, *Hematology: Pathophysiologic Basis for Clinical Practice* [3rd ed.]. Boston: Little, Brown & Co., 1993.)

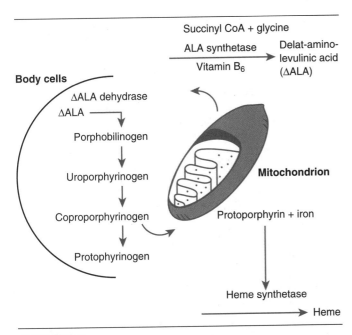

Body cells

Succinyl CoA + glycine

ALA synthetase
Vitamin B_6 → Delat-amino-levulinic acid (ΔALA)

ΔALA dehydrase
ΔALA →

Porphobilinogen

Uroporphyrinogen

Coproporphyrinogen

Protophyrinogen

Mitochondrion

Protoporphyrin + iron

Heme synthetase → Heme

FIGURE 5.6 Sites of heme synthesis.

which may be detected by testing the urine with Ehrlich's aldehyde reagent. In addition to increased urinary PBG, mild anemia and neurological changes may be associated with the porphyrias (Table 5.3).

The Role of Iron in Hemoglobin Synthesis

The physiology of iron metabolism is presented in Chapter 10. In relationship to the present discussion of hemoglobin synthesis, it is important to know that iron is delivered by a specific transport protein, **transferrin,** to the membrane of the immature cell. Iron in the ferric form (Fe^{3+}) is affixed to the cell membrane, and the transferrin is released back to the plasma. Most of the iron entering the cell is committed to hemoglobin synthesis and proceeds to the mitochondrion, where it is inserted into the protoporphyrin ring to form heme.

Excess iron accumulates as **ferritin aggregates** in the cytoplasm of immature erythrocytes. The amount of nonheme iron deposited depends on the ratio between the plasma iron level and the iron required by the cell.

TABLE 5.3 Clinical Classification of the Prophyrias

Pure neuropsychiatric	Mixed	Pure cutaneous
Acute intermittent	Variegate	Porphyria cutanea
Porphyria	Porphyria	Tarda
Plumboporphyria	Hereditary	Erythropoietic
	Coproporphyria	Protoprophyria
		Congenital
		Erythropoietic
		Porphyria

Globin Structure and Synthesis

Both the structure and the production of globin in the hemoglobin molecule are under genetic control. The specific sequences of amino acids are governed by the triplet code of DNA bases, which are genetically inherited. The rate of polypeptide synthesis is a function of the rate at which the DNA code is transcribed into messenger ribonucleic acid (mRNA). At least five genetic loci direct globin synthesis. Chromosomes 11 (non-alpha chain type) and 16 (alpha type) contain gene loci for globin synthesis.

The polypeptide chains of globin are produced, as are other body proteins, on the ribosomes. The alpha polypeptide chain unites with one of three other chains to form a dimer and ultimately a tetramer. In normal adult hemoglobin (hemoglobin A), these chains are two alpha and two beta chains.

Globin synthesis is highly coordinated with porphyrin synthesis. When globin synthesis is impaired, protoporphyrin synthesis is correspondingly reduced. Similarly, when porphyrin synthesis is impaired, excess globin is not produced. However, there is no such fine regulation of iron uptake with impairment of either protoporphyrin or globin synthesis. When globin production is deficient, iron accumulates in the cytoplasm of cells as ferritin aggregates. When porphyrin synthesis is impaired, the mitochondria become encrusted with iron, and some granules exist around the nucleus. These iron-containing granules in a nucleated erythrocyte are visible if the cell is stained with a special stain (Prussian blue stain). The cells are referred to as **sideroblasts** (refer to Chapter 10 for more details).

Normal Hemoglobin Types

In normal human development, several types of hemoglobin are produced. These hemoglobin types are hemoglobin A and a subfraction A_1; hemoglobin A_2; fetal hemoglobin; and embryonic hemoglobin. Each of these hemoglobin types has a distinctive composition of polypeptide chains (Table 5.4). Many other types of hemoglobin have been identified;

TABLE 5.4 Comparative Chain Composition of Hemoglobin Types

Hemoglobin Type	Symbol	Polypeptide (Globin) Chains
Embryonic Gower-1	$\zeta_2 \, \varepsilon_2$	2 zeta 2 epsilon
Gower-2	$\alpha_2 \, \varepsilon_2$	2 alpha 2 epsilon
Portland-1	$\zeta_2 \, \gamma_2$	2 zeta 2 gamma
Hemoglobin F	$\alpha_2 \, \gamma_2$	2 alpha 2 gamma
Hemoglobin A	$\alpha_2 \, \beta_2$	2 alpha 2 beta
Hemoglobin A_2	$\alpha_2 \, \delta_2$	2 alpha 2 delta

however, these are referred to as variant or abnormal hemoglobins.

Embryonic Hemoglobins

Embryonic hemoglobins are primitive hemoglobins formed by immature erythrocytes in the yolk sac. These hemoglobins include Gower I, Gower II, and Portland types. They are found in the human embryo and persist until approximately 12 weeks of gestation (Fig. 5.7). In these hemoglobins, the zeta chain is analogous to the alpha chain of fetal and adult hemoglobin and may combine with epsilon or gamma chains to form various embryonic hemoglobin types. The epsilon chain is analogous to gamma, beta, and delta chains.

Fetal Hemoglobin

Fetal hemoglobin (hemoglobin F) is the predominant hemoglobin variety in the fetus and the newborn. This hemoglobin type has two alpha and two gamma chains. The gamma chains have 146 amino acids, as do beta chains. However, gamma chains differ from beta chains. Two types of gamma chains exist, differing in only one amino acid. Either an alanine or a glycine may be present at amino acid position 136.

Fetal hemoglobin appears by the fifth week of gestation and persists for several months after birth. This hemoglobin type is associated with hepatic erythropoiesis. Although bone marrow erythropoiesis begins at the fourth month of gestation, the bone marrow does not establish itself as the primary hematopoietic organ until the end of the fifth or sixth month of gestation. Therefore, the synthesis of adult-type hemoglobin begins during fetal development, but the rate of synthesis is slow until the weeks just preceding birth. At birth, hemoglobin F accounts for 60% to 80% of the total hemoglobin, the remainder being adult-type hemoglobin A. Gradually, hemoglobin A replaces hemoglobin F in the circulating erythrocytes until the normal adult level of hemoglobin F (less than 2%) is attained. This process takes place until normal adult hemoglobin predominates, usually at about 6 months of age, although slight elevations may persist for 2 years. In abnormal cases, retention of hemoglobin F into adult life (15% to 30% of total hemoglobin) is referred to as **hereditary persistence** of fetal hemoglobin.

Glycosylated Hemoglobin (Hemoglobin A_1)

A subfraction of normal hemoglobin A is hemoglobin A_1. This subfraction can be termed **glycosylated hemoglobin** and includes the separate hemoglobin fractions A_{1a}, A_{1b}, and A_{1c}. This type of hemoglobin is formed during the maturation of the erythrocyte. Because proteins are vulnerable to modification after being synthesized by the ribosomes, this modification takes the form of glycosylation of hemoglobin in hyperglycemic persons. The formation of glycosylated hemoglobin is a slow, irreversible process that depends on the concentration of glucose in the body. Consequently, the concentration of glycosylated hemoglobin accurately reflects the patient's blood glucose level over the preceding weeks and has been recently used to monitor the control of diabetes.

Glycosylated hemoglobin is a stable hemoglobin and is structurally the same as hemoglobin A except for the *addition* of a carbohydrate group at the terminal valine of the beta chain. The concentration of hemoglobin A_1 is 3 to 6% in normal persons and 6% to 12% in both insulin-dependent and non–insulin-dependent diabetics.

Hemoglobin A

Although adult hemoglobin is predominantly of the A variety (95% to 97%), the A_2 type is also found in small quantities (2% to 3%). Hemoglobin A is composed of two alpha and two beta polypeptide chains. Hemoglobin A_2 is composed of two alpha and two delta chains. The delta chains differ from beta chains in eight of the 146 amino acids. Synthesis of delta chains begins during late fetal development, and the level of A_2 increases during the first year of life until the adult level is reached. The delta chains of hemoglobin A_2 are synthesized at only 1/40th the rate of beta chains. Therefore, the concentration of hemoglobin A_2 in a normal adult averages 2.5% of the total hemoglobin.

Variant Forms of Normal Hemoglobin

Carboxyhemoglobin, sulfhemoglobin, and methemoglobin are known as variant forms of normal hemoglobin. Unlike the abnormal hemoglobins with permanent structural rearrangements of the hemoglobin molecule, these variants are typified by differing from normal hemoglobin only by the molecule that replaces oxygen.

Carboxyhemoglobin

Hemoglobin has the capacity to combine with carbon monoxide in the same proportion as with oxygen, but the affinity

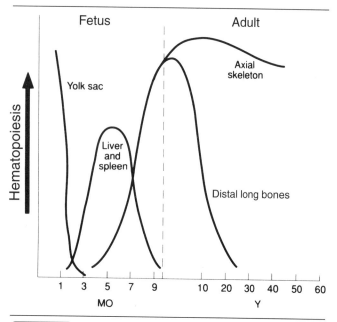

FIGURE 5.7 Hemoglobin development. Different types of hemoglobin are formed in different anatomical sites, progressing from the yolk sac to the red bone marrow. The yolk sac is the site of embryonic hemoglobin formation. The spleen and liver replace the yolk sac as the sites of cellular production of hemoglobin F. As the bones form, the red bone marrow takes over the production of red blood cells and hemoglobin A. Hemoglobin A consists of two beta and two alpha chains. (From R. S. Hillman and C. A. Finch, *Red Cell Atlas* [6th ed.]. Philadelphia: Davis, 1992.)

of the hemoglobin molecule for carbon monoxide is 210 times greater. This increased affinity results in the binding of carbon monoxide to hemoglobin to form carboxyhemoglobin even if the concentration of carbon monoxide is extremely low. The molecule forms an extremely stable compound, which renders the hemoglobin molecule useless for oxygen transport. A concentration of about 0.5% carboxyhemoglobin is produced by the normal degradation of hemoglobin. Slightly increased levels can be found in persons who smoke, and as a result of environmental pollution; increased levels may also be found in hemolytic anemia. Chronically increased levels can be associated with increased erythrocyte production. Levels of 20% to 30% carboxyhemoglobin saturation produce symptoms of dizziness, nausea, headache, and muscular weakness. Acute poisoning producing more than 40% saturation leads to rapid death.

Sulfhemoglobin

This variant of hemoglobin contains sulfur. In vitro and in the presence of oxygen, hemoglobin reacts with hydrogen sulfide to form a greenish derivative called sulfhemoglobin. The formation of this variant produces an irreversible change in the polypeptide chains of the hemoglobin molecule due to oxidant stress, and further change can result in denaturation and the precipitation of hemoglobin as **Heinz bodies.** Sulfhemoglobin cannot transport oxygen, but it can combine with carbon monoxide to form carboxysulfhemoglobin. Sulfhemoglobin can be formed by the action of certain oxidizing drugs such as phenacetin and sulfonamides on hemoglobin, in cases of bacteremia due to *Clostridium welchii*, and in enterogenous cyanosis. Concentrations of sulfhemoglobin in vivo are normally less than 1% and seldom exceed 10% of a patient's total hemoglobin. Elevated concentrations result in cyanosis but are usually otherwise asymptomatic.

Methemoglobin

This is a variant of hemoglobin, with iron in the ferric state, that is incapable of combining with oxygen. It can result from a metabolic defect (refer to Methemoglobin Reductase Pathway presented later in this chapter) or may occur because the structure of the hemoglobin molecule is abnormal due to the inheritance of an autosomal dominant trait. The genetically determined alteration in the amino acid composition of either alpha or beta globulin chains produces a hemoglobin molecule that has an enhanced tendency toward oxidation and a decreased susceptibility of the methemoglobin formed to reduction back to hemoglobin. Various forms of genetic alterations referred to as hemoglobin M disorders usually produce an asymptomatic cyanosis.

Normally, 2% methemoglobin is formed each day. At this concentration the abnormal hemoglobin is not harmful because the reduced ability of the erythrocytes to carry oxygen is insignificant. Higher concentrations of methemoglobin usually are avoided because of the presence of reducing systems. Cyanosis develops if methemoglobin levels exceed 10%; hypoxia develops if levels exceed 60%.

In addition to genetic reasons, increased methemoglobin production can result from environmental conditions such as exposure to certain drugs and oxidant chemicals. Once the offending agent is removed, methemoglobin disappears rapidly.

Infants are more susceptible to methemoglobin production because hemoglobin F is more easily converted to methemoglobin. In addition, the erythrocytes of infants are deficient in the required reducing enzymes. High nitrite quantities in food, water, or drugs can cause increased methemoglobin levels in infants.

Genetic Inheritance of Hemoglobin

Normal adult hemoglobin A is inherited in simple mendelian fashion. The genotype for this phenotype is A/A. Abnormalities of hemoglobin types may be seen in various hematological disorders; there are also approximately 350 variant types. Most defects in hemoglobin are related to either amino acid substitutions or diminished production of one of the polypeptide chains. Disorders referred to as **hemoglobinopathies** (discussed in detail in Chapter 13) represent disorders in which the production of normal adult hemoglobin is partly or completely suppressed, or partly or completely replaced by the production of one or more of the many variant hemoglobin types.

Abnormal hemoglobin such as that seen in sickle cell anemia results from mutant, codominant genes (see Chapter 3). Persons with this mutant gene may be homozygous (S/S) or heterozygous (S/A) for the trait. The sickle gene may occur with hemoglobin C, E, or D, giving rise to SC, SE, or SD disease. In the case of hemoglobin S, the defective molecule of the normal glutamic acid amino acid residue at the sixth position of the beta globin chain is replaced by a valine amino acid residue. This amino acid substitution results in erythrocytes that are sickled when deoxygenated hemoglobin S polymerizes and forms intracellular aggregates that deform the cell, and molecules of hemoglobin that are almost insoluble on deoxygenation. Altered solubility of the hemoglobin S molecule is due to the substitution of a nonpolar amino acid residue for a polar residue near the surface of the chain. In abnormal hemoglobin C, the normal glutamic acid amino acid residue at the sixth position on the beta globin is replaced by a lysine amino acid residue. A comparison of the defective beta chains with the normal sequence of amino acids in hemoglobin A is presented in Figure 5.8.

Analysis of Hemoglobin

Since the first hemoglobinopathy was described in 1910, several techniques have been developed to study hemoglobin. They include hemoglobin electrophoresis with various media, such as paper, cellulose acetate, or agar; solubility

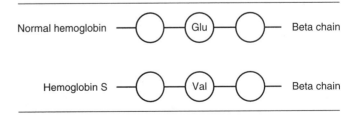

FIGURE 5.8 Comparison of normal and sickle hemoglobin molecules. Glu = glutamic acid; Val = valine.

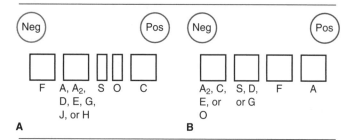

FIGURE 5.9 Hemoglobin electrophoresis by use of gel medium. Various types of hemoglobins migrate across an electrical field at different speeds. As depicted in the illustration, some variants have the same mobilities. Altering the pH of the medium changes the separation patterns. **A.** Citrate agar. **B.** Cellulose acetate, pH 8.6.

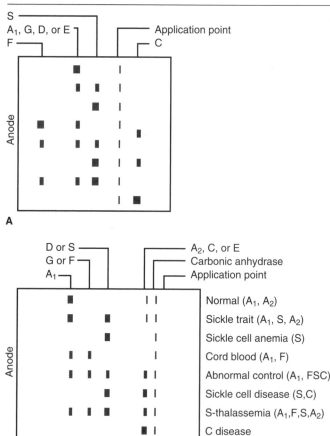

FIGURE 5.10 Hemoglobin electrophoresis. The mobilities and concentration of various hemoglobin fractions are depicted. The type of medium, such as citrate agar (**A**) and cellulose acetate (**B**), can alter the mobility patterns.

testing; and denaturation of hemoglobin through the use of acid or alkaline solutions (refer to Chapter 17). A method for the preliminary identification of abnormal hemoglobin is **electrophoresis** (Fig. 5.9).

Alkaline Electrophoresis

This method of separating hemoglobin fractions is based on the principle that hemoglobin molecules in an alkaline solution have a net negative charge and move toward the anode in an electrophoretic system. This screening procedure can separate hemoglobins A, F, S, and C and other variant hemoglobins (Fig. 5.10). Those with a greater electrophoretic mobility than hemoglobin A at pH 8.6 are classified as the **fast hemoglobins.** Examples of fast hemoglobins are hemoglobin Bart and the two fastest variants, hemoglobin H and hemoglobin I. Hemoglobin C is the slowest common hemoglobin.

Various media, such as paper, cellulose acetate, or starch blocks, and different buffers may be used for electrophoresis. These alternative methods vary in their efficiency of separation. For example, cellulose acetate at alkaline pH is rapid and reproducible. This technique separates the hemoglobin fractions S, F, A, C, and A₂.

Citrate Agar Electrophoresis

This process takes place at an acid pH. In this method, hemoglobins are separated on the basis of a complex interaction between hemoglobin, agar, and citrate buffer ions. Citrate agar separates hemoglobin fractions that migrate together on cellulose acetate. These fractions are hemoglobins S, D, G, C, E, and O. All hemoglobin specimens that show an abnormal electrophoretic pattern in alkaline media should undergo electrophoresis on acid citrate agar. The combined information allows for a complete identification of many variant hemoglobins.

Denaturation Procedures

A procedure commonly used to determine the amount of fetal blood that has mixed with maternal blood following delivery is the **Kleihauer-Betke** procedure (see Chapter 24). This test involves acid denaturation of hemoglobin. Fetal hemoglobin resists denaturation, while adult hemoglobin does not. Occasionally, intermediate (partially denatured) cells may be seen that are almost surely fetal hemoglobin-containing cells. Elevated levels of hemoglobin F can be seen in beta-thalassemia, a form of anemia, and paroxysmal nocturnal hemoglobinuria (PNH).

Chromatography

Quantitation of hemoglobin A₁ can be accomplished by cation exchange minicolumn chromatography. However, the results of this technique can be affected by several types of hemogoblin in addition to hemoglobin A₁. Cellulose acetate and citrate agar electrophoresis should be used in conjunction with cation exchange chromatography in order to eliminate the possibility of interference by hemoglobin variants. Other assay methods for glycosylated hemoglobin include high-pressure liquid chromatography (HPLC), radioimmunoassay (RIA), and colorimetric methods.

MEMBRANE CHARACTERISTICS AND METABOLIC ACTIVITIES OF ERYTHROCYTES

The mature erythrocyte has no nucleus or other organelles but is capable of existing in the blood circulation for an average of 120 days. However, the erythrocyte is more lim-

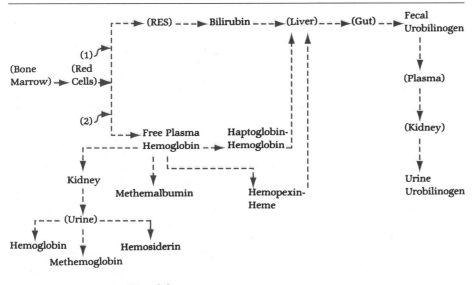

FIGURE 5.11 Pathway of erythrocyte glycolysis. RES = reticuloendothelial system. (From P. R. Reich, *Hematology: Physiopathologic Basis for Clinical Practice* [2nd ed.]. Boston: Little, Brown & Co., 1984.)

(1) Extravascular red cell breakdown
(2) Intravascular red cell breakdown

ited in metabolic activity than are other body cells. The cell has a limited ability to metabolize fatty acids and amino acids, and lacks mitochondria for oxidative metabolism. Energy for metabolic processes is generated almost exclusively through the breakdown of glucose. The overall pathway of erythrocyte glycolysis (Fig. 5.11) may be subdivided into the major anaerobic **Embden-Meyerhof** glycolytic pathway and three supplementary pathways, which act in different ways to maintain the function of hemoglobin. The Embden-Meyerhof pathway uses glucose and generates adenosine triphosphate (ATP). This pathway also is essential in maintaining pyridine nucleotides in a reduced state to support the methemoglobin reductase pathway and 2,3-diphosphoglycerate (2,3-DPG) synthesis, the Luebering-Rapaport pathway. In addition, the phosphogluconate pathway couples oxidative metabolism with pyridine nucleotide and glutathione reduction and protects erythrocytes from environmental oxidants. All of these processes (Table 5.5) are essential for the erythrocyte to transport oxygen and to maintain the physical characteristics required for survival in the blood circulation.

TABLE 5.5 Metabolic Pathways in the Erythrocyte

Metabolic Pathway	Function
Embden-Meyerhof pathway	Maintains cellular energy by generating ATP
Oxidative pathway or hexose-monophosphate shunt	Prevents denaturation of globin of the hemoglobin molecule by oxidation
Methemoglobin reductase pathway	Prevents oxidation of heme iron
Luebering-Rapaport pathway	Regulates oxygen affinity of hemoglobin

ATP = adenosine triphosphate.

Membrane Characteristics

The shape of the erythrocyte constantly changes as it moves through the circulation and performs extremely complex maneuvers. The cell is soft and pliable and can therefore move with ease through tissue capillaries and in the splenic microcirculation. The biconcave shape allows for maximum surface area and greatest flexibility.

The cellular membrane is composed of a protein-lipid bilayer (described in Chapter 3) with associated antigens. Antigens, such as those for type A or B and Rh type, are located on the outside or within the membrane. Antigens are chemically composed of oligosaccharides and glycoproteins. The membrane has a remarkable self-healing capacity. Injury to the cell may cause the production of viable fragments rather than intravascular hemoglobin leakage.

Cytoplasmic Characteristics

In addition to hemoglobin, the cytoplasmic contents of the erythrocyte include potassium ions in excess of the concentration of sodium ions, glucose, the intermediate products of glycolysis, and enzymes. The Embden-Meyerhof pathway uses about 90% of the erythrocyte's total glucose. Efficient cellular metabolism depends on long-lived enzymes. The enzymes synthesized during early cell development have to be sufficient to provide the energy needed for these processes:

1. Maintaining hemoglobin iron in an active ferrous (Fe^{2+}) state
2. Driving the cation pump needed to maintain intracellular sodium ion (Na^+) and potassium ion (K^+) concentrations despite the presence of a concentration gradient
3. Maintaining the sulfhydryl groups of globins, enzymes, and membranes in an active reduced state
4. Preserving the integrity of the membrane

If metabolic pathways are blocked or inadequate, the life span of the erythrocyte is reduced and hemolysis results. Defects in metabolism can include:

1. Failure to provide sufficient reduced glutathione, which protects other elements in the cell from oxidation
2. Insufficient energy-providing coenzymes such as reduced nicotinamide-adenine dinucleotide (NADH), nicotinamide-adenine dinucleotide phosphate hydrogenase (NADPH), and adenosine triphosphate (ATP)

The most common erythrocytic enzyme deficiency, which involves the Embden-Meyerhof glycolytic pathway, is a deficiency of **pyruvate kinase.** In newborn infants, the activity of phosphofructokinase, the rate-controlling enzyme in glycolysis, demonstrates decreased activity. This contributes to a decrease in glucose consumption, which in turn contributes to shortened erythrocyte survival. A deficiency of glucose-6-phosphate dehydrogenase (G6PD) limits the regeneration of NADPH, which renders the cell vulnerable to the oxidative denaturation of hemoglobin.

Metabolic Activities

Embden-Meyerhof Pathway

This glycolytic pathway (Fig. 5.12) is the major source of the essential cellular energy. In the breakdown of a molecule of glucose to lactate, two ATPs are consumed during the hexose portion of the pathway but four ATPs are generated at the triose level. This net gain of two ATPs provides the high-energy phosphates needed for maintenance of the erythrocyte's shape and flexibility, for maintenance of membrane lipids, and for driving the sodium-potassium pump and calcium flux. The essential role of ATP in erythrocyte physiology is demonstrated in at least two conditions: premature cell death in vivo because of a deficiency in ATP due to inherited defects in glycolysis, and the loss of viability that accompanies the depletion of ATP in vitro in stored blood for transfusion. The Embden-Meyerhof pathway also maintains pyridine nucleotides in a reduced state to permit their function in oxidation-reduction reactions within the cell.

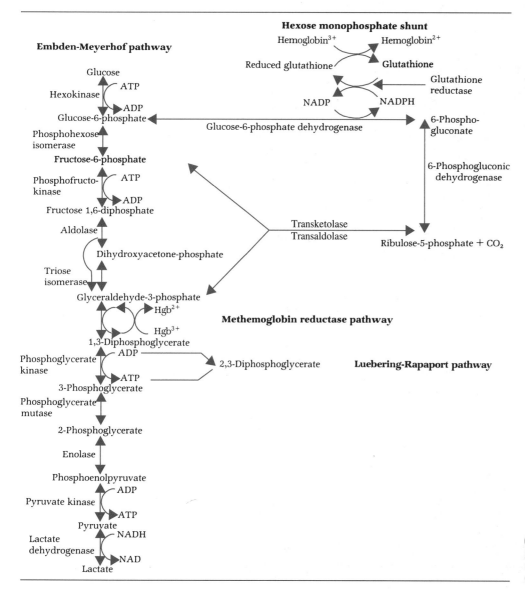

FIGURE 5.12 Embden-Meyerhof pathway, oxidative pathway or hexose monophosphate shunt, and methemoglobin reductase pathway.

Oxidative Pathway or Hexose Monophosphate Shunt

This energy system (see Fig. 5.12) couples oxidative catabolism of glucose with reduction of NADP (nicotinamide-adenine dinucleotide phosphate) to NADPH (the reduced form of NADP), which is subsequently required to reduce glutathione. The pathway's activity is increased with the increased oxidation of glutathione. When the pathway is defective, the amount of reduced glutathione becomes insufficient to neutralize oxidants. This causes denaturation of globin, which precipitates as aggregates referred to as **Heinz bodies** (discussed in Chapter 6). Cells containing Heinz bodies are ultimately phagocytized and destroyed by the mononuclear phagocyte cells of the spleen. Although it is minimal, some activity in the aerobic pathway is essential for normal erythrocyte survival.

Methemoglobin Reductase Pathway

The methemoglobin reductase pathway (see Fig. 5.12) is another important erythrocytic metabolic pathway that depends on the Embden-Meyerhof pathway for the reduced pyridine nucleotides that keep hemoglobin in a reduced state. Although the oxidative pathway, or hexose monophosphate shunt, is important in preventing denaturation of the globin of the hemoglobin molecule by oxidation, the function of the methemoglobin reductase pathway is to prevent the oxidation of **heme** iron. In the genetically inherited abnormalities in the amino acid sequence of the hemoglobin molecule, oxygen transport is affected by the oxidation of heme iron to methemoglobin.

Methemoglobin results from the oxidation of the reduced state (ferrous, Fe^{2+}) of heme to the trivalent (ferric, Fe^{3+}) form. In this form, hemoglobin can no longer combine reversibly with oxygen; therefore, the oxygen transport function of the molecule is lost. Maintenance of heme iron in a functional state (Fe^{2+}) requires the reducing action of NADH (the reduced form of nicotinamide-adenine dinucleotide), produced by the Embden-Meyerhof pathway, and the enzyme methemoglobin reductase. In the absence of this process, about 2% of the circulating hemoglobin is oxidized daily until 20% to 40% methemoglobin is present within the cell. Nonspecific reductants in the body are sufficient to keep the remaining hemoglobin reduced. A latent deficiency of methemoglobin reductase is compatible with the function of hemoglobin under normal conditions; however, high levels of methemoglobin can result when an afflicted person is challenged by an oxidant drug that denatures globin. **Methemoglobinemia,** an increased concentration of hemiglobin—a derivative of hemoglobin in which iron is oxidized to the ferric state—results from either an increased production of hemiglobin or decreased NAD-reductase activity. The condition may be hereditary or acquired.

Luebering-Rapaport Pathway

This pathway is important in the oxygen-carrying capability of erythrocytes. Because of this pathway, the erythrocyte has a built-in mechanism that is low in energy expenditure and is capable of regulating oxygen transport during conditions of hypoxia and disorders of acid-base balance. The Luebering-Rapaport pathway (Fig. 5.13) permits the accumulation of 2,3-DPG. Erythrocytic DPG is essential for maintaining

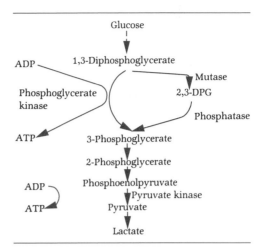

FIGURE 5.13 Luebering-Rapaport pathway. (From A. J. Bellingham and A. J. Grimes, "Red Cell 2,3-diphosphoglycerate." *Br. J. Haematol,* Vol. 25, No. 555, 1973.)

normal oxygen tension at a level necessary for oxygen transport, and it plays a regulator role in oxygen transport.

Regulation occurs in the following way: whenever the oxygen supply to the peripheral tissues is reduced, the proportion of oxygen extracted from the blood in the systemic capillaries increases. An increase in deoxyhemoglobin (deoxygenated hemoglobin) within the erythrocyte results in increased binding of DPG and stimulates glycolysis. This may result from a pH change within the cell and the consequent increase in total erythrocytic DPG and ATP. An increase in DPG and ATP produces a shift to the right in the oxygen dissociation curve.

In **acidosis,** erythrocytic glycolysis is reduced, available oxygen is increased, and 2,3-DPG falls to a level just sufficient to normalize the oxygen tension. In conditions of **alkalosis,** the converse reaction takes place.

Catabolism of Erythrocytes

Exceptions to the normal erythrocytic life span occur in premature infants, whose erythrocytes have a mean life span of only 35 to 50 days, and in fetuses, where the erythrocytes have an average life span of 60 to 70 days.

As an erythrocyte ages, the following processes occur:

1. The membrane becomes less flexible.
2. The concentration of cellular hemoglobin increases.
3. Enzyme activity, particularly glycolysis, diminishes.

When these changes have reached a critical point, the cell is no longer able to move through the microcirculation and is phagocytized. The spleen is the most active site for phagocytosis of aged cells because of its anatomy. Blood flow through the meshy splenic red cell pulp is slow, and the volume of plasma is reduced. This exposes aged or defective erythrocytes to phagocytosis. Intact erythrocytes return to the circulation via the small splenic venous sinusoids, where cell pliability is tested. The significant role of the spleen is demonstrated by the fact that erythrocytes with nuclear fragments (called **Howell-Jolly bodies**) and targeted erythrocytes (refer to Chapter 6) are seen after splenectomy.

Extravascular Catabolism

When an erythrocyte is phagocytized and digested by the macrophages of the reticuloendothelial system, the hemoglobin molecule is disassembled (Fig. 5.14). The resulting components are iron, protoporphyrin, and globin. Iron is transported in the plasma by transferrin in order to be recycled by the red bone marrow in the manufacture of new hemoglobin. Globin is catabolized in the liver into its constituent amino acids and enters the circulating amino acid pool. The porphyrin ring is broken at the alpha methene bridge by the heme oxidase enzyme. The alpha carbon leaves as carbon monoxide. The tetrapyrrole (bilirubin) resulting from the opened porphyrin ring is carried by plasma albumin to the liver, where it is conjugated to glucuronide and excreted in the bile. Both unconjugated (prehepatic) and conjugated (posthepatic) bilirubin are present in the plasma. Bilirubin glucuronide is excreted into the gut, converted by bacterial action, and excreted in the feces as stercobilinogen. A small amount of urobilinogen is reabsorbed into the blood circulation and excreted in the urine.

Intravascular Catabolism

Intravascular destruction is an alternate pathway for erythrocyte breakdown (Fig. 5.15). This process normally accounts for less than 10% of erythrocytic destruction. As the result of intravascular destruction, hemoglobin is released directly into the bloodstream and undergoes dissociation into alpha and beta dimers, which are quickly bound to the plasma

globulin **haptoglobin.** The formation of this large molecular haptoglobin-hemoglobin complex prevents urinary excretion of plasma hemoglobin. This stable complex is removed from the circulation by the hepatocytes, where it is processed by the cells in a manner similar to normal intact erythrocyte breakdown. Because haptoglobin is removed from the circulation as part of the haptoglobin-hemoglobin complex, the level of plasma haptoglobin decreases with hemolysis. Once plasma haptoglobin is depleted in the blood circulation, unbound hemoglobin alpha and beta dimers are rapidly filtered by the glomeruli in the kidneys, reabsorbed by the renal tubular cells, and converted to hemosiderin. The renal tubular uptake can process as much as 5 gm per day of filtered hemoglobin. Once the capacity for renal tubular uptake has been exceeded, free hemoglobin and methemoglobin begin to appear in the urine. The renal processing of filtered hemoglobin can produce:

1. Hemoglobin alone, if hemolysis is severe
2. Excretion of hemosiderin by itself
3. Excretion of both hemosiderin and hemoglobin; if desquamated tubular cells contain hemosiderin granules, this is evidence of a previous condition of hemoglobinemia.

Hemoglobin that is neither bound by haptoglobin nor directly excreted in the urine is oxidized to methemoglobin. The heme groups in methemoglobin are released and taken up by another transport protein, **hemopexin.** This complex is removed from the circulation by hepatocytes, and catabo-

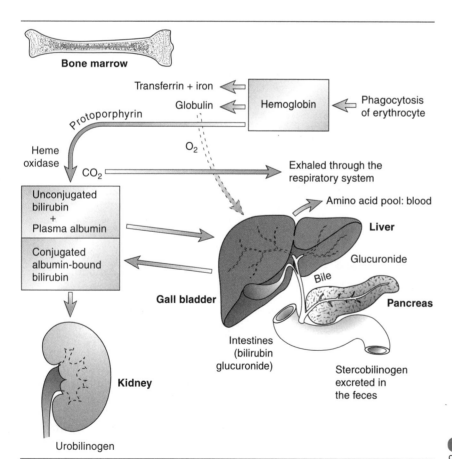

FIGURE 5.14 Extravascular catabolism of erythrocytes.

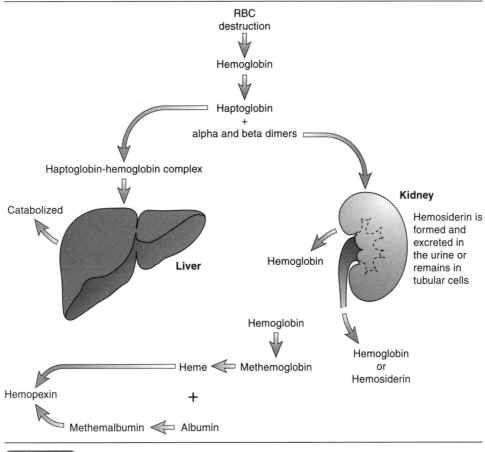

FIGURE 5.15 Intravascular catabolism of erythrocytes.

lized. Heme groups in excess of the hemopexin-binding capacity combine with albumin to form **methemalbumin** until more hemopexin is available. Once it is needed, hemopexin becomes available, and the complex is subsequently phagocytized by hepatocytes.

The combined depletion of haptoglobin and hemopexin and the presence of methemalbuminemia and hemosiderinuria can be seen in cases of intravascular hemolytic anemia and in intramarrow destruction of erythrocyte precursors. The presence of methemalbumin accompanied by hemopexin depletion *without* hemosiderinuria is associated with bleeding into the tissues, for example, intraabdominal bleeding in ectopic pregnancy.

MEASUREMENT OF ERYTHROCYTES

In evaluating erythrocytic disorders, it is necessary to have quantitative measurements of erythrocytes and evaluation of a peripheral blood smear as basic information. In this section, the erythrocyte indices of mean corpuscular volume, mean corpuscular hemoglobin, and mean corpuscular hemoglobin concentration are presented. The measurements of erythrocyte count, packed cell volume (hematocrit), and hemoglobin concentration may be performed manually (see Chapter 24). In Chapter 25, electronic methods of enumerating cells and additional measurements such as the red blood cell distribution width (RDW), including blood cell histo-

grams, are presented. Normal values for erythrocytes and related measurements appear in Table 5.6.

The erythrocyte indices are used to mathematically define cell size and the concentration of hemoglobin within the cell. They are:

1. Mean corpuscular volume (MCV)
2. Mean corpuscular hemoglobin (MCH)
3. Mean corpuscular hemoglobin concentration (MCHC)

Mean Corpuscular Volume

The MCV expresses the average volume of an erythrocyte. The formula is:

$$MCV = \frac{\text{patient's packed cell volume or hematocrit (L/L)}}{\text{erythrocyte count } (\times 10^{12}/L)} = fL.$$

Example: If the patient's hematocrit is 35%, or 0.35 L/L, and the erythrocyte count is $4.0 \times 10^{12}/L$, the MCV is determined thus:

$$MCV = \frac{0.35 \, L/L}{4.0 \times 10^{12}} = 87.5 \times 10^{-15} \, L = 87.5 \, fL^*$$

The normal value of MCV is 80 to 96 fL.

*One femtoliter (fL) = 10^{-15} L = 1 cubic micrometer (μm^3).

TABLE 5.6 Normal Values in the Measurement of Erythrocytes

Adult Values	
Packed cell volume	
Males	0.40–0.54 L/L
Females	0.38–0.47 L/L
Erythrocyte count	
Males	$4.6–6.2 \times 10^{12}$/L
Females	$4.2–5.4 \times 10^{12}$/L
Hemoglobin concentration	
Males	14.0–18.0 gm/dL
Females	11.5–16.0 gm/dL
Normal value of MCV	80–96 fL
Normal value of MCH	27–32 pg
Normal value of MCHC	32–36%
Representative Average Pediatric Values	
At birth	
Packed cell volume	0.56 L/L
Erythrocyte count	5.7×10^{12}/L
Hemoglobin concentration	21.5 gm/dL
MCV	106 fL
MCH	38 pg
At 6 years of age	
Packed cell volume	0.38 L/L
Erythrocyte count	4.7×10^{12}/L
Hemoglobin concentration	12.7 gm/dL
MCV	80 fL
MCH	27 pg
At 12 years of age	
Packed cell volume	0.40 L/L
Erythrocyte count	4.8×10^{12}/L
Hemoglobin concentration	13.4 gm/dL
MCV	81 fL
MCH	28 pg

Source: Adapted from P. L. Altman and D. S. Dittmer (eds.), *Blood and Other Body Fluids*, Bethesda, Md.: Federation of American Societies for Experimental Biology, 1961.

Mean Corpuscular Hemoglobin

The MCH expresses the average weight (content) of hemoglobin in an average erythrocyte. It is directly proportional to the amount of hemoglobin and the size of the erythrocyte. The formula is:

$$MCH = \frac{\text{hemoglobin} (\times 10 \text{ gm/dL})}{\text{erythrocyte count} (\times 10^{12}/L)} = pg$$

Example: If the patient's hemoglobin is 14 gm/dL and the erythrocyte count is 4×10^{12}/L, the MCH would equal:

$$MCH = \frac{140 \text{ gm/dL}}{4 \times 10^{12}/L} = 35 \times 10^{-12} \text{ gm} = 35 \text{ pg}†$$

The normal value of MCH is 27 to 32 pg.

†One picogram (pg) = 10–12 gm = 1 micromicrogram ($\mu\mu$g).

Mean Corpuscular Hemoglobin Concentration

The MCHC expresses the average concentration of hemoglobin per unit volume of erythrocytes. It is also defined as the ratio of the weight of hemoglobin to the volume of erythrocytes. The formula is:

$$MCHC = \frac{\text{hemoglobin} (\text{gm/dL})}{\text{packed cell volume or hematocrit (L/L)}} = gm/dL$$

Example: If the patient's hemoglobin is 14 gm/dL and the hematocrit is 45% or 0.45 L/L, the MCHC would equal:

$$MCHC = \frac{14 \text{ gm/dL}}{0.45 \text{ L/L}} = 31 \text{ gm/dL} = 31\%$$

The normal value of MCHC is 32 to 36%.

SUMMARY

The mature erythrocyte contains the respiratory protein hemoglobin. Hemoglobin is vital to the erythrocyte's major function, transport of oxygen and carbon dioxide.

Erythropoiesis

Erythropoiesis is the process of red blood cell production, which begins in the yolk sac of the embryo and ultimately continues throughout human life in the red bone marrow. Substances necessary for adequate erythropoiesis include amino acids (proteins), iron, vitamins B_{12} and B_6, folic acid, and the trace minerals cobalt and nickel. Deficiencies of any of these substances can produce defective erythropoiesis.

Erythropoietin, a glycoprotein synthesized mainly by the kidneys, is produced in response to tissue hypoxia. The action of this substance is responsible for stimulating erythropoiesis and a subsequent increase in circulating erythrocytes. Increased production of erythropoietin can produce a **secondary polycythemia.** Non–erythropoietin-related increases in erythrocytes can include the **relative polycythemias** or **polycythemia vera.**

Development and Maturation of Erythrocytes

Erythrocytes are rapidly maturing cells that undergo several mitotic divisions during the maturation process. After erythropoietin stimulation, the multipotential stem cell begins a series of maturational steps. The **rubriblast** is the first identifiable cell of this line, followed by the **prorubricyte, rubricyte, metarubricyte,** and **reticulocyte** stages in the bone marrow. Reticulocytes enter the circulating blood and fully mature into functional erythrocytes.

A defect in nuclear maturation can occur. This is referred to as megaloblastic maturation. In this condition, the nuclear maturation, which represents an impaired ability of the cell to synthesize DNA, lags behind the normally developing cytoplasm.

Reticulocytes represent the first nonnucleated stage in erythrocytic development. Although the nucleus has been lost from the cell by this stage, as long as RNA is present, synthesis of both protein and heme continues. The ultimate catabolism of RNA, ribosome disintegration, and loss of mitochondria mark the transition from the reticulocyte stage to full maturation of the erythrocyte. If erythropoietin stimulation produces increased numbers of immature reticulocytes in the blood circulation, these reticulocytes are referred to as "stress" or "shift" reticulocytes. Supravital stains, such as new methylene blue, are used to perform quantitative determinations of blood reticulocytes. Traditionally, the reticulocyte value is reported in a percentage. Additional mathematically derived methods of reporting reticulocytes have been developed; they include the corrected count and the RPI.

Characteristics and Properties of Hemoglobin

Normal adult hemoglobin (hemoglobin A) is the predominant type of hemoglobin. It consists of four iron-containing heme groups and four polypeptide chains: two alpha and two beta chains, containing 141 and 146 amino acids, respectively. The oxygen affinity of the hemoglobin molecule is regulated by the concentration of phosphates, particularly 2,3-DPG, which diminishes the molecule's affinity for oxygen. The oxygen dissociation curve is an expression of the affinity of hemoglobin for oxygen. Alterations in oxygen dissociation can be observed in the newborn, owing to the presence of fetal hemoglobin, which has an increased affinity for oxygen as well as a decreased level of 2,3-DPG.

Hemoglobin is synthesized during most of the erythrocytic maturation process. About 65% of the cell's hemoglobin is synthesized before the nucleus is lost, and the remaining 35% of hemoglobin is synthesized in the early reticulocyte.

The major components of hemoglobin are heme and globin. The red bone marrow and liver are the most predominant heme (porphyrin) producers. The synthesis of porphyrin, beginning with succinyl-coenzyme A (CoA), which precedes heme formation, takes place in the mitochondria until delta ALA is formed. Beginning with the condensation of two molecules of ALA, the next sequence of chemical reactions takes place in the cytoplasm. The final steps, the formation of protoporphyrin and the incorporation of iron into the molecule to form heme, take place once again in the mitochondria. The completed heme moiety consists of four pyrrole rings connected into a larger tetrapyrrole ring by methene bridges. Disorders of heme synthesis may be inherited (e.g., congenital erythropoietic porphyria) or acquired (e.g., lead poisoning, the porphyrias) defects.

Transferrin, a specific transport protein in the blood, delivers iron to the membrane of an immature erythrocyte. After the iron is affixed to the membrane, the transferrin is released back to the plasma. Excess iron accumulates as the compound **ferritin** in the cytoplasm of immature erythrocytes.

Both the structure and the production of globin are genetically determined and controlled by DNA. The polypeptide chains are synthesized, as are other proteins on the cytoplasmic ribosomes. Defects in either globin or porphyrin synthesis alter the synthesis of hemoglobin. A **sideroblast** is a nucleated erythrocyte in which iron deposits accumulate.

Several types of hemoglobin can be found during normal human growth and development: A, A_2, F, and embryonic forms. Abnormal types of hemoglobin, such as sickle cell hemoglobin, may be found. Adult hemoglobin is predominantly of the A type, although A_1 and A_2 are also found in small quantities. Fetal hemoglobin is the major hemoglobin in both the fetus and the newborn. Embryonic hemoglobins are the primitive hemoglobins found in the human embryo, and they persist until approximately 12 weeks of gestation. Variant forms of normal hemoglobin are carboxyhemoglobin, sulfhemoglobin, and methemoglobin.

Genetic defects related either to amino acid substitutions or to diminished production of one of the polypeptide chains are referred to as **hemoglobinopathies.** One of the best-known hemoglobinopathies is sickle cell anemia.

In order to identify and quantify normal and variant types of hemoglobins, several laboratory techniques have been developed. Two of the most popular are hemoglobin **electrophoresis** and the **Kleihauer-Betke** procedure. Other procedures include chromatography, HPLC, RIA, and colorimetric methods.

Membrane Characteristics and Metabolic Activities of Erythrocytes

Although it lacks a nucleus and other organelles, the mature erythrocyte is capable of surviving and functioning in the circulation for an average of 120 days. Energy for metabolic processes is generated almost exclusively by glycolysis through the anaerobic Embden-Meyerhof and supplementary pathways. In the **Embden-Meyerhof pathway,** the production of ATP provides the high energy needed to maintain membrane shape and flexibility through the maintenance of lipids, and for driving the sodium-potassium pump. The **oxidative pathway,** or **hexose monophosphate shunt,** couples oxidative metabolism with pyridine nucleotide and glutathione reduction. If a defect exists, the amount of reduced glutathione becomes insufficient to neutralize oxidants. This causes denaturation of globin, which precipitates as aggregates, **Heinz bodies.** The **methemoglobin reductase pathway** is essential to the prevention of oxidation of heme iron. Methemoglobin results from the conversion of the bivalent iron of heme to the trivalent forms. In this form, hemoglobin can no longer combine reversibly with oxygen; therefore, the oxygen transport function of the molecule is lost. The **Luebering-Rapaport pathway** is important to the oxygen-carrying capability of erythrocytes. Because of this pathway, the erythrocyte has a built-in mechanism that is low in energy requirements and is capable of regulating oxygen transport during conditions of hypoxia or disorders of acid-base balance. As the erythrocyte ages, the membrane becomes less flexible, with a loss of cell membrane; the concentration of cellular hemoglobin increases; and enzyme activity, particularly glycolysis, diminishes. When these changes reach a critical point, the erythrocyte is no longer able to move through the microcirculation and is phagocytized. When the erythrocyte is phagocytized and digested by the macrophages of the reticuloendothelial system, the hemoglobin molecule is disassembled. The resultant products are iron and globin. Iron is recycled back to the bone marrow by the plasma protein **transferrin.** Globin is catabolized in the liver into its constituent amino acids and enters the amino acid pool. The porphyrin ring is broken down by the enzyme heme oxidase, and the alpha carbon is lost as carbon monoxide. The tetrapyrrole (bilirubin) resulting from the opened porphyrin ring is carried by plasma albumin to the liver, where it is conjugated to glucuronide and excreted as bile. Both unconjugated and conjugated bilirubin are present in the plasma. Bilirubin glucuronide is excreted in the feces after conversion to stercobilinogen. A small amount of urobilinogen is excreted in the urine.

An alternate pathway for erythrocyte breakdown is intravascular destruction. Normally, this accounts for less than 10% of erythrocyte breakdown. As the result of intravascular destruction, hemoglobin is released directly into the bloodstream and undergoes dissociation into its alpha and beta dimers, which are quickly bound to the plasma globulin **haptoglobin** or excreted directly. Hemoglobin, which is neither bound by haptoglobin nor directly excreted in the urine, is oxidized to methemoglobin. In this oxidation process, heme groups are released and taken up by the transport protein **hemopexin.** If the hemopexin capacity is exceeded, heme groups combine with albumin to form methemalbumin, until more hemopexin becomes available.

Measurement of Erythrocytes

In the evaluation of erythrocytic disorders, it is necessary to have quantitative measurements of erythrocytes and a peripheral blood smear as basic information. Basic erythrocyte measurements include the erythrocyte count, packed cell volume (hematocrit), and hemoglobin concentrations. Several mathematically derived parameters based on these measurements are important to erythrocyte assessment. These parameters are the mean corpuscular volume (MCV), the mean corpuscular hemoglobin (MCH), and the mean corpuscular hemoglobin concentration (MCHC). Together, the MCV, MCH, and MCHC constitute the erythrocyte indices.

CASE STUDIES

CASE 1 The 6-month-old son of a 16-year-old mother was referred to the hospital laboratory by the well-baby clinic. The clinic's health officer noted that the baby was underweight and appeared pale. A complete blood cell (CBC) count was ordered.

Laboratory Data
The following determinations were obtained:

Hemoglobin 5.5 gm/dL
Hematocrit 0.23 L/L
Red blood cell (RBC) count 3.4 × 10¹²/L
Total white blood cell (WBC) count 12 × 10⁹/L

The differential leukocyte count revealed a normal distribution of leukocytes; however, the erythrocytes displayed a variety of morphological abnormalities.

Questions
1. What quantitative abnormalities were present in this baby's blood?
2. What are the MCV, MCH, and MCHC values, based on the data?
3. What type or types of abnormalities would be expected on the peripheral blood smear, on the basis of the erythrocyte indices?

Discussion
1. The baby's hemoglobin, hematocrit, and total erythrocyte count are all substantially below normal for a child of this age.
2. MCV, 67.6 fL; MCH, 16.2 pg; MCHC, 24%.
3. The indices demonstrate that the erythrocytes are smaller than normal and have a decreased amount of hemoglobin. These abnormalities should be very evident on the peripheral blood smear.

📖 **Diagnosis: Microcytic-hypochromic anemia**

CASE 2 A 30-year-old white man saw his family physician because of increasing fatigue over the previous few months. Physical examination revealed a pale but otherwise normal-appearing adult, although the liver and spleen appeared to be very slightly enlarged. The patient reported noticing that his first urine of the morning was occasionally dark brown. His physician ordered a CBC, urinalysis, and liver and spleen scan.

Laboratory Data
The following determinations were obtained:

Hemoglobin 8.5 gm/dL
Hematocrit 0.25 L/L
RBC count 2.6 × 10¹²/L
Total WBC count 4.4 × 10⁹/L

The differential leukocyte count revealed an increase in lymphocytes (60%), but the percentages of other leukocytes were within normal range. The urine demonstrated the presence of hemosiderin. A serum iron level and reticulocyte count were additionally requested. The total serum iron level was decreased, and the reticulocyte count was increased to 13%.

Questions
1. What is this patient's corrected reticulocyte count?
2. What is the RPI?
3. What type of defect was this patient suffering from?

Discussion
1. The corrected reticulocyte count was as follows:

$$\text{Reticulocyte count (\%)} \times \frac{\text{patient's hematocrit}}{\text{normal hematocrit}} = \%$$

$$0.13 \times \frac{0.25 \text{ L/L}}{0.45 \text{ L/L}} = 7.2\%$$

2. The RPI was as follows:

$$\frac{\text{corrected reticulocyte count in \%}}{\text{normal maturation time of 2 days}} = \frac{7.2}{2} = 3.6\%$$

3. The occasional presence of brown urine on early morning voiding is suggestive of hemolysis. Because these epi-

(continued)

sodes were described as intermittent by the patient, a diagnosis of paroxysmal nocturnal hemoglobinuria (PNH) would be suspected. That condition is a rare, acquired chronic hemolytic anemia. The episodes of intravascular hemolysis typically occur while the patient is asleep. During sleep, the blood pH decreases, making it easier for RBCs to lyse because of a membrane defect. This disorder represents an acquired erythrocytic membrane defect that renders one population of RBCs sensitive to lysis by normal plasma complement components.

Hemosiderinuria is an important diagnostic feature of this disorder. Demonstration of PNH in vitro depends on the lysis of PNH erythrocytes by complement. The sugar water screening test, or sucrose hemolysis test (see Chapter 24) is designed as a screening test for this purpose but is not specific enough. A positive screening test result should be followed up with the Ham test (acidified serum lysis test) before the diagnosis of PNH can be made. A leukocyte alkaline phosphatase cytochemical stain may also be of value because PNH is one of two disorders that show a decreased score. The other disorder is chronic myelogenous leukemia (discussed in Chapter 21).

✏ **Diagnosis: Paroxysmal nocturnal hemoglobinuria (PNH)**

CASE 3 An Rh-negative woman, 25 years old, was admitted to the hospital's maternity ward. After a prolonged and difficult labor, she delivered a full-term infant daughter. A cord blood sample was submitted to the blood bank for Rh testing; this is a routine procedure if the mother is Rh negative.

Laboratory Data
The baby's cord blood sample revealed that the baby was Rh (D+) positive.

Follow-up Testing
Because the mother had a long labor and there was evidence of greater-than-normal bleeding, her obstetrician ordered a Kleihauer-Betke test in order to determine whether one dose of immune globulin D would be sufficient to protect her from exposure to the baby's Rh-positive RBCs. A blood specimen was drawn from the mother. The figure shows a microscopic field of the Kleihauer-Betke results.

Questions
1. After examining the Kleihauer-Betke slide below, which cells are the baby's?

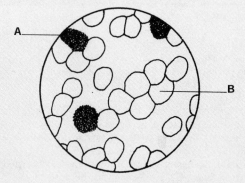

J. L. BENJAMIN

2. What accounts for the appearance of the baby's erythrocytes?
3. What is the significance of increased fetal cells in the maternal circulation?

Discussion
1. The dense-appearing cells (labeled A) are the erythrocytes containing fetal hemoglobin. The ghost cells (labeled B) contain adult hemoglobin A.
2. Cells containing hemoglobin F resist denaturation, but the cells containing adult hemoglobin are denatured. In all but rare cases in which hemoglobin F persists because of a hemoglobinopathy, increases in the number of fetal hemoglobin-containing cells are from the infant's blood and not from the mother's.
3. An increase in the number of fetal cells in the maternal circulation indicates that an increased amount of fetal blood crossed the placental barrier. If 2000 erythrocytes are counted, the percentage of fetal cells is multiplied by 50 to estimate the amount of fetal whole blood present in the maternal circulation. For example, if 1.5% fetal cells are counted and multiplied by 50, 75 mL of fetal-maternal hemorrhage has occurred.

✏ **Diagnosis: Increased fetal hemoglobin-containing erythrocytes in the maternal circulation**

CASE 4 An 18-month-old Puerto Rican boy had recently been brought to upstate New York from a poor neighborhood in New York City. His mother reported that he had been very cranky lately. She attributed this condition to teething. He had a habit of chewing on his favorite painted wooden toys, which were family heirlooms. He was referred to the hospital laboratory from the well-baby clinic because he was lethargic and pale. A CBC was ordered.

Laboratory Data
The following determinations were obtained:

Hemoglobin 6.5 gm/dL
Hematocrit 0.22 L/L
Total RBC count 3.0×10^{12}/L
Total WBC count 8.0×10^{9}/L

The peripheral blood smear revealed dense, dark-staining particles in some of the RBCs.

Questions
1. What are the erythrocyte indices in this patient?
2. Are any of the indices abnormal?
3. What are dark-staining granules in the erythrocytes? What is their origin?

Discussion
1. MCV, 73 fL; MCH, 21.7 pg; MCHC, 29.5%.
2. Normal ranges: MCV, 80 to 96 fL; MCH, 27 to 32 pg; MCHC, 32 to 36%.
3. The dark-staining granules were determined to be basophilic stippling (see Chapter 6), a condition that represents a defect in heme synthesis. In this child, the blood lead level was found to be increased.

✏ **Diagnosis: Lead poisoning. The probable etiology was the leaded paint on the child's toys.**

(continued)

CASE STUDIES *(continued)*

CASE 5 A 44-year-old Caucasian man consulted his primary care provider because of pain in his shoulder and fingers. The physical examination revealed no major abnormalities but his liver was slightly enlarged and tender. A CBC and blood chemistries were ordered.

Laboratory Data
Hemoglobin 13.5 gm/dL
Hematocrit 40%
Serum iron 37 μg/dL N=209 μg/dL
Serum transaminases slightly elevated
Serum ferritin 2430 ug/L (extremely elevated)
Serum transferrin saturation 95%

Followup laboratory data: A liver biopsy examination was performed. Tissue sections revealed fatty metamorphosis and an increase in fibrous tissue in portal areas consistent with early cirrhosis. Large amounts of parenchymal iron were noted with Prussian blue staining.

Questions
1. What is this patient's diagnosis based on the laboratory data?
2. What is the most common treatment for this disorder?
3. What is the cause of his medical condition?
4. Which laboratory assays are of the greatest value in establishing this diagnosis?

Discussion
1. The patient's diagnosis is hereditary hemochromatosis.
2. Therapeutic phlebotomy on a weekly basis is the usual treatment. In this case, the patient was phlebotomized weekly over a period of 10 months until his hematocrit reached 35% and iron saturation 15%. At that point, the therapeutic regimen was changed to phlebotomy every 2 to 3 months.
3. The cause of this patient's condition is hereditary hemochromatosis, a disorder described more than 100 years ago in western Europeans as "bronze diabetes." It is the most common autosomal-recessive genetic disease among whites with a tight linkage to the HLA-A locus on chromosome 6. Estimates of prevalence are that one in 10 to 20 whites carries the disease gene and that one in 400 are homozygotes at risk for developing the clinical syndrome.

   Hereditary hemochromatosis results from intestinal absorption of dietary iron in excess of bodily needs. The primary site for regulating iron absorption is in the cells of the duodenal mucosa.

   A patient destined to develop hemochromatosis begins early in life with a pattern of iron absorption that exceeds amounts appropriate to total body iron stores, and over the course of decades excess iron accumulates in various tissues and damages them. The disease pursues an insidious course and symptoms often do not occur until the fourth or fifth decade of life. Men are more frequently affected.
4. The single best screening test for hemochromatosis is serum transferrin saturation. The normal level is less than 50% and is generally about 30%.

Serum ferritin is generally viewed as an accurate reflection of body iron stores, but wide fluctuations in its value are often seen. In addition, serum ferritin is also an acute-phase reactant (protein) and is often elevated in conditions other than hereditary hemochromatosis.

Although abnormally high amounts of iron are absorbed into the circulation in patients with hemochromatosi, the total amount of transferrin decreases because, at least in part, high iron levels cause a decrease in transcription of the transferrin gene. Furthermore, transferrin is synthesized in the liver and levels of synthesis may decrease with the onset of liver disease. Thus, an increase in serum iron levels and a simultaneous decrease in transferrin levels combine to markedly increase transferrin saturation levels. If saturation levels are consistently greater than 62% without any overt hepatic disease that would contribute to a decrease in transferrin synthesis, the chances that the patient has hereditary hemochromatosis are greater than 90%. A liver biopsy confirms the diagnosis.

BIBLIOGRAPHY

Clinical Laboratory Reference. Tips on Technology—Hematology. Montvale, NJ: Medical Economics Publishing, 1985, p. 162.

Dubell, Jo Anne and Gerardo Perrotta. "Hemoglobin Raleigh and Glycosylated Hemoglobin." *Lab. Med.,* Vol. 15, No. 9, September, 1984, pp. 604–606.

Erslev, Allan J. "Erythropoietin." *N. Engl. J. Med.,* Vol. 324, No. 19, May 9, 1991, pp. 1339–1344.

Friedman, Ellen W. "Reticulocyte Counts: How to Use Them, What They Mean." *Diagn. Med.,* July, 1984, pp. 29–33.

Furlong, Maurice B. "Absolute Reticulocyte Count." Unpublished memo, Measurement of the Month, State University of New York, Upstate Medical Center, Syracuse, New York, April, 1973.

Groopman, J. E., J. Molina, and D. T. Scadden. "Hematopoietic Growth Factors." *N. Engl. J. Med.,* Vol. 321, No. 21, November 23, 1989, pp. 1449–1459.

Hillman, Robert S. and Clement A. Finch. *Red Cell Manual* (7th ed.). Philadelphia: Davis, 1996.

Hillman, Robert S. and Clement A. Finch. "The Misused Reticulocyte." *Br. J. Haematol.,* Vol. 17, 1969, pp. 313–315.

Insalaco, S. J. and Allen R. Potter. "Neonatal Transfusion Therapy." *Lab. Med.,* Vol. 16, No. 3, March, 1985, pp. 149–156.

Johnson, G. F. "Understanding Porphyrins and Porphyria: An Update." *Advance for Medical Laboratory Professionals,* Vol. 28, No. 11, Nov. 17, 1997, pp. 14–17.

Koepke, J. A. "Reticulocyte Count." *MLO,* June, 1995, p. 12.

Koepke, J. A. "Reference Values of Reticulocytes," *MLO,* Oct. 1992, p. 16.

Loftin, Eugene B. "Porphyrias: Demons in Disguise?" *Diagn. Med.,* October, 1984, pp. 21–30.

Miller, M. and G. M. Hutchins. "Hemochromatosis, Multiorgan Hemosiderosis, and Coronary Artery Disease," *JAMA,* Vol. 272, No. 3, July 20, 1994, pp. 231–233.

O'Connor, Barbara H. *A Color Atlas and Instruction Manual of Peripheral Blood Cell Morphology.* Baltimore: Williams & Wilkins, 1984, pp. 117–128.

Ortho Diagnostic Reporter. "Erythropoiesis." Vol. 2, No. 1. Raritan, NJ: Ortho Diagnostics, 1967, pp. 3–6.

Prouty, Hilda W. "Correcting the Reticulocyte Count." *Lab. Med.,* Vol. 10, No. 3, March, 1979, pp. 161–163.

Raphael, Stanley S. *Lynch's Medical Laboratory Technology.* Philadelphia: Saunders, 1983, p. 699.

Robinson, Stephen H. and Paul R. Reich. *Hematology: Pathophysiologic Basis for Clinical Practice* (3rd ed.). Boston: Little, Brown, 1993.

Romijn, J. A. "Erythropoietin in Anemia or Renal Failure in Sickle Cell Disease." *N. Engl. J. Med.,* Vol. 325, No. 16, October 17, 1991, p. 1175.

Thompson, F. L., J. S. Powers, and S. E. Graber. "Use of Recombinant Human Erythropoietin to Enhance Autologous Blood Donation in a Patient with Multiple Red Cell Allo-Antibodies and the Anemia of Chronic Disease." *Am J. Med.,* Vol. 90, March, 1991, pp. 398–400.

White, Patricia, Elizabeth Hendrick, and Mark Kolins. "Fetal-Maternal Hemorrhage Revisited." *Lab. Med.,* Vol. 16, No. 7, July, 1985, pp. 428–430.

REVIEW QUESTIONS

1. The progression of erythropoiesis from prenatal life to adulthood is:

   A. Yolk sac—red bone marrow—liver and spleen.
   B. Yolk sac—liver and spleen—red bone marrow.
   C. Red bone marrow—liver and spleen—yolk sac.
   D. Liver and spleen—yolk sac—red bone marrow.

2. Which of the following is (are) characteristic(s) of erythropoietin?

   A. A glycoprotein.   C. Secreted by the kidneys.
   B. Secreted by the liver.   D. All of the above.

3. Which of the following is a characteristic of erythropoietin?

   A. Produced primarily in the liver of the unborn.
   B. Gene for erythropoietin is found on chromosome 11.
   C. Most erythropoietin is secreted by the liver in adults.
   D. Cannot cross the placental barrier.

4. Stimulation of erythropoietin is caused by:

   A. Tissue hypoxia.   C. Inflammation.
   B. Hypervolemia.   D. Infection.

5. Increased erythropoietin production in secondary polycythemia can be due to:

   A. Chronic lung disease.   C. Renal neoplasms.
   B. Smoking.   D. All of the above.

6. Relative polycythemia exists when:

   A. Increased erythropoietin is produced.
   B. The total blood volume is expanded.
   C. The plasma volume is increased.
   D. The plasma volume is decreased.

7. The maturational sequences of an erythrocyte are:

   A. Rubriblast—prorubricyte—metarubricyte—rubricyte-reticulocyte.
   B. Rubriblast—prorubricyte—rubricyte—metarubricyte-reticulocyte.
   C. Pronormoblast—basophilic normoblast—polychromatic normoblast—orthochromic normoblast—reticulocyte.
   D. Both B and C.

8. What is the immature erythrocyte found in the bone marrow with the following characteristics? 12 to 17 μm in diameter, N:C of 4:1, nucleoli not usually apparent, basophilic cytoplasm.

   A. Rubriblast (pronormoblast).
   B. Reticulocyte.
   C. Metarubricyte (orthochromic normoblast).
   D. Prorubricyte (basophilic normoblast).

9. The nucleated erythrocyte with a reddish-pink cytoplasm and condensed chromatin pattern is a:

   A. Rubricyte (polychromatic normoblast).
   B. Basophilic normoblast (prorubricyte).
   C. Metarubricyte (orthochromic normoblast).
   D. Either B or C.

10. An erythrocyte remains in the reticulocyte stage in the circulating blood for:

    A. 1 day.   C. 3 days.
    B. 2.5 days.   D. 120 days.

11. In a Wright-stained peripheral blood film, the **reticulocyte** will have a blue appearance. This is referred to as:

    A. Megaloblastic maturation.
    B. Bluemia.
    C. Polychromatophilia.
    D. Erythroblastosis.

12. Which of the following is (are) characteristic(s) of megaloblastic maturation?

    A. Cells of some leukocytic cell lines are smaller than normal.
    B. Nuclear maturation lags behind cytoplasmic maturation.
    C. Cytoplasmic maturation lags behind nuclear maturation.
    D. Erythrocytes are smaller than normal.

13. In the reticulocyte stage of erythrocytic development:

    A. Nuclear chromatin becomes more condensed.
    B. RNA is catabolized and ribosomes disintegrate.
    C. Full hemoglobinization of the cell occurs.
    D. Both B and C.

14. On a Wright-stained peripheral blood smear, *stress* or *shift* reticulocytes are:

    A. Smaller than normal reticulocytes.
    B. About the same size as normal reticulocytes.
    C. Larger than normal reticulocytes.
    D. Noticeable because of a decreased blue tint.

15. The normal range for reticulocytes in adults is:

    A. 0 to 0.5%.   C. 0.5 to 1.5%.
    B. 0.5 to 1.0%.   D. 1.5 to 2.5%.

16. If a male patient has a reticulocyte count of 5.0% and a packed cell volume of 0.45 L/L, what is his *corrected* reticulocyte count?

    A. 2.5%.   C. 5.0%.
    B. 4.5%.   D. 10%.

17. If a male patient has a reticulocyte count of 6.0% and a packed cell volume of 0.45 L/L, what is his RPI?

    A. 1.5.   C. 4.5.
    B. 3.0.   D. 6.0.

18. Normal adult hemoglobin has:

    A. Two alpha and two delta chains.

    B. Three alpha and one beta chains.

    C. Two alpha and two beta chains.

    D. Two beta and two epsilon chains.

19. The number of heme groups in a hemoglobin molecule is:

    A. One.   C. Three.

    B. Two.   D. Four.

20. The presence of 2,3-DPG (2,3-diphosphoglycerate) ___ the oxygen affinity of the hemoglobin molecule.

    A. Increases.   C. Does not alter.

    B. Decreases.

21. After a molecule of hemoglobin gains the first two oxygen molecules, the molecule ___.

    A. Expels 2,3 DPG.

    B. Has decreased oxygen affinity.

    C. Becomes saturated with oxygen.

    D. Adds a molecule of oxygen to an alpha chain.

22. If normal adult (A$_1$) and fetal hemoglobin F are compared, fetal hemoglobin has ___ affinity for oxygen.

    A. Less.   C. A greater.

    B. The same.

23. Oxyhemoglobin is a ___ than deoxyhemoglobin.

    A. Weaker acid.

    B. Stronger acid.

24. Heme is synthesized predominantly in:

    A. The liver.   C. Mature erythrocytes.

    B. The red bone marrow.   D. Both A and B.

Questions 25 and 26: the initial condensation reaction in the synthesis of porphyrin preceding heme formation takes place in the (25)___ and requires (26)___.

25. _____   A. Liver.

                    B. Spleen.

                    C. Red bone marrow.

                    D. Mitochondria.

26. _____   A. Iron.

                    B. Vitamin B$_6$.

                    C. Vitamin B$_{12}$.

                    D. Vitamin D.

27. The final steps in heme synthesis, including the formation of protoporphyrin, take place in:

    A. A cell's nucleus.   C. The spleen.

    B. A cell's cytoplasm.   D. The mitochondria.

28. An acquired disorder of heme synthesis is:

    A. Congenital erythropoietic porphyria.

    B. Lead poisoning.

    C. Hemolytic anemia.

    D. A hemoglobinopathy.

29. The protein responsible for the transport of iron in hemoglobin synthesis is:

    A. Globin.   C. Oxyhemoglobin.

    B. Transferrin.   D. Ferritin.

Questions 30 and 31: if globin synthesis is insufficient in a person, iron accumulates in cell's (30)___ as (31)___ aggregates.

30. _____   A. Nucleus.

                    B. Cytoplasm.

                    C. Golgi apparatus.

                    D. Mitochondria.

31. _____   A. Transferrin.

                    B. Ferritin.

                    C. Albumin.

                    D. Iron.

Questions 32 and 33: when porphyrin synthesis is impaired, the (32)___ become encrusted with (33)___.

32. _____   A. Lysosomes.

                    B. Nucleoli.

                    C. Mitochondria.

                    D. Vacuoles.

33. _____   A. Protoporphyrin.

                    B. Hemoglobin.

                    C. Iron.

                    D. Delta-aminolevulinic acid.

34. Which of the following hemoglobin types is the major type of hemoglobin present in a normal adult?

    A. A.   C. A$_2$.

    B. S.   D. Bart.

35. The alkaline denaturation test detects the presence of:

    A. Hemoglobin A$_{1C}$.   C. Hemoglobin C.

    B. Hemoglobin F.   D. Hemoglobin S.

Questions 36 through 39: match the following hemoglobin types:

36. ___ A.   A. Two alpha and two delta chains.

37. ___ A$_2$.

38. ___ F.   B. Zeta chains and either epsilon or gamma chains.

39. ___ Embryonic.

                    C. Two alpha and two beta chains.

                    D. Two alpha and two gamma chains.

40. Fetal hemoglobin (hemoglobin F) persists until ___.

    A. A few days after birth.

    B. A few weeks after birth.

    C. Several months after birth.

    D. Adulthood.

41. Cellulose acetate at pH 8.6 separates the hemoglobin fractions:

    A. S.   C. A.

    B. H.   D. Both A and C.

42. If an alkaline (pH 8.6) electrophoresis is performed, hemoglobin E has the same mobility as:

    A. Hemoglobin S.   C. Hemoglobin A.

    B. Hemoglobin F.   D. Hemoglobin C.

43. The limited metabolic ability of erythrocytes is due to:

    A. The absence of RNA.
    B. The absence of ribosomes.
    C. No mitochondria for oxidative metabolism.
    D. The absence of DNA.

44. Which of the following statements is (are) true of the erythrocytic cytoplasmic contents?

    A. High in potassium ion.
    B. High in sodium ion.
    C. Contains glucose and enzymes necessary for glycolysis.
    D. Both A and C.

45. The Embden-Meyerhof glycolytic pathway produces ___% of the energy necessary for erythrocytic metabolism.

    A. 10.   C. 50.
    B. 20.   D. 90.

46. In erythrocytes, enzymes provide energy to:

    A. Maintain hemoglobin iron in its active ferrous state.
    B. Power the cation pump needed to maintain appropriate sodium-potassium concentration.
    C. Preserve the integrity of the cellular membrane.
    D. All of the above.

47. The end product of the Embden-Meyerhof pathway of glucose metabolism in the erythrocyte is:

    A. Pyruvate.   C. Glucose-6-phosphate.
    B. Lactate.   D. The trioses.

48. The net gain in ATPs in the Embden-Meyerhof glycolytic pathway is:

    A. One.   C. Four.
    B. Two.   D. Six.

49. The most common erythrocytic enzyme deficiency involving the Embden-Meyerhof glycolytic pathway is a deficiency of:

    A. ATPase.
    B. Pyruvate kinase.
    C. Glucose-6-phosphate dehydrogenase.
    D. Lactic dehydrogenase.

50. If a defect in the oxidative pathway (hexose monophosphate shunt) occurs, what will result?

    A. Insufficient amounts of reduced glutathione.
    B. Denaturation of globin.
    C. Precipitation of Heinz bodies.
    D. All of the above.

51. The function of the methemoglobin reductase pathway is to:

    A. Keep hemoglobin in a reduced state.
    B. Maintain ferrous iron in a functional state.
    C. Provide cellular energy.
    D. Control the rate of glycolysis.

52. The Luebering-Rapaport pathway:

    A. Permits the accumulation of 2,3-DPG.
    B. Promotes glycolysis.
    C. Produces cellular energy.
    D. Produces acidosis.

53. In conditions of acidosis:

    A. Erythrocytic glycolysis is reduced.
    B. Available oxygen is increased.
    C. DPG levels fall to a level sufficient to normalize oxygen tension.
    D. All of the above.

54. As the erythrocyte ages:

    A. The membrane becomes less flexible with loss of cell membrane.
    B. Cellular hemoglobin increases.
    C. Enzyme activity, particularly glycolysis, decreases.
    D. All of the above.

55. Erythrocytic catabolism produces the disassembling of hemoglobin followed by:

    A. Iron transported in the plasma by transferrin.
    B. Globin catabolized in the liver to amino acids and then entering the amino acid pool.
    C. Bilirubin formed from opened porphyrin ring and carried by plasma albumin to the liver, conjugated, and excreted in bile.
    D. All of the above.

56. Which of the following statements are true of the intravascular destruction of erythrocytes?

    A. It accounts for less than 10% of normal breakdown.
    B. Hemoglobin is released directly into blood.
    C. Alpha and beta dimers are converted to hemosiderin.
    D. All of the above.

57. The upper limit of the reference range of hemoglobin in an adult male is:

    A. 10.5 to 12.0 gm/dL.   C. 13.5 to 15.0 gm/dL.
    B. 12.5 to 14.0 gm/dL.   D. 14.5 to 18.0 gm/dL.

Questions 58 through 60: match the specific erythrocytic indices with the appropriate formula.

58. ___ MCV.

59. ___ MCH.

60. ___ MCHC.

A. Patient's packed cell volume or hematocrit (in L/L)/erythrocyte count ($\times 10^{12}$/L) = fL.

B. Hemoglobin (in gm/dL)/packed cell volume or hematocrit (in L/L) = gm/dL.

C. Hemoglobin ($\times 10$ gm/dL)/erythrocyte count ($\times 10^{12}$/L) = pg.

Questions 61 through 63: match the erythrocytic indices with the appropriate normal value.

61. ___ MCV.   A. 32 to 36%.

62. ___ MCH.   B. 27 to 32 pg.

63. ___ MCHC.   C. 80 to 96 fL.

6

Erythrocyte Morphology and Inclusions

OBJECTIVES

Erythrocytes: Normal and abnormal
- Name and describe the variations in the size of a mature erythrocyte.
- Describe the chemical causes of variation in cell size.
- Correlate at least one clinical condition with each of the erythrocytic size variations: anisocytosis, macrocytosis, and microcytosis.
- Explain the terms used when a mature erythrocyte assumes an irregular shape.
- Explain the chemical or physical reasons for differences in cell shape.
- Correlate at least one clinical condition with each of these erythrocytic shape variations: acanthocytes, blister cells, burr cells, crenated red cells, elliptocytes, keratocytes, knizocytes, leptocytes, poikilocytosis, pyknocytes, schistocytes, sickle cells, spherocytes, stomatocytes, and teardrops.
- Compare the chemical basis for differences in erythrocyte color on a stained blood smear.
- Describe the alterations in color that can be seen in an erythrocyte.
- Correlate at least one clinical condition with the conditions of hypochromia and polychromatophilia.

- Name and describe the appearance of inclusions that may be seen in a variety of abnormal conditions.
- Explain the cellular or chemical basis of inclusions.
- Correlate at least one clinical condition with the following erythrocyte inclusions: basophilic stippling, Cabot rings, Heinz bodies, hemoglobin C crystals, Howell-Jolly bodies, Pappenheimer bodies, and siderotic granules.
- Define the alterations in erythrocyte distribution that may be encountered when examining a blood smear.
- Briefly describe the chemical reasons for alterations in erythrocyte distribution on a peripheral blood smear.
- Name the clinical conditions associated with alterations in erythrocyte distribution on a blood smear.
- Name and describe the morphology of malaria, *Babesia*, and leishmania parasites on a peripheral blood smear.

ERYTHROCYTES: NORMAL AND ABNORMAL

Normal mature erythrocytes (discocytes) are biconcave and disc-shaped and lack a nucleus. Some variations in either size, shape, or color of erythrocytes may be seen on microscopic examination with a Wright or similar Romanowsky-type stain. In many disorders or disease states, erythrocytes may demonstrate variations in appearance or morphology as the result of pathological conditions.

The variations from normal can be classified as:

1. Variation in size
2. Variation in shape
3. Alteration in color
4. Inclusions in the erythrocyte
5. Alterations in the erythrocyte distribution on a peripheral blood smear

Some differences in appearance may be misleading. Alterations in appearance may be due to artifacts such as precipitated stain or proteins rather than an actual erythrocytic disorder. However, most erythrocyte deviations can be traced to specific chemical, physical, or cellular causes. This section discusses the appearance of erythrocytes on peripheral blood smears, the factors related to alterations in morphology, and the associated clinical disorders.

Types of Variations in Erythrocyte Size

A normal erythrocyte has an average diameter of 7.2 μm with a usual variation of 6.8 to 7.5 μm. The extreme size limits are generally considered to be 6.2 to 8.2 μm. This normal size is referred to as **normocytic.** Erythrocytes may be either larger than normal, **macrocytic,** or smaller than normal, **microcytic** (Fig. 6.1). Macrocytic erythrocytes exceed the 8.2-μm diameter limit, while microcytic erythrocytes are smaller than the average 6.2-μm diameter.

The general term used in hematology to denote an increased variation in cell size is **anisocytosis.** This term is nonspecific because it does not indicate the type of variation that is present. Anisocytosis is prominent in severe anemias.

The terms macrocytic, normocytic, and microcytic are the preferred terminology. Conditions in which a deviation from normal erythrocyte size occurs have a definite chemical or physiological basis. If more than one population of erythrocytes is present, such as following a transfusion of normocytic erythrocytes to a patient with many microcytic erythrocytes, more than one cell size may be present and the sizes of both populations should be recorded.

Macrocytosis is the result of a defect in either nuclear maturation or stimulated erythropoiesis. True macrocytes represent a nuclear maturation defect associated with a deficiency of either vitamin B_{12} or folate. These cells result from a disruption of the regular mitotic division in the bone marrow. Because of this defect, the cells appear as mature, enlarged erythrocytes in the circulating blood (Plate 8). The other type of macrocytosis is due to increased erythropoietin stimulation, which increases the synthesis of hemoglobin in developing cells. This disorder causes a premature release of reticulocytes into the blood circulation. These cells not only will appear to be macrocytic but also may be basophilic and slightly hypochromic on a peripheral smear.

Microcytosis (Plate 9) is associated with a decrease in hemoglobin synthesis. This decrease in hemoglobin content may be produced by a deficiency of iron, impaired globulin synthesis, or a mitochondrial abnormality affecting the synthesis of the heme unit of the hemoglobin molecule. Disorders in which microcytosis may occur include malabsorption syndrome, iron deficiency anemia, and in the case of variant hemoglobin types, the hemoglobinopathies.

Kinds of Variations in Erythrocyte Shape

The general term for mature erythrocytes that have a shape other than the normal round, biconcave appearance on a stained blood smear, or variations, is **poikilocytosis** (Plate 10). Poikilocytes can assume many shapes (Fig. 6.2), but they frequently resemble common objects such as eggs, pencils, and teardrops. Specific names have been given to many of these shapes. The names for specific kinds of poikilocytes include acanthocytes, blister cells, burr cells, crenated erythrocytes, echinocytes, elliptocytes, keratocytes, ovalocytes, pyknocytes, schistocytes, sickle cells, spiculated erythrocytes, spherocytes, stomatocytes, target cells, and teardrops. A newer nomenclature (Table 6.1) is preferred by many hematologists in place of the common names.

Deviation from the discoid shape of an erythrocyte represents a chemical or physical alteration of either the cellular membrane or the physical contents of the cell. In some cases, the exact mechanism is still unknown. However, recent research in cell biology has contributed to an increased knowledge of many of these mechanisms. Each of the poikilocyte types has distinctive features and may be found in increased numbers in specific hematological and nonhematological disorders (Table 6.2). The following paragraphs give a brief description of each.

Acanthocytes have multiple thorny, spike-like projections that are irregularly distributed around the cellular membrane and may vary in size. Unlike echinocytes, acanthocytes

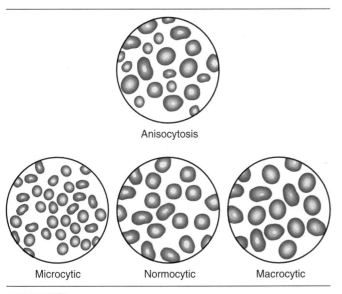

Anisocytosis

Microcytic · Normocytic · Macrocytic

FIGURE 6.1 Variations in erythrocyte size.

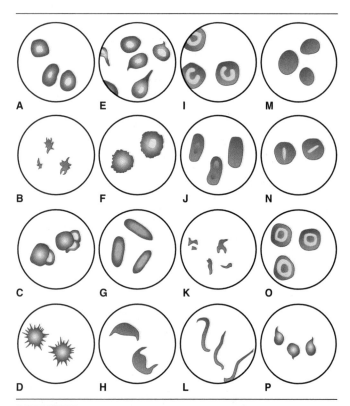

FIGURE 6.2 Variations in erythrocyte shape. A = normal red blood cells (RBCs) (discocytes); B = acanthocytes; C = blister cells; D = burr cells; E = poikilocytes; F = crenated RBCs (echinocytes); G = elliptocytes; H = helmet cells (schizocytes); I = leptocytes; J = oval macrocytes (megalocytes); K = schistocytes (schizocytes); L = sickle cells (drepanocytes); M = spherocytes; N = stomatocytes; O = target cells (codocytes); P = teardrops (dacryocytes).

TABLE 6.1 Erythrocyte Nomenclature

Common Terms	Synonyms (Greek Terminology)
Acanthocyte	Acanthocyte
Blister cell	
Burr cell	Echinocyte
Crenated erythrocyte	Echinocyte
Elliptocyte	Elliptocyte
Helmet cell	Schizocyte
Normal erythrocyte	Discocyte
Oval macrocyte	Megalocyte
Ovalocyte	Elliptocyte
Pyknocyte	
Schistocyte	Schizocyte
Sickle cell	Drepanocyte, meniscocyte
Spiculated erythrocyte	
Spherocyte	Spherocyte
Stomatocyte	Stomatocyte
Target cell	Codocyte
Teardrop	Dacryocyte
Keratocyte	
Knizocyte	
Leptocyte	

have few spicules. Acanthocytes are prevalent in two very different disorders: **abetalipoproteinemia,** a rare hereditary disorder, and spur cell anemia. In abetalipoproteinemia, acanthocytes represent an imbalance between erythrocyte and plasma lipids. The reason for this imbalance is that the patient does not absorb lipids in the small intestine. This results in decreased plasma lipids, which in turn produces a membrane defect. The loss of membrane integrity causes the cells to be more sensitive to external and internal forces. Acanthocytes are also found in cirrhosis of the liver with associated hemolytic anemia, following heparin administration, in hepatic hemangioma, in neonatal hepatitis, and postsplenectomy.

Blister cells are erythrocytes containing one or more vacuoles that resemble a blister on the skin. This cell has a markedly thinned area at the periphery or outer border of the cell membrane. The vacuoles may rupture. If rupturing does occur, distorted cells (**keratocytes**) and cell fragments (**schistocytes**) are produced. These cell alterations are found where there is damage to the membrane (e.g., severe burns). Blister cells result from the traumatic interaction of blood vessels and circulating blood such as fibrin deposits. Clinically, increased numbers can be seen as the result of pulmonary emboli in sickle cell anemia and microangiopathic hemolytic anemia.

Burr cells (echinocytes) are erythrocytes having one or more spiny projections of cellular membrane (Plate 11).

These cells are frequently elongated or assume irregular shapes such as a quarter-moon. Burr cells are less spherical than acanthocytes. In vitro, burr cells can be produced as artifacts. Pointed projections on the outer edge are uniformly shaped. These erythrocytes have decreased deformability. The deformability depends on a variety of factors such as the relationship of the surface area of the cell to its volume, the type of hemoglobin present, or the lipid characteristics. This decreased deformability produces increased red cell rigidity and premature destruction. Clinically, burr cells are increased in a variety of anemias, bleeding gastric ulcers, gastric carcinoma, peptic ulcers, renal insufficiency, pyruvate kinase deficiency, and uremia. They may also occur as artifacts.

Echinocytes (crenated erythrocytes) have short, scalloped, or spike-like projections that are regularly distributed around the cell membrane. The projections can vary in number and appearance. Crenation can occur as the result of the physical loss of intracorpuscular water (see Chapter 3 for the discussion on osmosis). No disease states are related to crenation, but this cellular distortion results from an osmotic imbalance.

Elliptocytes (Plate 12) are generally narrower and more elongated than megalocytes. These cells have a rod, cigar, or sausage shape. They represent a membrane defect where the membrane is radically affected and suffers a loss of integrity. Associated clinical disorders include hereditary elliptocytosis, anemias associated with malignancy, hemoglobin (Hb) C disease, hemolytic anemias (occasionally), iron deficiency anemia, pernicious anemia, sickle cell trait, and thalassemia.

TABLE 6.2 **Red Blood Cell (RBC) Morphology and Related Conditions**

RBC Morphology	Associated Clinical Conditions	RBC Morphology	Associated Clinical Conditions
Variation in Size		Pyknocytes	Acute, severe hemolytic anemias
Anisocytosis	Marked in severe anemias		G6PD deficiency
Macrocytes	Megaloblastic anemias and macro-cytic anemias (pernicious anemia and folic acid deficiency)		Hereditary lipoprotein deficiency
			May be seen in small numbers during the first 2–3 months of life as infantile pyknocytes
Microcytes	Iron deficiency anemia	Schistocytes (schizocytes)	Hemolytic anemias related to burns or prosthetic implants
	Hemoglobinopathies		Renal transplant rejection
Variation in Shape		Sickle cells (drepanocytes)	Sickle cell anemia
Acanthocytes	Abetalipoproteinemia	Spherocytes	ABO hemolytic disease of the newborn
	Cirrhosis of the liver with associated hemolytic anemia		Acquired hemolytic anemias
	Following heparin administration		Blood transfusion reactions
	Hepatic hemangioma		Congenital spherocytosis
	Neonatal hepatitis		DIC
	Postsplenectomy		Storage phenomenon producing microspherocytes in the recipient
Blister cells	An indication of pulmonary emboli in sickle cell anemia	Stomatocytes	Acute alcoholism
	Microangiopathic hemolytic anemia		Alcoholic cirrhosis
Burr cells (echinocytes)	A variety of anemias		Glutathione deficiency
	Bleeding gastric ulcers		Hereditary spherocytosis
	Gastric carcinoma		Infectious mononucleosis
	Peptic ulcers		Lead poisoning
	Renal insufficiency		Malignancies
	Pyruvate kinase deficiency		Thalassemia minor
	Uremia		Transiently accompanying a hemolytic anemia
Crenated RBCs (echinocytes)	Diseases—none	Target cells (codocytes)	Hemoglobinopathies: Hb C disease, S-C, S-S, sickle cell–thalassemia, thalassemia
	Result from osmotic imbalance		
Elliptocytes	Anemias associated with malignancy		Hemolytic anemias
	Hemoglobin C disease		Hepatic disease with or without jaundice
	Hemolytic anemias (occasionally)		Iron deficiency
	Hereditary elliptocytosis		Postsplenectomy
	Iron deficiency anemia		Artifact
	Pernicious anemia		
	Sickle cell trait		
	Thalassemia		
Keratocytes	Diffuse intravascular coagulation (DIC)	Teardrops (dacryocytes)	Homozygous β-thalassemia
			Myeloproliferative syndromes
Knizocytes	Hemolytic anemia, including hereditary spherocytosis		Pernicious anemia
			Severe anemias
Leptocytes	Hepatic disorders	*Alterations in Color*	
	Iron deficiency anemia	Hypochromia	Iron deficiency
	Thalassemia	Polychromatophilia	Rapid blood regeneration
Poikilocytosis	Hemolytic anemias		
	Myelofibrosis		
	Pernicious anemia		
	Thalassemia		

Helmet cells (schizocytes) are usually the larger scooped-out part of the cell (Plate 13) that remains after the rupturing of a blister cell and are formed due to the physical process of fragmentation. These cell fragments are formed in the spleen and intravascular fibrin clots. (See the discussion of schistocytes below for a description of related clinical disorders.)

Keratocytes are erythrocytes that are partially deformed but not cut. The spicules, resembling two horns, result from a ruptured vacuole. Usually the cell appears like a half-moon or spindle. These cells are seen in conditions such as disseminated (diffuse) intravascular coagulation (DIC).

Knizocytes resemble a pinched bottle. This abnormality is associated with the hemolytic anemias including hereditary spherocytosis.

Leptocytes resemble target cells (codocytes) but the inner, central portion is not completely detached from the outer membrane. This variation of the target cell is clinically associated with hepatic disorders, iron deficiency anemia, and thalassemia.

Oval macrocytes (megalocytes) have an oval or egg-like appearance (see Plate 8). Although these cells are similar in appearance to elliptocytes, megalocytes are macrocytic and have a fuller and rounder appearance. In contrast, elliptocytes tend to have a normal cell-size volume. Increases in this abnormality are seen in vitamin B_{12} and folate deficiencies and may be observed in erythrocytes that are in the reticulocyte stage.

Pyknocytes are distorted, contracted erythrocytes that are similar to burr cells. These cells are seen in acute, severe hemolytic anemia, glucose-6-phosphate dehydrogenase (G6PD) deficiency, and hereditary lipoprotein deficiency, and may be seen in small numbers during the first 2 to 3 months of life as infantile pyknocytes.

Schistocytes (schizocytes) are fragments of erythrocytes that are small and irregularly shaped. Because these cells are produced as the result of the breaking apart of an erythrocyte, the schistocyte is about half the size of a normal erythrocyte and may have a deeper-red appearance. Increased numbers of schistocytes can be seen in hemolytic anemias related to burns and prosthetic implants, and renal transplant rejections.

Sickle cells (drepanocytes) resemble a crescent (Plate 14). At least one of the ends of the cell must be pointed. Generally, the membrane is smooth and the cell stains uniformly throughout. Sickle cells result from the gelation of polymerized deoxygenated Hb S. Polymerization of Hb S is influenced by both lowered oxygen levels and decreased blood pH. A variety of chemical factors contribute to membrane changes in these cells. The influx of sodium ions and other metabolic changes produce an extremely increased level of intracellular calcium ions. Alterations in the cellular contents produce cell membrane rigidity. The presence of sickle cells is associated with sickle cell anemia.

Spherocytes are erythrocytes that have lost their normal biconcave shape (Plate 15). This type of cell has an extremely compact, round shape. It is usually smaller than 6 μm and has an intense orange-red color when stained. Spherocyte-like erythrocytes may appear as artifacts if a slide is examined at the thin end of a normal blood smear. Spherocytes occur as the ratio of surface area of the erythrocyte to the volume of the cell contents decreases due to the loss of cell membrane. This loss of cell membrane creates membrane instability. Membrane instability and the decreased deformability of the spherical cells lead to premature cell destruction. Spherocytes may be formed because of an inherited structural defect of the erythrocyte membrane or from direct physical trauma such as heat or chemical injury. Clinical disorders associated with spherocytes include acquired hemolytic anemia, blood transfusion reactions, congenital spherocytosis, and DIC. Microspherocytes are associated with ABO hemolytic disease of the newborn and a storage phenomenon that produces microspherocytes in the recipient of a blood transfusion.

Spiculated erythrocytes are irregularly contracted erythrocytes. Spiculated erythrocytes may also be referred to as burr cells, crenated cells, pyknocytes, spur cells, acanthocytes, and echinocytes. The terms **echinocyte** and **acanthocyte** are currently the preferred terms.

Stomatocytes have a slitlike opening that resembles a mouth. The slitlike opening is on one side of the cell. Stomatocytes result from increased sodium (Na^+) ion and decreased potassium (K^+) ion concentration within the cytoplasm of the erythrocyte. Clinical conditions associated with an increase in stomatocytes include acute alcoholism, alcoholic cirrhosis, glutathione deficiency, hereditary spherocytosis, infectious mononucleosis, lead poisoning, malignancies, thalassemia minor, and transiently accompanying hemolytic anemia. These cells can also be seen in hereditary stomatocytosis and Rh null disease, which both lack the Rh antigen complex.

Target cells (codocytes) are erythrocytes that resemble a shooting target (Plate 16). A central red bull's-eye is surrounded by a clear ring and then an outer red ring. The cells are thinner than normal, which may be due to an excessive ratio of membrane lipid to cell volume. Decreased intracellular volume in relationship to the membrane surface, as in thalassemia, may also account for thinner cells. In some instances, such as abnormal hemoglobins, the defect is related to a maldistribution of hemoglobin. In certain enzyme defects, cholesterol and phosphatidylcholine are abnormally increased within the erythrocyte and become incorporated into the membrane lipid. Clinically, target cells are seen in the hemoglobinopathies (Hb C disease, S-C and S-S disease, sickle cell-thalassemia, and thalassemia), hemolytic anemias, hepatic disease with or without jaundice, and iron deficiency anemia, as well as after a splenectomy. Laboratory-induced targeting can occur as an artifact.

Teardrop cells (dacryocytes) are usually smaller than normal erythrocytes (Plate 17). As the term implies, teardrop cells resemble tears. This cellular abnormality is associated with homozygous beta-thalassemia, myeloproliferative syndromes, pernicious anemia, and severe anemias.

Alterations in Erythrocyte Color

A normal erythrocyte has a moderately pinkish-red appearance with a lighter-colored center when stained with a conventional blood stain. The color reflects the amount of hemoglobin present in the cell. The lighter color in the middle, thinner portion of the cell does not normally exceed one third of the cell's diameter and is referred to as the "central pallor." Under these conditions the erythrocyte is referred to as **normochromic.** Normal and abnormal color variations reflect cytoplasmic chemical content.

The general term for a variation in the normal coloration is **anisochromia.** A more specific term, **hypochromia,** is more commonly used when the central pallor exceeds one third of the cell's diameter (Plate 18) or the cell has a pale overall appearance. In the case of hypochromia, inadequate iron stores result in a decrease in hemoglobin synthesis. Deficient hemoglobin content expresses itself as inadequate coloration or a lack of the typical red color associated with an erythrocyte on a peripheral smear. Hypochromia is clinically associated with iron deficiency anemia.

An alteration in the color of an erythrocyte may also reflect state of cell immaturity. The term **polychromatophilia** is used if a nonnucleated erythrocyte has a faintly blue-orange color (see Plate 7) when stained with Wright stain. This cell lacks the full amount of hemoglobin and the blue color is due to diffusely distributed residual RNA in the cytoplasm.

Usually, the polychromatophilic erythrocyte is larger than a mature erythrocyte. If stained with a supravital stain, a polychromatophilic erythrocyte would appear to have a threadlike netting within it and would be called a **reticulocyte.** Another term, **basophilic erythrocyte,** would be used if the cell stained an intense blue or blue-gray color without a pink cast. Increased numbers of polychromatophilic erythrocytes are associated with rapid blood regeneration and increased bone marrow activity.

Varieties of Erythrocyte Inclusions

Several types of inclusions can be seen in an erythrocyte stained with Wright stain. In addition to parasites such as malaria (discussed in the next section), substances that can be observed in peripheral blood smears include residual nucleic acids (DNA and RNA), aggregates of mitochondria, ribosomes, and iron particles. The nonparasitic inclusions include basophilic stippling (both a fine and coarse form), Cabot rings, Heinz bodies, Howell-Jolly bodies, Pappenheimer bodies, and siderotic granules.

Most inclusions are visible using Wright stain. However, some are only visible with other stains (Table 6.3). The inclusions are unique because they are composed of various biochemicals or organelles and are suggestive of specific abnormalities.

Basophilic stippling (fine) appears as tiny, round, solid-staining, dark-blue granules. The granules are usually evenly distributed throughout the cell and often require careful examination in order to detect them. Coarse basophilic stippling (Plate 19) is sometimes referred to as **punctate stippling.** These granules are larger than in the fine form and

are considered to be more serious in terms of pathological significance. Stippling represents granules composed of ribosomes and RNA that are precipitated during the process of staining of a blood smear. Stippling is associated clinically with disturbed erythropoiesis (defective or accelerated heme synthesis), lead poisoning, and severe anemias.

Cabot rings are ring-shaped, figure-eight, or loop-shaped structures. Occasionally, the inclusions may be formed of either double or multiple rings. These structures stain a red or reddish-purple color and have no internal structure. They may represent remnants of microtubules from the mitotic spindle. However, recent research suggests that these inclusions represent nuclear remnants or abnormal histone biosynthesis. Cabot rings can be seen in lead poisoning and pernicious anemia.

Crystals such as Hb C crystals appear as rodlike or angular opaque structures within some erythrocytes. These crystals are found in Hb C disease (Plate 20). Hb H bodies may be seen with a brilliant cresyl blue stain and appear as blue globules, with many in each erythrocyte. These precipitated bodies represent polymers of the beta chains of HB A.

Heinz bodies (Plate 21) are inclusions, 0.2 to 2.0 μm in size, that can be seen with a stain such as crystal violet or brilliant cresyl blue. They represent precipitated, denatured hemoglobin and are clinically associated with congenital hemolytic anemia, G6PD deficiency, hemolytic anemias secondary to drugs such as phenacetin, and some hemoglobinopathies.

Howell-Jolly bodies (Plate 22) are round, solid-staining, dark-blue to purple inclusions, 1 to 2 μm in size. If present, cells contain only one or two Howell-Jolly bodies. Although these inclusions are most frequently seen in mature erythrocytes that lack a nucleus, they may be seen in immature, nucleated erythrocytes. Howell-Jolly bodies are not seen in normal erythrocytes. They are nuclear remnants predominantly composed of DNA. Howell-Jolly bodies are believed to develop in periods of accelerated or abnormal erythropoiesis, because the spleen cannot keep up with "pitting" these remnants from the cell. The presence of Howell-Jolly bodies is associated with hemolytic anemias, pernicious anemia, postoperatively, and physiological atrophy of the spleen.

Pappenheimer bodies (siderotic granules) may be observed in Wright-stained smears as purple dots. These inclusions are infrequently seen in peripheral blood smears. Siderotic granules are dark-staining particles of iron in the erythrocyte that are visible with a special iron stain—Prussian blue. They appear as blue dots and represent ferric (Fe^{3+}) ions. Pappenheimer bodies (Plate 23) and siderotic granules are probably identical structures. Pappenheimer bodies are aggregates of mitochondria, ribosomes, and iron particles. Clinically, they are associated with iron-loading anemias, hyposplenism, and hemolytic anemias.

Alterations in Erythrocyte Distribution

Agglutination and rouleaux formation are two alterations in erythrocytic distribution that may be observed on a stained peripheral smear. **Agglutination,** or the clumping of erythrocytes, may be observed. **Rouleaux formation** (Plate 24), the arrangement of erythrocytes in groups that resemble stacks

TABLE 6.3 Staining Characteristics of Erythrocytes and Inclusions

Inclusion	Stain		
	Feulgen[a]	Supravital[b]	Wright
Basophilic stippling	Negative	Positive	Positive
Cabot rings	Negative	Negative	Positive
Howell-Jolly bodies	Positive	Positive	Positive
Polychromatophilia	Negative	Negative	Positive
Reticulocytes	Negative	Positive	Negative
Pappenheimer bodies	Negative	Positive	Positive
Heinz bodies[c]	Negative	Positive	Negative or positive

[a]Feulgen stain demonstrates the presence of DNA.

[b]Supravital stains, e.g., new methylene blue, or brilliant cresyl blue, demonstrate the presence of RNA.

[c]Can be demonstrated with crystal violet stain.

of coins, is usually present in the thick portions of normal blood smears. If the rouleaux exist in thin areas of the blood smear where the erythrocytes should just touch each other or barely overlap, pathological rouleaux are present.

True agglutination is due to the presence of antibodies reacting with antigens on the erythrocyte. Thus rouleaux formation is associated with the presence of cryoglobulins.

Parasitic Inclusions in Erythrocytes

Malaria

On a global basis, infection of red cells by protozoa is the most common cause of hemolytic anemia. Malaria alone has a prevalence of 490 million cases and in tropical Africa the annual mortality attributable to malaria infection exceeds 2.3 million. Malaria is usually the predominant type of parasitic infection that is included in the study of hematology.

Etiology

The modern tendency is to refer to the various types of malaria by the name of their causative agent: *Plasmodium vivax, P. falciparum, P. malariae,* and *P. ovale.* The life cycle of *Plasmodium* occurs in both humans and the mosquito.

The Disease Phase in the Mosquito

The disease cycle is initiated when a female mosquito of various species of anopheline mosquitoes bites an infected human. The infected blood of the person, which may contain male and female **gametocytes,** is drawn into the stomach of the mosquito. In the mosquito, the male or microgametocyte undergoes maturation and results in the production of **microgametes.** Concurrently, the female or macrogametocyte matures into a **macrogamete,** which may be fertilized by the microgamete to become a **zygote.** The active zygote is referred to as an **ookinete** and after constricting is referred to as an **oocyst.** The growth and development of the oocyte result in the production of a large number of threadlike **sporozoites,** which circulate throughout the body of the mosquito. The sporozoites that enter the salivary glands of the mosquito are ready to be inoculated into the next person bitten by the mosquito. The length of this cycle depends on factors such as the species of *Plasmodium* and the ambient temperature. It may range from as short as 8 days in *P. vivax* to as long as 35 days in *P. malariae.*

The Disease Phase in Humans

Sporozoites injected into the bloodstream of a human by an infected mosquito leave the circulatory system within a period of 40 minutes and invade the liver cells of the human host. In the cells of the liver, all four species undergo an **asexual** multiplication phase. This multiplication produces thousands of tiny **merozoites** in each infected cell. Subsequent rupture of the infected liver cells releases the merozoites into the circulation.

In the circulation, an **asexual cycle** takes place within the erythrocytes. This process, referred to as **schizogony,** results in the formation of 4 to 36 new parasites in each infected erythrocyte within 48 to 72 hours. At the end of this **schizogonic cycle,** the infected erythrocytes rupture, liberating merozoites, which in turn infect new erythrocytes.

Usually, after a patient has become clinically ill, gametocytes appear in circulating erythrocytes. Gametocytes, derived from merozoites, grow but do not divide, and finally form the male and female gametocytes. Gametocytes circulate in the blood for some time and if ingested by an appropriate species of mosquito undergo the **sexual cycle, gametogony,** which develops into **sporogony** in the mosquito.

Symptoms

There are usually no symptoms of malaria until several continuous life cycles have been completed. The simultaneous rupturing of erythrocytes liberates toxic products that characteristically produce chills followed by a fever in a few hours. A patient's temperature may rise to 104° to 105° F. The symptoms last from 4 to 6 hours and reoccur at regular intervals, depending on the species of malaria.

Laboratory Data

The diagnosis of malaria is based on the demonstration of the parasite in the blood (see Chapter 24 for the procedure). Many of the general morphological features are shared by all of the malarial species; however, differences (Plate 25) are usually sought in order to establish the species producing the illness (Table 6.4).

TABLE 6.4 **RBC Morphological Features of Malarial Species**

Plasmodium sp.	Size	Inclusions	Cytoplasm	Merozoites
P. vivax	Enlarged	Schüffner's dots	Blue discs with red nucleus Accolé forms Signet-ring forms	12–24
P. falciparum	Normal	Maurer's dots	Minute rings Two chromatin dots Accolé forms Gametes crescent-shaped	6–32
P. malariae	Normal	Ziemann's stippling	One ring with one dot	6–12
P. ovale	Enlarged	Schüffner's dots	One ring form	6–14

Plasmodium Vivax

P. vivax is the predominant species of malaria worldwide. It generally exhibits various stages in the asexual life cycle and many gametocytes in the blood. The stages of the asexual cycle found in the blood depend on when the blood specimen is taken in relation to the febrile cycle. In the first few hours after symptoms, the majority of infected erythrocytes will contain very early forms of the parasite, **trophozoites.** Giemsa-stained smears will reveal minute blue discs with a red nucleus within the pink cytoplasm of the erythrocyte. Sometimes the trophozoites are seen as crescent-shaped masses at the periphery of the erythrocyte (**accolé forms**). After this stage, an apparent vacuole forms in the blue cytoplasm of the parasite which pushes the nuclear chromatin to the edge of the cell. At this point, the parasite resembles a signet ring. Two or more ring forms may be present in an erythrocyte and they are usually large. Very active trophozoites may assume irregular forms within the erythrocyte.

Between 6 and 24 hours after the beginning of the cycle, the trophozoites grow to approximately half the size of the infected cell and granules of brownish pigment appear. Infected erythrocytes are usually enlarged and pale-staining. The cells may be irregularly shaped and may contain a number of fine red or pink granules known as **Schüffner's dots** or **granules.** The nature of Schuffner's dots is undetermined. Although Schuffner's dots may not always be seen, they can be seen in an erythrocyte infected from 15 to 20 hours or longer if the slide has been properly stained. If present, these inclusions are diagnostic of *P. vivax* or *P. ovale.*

During the second 24 hours of the asexual cycle, the erythrocyte continues to increase in overall size and the parasite nearly fills the entire cell. The single nucleus divides repeatedly. During the stages of division, the parasite is known as **schizont.** The cytoplasm finally segments to form separate small masses around each nucleus. The individual parasites thus produced are known as **merozoites** and on rupture of the infected cell at about 48 hours they are released to infect new erythrocytes. There may be 12 to 24 merozoites present.

Fully mature gametocytes fill the cell almost completely and contain more pigment. One can differentiate the microgametocytes and macrogametocytes morphologically. The nucleus of the macrogametocyte is dense, while that of the microgametocyte forms a pale, loose network.

All of the stages seen in thin films may also be found in thick-film preparations but the parasites appear somewhat distorted. Young trophozoites may be seen but *cannot* be distinguished from similar stages of *P. ovale* or *P. falciparum.* Gametocytes of *P. vivax, P. ovale,* and *P. malariae* are very similar in appearance. *P. malariae* are smaller and darker than the others and do *not* contain Schüffner's dots.

Plasmodium Falciparum

P. falciparum is almost entirely confined to the tropics and subtropics. Schizogony does not usually take place in peripheral blood. Young trophozoites and gametocytes are generally the only stages seen on the peripheral blood smear.

Young trophozoites are minute rings. Much more frequently than in other species, the ring may have two small chromatin dots. Multiple ring forms in a single erythrocyte are a common finding.

The gametocyte in *P. falciparum* is characteristic. It appears as an elongated crescentic or sausage-shaped structure. The ends of the gametocytes may be pointed or bluntly rounded and the remains of the erythrocyte may be seen in the concavity formed by the arched body of the parasite. Infected erythrocytes, which retain their original size, may develop a few irregular dark red- or pink-staining, rod- or wedge-shaped granules known as **Maurer's dots.**

In thick blood smears, many early trophozoites can be seen. Because these cells are delicate, they frequently collapse and assume various shapes such as a comma or swallow. Gametocytes are easily recognizable by their shape, which is similar to that seen in the thin film.

Plasmodium Malariae

P. malariae occurs primarily in subtropical and temperate areas where other species of malaria are found but is seen less frequently than *P. vivax* or *P. falciparum.* All stages of development can be observed on a peripheral blood smear. The asexual cycle of *P. malariae* occupies 72 hours as compared with approximately 48 hours in other species. Ring forms of *P. malariae* are not easily distinguished from those of *P. vivax.* Only one ring form is usually found per erythrocyte and this form generally contains only one chromatin dot. Infected cells are not enlarged. As the parasite grows, it may almost fill the erythrocyte prior to schizogony.

The schizont stage contains 6 to 12 merozoites. Generally, abundant numbers of hematin granules are present and the cytoplasm of the erythrocyte may contain dust-fine, pale-pink dots, called **Ziemann's stippling.** This stippling is seen only in heavily stained slides. Pigment is also produced in some quantity and is dark. The average number of merozoites is eight and they may be arranged symmetrically in a rosette form around a central mass of pigment. Typically, they are irregularly displaced within the mature schizont.

Gametocytes are difficult to distinguish from growing trophozoites. When they are mature, they may be slightly larger than the mature trophozoites, tend to be oval, and contain proportionately more pigment than trophozoites at all stages. Thick smears do not assume the amoeboid shapes seen in other species but usually appear as small dots of nuclear material with rounded or slightly elongated masses of cytoplasm. Older trophozoites are compact and the predominant color may be that of the abundant pigment.

Plasmodium Ovale

P. ovale is rather widely distributed in tropical Africa and replaces *P. vivax* in frequency on the West African coast. It has also been reported in South America and Asia. All stages of development may be present on the peripheral blood smear.

This form of *Plasmodium* is not as amoeboid as *P. vivax.* Infected erythrocytes may be enlarged and may be oval. Only one ring form is present in each erythrocyte and these ring forms contain only one chromatin dot.

There are 6 to 12 merozoites present in the schizont. The infected erythrocytes are enlarged and pale, and if properly stained, exhibit Schüffner's dots in all stages. The margins of infected cells are often ragged and the erythrocytes are distinctly elongated, ovoid, or irregular in shape.

Thick films appear similar to those of *P. vivax*. Schizonts are larger than those in *P. malariae* but with no more than 12 merozoites. Schüffner's dots can be observed.

Other Parasitic Inclusions

Several other types of parasites are associated with the blood. The family *Trypanosomatidae*, which includes the hemoflagellates, contains two genera that parasitize humans. These parasites may be seen in a variety of body locations: circulating blood, cardiac muscle, and cerebrospinal fluid. *Leishmania* is found primarily in the cells of the mononuclear phagocytic system and may at times be seen in the circulating blood in large mononuclear cells.

Babesiosis is an uncommon hemolytic disorder of the temperate North. It resembles *P. falciparum*. Babesiosis differs from malaria in that it is limited to erythrocytic propagation and sexual reproduction is not evident.

SUMMARY

Erythrocytes: Normal and Abnormal

Normal, mature erythrocytes lack a nucleus, average 7.2 μm in diameter, and assume a discoid shape. However, in many hematological and nonhematological conditions the red cell will deviate from its normal size, assume a variety of shapes, display color alterations, exhibit intracellular inclusions, or appear in an altered pattern of distribution. These characteristics are significant factors that can be observed during the examination of a peripheral blood film.

Variation in the overall size of an erythrocyte is referred to as anisocytosis. The two specific forms of anisocytosis are macrocytosis and microcytosis. An alteration in cellular shape is termed poikilocytosis. Poikilocytes may be named by a variety of common names that often refer to common objects such as teardrops. A more specific nomenclature for poikilocytes is becoming more widely used. The terms used in this newer nomenclature are acanthocyte, codocyte, dacryocyte, discocyte, drepanocyte, echinocyte, elliptocyte, keratocyte, knizocyte, leptocyte, megalocyte, schizocyte, spherocyte, and stomatocyte. Alterations in color reflect either an absence of iron (hypochromia) or cellular immaturity (polychromatophilia).

A variety of inclusions can be observed in abnormal erythrocytes when stained with Wright stain. These specific inclusions are termed basophilic stippling, Cabot rings, Howell-Jolly bodies, and Pappenheimer bodies (siderotic granules). The last significant erythrocyte characteristic that can be observed on a peripheral blood smear is an alteration in the distribution of red cells. These two abnormalities are true agglutination and rouleaux formation.

Alterations in erythrocyte morphology reflect chemical variances or physical abnormalities either of the red cell membrane itself or of its contents. Macrocytosis reflects either a nuclear maturational defect or stimulated erythropoiesis. Microcytosis is associated with a decrease in hemoglobin synthesis that can be produced by a deficiency of iron, impaired globulin synthesis, or a mitochondrial abnormality affecting the synthesis of heme.

Poikilocytosis may result from membrane defects caused by chemical alterations such as the decreased lipid in the cell membrane in acanthocytes. Chemical alterations in the red cell's content can produce poikilocytosis. Examples of content abnormalities include sickle cells (drepanocytes), which are produced by the gelation of hemoglobin, and stomatocytes, which result from increased sodium ion and decreased potassium ion within the cellular contents. Physical causes of poikilocytosis include schizocytes, which are produced by mechanical division of the red cell, and spherocytes, which experience a loss of cell membrane due to physical trauma such as heat.

Color variation in the erythrocyte ranges from abnormally pale hypochromic cells that are chemically deficient in iron to blue-orange-colored cells, polychromatophilic cells, that have distributed, residual RNA in the cytoplasm. Erythrocytic inclusions can represent parasitic infections such as malaria; DNA in Howell-Jolly bodies; RNA in basophilic stippling; aggregates of disintegrating ribosomes containing RNA in reticulocytes; nuclear remnants in Cabot rings; and aggregates of mitochondria, ribosomes, and iron particles in Pappenheimer bodies.

Maldistribution of red cells on a peripheral smear can be due to either warm- or cold-type antibodies. Chemically, antibodies are from the globulin fraction of proteins.

Parasitic Inclusions in Erythrocytes

Several types of parasites are associated with blood. On a global basis, infection of red blood cells by protozoa is the most common cause of hemolytic anemia. *P. vivax* is the predominant species of malaria worldwide. All of the stages of malaria infection that can be seen in thin films may also be found in thick-film preparations but the parasites appear somewhat distorted. Young trophozoites may be seen but *cannot* be distinguished from similar stages of *P. ovale* or *P. falciparum*. Gametocytes of *P. vivax*, *P. ovale*, and *P. malariae* are very similar in appearance. *P. malariae* are smaller and darker than the others and do *not* contain Schüffner's dots.

Other parasitic inclusions of red blood cells include *Leishmania* and *Babesia*.

BIBLIOGRAPHY

Costa, F. F. et al. "Linkage of Dominant Hereditary Spherocytosis to the Gene for the Erythrocyte Membrane-Skeleton Protein Ankyrin." *N. Engl. J. Med.*, Vol. 323, No. 15, October 11, 1990, p. 1046.

Creager, J. C. *Human Anatomy and Physiology*. Belmont, CA: Wadsworth, 1983.

Henry, J. B. (18th ed.). *Clinical Diagnosis and Management by Laboratory Methods*. Philadelphia: Saunders, 1997.

Hillman, R. S. and C. A. Finch. *Red Cell Manual* (7th ed.). Philadelphia: Davis, 1996.

Jandl, J. *Blood*. Boston: Little, Brown, 1987, pp. 192–204.

Kretchman, D. M. and B. S. Rogers. "Erythrocyte Shape Transformation Associated with Calcium Accumulation." *Am. J. Med. Technol.*, Vol. 47, No. 7, July, 1981, pp. 561–565.

Lackritz, E. M. et al. "Imported *Plasmodium falciparum* Malaria in American Travelers to Africa." *JAMA*, Vol. 265, No. 3, January 16, 1991, pp. 383–385.

Lehman, D. "Malaria and Other Bloodborne Parasites," *Advances for Medical Laboratory Professionals*, Vol. 28, No. 10, Oct. 7, 1997, pp. 19–21.

Marwick, C. "Long Struggle Continues to Find New Weapons Against an Old Foe—the Malaria Parasite." *JAMA*, Vol. 263, No. 20, May 23/30, 1990, p. 2718.

Mechanic, L. and A. Quiery. "Chloroquine-Resistant *Plasmodium falciparum*." *Lab. Med.*, Vol. 22, No. 3, March, 1991, pp. 167–169.

Miale, J. B. *Laboratory Medicine: Hematology* (6th ed.). St. Louis: Mosby, 1982.

Raphael, S. S. *Lynch's Medical Laboratory Technology* (4th ed.). Philadelphia: Saunders, 1983.

"Recommendations for the Prevention of Malaria Among Travelers." *JAMA*, Vol. 263, No. 20, May 23/30, 1990, pp. 2729–2740.

Scamurra, D. and F. R. Davey. "Anemias Associated With Spherocytic Erythrocytes." *Lab. Med.*, Vol. 16, No. 2, February, 1985, pp. 83–88.

White, N. J. "The Treatment of Malaria," *N. Engl. J. Med.*, Vol. 335, No. 11, Sept. 12, 1996, pp. 800–806.

REVIEW QUESTIONS

1. The average diameter of a normal erythrocyte is ___ μm.
   A. 5.2.
   B. 6.4.
   C. 7.2.
   D. 8.4.

Questions 2 through 5: match the following terms with the appropriate description.

2. ___ Macrocytic.
3. ___ Microcytic.
4. ___ Anisocytosis.
5. ___ Poikilocytosis.

A. Variation in erythrocyte size.
B. Larger than normal.
C. Smaller than normal.
D. Variation in erythrocyte shape.

Questions 6 through 9: match the common terms for erythrocytes with the equivalent nomenclature.

6. ___ Normal erythrocyte.
7. ___ Oval macrocyte.
8. ___ Target cell.
9. ___ Sickle cell.

A. Megalocyte.
B. Drepanocyte.
C. Codocyte.
D. Discocyte.

Questions 10 through 13: match the terms for erythrocytes with the appropriate morphological description.

10. ___ Echinocytes.
11. ___ Helmet cells.
12. ___ Schistocytes.
13. ___ Spherocytes.

A. Short, scalloped on spike-like projections that are regularly distributed around the cell.
B. Fragments of erythrocytes.
C. The scooped-out part of an erythrocyte that remains after a blister cell ruptures.
D. Compact round shape.

Questions 14 through 17: match the stated condition with the predominant erythrocyte type seen on a peripheral blood smear (use an answer only once).

14. ___ Associated with a defect in nuclear maturation.
15. ___ Associated with a decrease in hemoglobin synthesis.
16. ___ Represents an imbalance between erythrocytic and plasma lipids.
17. ___ Results from the gelation of polymerized deoxygenated Hb S.

A. Microcytes.
B. Sickle cells.
C. Macrocytes.
D. Acanthocytes.

18. Polychromatophilia is:
   A. A blue-colored erythrocyte when stained with Wright stain.
   B. Due to diffusely distributed RNA in the cytoplasm.
   C. Equivalent to a reticulocyte when stained with a supravital stain.
   D. All of the above.

Questions 19 through 22: match the following erythrocytic inclusions with the appropriate description.

19. ___ Basophilic stippling.
20. ___ Howell-Jolly bodies.
21. ___ Pappenheimer bodies.
22. ___ Heinz bodies.

A. DNA.
B. Precipitated denatured hemoglobin.
C. Granules composed of ribosomes and RNA.
D. Aggregates of iron, mitochondria, and ribosomes.

23. Which of the following is the term for erythrocytes resembling "a stack of coins" on thin sections of a peripheral blood smear?
   A. Anisocytosis.
   B. Poikilocytosis.
   C. Agglutination.
   D. Rouleaux formation.

Questions 24 through 27: match the following erythrocyte morphology with the appropriate clinical condition or disorder.

24. ___ Macrocytes.

25. ___ Microcytes.

26. ___ Acanthocytes.

27. ___ Echinocytes.

A. Iron deficiency anemia.

B. Abetalipoproteinemia.

C. Pernicious anemia.

D. No related disease state.

Questions 28 through 31: match the predominant erythrocyte morphology with the appropriate clinical condition or disorder.

28. ___ Leptocytes.

29. ___ Microspherocytes.

30. ___ Codocytes.

31. ___ Dacryocytes.

A. Hepatic disorders.

B. Hemolytic disease of the newborn.

C. Hemoglobinopathies.

D. Pernicious anemia.

Questions 32 through 35: match the following erythrocyte inclusions with the appropriate clinical condition or disorder.

32. ___ Basophilic stippling.

33. ___ Howell-Jolly bodies.

34. ___ Heinz bodies.

35. ___ Pappenheimer bodies.

A. Pernicious anemia.

B. G6PD deficiency.

C. Iron loading anemia.

D. Lead poisoning.

Questions 36 through 39: match the appropriate species of malaria with one of the following characteristics.

36. ___ *Plasmodium vivax.*

37. ___ *Plasmodium falciparum.*

38. ___ *Plasmodium malariae.*

39. ___ *Plasmodium ovale.*

A. The schizont contains 6 to 12 merozoites; generally abundant in hematin granules; may contain Zeimann's stippling.

B. The most predominant species worldwide; 12 to 24 merozoites, may contain Schuffner's granules.

C. Infected erythrocytes may be enlarged and oval-shaped; may contain Schuffner's dots; 6 to 14 merozoites in the schizont.

D. Young trophozoites and gametocytes are generally the only stage seen in peripheral blood; gametocytes appear as crescent or sausage-shaped structures in erythrocytes; Maurer's dots may be present.

Classification and Laboratory Assessment of Anemias

OBJECTIVES

Causes of anemia
- Define the term **anemia**, based on a physiological description.
- Name the three causes of anemia.
- Explain some of the factors contributing to anemia.

Clinical signs and symptoms of anemia
- State what causes the clinical signs and symptoms of anemia.
- Briefly describe the usual complaints of an anemic patient.

Classification of anemias
- Describe the organization of anemias according to erythrocyte size and explain the limitation of such a system.

- Briefly explain the advantage of the categories of anemia using a pathophysiological basis.

Laboratory assessment of anemias
- List the three laboratory manifestations of an anemia.
- Explain the grading system used to describe erythrocyte abnormalities on a peripheral blood film.
- Name the tests usually performed in the hematology laboratory to assist in the establishment of a specific anemia diagnosis.
- List the tests usually performed in other sections of the clinical laboratory that may be of assistance in establishing a specific anemia diagnosis.

CAUSES OF ANEMIA

Anemia is considered to be present if the hemoglobin concentration of the red blood cells or the packed cell volume of red blood cells (hematocrit) is below the lower limit of the 95% reference interval for the individual's age, sex, and geographic location (see inside cover).

The causes of anemia fall into three major pathophysiologic categories: blood loss, impaired red cell production, and accelerated red cell destruction (hemolysis in excess of the ability of the marrow to replace these losses.

Anemia may be a sign of an underlying disorder. Dilutional anemia with normal or increased total red cell mass may occur with pregnancy, macroglobulinemia, and splenomegaly. Some anemias have more than one pathogenetic mechanism and go through more than one morphologic state, such as blood loss anemia.

CLINICAL SIGNS AND SYMPTOMS OF ANEMIA

The clinical signs and symptoms of anemia result from diminished delivery of oxygen to the tissues. Signs and symptoms of anemia are related to the lowered hemoglobin concentration and blood volume.

In addition, clinical signs reflect the rate of reduction of hemoglobin and blood volume. If anemia develops slowly in a patient who is not otherwise severely ill, a hemoglobin concentration of as low as 6gm/dL may develop without producing any discomfort or physical signs if the patient is sedentary.

The usual complaints of an anemic patient are easy fatigability and dyspnea on exertion. Other general manifestations can include vertigo, faintness, headache, and heart palpitations. The most common physical expressions of anemia are pallor, low blood pressure, a slight fever, and some edema. In addition to these general signs and symptoms, particular clinical findings may be characteristically associated with a specific type of anemia.

CLASSIFICATION OF ANEMIAS

Many different types of anemias exist with many causes and manifestations.

Categories and Occurrence of Anemias

In an attempt to organize the anemias into understandable units, several classification schemes have been proposed. These classifications group anemias based on erythrocyte morphology, physiology, or probable etiology.

The method based on red cell morphology, which was originally proposed by Wintrobe, categorizes anemias by the size of the erythrocytes. Anemia also may be classified by red cell morphology as **macrocytic, normocytic,** or **microcytic** (see Laboratory Assessment of Anemias). The major limitation of such a classification is that it tells nothing about the etiology or reason for the anemia.

Several schemes have been proposed to categorize anemias by etiology. None of these classifications is entirely satisfactory because within each classification the various subdivisions are not completely inclusive. However, the physiological system has merit, since it describes the basic mechanism or probable mechanism responsible for the anemia.

Although many classification schemes exist, a classification system that divides the major pathophysiological characteristics into three major categories is easier to understand than other systems. The three major categories in this system are accelerated erythrocyte destruction, blood loss, and impaired red blood cell production. A modified organizational approach to this classification system is used in this chapter (Table 7.1) in order to discuss the more frequent types of anemia.

Although the incidence of certain anemias varies within different geographic areas of the world and among specific populations, some forms of anemia are generally more common than others. The most frequent forms of anemia result from either blood loss or iron deficiency conditions.

LABORATORY ASSESSMENT OF ANEMIAS

The laboratory investigation of anemias involves the quantitative and semiquantitative measurements of erythrocytes and supplementary testing of blood and body fluids. The results of these analyses provide the foundation for both the diagnosis and treatment of anemia. In this section, the reader should become familiar with basic measurements associated with erythrocytes, various conditions and diseases that produce morphological alterations, and correlated testing that is necessary in order to categorize an anemia.

Quantitative Measurements of Anemia

Anemia is physiologically defined as a condition in which the circulating blood lacks the ability to adequately oxygenate body tissues. The three major laboratory manifestations of anemia include:

1. A decreased hemoglobin concentration
2. A reduced packed cell volume (microhematocrit) level
3. A decreased erythrocyte concentration

In addition to the direct measurement of hemoglobin, packed cell volume (microhematocrit), and erythrocyte count (see Chapter 24), a variety of other measurements or

TABLE 7.1　**Categories of Anemia**

1. Blood loss
   A. Acute
   B. Chronic
2. Impaired production
   A. Aplastic
   B. Iron deficiency
   C. Sideroblastic anemia
   D. Anemia of chronic disease
   E. Megaloblastic
3. Hemolytic
   A. Inherited defects
   B. Acquired disorders
4. Hemolytic-hemoglobin disorders

calculations can yield additional information. These assessments include:

1. Red blood cell indices (see Chapter 5)
2. The red cell histogram (see Chapter 25)
3. Red cell distribution width (RDW) or red cell morphology index (RCMI) (see Chapter 25)

Semiquantitative Grading of Erythrocyte Morphology

Direct observation of a peripheral blood smear (Fig. 7.1) for abnormalities in erythrocytic morphology or immature erythrocytes (described in Chapter 5) can yield additional information. In addition to the identification of erythrocyte abnormalities, erythrocyte morphology may be determined semiquantitatively in order to reflect the severity of the abnormalities.

Erythrocyte changes (Fig. 7.2) are commonly reported using either descriptive terms such as **moderate** or **marked** or grades on a numerical scale such as 1+, 2+, 3+, or 4+. The characteristics of such a grading scale may vary from one laboratory to another but will generally conform to the scale as presented in Table 7.2.

Supplementary Assessment of Anemias

Other procedures that support the diagnostic process of identifying an anemia may be needed. Some of these assays are performed in the hematology laboratory and others may be performed in another section of the clinical laboratory. A bone marrow examination (see Chapter 24) may be performed and may reveal an abnormal ratio of leukocytes

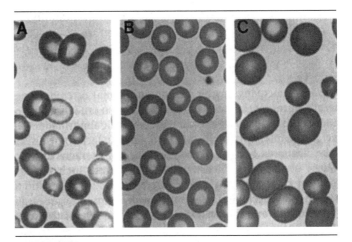

FIGURE 7.2 Red cell size changes as detected by morphology. When pronounced, microcytosis and hypochromia (**A**) and macrocytosis (**C**) are readily distinguishable from normocytic, normochromic red cells (**B**). The blood smear can be more sensitive than the MCV by revealing a minor population of either smaller or larger cells that have little effect on the MCV. (From R. S. Hillman and C. A. Finch, *Red Cell Manual* [7th ed.]. Philadelphia: Davis, 1996.)

to erythrocytes, the myeloid-erythroid (M:E) ratio. Other maturational irregularities or unusual cellular elements may be observed. The following procedures (see Chapter 24 for additional details) may provide supplementary information:

Acid hemolysis test
Autohemolysis test
Donath-Landsteiner (direct and indirect) test
Fetal hemoglobin (Hb F) concentration
Malarial smears
Osmotic fragility test
Platelet count
Reticulocyte count
Sickle cell testing
Glucose-6-phosphate dehydrogenase (G6PD) assay
Hemoglobin electrophoresis

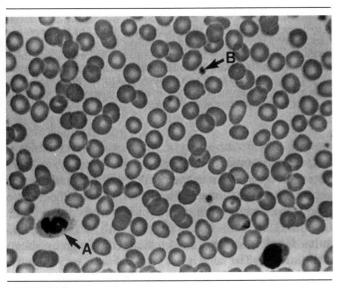

FIGURE 7.1 Blood smear morphology. The best area on a blood smear for the examination of red cell morphology is where the red cells are barely touching but not overlapping. Under low-power magnification, it is possible to evaluate the relative frequency of white blood cells (*arrow A*) and platelets (*arrow B*) in relationship to the number of red blood cells. There should be approximately one white cell for every 500 to 1000 red cells and one platelet for every 5 to 10 red cells. (From R. S. Hillman and C. A. Finch, *Red Cell Manual* [7th ed.]. Philadelphia: Davis, 1996.)

TABLE 7.2 Grading of Erythrocyte Morphology

Numerical Scale	Description
0	Normal appearance or slight variation in erythrocytes
1+	Only a small population of erythrocytes displays a particular abnormality; the terms **slightly increased** or **few** would be comparable
2+	More than occasional numbers of abnormal erythrocytes can be seen in a microscopic field; an equivalent descriptive term is **moderately increased**
3+	Severe increase in abnormal erythrocytes in each microscopic field; an equivalent descriptive term is **many**
4+	The most severe state of erythrocytic abnormality, with the abnormality prevalent throughout each microscopic field; comparable terms are **marked** or **marked increase**

Additional procedures may be of assistance in identifying specific types of anemia but are usually performed in other sections of the clinical laboratory. These procedures include:

Antibody screening and identification tests
Direct antiglobulin (AHG) test
Measurements of bilirubin levels
Folic acid assay
Measurement of haptoglobin level
Lactic dehydrogenase (LDH) determination
Serum iron and total iron-binding capacity (TIBC)
Vitamin B_{12} assay
Gastric analysis
Occult blood testing
Urobilinogen screening

BIBLIOGRAPHY

Hillman, R. S. and C. A. Finch. *Red Cell Manual* (7th ed.). Philadelphia: F. A. Davis, 1996.

Jandl, J. R. *Blood* (2nd ed.). Boston: Little, Brown & Co., 1996.

Pansky, B. *Dynamic Anatomy and Physiology.* New York: Macmillan, 1975.

Soloway, H. B. and J. B. Peter. "Interpretation of Tests." *Diagn. Med.,* Vol. 8, No. 4, April, 1985, pp. 10–11.

Wallach, J. *Interpretation of Diagnostic Tests* (5th ed.). Boston: Little, Brown & Co, 1982.

REVIEW QUESTIONS

1. The causes of anemia include:
   A. Blood loss.
   B. Impaired red cell production.
   C. Accelerated red cell destruction.
   D. All of the above.

2. The clinical signs and symptoms of anemia can result from:
   A. Diminished delivery of oxygen to the tissues.
   B. Lowered hemoglobin concentration.
   C. Increased blood volume.
   D. Both A and B.

3. Which of the following is a significant laboratory finding in anemia?
   A. Decreased hemoglobin.
   B. Increased packed cell volume.
   C. Increased erythrocyte count.
   D. Normal erythrocyte indices.

4. If you are grading changes in erythrocytic size or shape using a scale of 0 to 4+ and *many* erythrocytes deviate from normal per microscopic field, the typical score would be:
   A. 1+.   C. 3+.
   B. 2+.   D. 4+.

5. Anemias can be categorized into:
   A. Hemolytic types.
   B. Blood loss types.
   C. Impaired production types.
   D. All of the above.

Acute and Chronic Blood Loss Anemias

OBJECTIVES

Acute bood loss
- Describe the etiology and physiology of acute blood loss.
- Explain the significant hematological laboratory findings in acute blood loss.

Chronic blood loss
- Describe the etiology and physiology of chronic blood loss.

- Explain the significant hematological laboratory findings in chronic blood loss.

Case studies
- Apply the laboratory data to the stated case studies and discuss the implications of these cases for the study of hematology.

ACUTE BLOOD LOSS ANEMIA

Etiology

The acute loss of blood is usually associated with traumatic conditions such as an accident or severe injury. Occasionally, acute blood loss may occur during or after surgery.

Physiology

An acute blood loss does not produce an immediate anemia. A severe hemorrhage or rapid blood loss amounting to more than 20% of the circulating blood volume reduces an individual's total blood volume and produces a condition of shock and related cardiovascular problems. Even if enough hemoglobin remains in the circulation, an oxygen impairment can exist due to the circulatory failure. However, severe acute bleeding can be fatal as a result of collapse of the circulatory system; immediate expansion of the blood volume is required (Table 8.1).

In acute blood loss, the body itself adjusts to the situation by expanding the circulatory volume, which produces the subsequent anemia. Fluid from the extravascular spaces enters the blood circulation and has a diluting effect on the remaining cells.

Laboratory Findings

Hematological findings are very different in the patient who has experienced an acute bleeding episode within the past 24 to 48 hours compared with a patient who has suffered from chronic bleeding for several months. Table 8.2 presents a profile of the typical findings in each case.

The earliest hematological change in acute blood loss is a transient fall in the platelet count, which may rise to elevated levels within an hour. The next change is the development of neutrophilic leukocytosis (from 10 to 35 $\times$ 10^9/L) with a shift to the left. The hemoglobin and hematocrit do not fall immediately but fall as tissue fluids move into the blood circulation. It can be 48 or 72 hours after the hemorrhage until the full extent of the red cell loss is apparent.

Assuming that the patient with acute bleeding was

TABLE 8.1 Signs and Symptoms of Acute Blood Loss

Less than 1000 mL (<20% total blood volume)	No signs and symptoms; occasional vasovagal
Greater than 1000 mL (>20% total blood volume)	Orthostatic hypotension (decreased blood pressure)
More than 1500 mL (>30% total blood volume)	Decreased resting (supine) blood pressure; anxiety or restlessness
More than 2000 mL (>40% total blood volume)	Hypovolemic shock; air hunger; disorientation; diaphoresis

Source: Modified from Hillman, R. S. and C. A. Finch. *Red Cell Manual* (7th ed.). Philadelphia: F. A. Davis, 1996.

TABLE 8.2 Blood Loss Anemia

	Acute (24 hours)	Chronic (months)
Etiology	Trauma	GI tract Menstruation Urinary tract
Blood volume disruption	Yes	No
Iron deficiency	No	Yes
Hematocrit (packed cell volume)	Usually normal	Decreased
White blood cell count	Increased	Normal
Platelets	Increased	Normal
Reticulocytes	Normal	Increased

healthy before the episode, the peripheral blood film at 24 hours should be essentially normochromic and normocytic with normal red blood cell indices (MCV, MCH, and MCHC). When an increased number of reticulocytes reach the circulating blood because of increased erythropoiesis, a transient macrocytosis develops. This phenomenon takes place beginning about 3 to 5 days after the blood loss and reaches a maximum around 10 days later.

It takes about 2 to 4 days after the blood loss for the total white blood cell count to return to normal, and about 2 weeks for the morphological changes to disappear. The return of the red cell profile to previous values takes longer.

CHRONIC BLOOD LOSS ANEMIA

Etiology

Chronic blood loss is frequently associated with disorders of the gastrointestinal (GI) tract, although chronic blood loss may be related to heavy menstruation in women or urinary tract abnormalities.

In chronic anemias, blood loss of small amounts occurs over an extended period of time, usually months. The chronic and continual loss of small volumes of blood does not disrupt the blood volume.

If blood is lost in small amounts over an extended period of time, both the clinical and hematological features seen in acute bleeding are absent. Regeneration of red blood cells occurs at a slower rate. The reticulocyte count may be normal or only slightly increased.

A noticeable anemia does not usually develop until after storage iron is depleted. At first, the anemia is normochromic and normocytic. Gradually, the chronic bleeding results in an iron deficiency and the newly formed cells are morphologically hypochromic and microcytic. The white blood cell count is normal or slightly decreased. Platelets are commonly increased, and only later, in severe iron deficiency, are they likely to be decreased.

SUMMARY

Acute blood loss is usually associated with traumatic conditions or during or after surgery. It does not produce an immediate anemia. A severe hemorrhage reduces an individual's total blood volume and can be fatal due to the collapse of the circulatory system.

In acute blood loss, the body itself attempts to adjust to the situation by expanding the circulatory volume, which produces the subsequent anemia. Fluid from the extravascular spaces enters the blood circulation and has a diluting effect on the remaining cells.

The earliest hematological change in acute blood loss is a transient fall in the platelet count, which may rise to elevated levels within an hour. The next change is the development of neutrophilic leukocytosis with a shift to the left. The hemoglobin and hematocrit do not fall immediately. It can be 48 or 72 hours after the hemorrhage until the full extent of the red cell loss is apparent.

Chronic blood loss lacks both the clinical and hematological features seen in acute bleeding. A noticeable anemia does not usually develop until after storage iron is depleted. In time, the peripheral blood smear becomes hypochromic and microcytic.

CASE STUDIES

CASE 1 A 38-year-old white woman was treated in the emergency room for severe lacerations and possible abdominal injuries sustained in an automobile accident. She was admitted to the hospital for observation and further evaluation. On admission, a complete blood count (CBC), urinalysis, and radiograph series were ordered.

Laboratory Data
Her CBC results were as follows:

Hemoglobin 10.5 gm/dL
Hct 0.34 L/L
Red blood cell (RBC) 3.8×10^{12}/L
White blood cell (WBC) 12.0×10^9/L

The RBC indices were as follows:

MCV 89.6 fL
MCH 27.6 pg
MCHC 31%

The peripheral blood smear showed essentially normal RBC morphology and platelet distribution.

Forty-eight hours after admission, a stat repeat CBC was ordered. The results were as follows:

Hemoglobin 8.0 gm/dL
Hct 0.26 L/L
RBC 2.9×10^{12}/L
WBC 15.5×10^9/L

The RBC indices were all within their normal ranges. A peripheral blood smear showed normal RBC morphology, although some polychromatophilia was noted. The distribution of platelets had increased. A follow-up platelet count was 0.60×10^{12}/L.

Subsequently, the patient was typed and cross-matched for 6 units of blood. Two units of whole blood cells were administered immediately. An emergency laparotomy revealed that the patient had injuries to both the liver and spleen.

Questions
1. Why was the patient's hemoglobin and Hct normal on admission, but decreased after 48 hours?
2. What is the significance of this patient's increased leukocyte (WBC) and thrombocyte (platelet) count?
3. What is the reason for the polychromatophilia noted on the 48-hour peripheral blood film?

Discussion
1. The body adjusts to severe hemorrhaging by expanding the circulating volume at the expense of the extravascular fluid. This volume adjustment produces a delayed anemia. As the extravascular fluid enters the bloodstream, it dilutes the RBCs. The hemoglobin and Hct become decreased after 48 to 72 hours in such cases.
2. In acute blood loss, the platelets and circulating granulocytes increase within a few hours. Immature WBCs may also be seen. Increased leukocytes and platelets are a normal body response to stress. The body continually strives to maintain homeostasis.
3. Acute blood loss immediately begins to stimulate a healthy, normal bone marrow. Reticulocytosis becomes apparent within 24 hours, and peaks at 7 to 10 days after severe blood loss. When erythrocyte restoration is completed, reticulocytosis ceases. Reticulocytes are seen as polychromasia, or polychromatophilic RBCs when the RBCs are stained with Wright stain. A supervital stain such as new methylene blue needs to be used to visibly demonstrate reticulocytes in erythrocytes.

✏ Diagnosis: Acute blood loss

CASE 2 A 55-year-old white male college professor had been experiencing fatigue and shortness of breath when walking over the last several months. Getting more sleep at night did not help. He reported eating a balanced diet of fruits, vegetables, meat, and dairy products.

Upon physical examination, he appeared slightly pale but had no other abnormalities. His primary care physician ordered a complete blood count, urinalysis, and fecal occult blood (×3) tests.

Laboratory Data
Laboratory findings were as follows:

Hemoglobin 12.5 gm/dL
Hematocrit 0.32 L/L
Red blood cell (RBC) 4.2×10^{12}/L
White blood cell (WBC) count within normal limits
RBC indices: MCV 42 fL
MCH 29.7 pg
Urinalysis: normal findings
Fecal occult blood (×3) positive

Questions
1. What is the most likely cause of this patient's anemia?
2. What type of red cell morphology would be expected on a peripheral blood smear?
3. What follow-up tests should be conducted?

Discussion
1. The most likely cause of this patient's anemia is chronic blood loss. The source of the bleeding could be the gastrointestinal tract in view of the fact that he had a positive test for fecal blood.

(continued)

CASE STUDIES (*continued*)

2. Hypochromic, microcytic red blood cells would be expected on his peripheral blood smear.
3. The source of the fecal bleeding needs to be located. In this case, the patient had a follow-up colonoscopy that revealed a number of non-malignant, bleeding polyps.

✏️ **Diagnosis: Chronic blood loss**

BIBLIOGRAPHY

Hillman, R. S. and C. A. Finch. *Red Cell Manual* (7th ed.). Philadelphia: F. A. Davis, 1996.
Jandl, J. H. *Blood*. Boston: Little, Brown & Co., 1996.

REVIEW QUESTIONS

Questions 1 through 5: match the following characteristics with either A or B.

1. ___ Disorders of the gastrointestinal system or heavy menstruation.

2. ___ Increased thrombocytes (platelets).

3. ___ Traumatic conditions.

4. ___ Does *not* disrupt the blood volume.

5. ___ Results in an iron deficiency and a hypochromic/microcytic erythrocyte morphology on a peripheral blood smear.

A. Acute blood loss.

B. Chronic blood loss.

6. The erythrocyte morphology associated with anemia in an otherwise healthy individual due to acute blood loss is usually:

A. Microcytic.
B. Megaloblastic.
C. Normochromic.
D. Hypochromic.

7. Anemia due to chronic blood loss is characterized by:

A. Hypochromic, microcytic erythrocytes.
B. Decreased packed cell volume.
C. Increased platelets.
D. Both A & B

Aplastic and Related Anemias

OBJECTIVES

Aplastic anemia

- Describe the major characteristics of aplastic anemia.
- Name the major form of aplastic anemia.
- Define the term **iatrogenic**.
- List at least three iatrogenic substances that can cause aplastic anemia.
- Name at least four types of viral infection that have been associated with aplastic anemia.
- Briefly describe how the immune process causes aplastic anemia.
- Name the three phases of development of aplastic anemia.
- Describe the clinical features of aplastic anemia.
- Discuss the laboratory findings in aplastic anemia.
- Explain how the laboratory findings in aplastic anemia manifest themselves after acute radiation exposure.
- Discuss the role of bone marrow transplantation in the treatment of aplastic anemia.

Fanconi's anemia

- Describe the mode of inheritance of Fanconi's anemia.
- Explain the clinical signs and symptoms of Fanconi's anemia.
- Name one treatment for Fanconi's anemia.

- Compare the relationship between familial aplastic anemia and Fanconi anemia.
- Describe the laboratory features of familial aplastic anemia.

Related aplastic anemia

- Name three causes and examples of red cell aplasia.
- Identify the cause of pure red cell aplasia.
- Compare acquired pure red cell aplasia to chronic red cell aplasia.
- Describe the characteristics of Diamond-Blackfan syndrome, including the nature of the defect.
- Discuss the characteristics of transient erythroblastopenia of childhood.
- Name four types of congenital dyserythropoietic anemia.
- Describe characteristics of congenital dyserythropoietic anemia.
- Explain the laboratory findings in congenital dyserythropoietic anemia.

Case study

- Apply the laboratory data to the stated case study and discuss the implications of this case to the study of hematology.

APLASTIC ANEMIA

Impaired erythrocyte production can be caused by a variety of factors. Aplastic anemia is one of a group of disorders, known as hypoproliferative disorders, that are characterized by reduced growth or production of blood cells. The other anemias in this category include those caused by deficiencies of erythropoietin (Chapter 5), iron (Chapter 10), and folic acid and vitamin B_{12} (Chapter 11).

Etiology

Aplastic anemia was first described by Paul Ehrlich in 1888 from an autopsy of a young pregnant woman. It differs from agranulocytosis and pure red-cell aplasia, which involve only granulocyte and erythrocyte production, respectively; from myelodysplasia (Chapter 22), in which marrow morphology is abnormal and chromosomal abnormalities are common; and from Fanconi's anemia, in which aplastic anemia is inherited. In all these disorders, the immune system may influence hematopoiesis.

The major form of aplastic anemia is idiopathic (up to 70% of cases in the United States and Europe). Idiopathic aplastic anemia occurs in patients with no established history of chemical or drug exposure or viral infection. Other forms of aplastic anemia are iatrogenic and constitutional aplastic anemia. The term **constitutional aplastic anemia** designates individuals with a congenital or genetic predisposition to bone marrow failure (see Fanconi's anemia later in this chapter).

The other forms of aplastic anemia are considered secondary to etiologic agents that are drug-related (iatrogenic) and chemically related. Aplastic anemia is iatrogenic when the transient marrow failure follows cytotoxic chemotherapy or radiotherapy. Certain chemical or physical agents directly injure both proliferating and quiescent hematopoietic cells, leading to damage to DNA and ultimately to apoptosis. Drug-related and chemically related aplastic anemias account for 11% to 20% of all cases (Table 9.1). Ionizing radiation has been well-documented as a cause of aplastic anemia. In addition, a variety of antigens—derived from chemicals, viruses, and perhaps altered self-antigens—have been inferred from clinical histories to initiate the immune process, but the precise nature of the antigenic stimulus has not been identified.

Iatrogenic agents include:

1. Benzene and benzene derivatives
2. Trinitrotoluene
3. Insecticides and weed killers
4. Inorganic arsenic
5. Antimetabolites (antifolate compounds and analogues of purines and pyrimidines)
6. Antibiotics

Benzene

Patients with community-acquired aplastic anemia rarely have a history of exposure to any substance that is toxic to the bone marrow, and even benzene is now infrequently associated with aplastic anemia in developed countries. However, exposure to burning oil wells in Kuwait during

TABLE 9.1 An Etiologic Classification of Aplastic Anemia*

Direct Toxicity
 Iatrogenic causes
  Radiation
  Chemotherapy
 Benzene
 Intermediate metabolites of some common drugs

Immune-mediated Causes
 Iatrogenic causes
  Transfusion-associated graft-versus-host disease
 Eosinophilic fasciitis
 Hepatitis-associated disease
 Pregnancy
 Intermediate metabolites of some common drugs
 Idiopathic aplastic anemia

*Boldface type indicates relatively well-established mechanisms.

the Gulf war led to the development of aplastic anemia in at least one patient.

Burning gasoline aerosolizes many pollutants, one of which is benzene. Benzene can be metabolized in the liver to a series of phenolic and open-ring structures, including hydroquinones, which can inhibit the maturation and amplification of bone marrow stem and blast cells. In addition, the metabolites of benzene alter the function of stromal cells in the bone marrow so that they cannot adequately support the growth and differentiation of hematopoietic cells. The net result can be aplastic anemia which does not typically develop until several years after exposure to benzene.

Drugs

Drugs have been associated with aplastic anemia. But unlike anticancer agents and benzene, which at sufficient doses regularly result in marrow aplasia, idiosyncratic reactions to drugs are infrequent. However, the antibiotic chloramphenicol leads the list of antibodies that annually produce cases of aplastic anemia if not prescribed properly. In Europe and Israel in the 1980s, about 25 percent of cases of aplastic anemia were attributed to drugs. Depending on the extent of damage, some cases of chemically induced aplastic anemia are reversible.

Other drugs that can produce aplastic anemia, depending on the dosage and duration of consumption, include tetracyclines, organic arsenicals, phenylbutazone, trimethadione, and methylphenylethylhydantoin.

Infections

Infections can also be responsible for acquired cases of aplastic anemia. Viral infections, particularly hepatitis B, hepatitis C, measles, Epstein-Barr virus, and cytomegalovirus have been implicated. The mechanism associated with the induction of aplastic anemia subsequent to viral infection includes the possibility of drug exposure during treatment, direct stem cell damage by the virus, depressed hematopoiesis by the viral genome, and virus-induced autoimmune damage.

In addition, viral infections may be only secondary to bone marrow aplasia.

Hepatitis-associated aplastic anemia is a variant of aplastic anemia in which aplastic anemia follows an acute attack of hepatitis. Severe pancytopenia can occasionally occur 1 to 2 months after an episode of apparent viral hepatitis. The stereotypical syndrome of posthepatitis aplasia would seem to offer the opportunity to identify a specific infectious cause of aplastic anemia. In most patients, the hepatitis is non-A, non-B, non-C, and non-G. The hepatitis of the hepatitis-associated aplastic anemia does not appear to be caused by any of the known hepatitis viruses. Several features of the syndrome suggest that it is mediated by immunopathologic mechanisms. Although aplastic anemia is a rare sequela of hepatitis, there is a striking relationship between fulminant seronegative hepatitis and aplastic anemia. Epidemiologic studies suggest the involvement of an enteric microbial agent in the causation of aplastic anemia. Aplastic anemia is not only more common in the Far East (4 to 10 percent in the Far East compared to 2 to 5 percent of cases of aplastic anemia in the West) where hepatitis viruses are prevalent, but is also associated with poverty, rice farming, and past (but not recent) exposure to hepatitis A.

Hepatitis-associated aplastic anemia is often fatal if untreated. If an HLA-matched related donor is not available for bone marrow transplantation, immunosuppressive treatment is given.

Pathophysiology

The sudden appearance of aplastic anemia or pure red cell aplasia is often caused by an immune process, either antibodies directed against the stem cell or a cellular immune mechanism (T lymphocytes) that suppresses stem cell proliferation. Cellular immune suppression may occur transiently with certain viral infections such as parvovirus or as a result of drug action. Pure red cell aplasia is often associated with thymomas.

Hematopoietic failure may occur at any level in the differentiation of bone marrow precursor cells. There may be insufficient or defective pluripotent stem cells (CFU-S) or committed stem cells (CFU-C). The microenvironment may be unable to provide for the normal development of hematopoietic cells. The appropriate humoral and cellular stimulators for hematopoiesis may be absent. In addition, bone marrow failure could result from excessive suppression of hematopoiesis by T lymphocytes or macrophages. Finally, stem cells could interact among themselves with one clone inhibiting the growth of another. In most cases of aplastic anemia, it is likely that damage to the hematopoietic stem cell by a known or unknown agent in some way alters the ability of the cell to proliferate or differentiate.

In most patients with acquired aplastic anemia, bone marrow failure results from immunologically mediated, tissue-specific organ destruction. The course of the disease can be separated into distinct phases (Table 9.2). The bone marrow is unlikely to recover spontaneously and most patients die of infection or bleeding complications within a few years.

A model for the interaction between the immune system and hematopoietic cells in patients with aplastic anemia has been developed from laboratory observations (Fig. 9.1). An early experiment showed that mononuclear cells from the blood and marrow of patients with aplastic anemia sup-

TABLE 9.2	Phases of Aplastic Anemia
Phase 1 Onset of Disease	After an initiating event, e.g., viral infection, the hematopoietic compartment is destroyed by the immune system. Small numbers of surviving stem cells support adequate hematopoiesis for some time, but eventually the circulating cell counts become very low and clinical symptoms appear.
Phase 2 Recovery	Either a partial response or a complete response can occur, at least initially, without increased numbers of stem cells. In a minority of patients, the primitive-cell compartment appears to repopulate over time by the process of self-renewal of stem cells.
Phase 3 Late Disease	Years after recovery, blood counts may fall as a relapse of pancytopenia occurs, or an abnormal clone of stem cells may emerge, leading to a new diagnosis of paroxysmal nocturnal hemoglobinuria (PNH), myelodysplasia (MDS), or acute myelogenous leukemia (AML).

pressed hematopoietic colony formation by normal marrow cells; the removal of T cells from patients' samples sometimes improved in vitro colony formation by the affected marrow. Blood and marrow from patients also contained increased numbers of activated cytotoxic lymphocytes, and the activity and numbers of these cells decreased with successful antithymocyte globulin therapy. Interferon-alpha and tumor necrosis factor suppress the proliferation of early and late hematopoietic progenitor cells and stem cells. This suppression is greater when the interferon-alpha and tumor necrosis factor are secreted into the marrow microenvironment than when they are added to cultured cells.

The immunologic events that precede the destruction of hematopoietic cells are not as clear as the mechanism of suppression of proliferation (Fig. 9.2). Involvement of lymphocytes of the CD4 or helper class has been inferred from overrepresentation of the class II histocompatibility antigen HLA-DR2 in white patients and a more specific haplotype has been linked to the disorder in Japanese patients. But both the dysregulatory events that lead to loss of tolerance and to autoimmune destruction of hematopoietic cells and the initial antigen exposure that triggers immune system activation are unknown.

Laboratory studies of patients' lymphocytes and their products support the concept of pathophysiologic roles for lymphocytes and lymphokines in the destruction of hematopoietic cells. Alpha-interferon expression is prevalent in acquired aplastic anemia and may be a specific marker of this disease. Local production of this inhibitory lymphokine in the target organ, the bone marrow, may be important in mediating aplastic anemia. Measurement of this lymphokine's message may be useful in distinguishing acquired aplastic anemia from other forms of bone marrow failure.

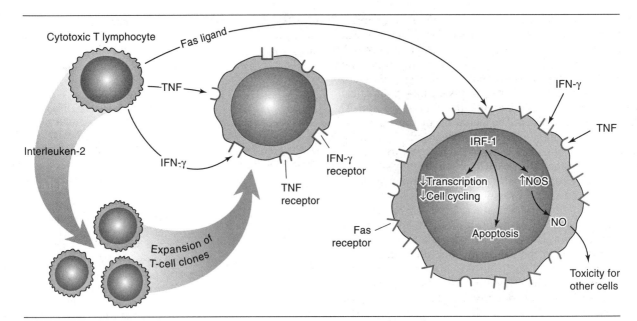

FIGURE 9.1 Immune destruction of blood cell production. Hematopoietic cell targets are affected by many factors. Activated cytotoxic T lymphocytes play a major role in tissue damage, partially through secreted cytokines like interferon-gamma (IFN-γ) and tumor necrosis factor (TNF). Increased production of interleukin-2 (IL-2) leads to polyclonal expansion of T cells. However, activation of the Fas receptor leads to apoptosis in target cells. Some effects of IFN-γ are mediated through interferon regulatory factor 1 (IRF-1), which inhibits the transcription of cellular genes and entry into the cell cycle. IFN-γ is a potent inducer of many cellular genes, including inducible nitric oxide synthase (NOS), and production of the toxic gas nitric oxide (NO) may further diffuse toxic effect. In addition, direct cell–cell interactions between lymphocytes and targets probably occur. (Young, N. S. and J. Maciejewski. "The Pathophysiology of Acquired Aplastic Anemia." *N. Engl. J. Med.,* Vol. 336, No. 19, May 8, 1997, p. 1368.)

Clinical Features

Aplastic anemia is characterized by total bone marrow failure with a reduction in circulating levels of red blood cells, white blood cells, and platelets. It is not a common disease.

The clinical course may be acute and fulminating, with profound pancytopenia and a rapid progression to death, or the disorder may have an insidious onset and a chronic course. The signs and symptoms depend on the degree of the deficiencies and include bleeding from thrombocytopenia, infection from neutropenia, and signs and symptoms of anemia. Splenomegaly and lymphadenopathy are absent.

Recent studies have shown that long-term survivors of acquired aplastic anemia may be at high risk for subsequent malignant diseases or late clonal hematologic diseases, often years after successful immunosuppressive therapy. Paroxysmal nocturnal hemoglobinuria (PNH) occurs in approximately 9% of patients, and myelodysplasia and acute myelogenous leukemia occur at a cumulative incidence rate of about 16% 10 years after treatment. The incidence of solid tumors is similarly increased after immunosuppression and after bone marrow transplantation. One hypothesis has postulated that aplastic anemia is primarily a preleukemic condition.

Laboratory Findings

Aplastic anemia is due to damage or destruction of the hemopoietic tissue of the bone marrow that results in deficient production of blood cells. If all of the cell lines (erythrocytic, leukocytic, and thrombocytic) are affected, the disorder is referred to as **pancytopenia.** However, if only one cell line is involved, it is usually the erythrocytic cells.

A diagnosis of severe aplastic anemia is made when at least two of the three peripheral blood values fall below critical levels: granulocytes less than 0.5×10^9/L; platelets less than 20×10^9/L, or reticulocytes less than 0.6%. The bone marrow is either markedly or moderately hypocellular with less than 30% of residual hematopoietic cells. Most severely affected patients have neutrophil counts of less than 200×10^9/L, platelet counts of <20×10^9/L, or reticulocyte counts of <0.6%.

Red blood cells usually are normochromic and normocytic. In some cases, there may be varying degrees of anisocytosis and poikilocytosis or macrocytosis. The RDW is normal in nontransfused patients. Leukopenia with a marked decrease in granulocytes and a relative lymphocytosis are noticeable. Thrombocytopenia is typically present. Serum iron usually is increased; this is a valuable early sign of erythroid hypoplasia and reflects the decreased plasma iron turnover. In addition, the erythrocyte use of iron is decreased. Both effective and total erythropoiesis are decreased in aplastic anemia.

The bone marrow reveals very few early erythroid and myeloid cells at any stage of differentiation, and megakaryocytes are scanty if present at all. Primitive progenitor and stem cells, which normally constitute about 1% of marrow cells, cannot be identified by their appearance.

If acute exposure to radiation is the inciting agent, the

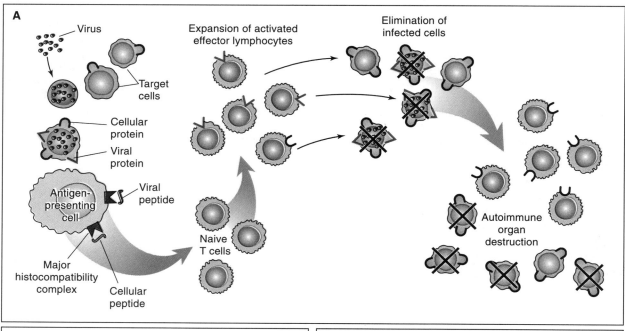

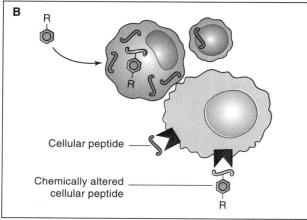

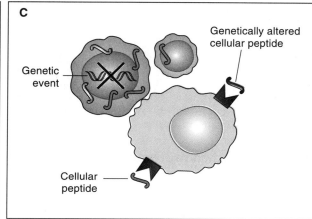

FIGURE 9.2 Destruction of bone marrow initiated by antigenic stimulation. **A.** Viral infection of hematopoietic cells with subsequent immune response results in the destruction of infected cells. This process is initiated with the production of viral proteins and the excessive or aberrant production of normal cellular proteins, which are released, and are taken up by antigen-presenting cells. The proteins are processed into peptides in the antigen-presenting cells, and then form complexes with major histocompatibility complex molecules that are then presented to naive T cells. Infected cells are subsequently destroyed. Rarely, the lymphocyte response persists and affects normal cells, resulting in autoimmune organ destruction. **B.** Drug-induced aplastic anemia may occur in a process similar to viral infection of hematopoietic cells after reactive drug metabolites, formed in marrow cells, bind to cellular proteins. This leads the immune system to recognize the complex as foreign and the destructive sequence is initiated. **C.** A product of a chromosomal translocation or an oncogene may also initiate a T-cell response that expands to include nonmalignant cells, which leads to marrow hypocellularity in myelodysplasia by a sequence similar to viral and drug-induced processes. (Young, N. S. and J. Maciejewski. "The Pathophysiology of Acquired Aplastic Anemia." *N. Engl. J. Med.,* Vol. 336, No. 19, May 8, 1997, p. 1369.)

production of new red blood cells (reticulocyte count) falls, but the red blood cells decline slowly because of their long survival. Within the first few hours, there is a neutrophilic leukocytosis due to a shift from marginal and probably marrow storage pools. A fall in lymphocytes occurs after the first day and is responsible for the early leukopenia. After five days or so, granulocytes begin to fall. The platelets

decrease later. Platelets are often the last to return to normal in the recovery phase.

Treatment

Aplastic anemia responds to immunosuppressive therapy, but the limitations to success in treating this disease, like

others, appear to be the degree of organ destruction, the capacity for tissue regeneration, and perhaps most important, a pharmacology that is inadequate to control a misdirected and extraordinarily potent immune response.

The prognosis for patients with aplastic anemia is poor with a high mortality rate. Complications include infection, bleeding, and problems of iron overload from repeated transfusion. In the past, more than 70% of patients died within 5 years, but modern treatment protocols such as immunosuppressive therapy and bone marrow transplantation have improved patient prognosis. However, bone marrow transplantation is not the therapeutic answer for most patients. Even with the use of matched sibling donors and a large pool of nonrelated matched donors, less than 50% of patients receive transplants. Bone marrow transplantation is recommended in younger patients who have an identical twin donor or an HLA-matched donor. Two-year survival rates are reported to be 60% to 70%, with 5% to 15% of patients not surviving the transplant procedure. Immunosuppressive therapy, particularly ATG (antithymocyte globulin) and ATDLG (antithoracic duct lymphocytic globulin), has been shown to be effective in more than 50% of patients over 40 years of age.

FANCONI'S ANEMIA

Fanconi's anemia is the best-described congenital form of aplastic anemia. It is inherited through an autosomal recessive mode. Chromosomal analysis usually reveals frequent chromatid breaks, gaps, rearrangements, reduplications, and exchanges. Fanconi's anemia is twice as common in males as females and can be confused with pure red cell aplasia and thrombocytopenia-absent radius (TAR) syndrome.

Clinical Signs and Symptoms

Clinical signs and symptoms of Fanconi's anemia commonly include skin hyperpigmentation (café-au-lait spots) and short stature. Other manifestations can include skeletal disorders (aplasia or hypoplasia of the thumb), renal malformations, microcephaly, mental retardation, and strabismus. Among patients with congenital malformations, only 28% were given a diagnosis before the onset of hematologic manifestations. Progressive pancytopenia usually becomes apparent by the age of 5 years. If moderate to severe pancytopenia is present, the hemoglobin concentration is between 5 to 6 gm/dL at diagnosis. In addition, there is a predisposition to neoplasia and nonhematopoietic developmental anomalies. Susceptibility to an immune cytokine may be a marker of the genetic defect.

Hypersensitivity to the clastogenic effect of DNA-cross-linking agents such as diepoxybutane acts as a diagnostic indicator of the genotype of Fanconi's anemia, both prenatally and postnatally. Prenatal HLA typing has made it possible to ascertain whether a fetus is HLA-identical to an affected sibling.

Therapy

Therapy includes bone marrow transplantation in order to ward off hemorrhage and infection. A successful case has been reported of hematopoietic reconstitution in a boy who received cryopreserved umbilical-cord blood from a sister shown by prenatal testing to be unaffected by the disorder, to have a normal karyotype, and to be HLA-identical to the patient. A pretransplantation conditioning procedure developed specifically for the treatment of such patients makes use of the hypersensitivity of abnormal cells to alkylating agents that cross-link DNA and to irradiation.

There is an increased incidence of malignancy, including acute leukemia, in patients with Fanconi's anemia. However, therapeutic measures are not always successful and most patients die by their mid-to-late teens.

Familial aplastic anemia is a subset of Fanconi's anemia with a low incidence of congenital abnormalities. Some patients may have a relative with classic Fanconi's anemia. The age of diagnosis varies from younger than 1 year to 77 years of age. A few children present with bleeding manifestations secondary to amegkaryocytic thrombocytopenia. As their disease progresses, they develop a pancytopenia and a hypocellular bone marrow.

Patients may have pancytopenia and a hypocellular marrow without major developmental anomalies. In some cases, there may be skin hyperpigmentation or stunted growth.

RELATED DISORDERS

Hypoproliferation of the erythroid elements, without corresponding decreases in other cell lines, is characteristic of pure red cell aplasia. Pure red cell aplasia exists in three forms; however, a number of variant and intermediate forms have been recognized. These established causes and examples of red cell aplasia are:

Congenital—Diamond-Blackfan syndrome
Acquired chronic—idiopathic, associated with thymoma and lymphoma
Acute (transient)—parvovirus, other infections, drugs, riboflavin deficiency

Pure Red Cell Aplasia

This is a disorder primarily involving disturbed erythropoiesis. Immune suppression of erythropoiesis is believed to play a role in this form of red cell aplasia. An immune system etiology is supported by the fact that some patients respond to steroid treatment. Patients with pure red cell aplasia have antibodies against erythroid precursor cells and lymphocytes capable of inhibiting erythropoiesis.

Erythroid precursors are absent from the bone marrow and evidence of hemolysis or hemorrhage is not present in red cell aplasia. The level of serum erythropoietin is usually increased. An aplastic crisis can develop in some patients with hemolytic anemia and concomitant infection. Other causes of acquired red cell aplasia include malnutrition and neoplasia. Thymoma (tumor of the thymus gland) is a frequent finding.

Acquired pure red cell aplasia characterized by selective failure of red blood cell production rarely occurs in middle-aged adults. Reticulocytopenia and a cellular marrow devoid of all but the most primitive erythroid precursors are characteristic. Leukocyte and platelet production are normal.

About half of the reported cases have been associated with thymoma, usually a noninvasive spindle cell type. Only 5% to 10% of patients with thymoma have the anemia. Remission of the anemia occurs in about one fourth of the cases following surgical removal of the thymoma.

Chronic acquired red cell aplasia has been associated with other conditions, such as drugs, collagen vascular disorders, or lymphoproliferative disorders. Most of these anemias appear to be part of a spectrum of autoimmune cytopenias in which the target cells are either erythroid stem cells or normoblasts. In some patients, antibodies that react with these cells have been identified. Corticosteroids and immunosuppressive drugs have been used as therapy, but less than 50% of patients achieve satisfactory remission.

Diamond-Blackfan Syndrome

Diamond-Blackfan syndrome, also known as congenital hypoplastic anemia, is a rare congenital form of red cell aplasia. This disorder is believed to result from a defective stem cell, probably the committed erythroid stem cell, BFU-E.

The disorder is characterized by a slowly progressive and refractory anemia, with no concurrent leukopenia or thrombocytopenia. It manifests itself in early infancy. Inheritance is probably dominant. Although the chromosomal karyotype is normal, patients can exhibit a wide range of congenital defects. Spontaneous remission occurs in about one fourth of patients.

The severe anemia is normochromic and slightly macrocytic; reticulocyte level is low; leukocytes are normal or slightly decreased; platelets are normal or increased; and the marrow usually shows a reduction in all developing erythroid cells but normal granulocytic and megakaryocytic cell lines. In a small number of cases, residual erythroid precursors are detected. These precursors are mostly pronormoblasts. Fetal hemoglobin is elevated (5% to 25%) to a degree not expected for the patient's age, and the I antigen is often present. These findings contrast with those of transient arrest of erythropoiesis (TEC).

The defect appears to be in the erythroid-committed progenitor cells. CFU-Es and BFU-Es are decreased in the marrow, and BFU-Es, which normally circulate, are absent or decreased in the blood. In addition, these progenitor cells fail to respond in in vitro culture systems to normal T cells and to usual levels of EPO, suggesting a qualitative defect.

About 75% of patients respond at least partially to steroids and overall long-term survival is about 65%, although many patients require long-time steroid use.

Transient Erythroblastopenia of Childhood

Transient erythroblastopenia of childhood (TEC) occurs in previously healthy children, usually younger than 8 years of age, with most cases occurring between the ages of 1 and 3 years. A history of a viral infection within the past 3 months is frequent. It is usually self-limited, with recovery occurring within 1 or 2 months without therapy. The pathogenesis appears to involve humoral inhibition of erythropoiesis or decreased stem cells in many of the patients who have been studied, but parvovirus is not a cause. Erythroid marrow recovery is usually 1 to 2 weeks after onset.

TEC is characterized by a moderate to severe normocytic anemia and severe reticulocytopenia. The bone marrow generally is normocellular and shows virtual absence of erythroid precursors, except for a few early forms.

Congenital Dyserythropoietic Anemia

Four types of congenital dyserythropoietic anemia (CDA) have been identified. They are characterized by indirect hyperbilirubinemia, ineffective erythropoiesis, and peculiarly shaped multinuclear erythroblasts. Type 1 patients demonstrate a mildly macrocytic anemia with prominent anisocytosis and poikilocytosis. This form is apparent at birth and is not a threat to life. Type 2 (the most common type of CDA) CDA patients have a positive acidified serum test. Their erythrocytes are similar to those of patients with paroxysmal nocturnal hemoglobinuria (PNH) because the red cells in both abnormalities are susceptible to hemolysis in acidified normal serum. However, type 2 CDA red cells differ from PNH red cells because they fail to hemolyze in the sugar water test and react strongly with both anti-i and anti-I. Type 3 CDA is similar to type 1 because patients frequently demonstrate giant multinucleated erythroblasts. Megaloblastic changes are not prominent and the red cells are not susceptible to lysis by acidified normal serum. A proposed type 4 classification exists. It is similar to type 2 but differs, in part, because of the lack of serologic abnormalities.

Physiology

The pathogenesis of the bone marrow failure is not entirely certain. One hypothesis states that a foreign agent, such as a drug or virus, may enter the body and attach itself to the pluripotent hemopoietic stem cells. This attachment may then provoke the body into defending itself against what is perceived as a foreign body. The patient's own body defense mechanism may destroy the stem cells. In addition, cellular and humoral abnormalities in hematopoietic regulation and an altered marrow microenvironment have been implicated as possible factors in aplastic anemia.

Laboratory Findings

If all cell lines are involved, the patient will have a decreased hemoglobin, hematocrit (Hct or packed cell volume), and red cell count with decreased leukocyte and platelet counts. If only the red cell line is affected, only the hemoglobin, Hct, and red cell count will be affected. If a bone marrow examination is performed, the erythroid cell line and perhaps the leukocyte and thrombocyte cell lines will all demonstrate a lack of maturational activity.

SUMMARY

Aplastic anemia is one of a group of disorders, known as hypoproliferative disorders, that are characterized by reduced growth or production of blood cells. The other anemias in this category include those caused by deficiencies of erythropoietin, iron, and folic acid and vitamin B_{12}.

Aplastic anemia differs from agranulocytosis and pure

red cell aplasia, which involve only granulocyte and erythro-cyte production, respectively; from myelodysplasia, in which marrow morphology is abnormal and chromosomal abnor-malities are common; and from Fanconi's anemia, in which aplastic anemia is inherited. In all these disorders, however, the immune system may influence hematopoiesis.

The major form of aplastic anemia is idiopathic. Idiopathic aplastic anemia occurs in patients with no established history of chemical or drug exposure or viral infection. Other forms of aplastic anemia are iatrogenic and constitutional aplas-tic anemia.

The sudden appearance of aplastic anemia or pure red cell aplasia is often caused by an immune process, either antibodies directed against the stem cell or a cellular immune mechanism (T lymphocytes) that suppresses stem cell prolif-eration. Cellular immune suppression may occur transiently with certain viral infections such as parvovirus or as a result of drug action. Pure red cell aplasia is often associated with thymomas.

Hematopoietic failure may occur at any level in the differ-entiation of bone marrow precursor cells. In most patients with acquired aplastic anemia, bone marrow failure results from immunologically mediated, tissue-specific organ de-struction.

Aplastic anemia is characterized by total bone marrow failure with a reduction in circulating levels of red blood cells, white blood cells, and platelets. It is not a common disease. The clinical course may be acute and fulminating, with profound pancytopenia and a rapid progression to death, or the disorder may have an insidious onset and a chronic course, involving bleeding from thrombocytopenia, infection from neutropenia, and signs and symptoms of ane-mia. Recent studies have shown that long-term survivors of acquired aplastic anemia may be at high risk for subsequent malignant diseases.

If all of the cell lines (erythrocytic, leukocytic, and throm-bocytic) are affected, the disorder is referred to as **pancytope-nia.** However, if only one cell line is involved, it is usually the erythrocytic cells. A diagnosis of severe aplastic anemia is made when at least two of the three peripheral blood values fall below critical values: granulocytes less than 0.5×10^9/L, platelets less than 20×10^9/L, and reticulocytes less than 0.6%.

Aplastic anemia responds to immunosuppressive ther-apy; ATG (antithymocyte globulin) and ATDLG (antitho-racic duct lymphocytic globulin) have been shown to be effective in more than 50% of patients over 40 years of age. But success in treating this disease appears to be related the degree of organ destruction, the capacity for tissue regenera-tion, and drug treatment. The prognosis for patients with aplastic anemia is poor, with a high mortality rate. Complica-tions include infection, bleeding, and problems of iron over-load from repeated transfusion. Even in the best of circum-stances, bone marrow transplantation is not the therapeutic answer for most patients.

Fanconi's anemia is the best-described congenital form of aplastic anemia. Progressive pancytopenia usually becomes apparent by the age of 5 years. If moderate to severe pancyto-penia is present, the hemoglobin concentration is between 5 to 6 gm/dL at diagnosis. In addition, there is a predisposi-tion to neoplasia and nonhematopoietic developmental anomalies, including acute leukemia, in patients with Fan-coni's anemia. Most patients die by their mid-to-late teens.

Related disorders include hypoproliferation of the ery-throid elements, e.g., pure red cell aplasia. Pure red cell aplasia exists in three forms. Intermediate forms include Diamond-Blackfan syndrome, acquired chronic, and acute transient forms.

Pure red cell aplasia is a disorder primarily involving disturbed erythropoiesis. Patients with pure red cell aplasia have antibodies against erythroid precursor cells and lym-phocytes capable of inhibiting erythropoiesis. Acquired pure red cell aplasia characterized by selective failure of red blood cell production occurs rarely in middle-aged adults. Chronic acquired red cell aplasia has been associated with other conditions, such as drugs, collagen vascular disorders, or lymphoproliferative disorders.

Diamond-Blackfan syndrome is a disorder believed to result from a defective stem cell, probably the committed erythroid stem cell, BFU-E. Transient erythroblastopenia of childhood (TEC) is usually self-limited with recovery oc-curring within 1 or 2 months without therapy. The pathogen-esis appears to involve humoral inhibition of erythropoiesis or decreased stem cells in many of the patients.

Four types of congenital dyserythropoietic anemia (CDA) have been identified. Type 1 patients demonstrate a mildly macrocytic anemia with prominent anisocytosis and poikilo-cytosis. Type 2 CDA patients have a positive acidified serum test. Their erythrocytes are similar to those of patients with paroxysmal nocturnal hemoglobinuria (PNH) because the red cells are also susceptible to hemolysis in acidified normal serum. However, type 2 CDA red cells differ from PNH red cells because they fail to hemolyze in the sugar water test. Type 3 CDA is similar to type 1 because patients frequently demonstrate giant multinucleated erythroblasts. Megalo-blastic changes are not prominent and the red cells are not susceptible to lysis by acidified normal serum. A proposed type 4 classification exists.

The pathogenesis of the bone marrow failure is not en-tirely certain. If all cell lines are involved, the patient will have a decreased hemoglobin, hematocrit (Hct or packed cell volume), and red cell count with decreased leukocyte and platelet counts. If only the red cell line is affected, only the hemoglobin, Hct, and red cell count will be affected. If a bone marrow examination is performed, the erythroid cell line and perhaps the leukocyte and thrombocyte cell lines will all demonstrate a lack of maturational activity.

CASE STUDY

CASE 1 A 22-year-old white woman was admitted to the hospital because of severe menstrual bleeding. She had nu-merous petechiae and some purpura. The patient was a reli-gious missionary who had recently returned from a 2-year as-signment in Haiti. Six months ago, she had developed a severe respiratory infection. She was treated by a local Hai-

(continued)

tian physician at that time, but was not hospitalized due to the lack of medical facilities on the island. She had refused to return home for further treatment at that time.

Initially, she received a cephalosporin-type antibiotic, but later received chloramphenicol because her symptoms persisted. At the time of admission she showed no evidence of a respiratory disorder. However, she had recently discontinued the chloramphenicol that she had taken continuously for 5 months.

On admission, the following tests were ordered: CBC, platelet count, cold agglutinin antibody screen, urinalysis, and chest radiograph.

Laboratory Data
The results of the tests were as follows:

Hemoglobin 5.5 gm/dL
Hct 0.18 L/L
RBC 1.85 × 10^{12}/L

The RBC indices were as follows:

MCV 97.2 fL
MCH 29.7 pg
MCHC 31%

Her WBC count was 2.1 × 10^9/L. On the peripheral blood smear the RBCs had a normochromic, normocytic appearance. Platelets were severely diminished on the blood film. Her platelet count was 6.5 × 10^9/L. The screening test for cold agglutinins was negative. Normal results were obtained on the urinalysis.

Thirty-six hours after admission the patient died due to a massive cerebral hemorrhage. Tests performed on specimens obtained on autopsy revealed that the patient's bone marrow showed an almost total absence of hematopoiesis. A blood culture was positive for the gram-negative rod *Proteus vulgaris*.

Questions
1. What is the most likely cause of this patient's pancytopenia?
2. How do certain drugs affect the body's cellular elements?
3. What caused the patient's death?

Discussion
1. This patient's reduced erythrocytes, leukocytes, and thrombocytes (pancytopenia) had probably been induced by the drug chloramphenicol. Certain drugs depress bone marrow activity at a critical dosage level. Chloramphenicol is most notorious for its depression of hematopoiesis. The patient's prolonged use of this drug with its known high tissue toxicity index undoubtedly produced this bone marrow failure.
2. Various types of antibiotics function in different ways in the human body. Penicillin, for example, inhibits the cell wall synthesis of peptidoglycans, which constitute the major cell wall chemical in gram-positive microorganisms. Many antibiotics interfere with protein synthesis. In the case of chloramphenicol, the specific in vivo action is unclear. However, in vitro studies have demonstrated that chloramphenicol inhibits protein synthesis and mitochondrial synthetic activity.
3. This patient died from bacteremia (septicemia) due to the gram-negative microorganism *P. vulgaris*. Because the patient's body defenses had been severely compromised due to the effects of chloramphenicol, she was unable to effectively ward off a massive bacterial infection.

> ✏️ **Diagnosis: Drug-induced aplastic anemia**

BIBLIOGRAPHY

Alter, B. P. and N. S. Young. "Bone marrow failure syndromes," in Nathan, D. G. and F. A. Oski (eds.). *Hematology of Infancy and Childhood* (4th ed.). Philadelphia: Saunders, 1993, p. 216.

Bluhm, R. et al. "Aplastic Anemia Associated With Canthaxanthin Ingested for 'Tanning' Purposes." *JAMA*, Vol. 264, No. 9, September 5, 1990, pp. 1141–1142.

Brown, K. E. et al. "Hepatitis-Associated Aplastic Anemia." *N. Engl. J. Med.*, Vol. 336, No. 15, April 10, 1997, 1059–1064.

Browne, P. V. et al. "Donor-Cell Leukemia After Bone Marrow Transplantation for Severe Aplastic Anemia." *N. Engl. J. Med.*, Vol. 325, No. 10, September 5, 1991, pp. 710–713.

Frickhofen, N. et al. "Treatment of Aplastic Anemia With Antilymphocyte Globulin and Methylprednisone With or Without Cyclosporine." *N. Engl. J. Med.*, Vol. 324, No. 19, May 9, 1991, pp. 1297–1304.

Giampietro, P. F. and J. G. Davis. "Fanconi Anemia." *N. Engl. J. Med.*, Vol. 330, No. 10, March 10, 1994, pp. 720–721.

Gluckman, E. et al. "Hematopoietic Reconstitution in a Patient With Fanconi's Anemia by Means of Umbilical-Cord Blood From an HLA-Identical Sibling." *N. Engl. J. Med.*, Vol. 321, No. 17, Oct. 26, 1989, pp. 1174–1178.

Hillman, R. S. and C. A. Finch. *Red Cell Manual* (7th ed.). Philadelphia: F. A. Davis, 1996.

Jandl, J. H. *Blood* (2nd ed.). Boston: Little, Brown & Co, 1996.

Nistico, A. and N. S. Young. "Gamma-Interferon Gene Expression in the Bone Marrow of Patients With Aplastic Anemia." *Annals of Internal Medicine*, Vol. 120, No. 6, March 15, 1994, pp. 463–469.

Socie, G. et al. "Malignant Tumors Occurring After Treatment of Aplastic Anemia." *N. Engl. J. Med.*, Vol. 329, No. 16, Oct. 14, 1993, pp. 1152–1157.

Stern, M. A., J. Eckman, and M. K. Offermann. "Aplastic Anemia After Exposure to Burning Oil." *N. Engl. J. Med.*, Vol. 331, No. 1, July 7, 1994, p. 58.

Thomas, E. D. and R. Storb. "Acquired Severe Aplastic Anemia: Progress and Perplexity." *Blood*, Vol. 64, No. 2, August, 1984, pp. 325–328.

Young, N. S. and J. Maciejewski. "The Pathophysiology of Acquired Aplastic Anemia." *N. Engl. J. Med.*, Vol. 336, No. 19, May 8, 1997, pp. 1365–1372.

REVIEW QUESTIONS

1. An acquired aplastic anemia may be caused by:
   A. Benzene or benzene derivatives.
   B. Ionizing radiation and vitamin B_{12}.
   C. Purine or pyrimidine analogues.
   D. All of the above.

2. The sudden appearance of aplastic anemia or pure red cell aplasia is often caused by:
   A. A hemolytic process.
   B. An immune process.
   C. Acute leukemias.
   D. Chronic leukemias.

3. Aplastic anemia can occur years before a diagnosis of ___ is made.
   A. Paroxysmal nocturnal hemoglobinuria.
   B. Myelodysplasia.
   C. Acute myelogenous leukemia.
   D. All of the above.

4. If a patient with aplastic anemia is referred to as exhibiting pancytopenia, which cell lines are affected?
   A. Erythrocytes.
   B. Leukocytes.
   C. Thrombocytes.
   D. All of the above.

Questions 5 to 8: match the following.

5. ___ Fanconi's anemia.

6. ___ Familial aplastic anemia.

7. ___ Pure red cell anemia.

8. ___ Diamond-Blackfan syndrome.

A. A subset of Fanconi's anemia.

B. A rare congenital form of red cell aplasia.

C. Is characterized by selective failure of red blood cell production.

D. The best-described congenital form of aplastic anemia.

10

Hypochromic Anemias and Disorders of Iron Metabolism

Iron deficiency anemia
Etiology
Epidemiology
Physiology
Clinical signs and symptoms
Laboratory characteristics
Sideroblastic anemia
Etiology
Physiology

Laboratory characteristics
Anemia of chronic diseases
Etiology
Pathophysiology
Laboratory characteristics
Summary
Case studies
Bibliography
Review questions

OBJECTIVES

Iron deficiency anemia
- Name four conditions that can contribute to iron deficiency anemia.
- Name three of the most common groups vulnerable to iron deficiency anemia.
- Describe the physiology of iron metabolism, including the iron needs of children and normal dietary sources.
- Characterize the signs and symptoms of iron deficiency anemia.
- Explain the value of soluble transferrin receptors.

Sideroblastic anemia
- Name five causes of sideroblastic anemia.
- Describe the pathophysiology of sideroblastic anemia.

- Explain the remarkable laboratory characteristics of sideroblastic anemia.

Anemia of chronic diseases
- Describe the etiological basis of anemia of chronic diseases.
- Explain the cause of anemia of chronic diseases.
- Discuss the laboratory characteristics of anemia of chronic diseases.

Case study
- Apply knowledge of etiology, pathophysiology, and laboratory findings to case studies of iron deficiency and anemia of chronic diseases.

IRON DEFICIENCY ANEMIA

Etiology

Although an individual's need for dietary iron is small and will only manifest itself after iron storage sites in the body have been depleted, iron deficiency anemia is one of the most frequently encountered types of anemia.

An iron deficiency anemia may result from, at least, four conditions (Table 10.1). These conditions are

1. Nutritional deficiency where not enough iron is consumed to meet the normal, daily required amount of iron, for example, fad diets and an imbalanced vegetarian diet
2. Faulty or incomplete iron absorption, for example, achlorhydria in certain disorders or following gastric resection; chronic diarrhea associated with disorders such as celiac disease, sprue, or resection of the small bowel; and the absence of factors needed for iron absorption
3. An increased demand for iron that is not met, such as during pregnancy, the growth years, or periods of increased blood regeneration
4. Excessive loss of iron, for example, due to acute or chronic hemorrhage or heavy menstruation. Adult males and postmenopausal females with iron deficiency must be evaluated for abnormal occult bleeding, especially gastrointestinal (GI) bleeding.

An iron deficiency may result from several other less commonly occurring conditions: a disorder of iron utilization, **sideroblastic anemia;** selected hemoglobinopathies; anemia related to chronic disorders; chronic inflammation; parasitic infections such as hookworm; and a deficiency of the plasma iron transporting protein **transferrin.**

Epidemiology

Although a high prevalence of iron deficiency existed in the 1960s in the U.S. population, intensified efforts to combat iron deficiency in this country appear to have successfully reduced anemia in some vulnerable age subgroups, such as infants. However, iron deficiency still remains common in

TABLE 10.1 Causes of Iron Deficiency Anemia

1. Decreased iron intake
   a. Cereal-rich, meat-poor diets
   b. Food fadists
   c. Elderly and indigent
   d. Malabsorption
 	
2. Faulty or incomplete iron absorption
   a. Celiac disease
   b. Sprue
   c. Resection of small bowel
   d. Absence of factors needed to absorb iron
 	
3. Increased iron utilization
   a. Postnatal growth spurt
   b. Adolescent growth spurt
	4A. Iron loss (pathological)
	   a. GI bleeding
	   b. Urogenital bleeding
	   c. Pulmonary hemosiderosis
	   d. Intravascular hemolysis
	   e. Malignancy (e.g., colon cancer)
	
	4B. Iron loss (physiological)
	   a. Menstruation
	   b. Pregnancy

TABLE 10.2 Prevalence of Iron Deficiency and Iron Deficiency Anemia All Races, NHANES III 1988–1994

Sex & Age	Iron Deficiency (%)	Iron Deficiency Anemia (%)
Both Sexes		
1–2	9	3*
3–5	3	<1
6–11	2	<1
Females		
12–15	9	2*
16–19	11*	3*
20–49	11	5*
50–69	5	2
70 and over	7*	2*
Males		
12–15	1	<1
16–19	<1	<1
20–49	<1	<1
50–69	2	1
70 and over	4	2

*Prevalence in nonblacks is 1% lower than prevalence in all races.

NHANES = National Health and Nutrition Examination Survey.

Source: Looker, A. C. et al. "Prevalence of Iron Deficiency in the United States." *JAMA,* Vol. 277, No. 12, March 26, 1997, p. 975.

toddlers, adolescent girls, and women of childbearing age (Tables 10.2 and 10.3).

Physiology

Humans have 35 to 50 mg of iron per kilogram of body weight. The average adult has 3.5 to 5.0 gm of total iron. Normal iron loss is very small, amounting to less than 1 mg/day. Iron is lost from the body through exfoliation of intestinal epithelial and skin cells, the bile, and through urinary excretion. To compensate for this loss, the adult male has a replacement iron need of 1 mg/day. However, additional iron is needed during the growth years, pregnancy, and lactation. Some women require supplementary iron due to heavy menstrual blood loss. Seventy percent of iron is functional or essential and 30% is stored or nonessential iron. Most functional iron is incorporated into the hemoglobin molecules of erythrocytes and is recycled.

Iron Needs in Infants and Children

In the normal infant at term, iron stores are adequate to maintain iron sufficiency for approximately 4 months of postnatal growth. In the premature infant, total body iron is lower than in the full-term newborn, although the proportion of iron to body weight is similar. Premature infants have a faster rate of postnatal growth than infants born at term, so unless the diet is supplemented with iron, they become iron-depleted more rapidly than full-term infants. Iron deficiency can develop by 2 to 3 months of age in

TABLE 10.3 Hemoglobin Cutoff Values

Sex & Age	G/L
Both Sexes	
1–2	7.34
3–5	7.57
6–11	7.92
Females	
12–15	9.27
16–19	8.21
20–49	9.12
50–69	9.82
70 and over	10.68
Males	
12–15	10.0
16–19	10.03
20–49	9.68
50–69	10.64
70 and over	12.87

premature infants. Iron intake must supplement the approximately 75 mg of iron per kilogram of body weight that is present at birth. Iron losses from the body are small and relatively constant except during episodes of diarrhea or during the feeding of whole cow's milk, when iron losses may be increased. About two thirds of iron losses in infancy occur when cells are extruded from the intestinal mucosa and the remainder when cells are shed from the skin and urinary tract. In the normal infant, these losses average approximately 20 μg per kilogram per day. An infant who weighs 3 kg at birth and 10 kg at 1 month will require approximately 270 to 280 mg of additional iron during the first year of life.

Breast milk and cow's milk both contain about 0.5 to 1.0 mg of iron per liter, but its bioavailability differs markedly. The absorption of iron from breast milk is uniquely high, about 50% on average, and tends to compensate for its low concentration. In contrast, only about 10% of iron in whole cow's milk is absorbed. About 4% of iron is absorbed from iron-fortified cow's-milk formulas that contain 12 mg of iron per liter. Reasons for high bioavailability of iron in breast milk are unknown.

Dietary Iron

There are two broad types of dietary iron. About 90% of iron from food is in the form of iron salts and is referred to as non-heme iron. The extent to which this type of iron is absorbed is highly variable and depends both on the person's iron status and on the other components of the diet. The other 10% of dietary iron is in the form of heme iron, which is derived primarily from the hemoglobin and myoglobin of meat. Heme iron is well absorbed, and its absorption is less strongly influenced by the person's iron stores or the other constituents of the diet. There is little meat in the diet of most infants, therefore, most of their dietary iron is non-heme, and their intake is highly influenced by other dietary factors. Ascorbic acid enhances the absorption of non-heme iron, as do meat meat, fish, and poultry. Inhibitors of absorption include bran, polyphenols, oxalates, phytates, vegetable fiber, the tannin in tea, and phosphates. Heme iron itself promotes the absorption of non-heme iron. For example, adults absorb approximately four times as much non-heme iron from a mixed meal when the principal protein source is meat, fish, or chicken than when it is milk, cheese, other dairy products, or eggs. The beverage is also important. Orange juice doubles the absorption of non-heme iron from the entire meal, whereas tea decreases it by 75%.

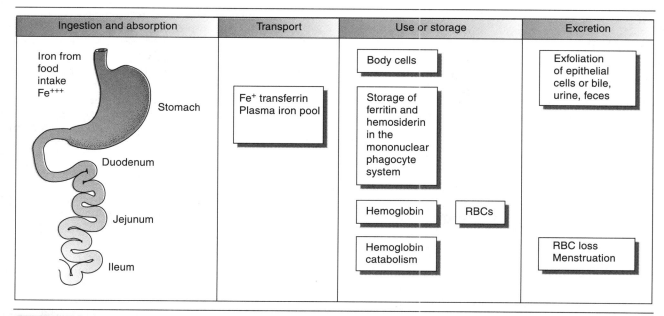

FIGURE 10.1 Iron physiology.

Following the oral intake of iron (Fig. 10.1) in the ferric (Fe^{3+}) state, stomach secretions reduce the iron to the ferrous (Fe^{2+}) state. These stomach secretions, referred to as reducing agents, include glutathione, ascorbic acid, and sulfhydril groups of proteins and digestion products. Gastric juice plays an important but poorly understood role in promoting absorption. The low pH of gastric juice makes iron available from hemoglobin-containing meat in the diet and other sources. However, very little iron is absorbed by the stomach.

Most of the iron passes from the stomach to the duodenum and upper jejunum, where it can be readily absorbed. Absorption by the GI epithelial cells is finely tuned to admit just enough iron to cover losses, without permitting either excess or deficiency of body iron to develop. Absorption normally admits about 5% to 10% of a total dietary intake of 10 to 20 mg/day.

Most absorbed iron becomes attached to the plasma protein transferrin, which is formed in the liver. Transferrin, a beta globulin, is a glycoprotein. Transferrin chelates iron within the intestinal lumen and shuttles it into the mucosal cells of the small intestine.

The internal iron transport of most mammals consists of transferrin transport of iron between donating tissues and transmembrane transferrin receptors, designed to procure iron for the cell. The cellular uptake of iron begins with the binding of the transferrin-iron complex to a specific receptor. Under normal circumstances, the iron required for cellular metabolism is acquired via transferrin receptors. Cells of different organ systems show considerable differences in the concentration of cellular transferrin receptors, the highest concentrations being found in cells of organs with the highest requirements, such as the hemoglobin synthesizing erythroid bone marrow cells and placental trophoblasts. The concentration of cell surface transferrin receptors is carefully regulated by transferrin receptor mRNA according to the internal iron content of the cell and its individual iron requirements. Iron-deficient cells contain increased numbers of receptors, while receptor numbers are downregulated in iron-replete cells.

Circulating transferrin receptor concentrations do not differ between healthy males and females, although concentrations are slightly higher in blacks than nonblacks. Concentrations vary in populations living at different altitudes, the higher concentrations occurring at higher altitudes.

Circulating transferrin receptor concentrations increase in tissue iron deficiency, reflecting the degree of iron deficiency in the erythroid precursors of the marrow. When iron stores decline, serum ferritin concentrations drop until iron stores are depleted, at which time the ferritin concentration falls below the lower limit of the reference interval. With further iron loss, and as iron-deficient erythropoiesis begins, circulating transferrin receptor concentrations begin to increase and continue to so as the severity of iron-deficient erythropoiesis increases, reflecting the increasing number of receptors on the erythroid cells of the bone marrow. The ratio of transferrin receptor to ferritin displays an inverse linear relationship to iron status, covering the spectrum from usual iron stores in health to substantial functional iron deficiency. The measurement of transferrin receptors is especially valuable in physiological conditions in which iron stores are depleted, making it difficult to clearly distinguish iron-deficient erythropoiesis from depleted iron stores. Such situations are commonly encountered in childhood and adolescence and during pregnancy, when iron stores are uniformly low to absent but iron-deficient erythropoiesis is not necessarily present.

Intracellular migration of transferrin-iron complexes produces an invagination of the cell membrane that results in a vacuole. Iron is subsequently released, and the transferrin is returned to the plasma to resume iron transport once again.

Any remaining iron is retained in the cells, where it combines with the protein apoferritin to form ferritin. Ferritin also occurs in hepatic parenchymal cells and reticuloendothelial cells of the bone marrow, liver, and spleen. If the amount of apoferritin is insufficient, the remaining iron will be deposited in tissues as hemosiderin. Hemosiderin represents an iron reserve. Ferritin and hemosiderin, chiefly in reticuloendothelial tissues, form the bulk of the iron reserve. Iron is taken from these storage deposits and transported back to erythroid precursors by transferrin.

The first line of iron supply is the mononuclear phagocyte system. In iron deficiency, any increase in iron supply must come from the GI tract, since body tissues are already depleted of storage iron. At the time that iron has been depleted from these iron stores, an iron deficiency will manifest itself.

Clinical Signs and Symptoms

Papilledema may be caused by iron deficiency anemia. The mechanism may be related to abnormal hemodynamics, as in other states of increased blood flow to the brain. Anemia may lead to reversible bulging of the fontanelles in infants with iron deficiency, rather than papilledema. Patients with iron deficieny anemia and headache should undergo a careful examination of the optic fundi to rule out papilledema, since this can lead to visual loss if left untreated.

Iron deficiency anemia in children is associated with psychomotor and mental impairment in the first 2 years of life. Currently, 35% of American children demonstrate evidence of iron insufficiency, 7% have iron deficiency without anemia, and 10% have iron deficiency anemia.

Pica, the compulsive ingestion of nonnutritive substances, e.g., ice, wooden toothpicks, chalk, or dirt, has a well-documented association with iron deficiency. It may be a habit that induces iron deficiency by replacing dietary iron sources or inhibiting the absorption or iron. But considerable evidence suggests that iron deficiency is usually the primary event and pica a consequence. Pica may occur in as many as half of iron-deficient patients.

Laboratory Characteristics

A typical iron deficiency anemia will exhibit the following laboratory characteristics. The hemoglobin and Hct are both decreased, whereas the red cell count may be normal initially, but will decrease as the iron deficiency state continues. The red cell indices demonstrate a decreased mean corpuscular volume (MCV), mean corpuscular hemoglobin (MCH), and mean corpuscular hemoglobin concentration (MCHC) (Table 10.4).

Examination of the blood film in this anemia characteristically reveals a hypochromic, microcytic pattern. Although

TABLE 10.4 Four Sequential Phases of Iron Deficiency

I. Decrease in storage iron
   Decreased tissue iron
   Decreased marrow iron
   Decreased serum ferritin level
   Increased transferrin level

II. Decrease in iron for erythropoiesis
   Decreased MCV
   Decreased MCH
   Decreased transferrin saturation
   Increased free erythrocyte protoporphyrin

III. Decrease in peripheral blood hemoglobin
   Decreased hemoglobin
   Decreased hematocrit

IV. Decrease in peripheral tissue oxygen delivery
   Clinical symptoms
   Clinical signs

Source: Bick, R. L. and W. F. Baker. "Iron Deficiency Anemia." *Lab. Med.,* Vol. 21, No. 10, October 1990, p. 646.

TABLE 10.6 Laboratory Findings in Iron Deficiency Anemia

Serum iron	Marked decrease
Total iron-binding capacity (TIBC)	Increased
Percent saturation	Marked decrease
Serum ferritin	Decreased

ferrin saturation provide little additional diagnostic value over ferritin. However, because ferritin is an acute-phase reactant, diagnosis of iron deficiency in hospitalized or ill patients can be difficult, as such patients may have normal or increased ferritin values even when iron deficient. The low sensitivity of ferritin for iron deficiency in these patients may require a bone marrow biopsy or a trial of iron therapy to differentiate iron deficiency from other causes of anemia.

A newer test is **soluble transferrin receptor (sTfR).** The complete transferrin receptor is a membrane-bound protein which captures transferrin with its two iron atoms from extracellular fluid. A fragment of TfR finds its way into serum, and appears to reflect production of TfR in the body. As the supply of transferrin-bound iron declines, hungry cells produce more TfR which results in a higher serum concentration of the fragment. An apparent, and potentially major advantage, is the ability of sTfR to differentiate iron deficiency anemia from anemia of chronic diseases (ACD). The use of sTfR, in conjunction with ferritin and reticulocyte index, could reduce the need for bone marrow examinations to confirm iron deficiency or differentiate it from ACD. Commercial test kits are beginning to appear.

Soluble transferrin receptor (sTfR), a truncated form of the membrane-associated transferrin receptor, has been reported to be an indicator of iron deficiency and is not an acute-phase reactant. Therefore, it has been proposed as a laboratory test to identify iron deficiency in hospitalized and chronically ill patients. This could reduce the need for a bone marrow biopsy or trial of iron therapy.

Ferritin detects deficient iron stores; sTfR detects increased erytropoiesis. StfR is not superior to ferritin for the routine clinical evaluation of patients with suspected iron deficiency.

When total body iron is low, transferrin levels increase, but the relative and absolute amounts of serum iron decline. Low serum iron levels, some down to 10 to 15 gm/dL, characterize iron deficiency. The percent saturation is ex-

this anemia may initially be normochromic or normocytic, or may only have some anisocytosis and hypochromia, a full manifestation of the anemia will exhibit both the hypochromic and the microcytic red cell patterns (Table 10.5).

Other hematological findings related to the anemia include the following: platelets are usually normal but may be increased following acute blood loss; the leukocyte count is usually normal; the reticulocyte count is decreased or normal; and osmotic fragility is normal or decreased. A bone marrow examination reveals a marked decrease in stainable iron and erythroid hyperplasia.

Clinical chemistry analysis to assess the iron status includes serum iron, total iron-binding capacity, percent saturation, and serum ferritin. The results of these assays are demonstrated in Table 10.6.

Transferrin saturation alone can be very misleading. Conditions associated with increased serum ferritin include infection, malignancy, iron overload, inflammation, and liver disease.

Serum ferritin is currently the accepted laboratory test for diagnosing iron deficiency. A ferritin value of 12 μg/L or less is a highly specific indicator of iron deficiency. Other commonly used laboratory tests such as serum iron, total iron-binding capacity, mean corpuscular volume, and trans-

TABLE 10.5 Differential Diagnosis of Microcytic, Hypochromic Anemia

	Iron Deficiency Anemia	β-thal Trait	ACD	Sideroblastic Anemia
Serum iron	Marked decrease	Normal	Decreased	Increased
TIBC	Increased	Normal	Decreased	Normal
Serum ferritin	Decreased	Normal	Increased	Increased
Red cell protoporphyrin	Increased	Normal	Increased	Increased or normal
Hemoglobin A$_2$	Decreased	Increased	Normal	Decreased

tremely low because more transferrin is available for less iron. Iron turnover and the percentage of serum iron used in red cell production increase as a way of getting the most possible mileage out of the little iron that is available.

The main value of the transferrin receptor assay is in the differential diagnosis of microcytic anemias. Assay of transferrin receptor with calculation of the transferrin receptor:ferritin ratio is a useful addition to this evaluation. Because circulating transferrin receptors do not increase in anemia secondary to inflammatory disorders, they are helpful for distinguishing ACD from iron deficiency anemia. In situations where iron deficiency anemia coexists with ACD, transferrin receptor concentrations increase secondary to the underlying iron deficiency. With serum ferritin concentrations greater than 30 $\mu g/L$ in patients with frank inflammatory disease, measurement of circulating transferrin receptor is warranted to exclude concurrent iron deficiency. Transferrin receptor concentrations are also increased in other causes of microcytic anemia, including sideroblastic anemia and the thalassemias; however, these diseases can be distinguished from iron deficiency anemia by ferritin concentrations being within the reference interval or greater.

SIDEROBLASTIC ANEMIA

Sideroblastic anemia is anemia associated with mitochondrial iron loading in marrow erythroid precursors (ringed sideroblasts) and ineffective erythropoiesis.

Causes of sideroblastic anemia include:

Congenital defect: hereditary sex-linked (primarily males); autosomal
Acquired defect: primary (one of the myelodysplastic syndromes); may evolve into acute myelogenous leukemia
Association with malignant marrow disorders: acute myelogenous leukemia, polycythemia vera, myeloma, myelodysplastic syndromes
Secondary to drugs: INH, chloramphenicol, after chemotherapy; toxins, including alcohol, and chronic lead poisoning

Diagnosis of sideroblastic anemia is based on variable red cell indices with a microcytic, hypochromic component of red cells on review of the peripheral smear; increased serum iron and serum ferritin; and characteristic ringed sideroblasts on iron stain of bone marrow aspirate.

Treatment is pyridoxine trial in pharmacologic doses. This approach is usually ineffective in acquired forms, but a significant number of patients with the sex-linked hereditary forms will respond. Other approaches include removing offending drugs or toxins and providing supportive care, such as blood product support and iron chelation as indicated. Chemotherapy may also be used if the condition evolves into acute myelogenous leukemia.

Etiology

Sideroblastic anemias are associated with a variety of causes:

1. Drugs, for example, isoniazid, chloramphenicol, alcohol, and cytotoxic drugs
2. Diseases, for example, hematological, neoplastic, and inflammatory
3. Miscellaneous disorders, for example, uremia, thyrotoxicosis, and porphyria
4. Hereditary factors
5. Idiopathic origin

Hereditary and idiopathic types of sideroblastic anemia may be pyridoxine-responsive or refractory.

Physiology

In this type of anemia, the body has adequate iron but is unable to incorporate it into hemoglobin synthesis. The iron enters the developing erythrocyte but then accumulates in the perinuclear mitochondria of metarubricytes (normoblasts). An established heme enzyme abnormality in sideroblastic anemia is a decrease in the activity of delta-aminolevulinic acid (delta-ALA) synthetase. Ringed sideroblasts are formed by mitochondria containing accumulated nonferritin iron that circles the normoblast (metarubricyte) nucleus. A Prussian blue stain reveals the iron as blue deposits circling the nucleus. Iron is normally deposited diffusely throughout the cytoplasm. Other forms of this anemia are associated with the administration of drugs or disease onset. If drugs are implicated, the drugs interfere with the activity of heme enzymes.

Laboratory Characteristics

Iron granules can be seen on bone marrow preparations stained for iron. Some of the granules may encircle the nucleus, particularly of metarubricytes (normoblasts), to form **ringed sideroblasts**. There is increased erythropoietic activity in the bone marrow. Thus, the marrow is hypercellular, but the number of circulating reticulocytes is not elevated. The mature, nonnucleated erythrocytes are generally hypochromic with normocytic and/or microcytic erythrocytes.

In hereditary types of sideroblastic anemia, a severe anemia is seen. The erythrocytes display marked hypochromia and microcytosis, target cells, basophilic stippling, and dimorphic red blood cell populations, although the leukocytes and platelets are usually normal. From 10% to 40% of the nucleated erythrocytes in the bone marrow are ringed sideroblasts. Megaloblastic changes in the marrow indicate complicating folate deficiency. In hereditary cases, transferrin saturation is high, and less than 50% of patients respond to pyridoxine therapy.

Idiopathic refractory types of sideroblastic anemia usually display moderate anemia. The peripheral blood is normocytic or macrocytic, with a small population of hypochromic erythrocytes. Some patients have marked stippling in the erythrocytes. The leukocytes and platelets are usually normal. The bone marrow demonstrates erythroid hyperplasia, with 45% to 95% of the nucleated erythrocytes being ringed sideroblasts. In 20% of patients, megaloblastic changes suggest a complicating folate deficiency. Transferrin saturation levels are increased (greater than 90%) in about one third of patients and serum ferritin levels are also increased with his form of anemia. Acute leukemia develops in approximately 10% of patients.

ANEMIA OF CHRONIC DISEASES

Etiology

The anemia that results from long- or short-term inflammation is commonly referred to as the anemia of chronic diseases or disorders (ACD). Many chronic diseases are not accompanied by anemia, e.g., diabetes, and many patients with chronic disease have anemia but do not have the type of anemia under discussion. It is important to exclude iron, folate, and cobalamin deficiencies and hemolysis before diagnosing a chronically ill patient as having the type of anemia that results from inflammation. A variety of anemias that are characterized as chronic nonhematological diseases with surplus storage iron and increased macrophage-ingested iron are classified as anemias of chronic diseases. ACD is the term that is used to describe the anemia associated with inflammation, chronic infection, and malignancy. Half of these are due to subacute or chronic infections, such as tuberculosis, lung abscess, and bacterial endocarditis. Other cases may be due to neoplasms, rheumatoid arthritis, rheumatic fever, systemic lupus erythematosus (SLE), uremia, and chronic liver disease.

Pathophysiology

ACD is not related to any nutritional deficiency. ACD is associated with and is caused by one or more of the many biochemical changes that occur during inflammation. The life span of erythrocytes is mildly shortened in this disorder, but this mechanism is not a major factor in the development of anemia. The main defect is probably the result of a failure of erythropoiesis, and it is likely that one or more of the following mediators are significant suppressors of erythropoiesis: tumor necrosis factor, interferons alpha and gamma, and interleukin-1.

Several mechanisms have been proposed as being induced by the inflammatory response in ACD. Anemia can result from

1. Blockage of the release of iron from macrophages for recycling in heme synthesis, which results in a decreased flow of iron to the bone marrow
2. Decreased erythropoietin production (although not caused by erythropoietin deficiency, the erythropoietin response may be blunted in this condition)
3. Suppression of erythropoiesis by cytokines from activated macrophages and lymphocytes
4. Decreased erythrocyte survival time; in some patients, the average erythrocyte survival time is 90 days

Laboratory Characteristics

Anemia is usually mild, but in some cases (e.g., uremia) the hemoglobin may be as low as 5 gm/dL. The peripheral blood smears usually show normochromic and normocytic erythrocytes; however, one fourth to one third of patients display hypochromic and microcytic erythrocytes. In patients with abnormal red cell morphology, it is less marked than in iron deficiency anemia. The total leukocyte count is consistent with the type and degree of infection present in the patient; the platelets are normal in quantity. In the bone marrow, hemosiderin is increased or normal; sideroblasts are decreased. The reticulocyte count is usually <2%.

Abnormalities in iron metabolism are associated with this disorder. Serum iron levels and transferrin (iron-binding capacity) are decreased. The total iron-binding capacity and transferrin saturation levels are decreased or normal. It is confusing to rely on the percentage of saturation of the iron-binding capacity to distinguish between iron deficiency and inflammation. The percentage of saturation may be very low in inflammation with abundant iron in the marrow. Total serum iron-binding capacity is superior to the percentage of saturation as an indicator of iron deficiency. If the total iron-binding capacity is increased, iron deficiency anemia must be ruled out. Serum ferritin levels are variable.

SUMMARY

Iron Deficiency Anemia

Although an individual's need for dietary iron is small and will only manifest itself after iron storage sites in the body have been depleted, iron deficiency anemia is one of the most frequently encountered types of anemia.

An iron deficiency anemia may result from nutritional deficiency, faulty or incomplete iron absorption, increased demand for iron that is not met, or excessive loss of iron. An iron deficiency may result from several other less commonly occurring conditions: a disorder of iron utilization, **sideroblastic anemia;** selected hemoglobinopathies; anemia related to chronic disorders; chronic inflammation; parasitic infections such as hookworm; and a deficiency of the plasma iron transporting protein **transferrin.**

Humans have 35 to 50 mg of iron per kilogram of body weight. The average adult has 3.5 to 5.0 gm of total iron. Normal iron loss is very small, amounting to less than 1 mg/day. Iron is lost from the body through exfoliation of intestinal epithelial and skin cells, the bile, and through urinary excretion. To compensate for this loss, the adult male has a replacement iron need of 1 mg/day. However, additional iron is needed during the growth years, pregnancy, and lactation. Some women require supplementary iron due to heavy menstrual blood loss. Seventy percent of iron is functional or essential and 30% is stored or nonessential iron. Most functional iron is incorporated into the hemoglobin molecules of erythrocytes and is recycled.

In the normal infant at term, iron stores are adequate to maintain iron sufficiency for approximately 4 months of postnatal growth. In the premature infant, total body iron is lower than in the full-term newborn, although the proportion of iron to body weight is similar. Iron deficiency can develop by 2 to 3 months of age in premature infants. Iron intake must supplement the approximately 75 mg of iron per kilogram of body weight that is present at birth.

There are two broad types of dietary iron. About 90% of iron from food is in the form of iron salts and is referred to as non-heme iron. The other 10% of dietary iron is in the form of heme iron, which is derived primarily from the hemoglobin and myoglobin of meat.

Iron deficiency anemia in children is associated with psychomotor and mental impairment in the first 2 years of life. Currently, 35% of American children demonstrate evidence of iron insufficiency, 7% have iron deficiency without anemia, and 10% have iron deficiency anemia. Pica, the compulsive ingestion of nonnutritive substances, e.g., ice, wooden toothpicks, chalk, or dirt, has a well-documented association with iron deficiency.

A typical iron deficiency anemia will exhibit the following laboratory characteristics: the hemoglobin and Hct are both decreased, whereas the red cell count may be normal initially, but will decrease as the iron deficiency state continues; and the red cell indices demonstrate a decreased mean corpuscular volume (MCV), mean corpuscular hemoglobin (MCH), and mean corpuscular hemoglobin concentration (MCHC).

Examination of the blood film in this anemia characteristically reveals a hypochromic, microcytic pattern. Although this anemia may initially be normochromic or normocytic, or may only have some anisocytosis and hypochromia, a full manifestation of the anemia will exhibit both the hypochromic and the microcytic red cell patterns.

Serum ferritin is currently the accepted laboratory test for diagnosing iron deficiency, and a ferritin value of 12 μg/L or less is a highly specific indicator of iron deficiency. A newer test is soluble transferrin receptor (sTfR). Ferritin detects deficient iron stores; sTfR detects increased erythropoiesis. StfR is not superior to ferritin for the routine clinical evaluation of patients with suspected iron deficiency.

Sideroblastic Anemia

Sideroblastic anemia is an anemia associated with mitochondrial iron loading in marrow erythroid precursors (ringed sideroblasts) and ineffective erythropoiesis. It can be congenital or acquired.

Anemia of Chronic Diseases

Anemia of chronic diseases (ACD) result from long- or short-term inflammation. ACD is the term that is used to describe the anemia associated with inflammation, chronic infection, and malignancy.

ACD is not related to any nutritional deficiency. ACD is associated with and is caused by one or more of the many biochemical changes that occur during inflammation. The life span of erythrocytes is mildly shortened in this disorder, but this mechanism is not a major factor in the development of anemia. The main defect is probably the result of a failure of erythropoiesis, and it is likely that one or more of the following mediators are significant suppressors of erythropoiesis: tumor necrosis factor, interferons alpha and gamma, and interleukin-1.

CASE STUDIES

CASE 1 A 10-month-old Central American child was referred to the laboratory for testing after being seen by a pediatrician. The phlebotomist noticed that the child was very pale and listless. The following tests were ordered: CBC, platelet count, reticulocyte count, total serum iron and iron-binding capacity (TIBC), and a stool examination for occult blood, ova, and parasites. The results were as follows:

Hemoglobin 5.6 gm/dL
Hct 0.24 L/L
RBC 3.5×10^{12}/L
WBC 10.5×10^9/L

The RBC indices were as follows:

MCV 68.6 fL
MCH 16 pg
MCHC 23%

The peripheral blood smear revealed marked anisocytosis, microcytosis, hypochromia, and poikilocytosis. A normal distribution of platelets was present. Additional laboratory findings were as follows:

Platelet count 200×10^9/L
Reticulocyte count 0.5%
Total serum bilirubin 0.9 mg/dL
Serum iron 40 μg/dL
TIBC 465 μg/dL
Percent saturation of transferrin 8.6%

A stool examination was negative for occult blood, ova, and parasites.

Questions
1. What category of anemia is suggested by the morphology of the RBCs on the peripheral blood smear?
2. What laboratory assays would be of additional value in establishing the diagnosis?
3. What is the most probable cause of the patient's anemia?

Discussion
1. The demonstration of hypochromic, microcytic erythrocytes in a peripheral blood film suggests iron deficiency anemia.
2. The RBC indices revealed both a decreased MCV and MCH. These findings support the RBC morphology observations of microcytosis and hypochromia. Several follow-up laboratory assays were of value in establishing the etiology of this patient's anemia. These tests were the serum iron, TIBC, and percent saturation. A decreased serum iron and percent saturation were present, along with an increased TIBC. The serum bilirubin and reticulocyte count were normal. No evidence of bleeding or parasitic infections was detected.
3. The most probable cause of this patient's anemia was a deficiency of iron. The laboratory findings demonstrated an iron deficit with no evidence of either hemolysis or blood loss. Small children are among the most frequent victims of inadequate dietary iron. The newborn begins life with 350 to 500 mg of iron. A daily intake of 1 mg/kg (2.2 lb) of body weight is needed during infancy in order to keep pace with growth. Some iron-poor foods, such as milk, never become useful sources for the absorption of iron.

(continued)

Children in underdeveloped countries frequently suffer from a combination of poor diet and parasitic infections. With a diet consisting largely of milk and unsupplemented with fortified food products during the early years of development, iron deficiency anemia is a frequent by-product.

Diagnosis: Iron deficiency anemia

CASE 2 A 75-year-old woman started feeling a bit weak. The patient reported limited red meat intake. A cholecystectomy was performed at age 60 and some bowel was removed. The patient has occasional diarrhea but considers this a minor inconvenience. The patient has experienced some bilateral loss of sensation in the feet and a tingling which was getting worse and more frequent over the last few months. She takes over-the-counter medications and her husband's pills for indigestion. The patient complained of arthritis; she has been taking nonsteroidal anti-inflammatory drugs for 5 years, and she has started on low-dose thotrexate for arthritis flare-ups.

The physician is certain that she is anemic and requests a CBC and differential, Iron, TIBC, and % Sat/ferritin.

No malignancies or GI bleeding are noted. Blood loss from the GI tract has been ruled out. Profound atrophic gastritis with patches of inflammation is noted, as is *Helicobacter pylori* at stomach biopsy study.

Laboratory Data
Hemoglobin: 10 gm/dL (12 gm/dL)
Hematocrit: 33% (36–45%)
MCV: 83 fL (81–98fL)
RDW: 17.5 (11.5–14.5)
Iron: 25µg/dL (50–170 dL)
TIBC: 250 µg/dL (250–450 µg/dL)
% Sat: 10% (15–50%)
Ferritin: 45 µg/L (12–120 µg/L)
Serum folate: 4 ng/mL (3–16 ng/mL)
RBC folate: 100 ng/mL (130–628 ng/mL)
Vitamin B_{12}: 100 pg/mL (200–900 pg/mL)

Question
1. Is ferritin a reliable laboratory indicator of iron stores?

Discussion
Ferritin is an iron-storage molecule. The amount in serum reflects iron storage: every 1 µg/L indicates (very roughly) 10 mg of body stores. Concern about the use of this indicator in the elderly arises because a range of inflammatory diseases increase ferritin; therefore, its concentration no longer reflects iron stores. Ferritin acts as an "acute phase" reactant. In this case, the increased ferritin was due to the inflammation of rheumatoid arthritis, illustrating the diagnostic pitfall of placing too much faith in ferritin.

Atrophic gastritis is common in the elderly and is almost certainly due to some extent to *H. pylori*.

Follow-up: The patient was placed on the usual course of IM B_{12} and oral folate, 1 mg/day. The following were the laboratory results at her 3-month follow-up:

Hemoglobin: 11 g/dL
MCV: 75fL
TIBC: 500 µg/dL
RDW: 15
Ferritin: 8 µg/L
Iron: 35 µg/dL

% Sat: 7%
Bone marrow ordered for refractory anemia

Diagnostic Problems
This case presented some challenging diagnostic problems:

The patient had an extremely elevated RDW, which suggested a mixed red cell population.
A mixed B_{12}/iron deficiency is well recognized in the literature but seldom considered in practice. Note the normal MCV which became microcytic when the B_{12} deficiency was corrected.
A microbiological component to nutritional deficiency. *H. pylori* is very common in the elderly and, ulcers or no ulcers, requires consideration. Biopsy is not necessary for reasonably reliable identification of affected persons; serologic tests are available. However, after the gastric damage has been done, nutritional support may be necessary.
Nonresponse to a particular form of oral iron supplement, which could involve gastric pH, bowel loss or disease, malabsorption secondary to B_{12} deficiency, or other components of her diet which reduce iron absorption

Diagnosis: Iron deficiency and vitamin B_{12} deficiency anemia

BIBLIOGRAPHY

Bacon, B. R. "Causes of Iron Overload." *N. Engl. J. Med.,* Vol. 326, No. 2, January 9, 1992, pp. 126–127.

Bick, R. L. and W. F. Baker. "Iron Deficiency Anemia." *Laboratory Medicine,* Vol. 21, No. 10, October, 1990, pp. 641–648.

Gordeuk, V. et al. "Iron Overload in Africa." *N. Engl. J. Med.,* Vol. 326, No. 2, January 9, 1992, pp. 95–100.

Huebers, H. A. and C. A. Finch. "Transferrin: Physiologic Behavior and Clinical Implications." *Blood,* Vol. 64, No. 4, October, 1984, pp. 763–767.

Khumalo, H. et al. "Serum Transferrin Receptors Are Decreased in the Presence of Iron Overload." *Clinical Chemistry,* Vol. 44, No. 1, 1998, pp. 40–44.

Looker, A. C. et al. "Prevalence of Iron Deficiency in the United States." *JAMA,* Vol. 277, No. 12, March 26, 1997, pp. 973–976.

Mast, A. E. et al. "Clinical Utility of the Soluble Transferrin Receptor and Comparison With Serum Ferritin in Several Populations." *Clinical Chemistry,* Vol. 44, No. 1, 1998, pp. 45–51.

Moore, D. F. and D. A. Sears. "Pica, Iron Deficiency, and the Medical History." *Am. J. Med.,* Vol. 97, October, 1994, pp. 390–393.

Muta, K. et al. "Erythroblast Transferrin Receptors and Transferrin Kinetics in Iron Deficiency and Various Anemias." *A. J. Hematol.,* Vol. 25, No. 2, June, 1987, pp. 155–163.

Oski, F. A. "Iron Deficiency in Infancy and Childhood," *N. Engl. J. Med.,* Vol. 329, No. 3, July 15, 1993, pp. 190–193.

Schilling, R. F. "Anemia of Chronic Disease: A Misnomer." *Ann. Intern. Med.,* Vol. 115, No. 7, October 1, 1991, pp. 572–573.

Skikne, B. S. "Circulating Transferrin Receptor Assay—Coming of Age." Clinical Chemistry, Vol. 44, No. 1, 1998, pp. 7–9.

Statland, B. E. "Ferritin vs. Iron, Tips on Technology." *Med. Lab. Observer,* Vol. 21, No. 8, August, 1989, pp. 11–12.

Tsang, C. W. et al. "Hematologic Indices in an Older Population Sample: Derivation of Healthy Reference Values." *Clinical Chemistry,* Vol. 44, No. 1, 1998, pp. 96–101.

Walter, T. "Iron Deficiency Anemia: Adverse Effects on Infant Psychomotor Development." *Pediatrics,* Vol. 84, No. 1, July, 1989, pp. 7–17.

REVIEW QUESTIONS

1. The etiology of iron deficiency anemia is:
   A. Nutritional deficiency.
   B. Faulty iron absorption.
   C. Excessive loss of iron.
   D. All of the above.

2. Iron deficiency is still common in:
   A. Toddlers.
   B. Adolescent girls.
   C. Women of childbearing age.
   D. All of the above.

Questions 3 through 7: match the following categories with an appropriate example.

3. ___ Decreased iron intake.   A. Sprue.

4. ___ Faulty iron absorption.   B. Colon cancer.

5. ___ Pathological iron loss.   C. Adolescent growth spurt.

6. ___ Physiological iron loss.   D. Menstruation.

7. ___ Increased iron utilization.   E. Meat-poor diet.

8. The average adult has ___ g of total iron.
   A. 0.2–1.4   C. 3.5–5.0
   B. 1.5–3.4   D. 5.1–10.0

9. Most functional iron in humans is found in:
   A. The bone marrow.
   B. The liver.
   C. Hemoglobin molecules of RBCs.
   D. Free hemoglobin in the circulation.

Questions 10 and 11: about *(10)* ___% of iron from food is in the form of *(11)* ___ iron.

10. A. 25   11. A. Non-heme
    B. 50   B. Heme
    C. 70
    D. 90

12. Most ingested iron is absorbed into the body in the:
    A. Stomach and duodenum.
    B. Duodenum and upper jejunum.
    C. Ileum and duodenum.
    D. Upper jejunum and ileum.

13. Transferrin represents a:
    A. Storage form of iron.
    B. Beta globulin that moves iron.
    C. Glycoprotein that moves iron.
    D. Both B and C.

14. In iron deficiency anemia, the erythrocytic indices are typically:
    A. MCV increased, MCH decreased, and MCHC decreased.
    B. MCV decreased, MCH decreased, and MCHC decreased.
    C. MCV decreased, MCH increased, and MCHC decreased.
    D. MCV decreased, MCH decreased, and MCHC normal.

15. The peripherial blood smear demonstrates ___ red blood cells in iron deficiency anemia
    A. Microcytic, hypochromic
    B. Macrocytic, hypochromic
    C. Macrocytic and spherocytic
    D. Either A or B

16. In iron deficiency anemia the:
    A. Serum iron is severely decreased and the total iron-binding capacity (TIBC) is increased.
    B. Serum iron is decreased and the TIBC is normal.
    C. Serum iron is normal and the TIBC is normal.
    D. Serum iron is increased and the TIBC is normal.

17. Sideroblastic anemia can be caused by:
    A. Congenital (chromosomal) defect.
    B. Drugs (e.g., chloramphenicol).
    C. Association with malignant disorders (e.g., acute myelogenous leukemia).
    D. All of the above.

18. A common feature of sideroblastic anemia is:
    A. Ringed sideroblasts.
    B. Decreased serum iron.
    C. Decreased serum ferritin.
    D. Macrocytic red blood cells.

19. Anemias of chronic diseases can be caused by:
    A. Inflammation.
    B. Infection.
    C. Malignancy.
    D. All of the above.

20. The typical peripheral blood film of a patient with anemia of chronic disease reveals ___ red blood cells.
    A. Microcytic, hypochromic.
    B. Macrocytic, hypochromic.
    C. Normocytic, normochromic.
    D. Many spherocytes.

11

Megaloblastic Anemias

OBJECTIVES

Megaloblastic anemias

- List four causes of vitamin B_{12} deficiency.
- List three causes of folic acid deficiency.
- Briefly describe the epidemiology of pernicious anemia.
- Explain the physiology, including the immune nature, of pernicious anemia.
- Describe the clinical signs and symptoms of pernicious anemia.
- Delineate the laboratory findings in pernicious anemia.

- Explain the usual management and therapy for pernicious anemia.
- Compare megaloblastic anemia due to folic acid deficiency to pernicious anemia.

Case study

- Apply knowledge of etiology, epidemiology, physiology, clinical signs and symptoms, laboratory findings, and management therapy to the case studies.

MEGALOBLASTIC ANEMIAS

Megaloblastic anemias can be classified into two major categories based on etiology. The major divisions are vitamin B_{12} deficiencies and folic acid deficiencies.

The term **megaloblastic** refers to the abnormal marrow erythrocyte precursor seen in processes, such as pernicious anemia, associated with altered DNA synthesis. Macrocytes can occur in the absence of a megaloblastic process. For example, an increased mean corpuscular volume (MCV) can result simply from an increase in the number of circulating reticulocytes, which are larger than mature erythrocytes.

The most common causes of megaloblastic anemia are acquired, although congenital forms exist. Deficiencies in cobalamin, folate, or both account for the majority of cases. The most common disorder of cobalamin deficiency is pernicious anemia. Less common manifestations include postgastrectomy, inflammatory disorders of the terminal ileum, and infestation with fish tapeworm *Diphyllobothrium latum*. Folic acid deficiency is usually due to inadequate dietary intake.

Red blood cells in megaloblastic anemias (Plate 26) have an abnormal nuclear maturation and imbalance between nuclear and cytoplasmic maturation. The absence of vitamin B_{12} or folates impairs DNA synthesis, which slows nuclear replication and delays each step of maturation. The premitotic interval is prolonged. This results in a large nucleus, increased cytoplasmic RNA, and early synthesis of hemoglobin. Many cells never undergo mitosis and breakdown in the bone marrow, producing extremely increased levels of serum LDH. This deficiency can impair maturation in myelogenous white blood cells and megakaryocytes, producing leukopenia with neutrophilic hypersegmentation and thrombocytopenia. Megakaryocyte fragments and giant platelets may be seen on peripheral blood smears. Megaloblastic anemias such as pernicious anemia are also characterized by active intramedullary hemolysis. In addition to hematologic manifestations, neuropsychiatric disturbances, such as peripheral neuropathy or depression, are also common with cobalamin or folate deficiency and may occur in the absence of significant hematologic manifestations. These neuropsychiatric conditions are reversible if treated promptly by cobalamin or folate replenishment.

Usually, the measurement of of serum cobalamin or folate levels will be sufficient to make the diagnosis. Inherited enzyme deficiencies are rare causes of megaloblastic anemia.

Etiology

Megaloblastic anemia due to vitamin B_{12} deficiency is associated with:

1. Increased utilization of vitamin B_{12} due to parasitic infections such as *Diphyllobothrium latum* (tapeworm) and pathogenic bacteria in disorders such as diverticulitis and small-bowel stricture
2. Malabsorption syndrome due to gastric resection, gastric carcinoma, and some forms of celiac disease or sprue
3. Nutritional deficiency or diminished supply of vitamin B_{12} in such disorders such as kwashiorkor
4. Pernicious anemia

Megaloblastic anemia caused by folic acid deficiency is associated with:

1. Abnormal absorption due to celiac disease or sprue
2. Increased utilization caused by pregnancy or some acute leukemias
3. Treatment with antimetabolites that act as folic acid antagonists

Epidemiology

Research studies have recently documented that 1.9% of persons more than 60 years old have undiagnosed pernicious anemia. Earlier studies suggested that pernicious anemia is restricted to Northern Europeans; however, newer studies report the disease in both blacks and Latin Americans. The median age at diagnosis is 60 years. Slightly more women than men are affected.

Although the disease is silent for a span of 20 to 30 years until the end stage, the underlying gastric lesion can be predicted many years before anemia develops. The underlying gastritis that causes pernicious anemia is immunologically related to an autoantibody to intrinsic factor, a serum inhibitor of intrinsic factor, and autoantibodies to parietal cells.

A genetic predisposition to pernicious anemia is suggested by the clustering of the disease and of gastric autoantibodies in families, and by the association of the disease and gastric autoantibodies with the autoimmune endocrinopathies. About 20% of the relatives of patients with pernicious anemia have pernicious anemia. These relatives, especially first-degree female relatives, also have a higher frequency of gastric autoantibodies than normal subjects. In contrast to some other autoimmune diseases, there is little evidence of an association between pernicious anemia and particular molecules of the major histocompatibility complex.

Pernicious anemia may be associated with autoimmune endocrinopathies and antireceptor autoimmune disease. These diseases include chronic autoimmune thyroiditis (Hashimoto's thyroiditis), insulin-dependent diabetes mellitus, Addison's disease, primary ovarian failure, primary hypoparathyroidism, Graves' disease, and myasthenia gravis.

Physiology

Normal red cell maturation is dependent on many hematological factors, two of which are the vitamin B_{12} coenzymes (also called cobalamin) and folates. Megaloblastic dyspoiesis occurs when one of these factors is absent.

Vitamin B_{12} and a variety of structurally similar compounds known as cobalamin analogues that lack the functional coenzyme activity of the vitamin occur in nature as a product of certain microorganisms. It becomes available to humans through the food chain. About one third of the body's average total of 5000 μg is stored in the liver. The average loss of vitamin B_{12} is about 5 μg/day. The daily average adult requires about 5 μg of vitamin B_{12} per day to balance this loss, with a greater need during unusual periods such as pregnancy. A normal diet contains 5 to 30 μg.

Folates are abundant in yeast, many leafy vegetables, and

TABLE 11.1 Vitamin B$_{12}$ (Cobalamin)–Binding Proteins

Binding Protein	Source	Function	Membrane Receptors
Intrinsic factor	Stomach	Intestinal absorption	Ileal enterocytes
Transcobalamin II	Liver, other tissues	Delivery to cells	Many cells
R proteins	Leukocytes, other tissues	Excretion, storage	Liver cells

organ meats such as liver and kidneys. An ample amount of folate is present in most well-balanced diets. The human body stores little folic acid. Storage amounts would last about 3 to 4 months if a complete absence of dietary folates existed. However, a chronically inadequate diet can produce folic acid deficiency anemia. In addition to a poor diet, alcohol is the most common pharmacological cause of folic acid deficiency. However, folic acid antagonists, such as certain drugs used to treat leukemias and oral contraceptives, appear to reduce the absorption of folic acid.

Vitamin B$_{12}$ (Cobalamin) Transport

Cobalamin transport is mediated by three different binding proteins (Table 11.1) that are capable of binding the vitamin at its required physiological concentrations: **intrinsic factor, transcobalamin II,** and the **R proteins.**

Intrinsic factor (IF), a glycoprotein, is synthesized and secreted by the parietal cells of the mucosa in the fundus region of the stomach in several mammalian species including humans. In health, the amounts of IF secreted by the stomach greatly exceed the quantities required to bind ingested cobalamin in its coenzyme forms. At a very acidic pH, cobalamin splits from dietary protein and combines with IF to form a vitamin-IF complex (Fig. 11.1). Binding by IF

is extraordinarily specific and is lost with even slight changes in the cobalamin molecule. This complex is stable and remains unabsorbed until it reaches the ileum. In the ileum, the vitamin-IF complex attaches to specific receptor sites present only on the outer surface of microvillus membranes of ileal enterocytes.

The release of this complex from the mucosal cells with subsequent transport to the tissues depends on transcobalamin II (TC II). TC II is a plasma polypeptide synthesized by the liver and probably several other tissues. Like IF, TC II, which turns over very rapidly in the plasma, acts as the acceptor and principal carrier of the vitamin to the liver and other tissues. Receptors for TC II are observed on the plasma membranes of a wide variety of cells. TC II is also capable of binding a few unusual cobalamin analogues, and it stimulates cobalamin uptake by reticulocytes.

The R proteins comprise an antigenically cross-reactive group of cobalamin-binding glycoproteins. The R proteins bind cobalamin and various cobalamin analogues. Their function is unknown but they appear to serve as storage sites and as a means of eliminating excess cobalamin and unwanted analogues from the blood circulation through receptor sites on liver cells. R proteins are produced by leukocytes and perhaps other tissues. They are present in plasma as transcobalamin I and transcobalamin III, as well

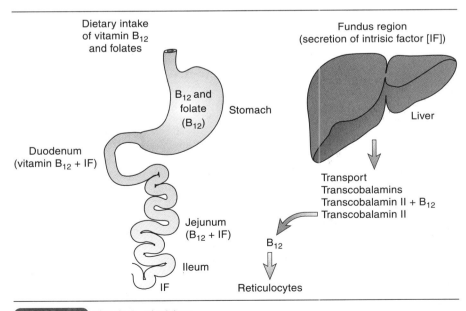

FIGURE 11.1 Vitamin B$_{12}$ physiology.

as in saliva, milk, and other body fluids. Transcobalamin I probably serves only as a backup transport system for endogenous cobalamin. Endogenous vitamin is synthesized in the human GI tract by bacterial action, but none is adsorbed.

Vitamin B$_{12}$ (Cobalamin) and Folic Acid Deficiencies

In addition to dietary and other causes of deficiencies of cobalamin (Table 11.2), a deficiency of TC II can produce a vitamin deficiency. Folic acid deficiencies appear to be less

TABLE 11.2   Cobalamin Deficiency

Dietary
Malnutrition
Veganism
Breast-fed infants of vegan mothers

Malabsorption
Gastric
    Pernicious anemia
        Autoimmune with antibody against IF and parietal cells
        Food-associated cobalamin malabsorption
        Congenital decreased or production of abnormal IF
    Destruction by caustic substances (lye)
    Gastric resection

Intestinal
Crohn's disease, tuberculosis, other granulomatous diseases
Tropical sprue
Ileal resection or irradiation
Stagnant loop syndrome
Pancreatic malabsorption
Lymphoma
Amyloidosis
Drugs
    Metformin
    Neomycin
    Para-aminosalicylic acid
    Alcohol
    Colchicine
    Potassium chloride
Diphyllobothrium latum infestation
Imerslund-Grasbeck syndrome

Impaired Utilization
Nitrous oxide anesthesia
Transcobalamin II deficiency or abnormality
Homocystinuria with methylmalonic aciduria

Increased Demand
Pregnancy
Chronic hemolytic anemia
Multiple myeloma or other neoplasms
Myeloproliferative diseases
Hyperthyroidism

Source: Scates, S. and J. Glaspy. "The Macrocytic Anemias." *Lab. Med.*, Vol. 21, No. 11, November, 1990, p. 737.

related to transport, but are typically associated with conditions of either dietary inadequacy or malabsorption syndromes.

In pernicious anemia, the deficiency is caused by reduced IF secondary to gastric atrophy. In the majority of cases of pernicious anemia, anti-IFs or antibodies to parietal cells (large cells on the margin of the peptic glands of the stomach) have been reported. Most authorities consider the demonstration of these antibodies to support the theory that pernicious anemia is an autoimmune disorder. The presence of IF-blocking antibodies is diagnostic of pernicious anemia.

Clinical Signs and Symptoms

Pernicious anemia is frequently seen in those of Northern European ancestry, with clinical presentation during the fourth or fifth decade of life.

Acquired megaloblastic anemias tend to have a very insidious onset, with symptoms that may have been present for years before the diagnosis is made. Because of the pivotal role of cobalamin in metabolism, multiple organ systems can be affected in pernicious anemia.

Patients may notice changes in their skin color to a lemon-yellow appearance. The nailbeds, skin creases, and periorbital areas may become hyperpigmented owing to melanin deposition. Angular cheilitis (cracking at the corners of the mouth), dyspepsia, and diarrhea can occur. Glossitis and a painful tongue are frequently observed.

Early graying of the hair can be seen. Patients may complain of tiredness, dyspnea on exertion, vertigo, or tinnitus secondary to anemia. Congestive heart failure, angina, or palpitations may be noted. Neurologic and cognitive abnormalities may be seen in cobalamin deficiency. Paresthesias, loss of balance, visual changes, paraplegia, memory loss, dementia, and other psychiatric disturbances have been described. The degree to which these symptoms are present may not be correlated with the degree of anemia. If the disease is severe, infection, bleeding, or bruising may occur due to granulocytopenia.

Laboratory Findings

Pernicious anemia, the most common megaloblastic anemia, is a prototype of the entire group. The hematological picture is the same whether the cause is vitamin B$_{12}$ or folic acid deficiency. However, supporting laboratory assays will differ for the various megaloblastic anemias.

The hemoglobin and red cell count are usually extremely low in this anemia. However, the Hct (packed cell volume) may not reflect the actual decrease in erythrocytes because of the enlarged size of the red cells. This increase in red cell size is typically reflected in the MCV, which may be as high as 130 fL. The MCH varies, but is usually increased in 90% of cases. Concurrent conditions that decrease the MCV, such as thalassemia or iron deficiency, may cause the MCV to be normal. The MCH concentration (MCHC) is usually normal. In this anemia, platelet counts are usually moderately decreased. The total white blood cell count will classically demonstrate a leukopenia, particularly a neutropenia.

Examination of a peripheral blood smear will reveal a moderate to marked anisocytosis and poikilocytosis with many macrocytic, ovalocytic red cells. Erythroid precursors, notably metarubricytes, may also be observed. Red cell inclusions such as basophilic stippling, Howell-Jolly bodies, and Cabot rings may be observed. Abnormalities in the leukocytes may include hypersegmented (more than 4 lobes) neutrophils and an increase in the percentage of eosinophils (eosinophilia). Platelets are also typically decreased in number.

The reticulocyte count is less than 1% in untreated pernicious anemia and is low for the degree of anemia. However, subsequent to vitamin B_{12} treatment, assuming that the patient does not have antibodies against IF, the reticulocyte count can increase up to 25% in 5 to 8 days.

Pancytopenia may be seen in advanced cases. In severe anemia with a hematocrit of less than 20%, promegaloblasts and nucleated erythrocytes may be seen, due to extramedullary hematopoiesis in the spleen and very early marrow release. A dimorphic population of red cells may be present with concurrent iron deficiency. The red cell distribution width is high.

The bone marrow is usually hypercellular with megaloblastic changes in either the erythroid line or all lines, but it can be hypocellular and mimic aplastic anemia. Erythrocyte precursors are enlarged with a decreased nuclear-cytoplasmic ratio. Nuclear-cytoplasmic asynchrony, with relative immaturity of the nucleoplasm, is typical. Changes give red cells a dysplastic appearance, and a mistaken diagnosis of myelodysplastic syndrome can be made. Granulocytic precursors may also display nuclear-cytoplasmic dissociation and enlargement. Characteristically, giant metamyelocytes with large, incompletely segmented nuclei are seen. The number of mitoses are increased and the M:E ratio is diminished to 1:1 or less. Iron stores are increased, unless iron deficiency is coincidentally present.

Clinical chemistry assays that are of value in the diagnosis of pernicious anemia include:

Serum haptoglobin-binding capacity—decreased
Gastric analysis (histamine)—achlorhydria
Serum vitamin B_{12}—decreased
Folate—normal
Serum iron—increased
Total iron-binding capacity—normal or decreased
Percent transferrin—increased
Serum lactic dehydrogenase isoenzymes 1 and 2—markedly increased
Unconjugated bilirubin—increased
Urinary methylmalonic acid and homocysteine levels—elevated

Achlorhydria, decreased serum vitamin B_{12}, and an extremely elevated LDH, isoenzymes 1 and 2, are extremely important diagnostic findings in pernicious anemia. The LDH isoenzymes 1 and 2 and unconjugated bilirubin are elevated owing to intramedullary hemolysis. Uric acid levels are low secondary to decreased DNA synthesis.

Achlorhydria, the absence of hydrochloric acid (HCl) in the stomach, is an important finding in pernicious anemia. An absence of free HCl in gastric fluid after histamine stimulation is a universal feature of this form of megaloblastic anemia. Achlorhydria results from atrophy of the parietal cells of the stomach. The LDH is markedly increased owing to the increased intramedullary destruction of megaloblastic bone marrow cells. Folic acid deficiency anemias present the same erythrocytic picture as pernicious anemia. A comparison of selected laboratory findings in disorders representing an impaired production of erythrocytes is presented in Table 11.3.

Diagnosis of cobalamin deficiency is usually made by measuring the amount of the substance in plasma using either a microbiologic assay or radiodilution. Radiodilution assays can use either R proteins, such as gastric R binder, or intrinsic factor as binding agents. R protein will bind analogues of cobalamin, thus the assays utilizing IF are more specific. If cobalamin deficiency is suspected, it becomes

TABLE 11.3 Comparison of Selected Laboratory Findings in Various Types of Anemia

Disorder	Test	Result
Aplastic anemia (Chapter 9)	Hemoglobin	Severely decreased
	PCV	Severely decreased
	Erythrocyte count	Severely decreased
	WBC count	Severely decreased
	Platelet count	Severely decreased
	MCV	Normal
	Serum iron	N/A
	TIBC	N/A
	Percent saturation	N/A
	Serum ferritin	N/A
Iron deficiency anemia (Chapter 10)	Hemoglobin	Decreased
	PCV	Decreased
	Erythrocyte count	Decreased
	WBC count	Normal
	Platelet count	Normal
	MCV	Decreased
	Serum iron	Severely decreased
	TIBC	Increased
	Percent saturation	Severely decreased
	Serum ferritin	Decreased
Anemia of chronic diseases (Chapter 10)	Hemoglobin	Decreased
	WBC count	Variable
	MCV	Usually normal
	MCH	Usually normal
	Platelet count	Normal
	Serum iron	Decreased
	TIBC	Decreased or normal
	Percent saturation	Decreased or normal
	Serum ferritin	Variable
Megaloblastic anemia (Chapter 11)	Hemoglobin	Severely decreased
	PCV	Severely decreased
	Erythrocyte count	Decreased
	WBC count	Slightly decreased
	Platelet count	Slightly decreased or normal
	MCV	Increased
	Serum iron	Increased
	TIBC	Normal or decreased
	Percent saturation	Increased
	Serum ferritin	Increased

PCV = packed cell volume; WBC = white blood cell (leukocyte) count; MCH = mean corpuscular hemoglobin; MCV = mean corpuscular volume; TIBC = total iron-binding capacity; N/A = not applicable.

important to determine the source of the deficiency. Schilling's test is the first test normally done. In this test, 1 mg of unlabeled cobalamin is administered parenterally to saturate TC I, II, and III. The patient is then given 1 μg of ^{57}Co-labeled cobalamin orally, and urine is collected for 48 hours. If less than 10% of the oral dose is retrieved in the urine, the patient has not absorbed the cobalamin, and the test is repeated in the presence of oral IF. If the yield of radioactive cobalamin in the urine increases to more than 10%, the findings are consistent with a lack of normal intrinsic factor activity. If the yield of cobalamin remains low, this is consistent with a decrease in absorption from the terminal ileum, for instance. If the test results are normal in the face of documented low serum cobalamin levels, protein-bound cobalamin can be used in the test to rule out food-bound cobalamin malabsorption, which may appear early in the development of pernicious anemia. A variety of conditions can cause false-positive or false-negative results.

Monitoring Therapy

A response to successful treatment with cobalamin or folate begins within 8 to 12 hours in the bone marrow, with resolution of megaloblastic hematopoiesis. The reticulocyte count begins to increase 2 to 3 days after treatment and peaks in 5 to 8 days; higher and later peaks occur in more severe anemia. The hematocrit begins to increase in approximately 1 week. Resolution of neurologic abnormalities is dependent on the duration of loss. Most neurologic symptoms will show maximal improvement within 6 months of initiation of therapy. Serum iron levels will begin to fall within 24 hours of successful treatment, but the patient must be observed over the next 2 to 3 weeks.

SUMMARY

Megaloblastic anemias can be classified into vitamin B$_{12}$ deficiencies and folic acid deficiencies.

Earlier studies suggested that pernicious anemia is restricted to Northern Europeans; however, newer studies report the disease in both blacks and Latin Americans. The median age at diagnosis is 60 years. Slightly more women than men are affected.

The term **megaloblastic** refers to the abnormal marrow erythrocyte precursor seen in processes, such as pernicious anemia, associated with altered DNA synthesis. Macrocytosis can occur in the absence of a megaloblastic process. For example, an increased MCV can result simply from an increase in the number of circulating reticulocytes, which are larger than mature erythrocytes. The most common disorder of cobalamin deficiency is pernicious anemia.

Pernicious anemia is immunologically related to an autoantibody to intrinsic factor, a serum inhibitor of intrinsic factor, and autoantibodies to parietal cells. A genetic predisposition to pernicious anemia is suggested by the clustering of the disease and of gastric autoantibodies in families, and by the association of the disease and gastric autoantibodies with autoimmune endocrinopathies.

Normal red cell maturation is dependent on many hematological factors, two of which are the vitamin B$_{12}$ coenzymes

(also called cobalamin) and folates. Macrocytic anemias and megaloblastic dyspoiesis occur when one of these factors is absent.

Red blood cells in megaloblastic anemia have an abnormal nuclear maturation and imbalance between nuclear and cytoplasmic maturation. The absence of vitamin B$_{12}$ or folates impairs DNA synthesis, which slows nuclear replication and delays each step of maturation. The premitotic interval is prolonged. This results in a large nucleus, increased cytoplasmic RNA, and early synthesis of hemoglobin. Many cells never undergo mitosis and breakdown in the bone marrow producing extremely increased levels of serum LDH.

In addition to dietary and other causes of deficiencies of cobalamin, a deficiency of TC II can produce a vitamin deficiency. Folic acid deficiencies appear to be less related to transport, but are typically associated with conditions of either dietary inadequacy or malabsorption syndromes.

In pernicious anemia, the deficiency is caused by reduced IF secondary to gastric atrophy. In the majority of cases of pernicious anemia, anti-IFs or antibodies to parietal cells (large cells on the margin of the peptic glands of the stomach) have been reported. Most authorities consider the demonstration of these antibodies to support the theory that pernicious anemia is an autoimmune disorder. The presence of IF-blocking antibodies is diagnostic of pernicious anemia.

Pernicious anemia is frequently seen in those of Northern European ancestry, with clinical presentation during the fourth or fifth decade of life.

Pernicious anemia, the most common megaloblastic anemia, is a prototype of the entire group. The hematological picture is the same whether the cause is vitamin B$_{12}$ or folic acid deficiency. However, supporting laboratory assays will differ for the various megaloblastic anemias.

CASE STUDY

CASE 1 A 50-year-old white woman had seen her physician, and reported having no energy and feeling tired all of the time. She also reported experiencing a mild pain in the abdominal region. The physician ordered a routine CBC.

Laboratory Data
The results of the blood count were as follows:

Hemoglobin 6.2 gm/dL
Hct 0.22 L/L
RBC 1.7 × 10^{12}/L
WBC 4.0 × 10^9/L

Her RBC indices were as follows:

MCV 129.4 fL
MCH 36.5 pg
MCHC 28%

The peripheral blood smear revealed anisocytosis, poikilocytosis, 3+ macrocytes, polychromatophilia, two nucleated RBCs (metarubricytes), rare Howell-Jolly bodies, and basophilic stippling. The platelet distribution appeared to be slightly decreased.

(continued)

On receipt of the laboratory data, the physician ordered the following additional tests: vitamin B_{12} and folate assays, reticulocyte count, serum iron and TIBC, serum bilirubin, and serum LDH. A fecal examination for occult blood was additionally ordered. The results of the tests were as follows:

Vitamin B_{12} 121 pmol/L (decreased)
Serum folate level normal
Reticulocyte count 0.4%
Serum iron and TIBC normal
Serum bilirubin 1.8 mg/dL (slightly increased)
Serum LDH over 3000 units (markedly increased)

The test for occult blood was negative, and a gastric analysis demonstrated an absence of hydrochloric acid.

Questions
1. What category of anemia is suggested by the hematological findings in this case?
2. What specific kind of anemia can be diagnosed based on the laboratory findings?
3. What is the etiology and physiological process in this anemia?

Discussion
1. The increased RBC size as seen on the peripheral blood (macrocytes) and the increased MCV indicate a macrocytic-megaloblastic-type anemia.
2. The two most common megaloblastic anemias are pernicious anemia and folic acid deficiency. Supporting laboratory assays can differentiate between these two types of anemia. In this case, a decreased vitamin B_{12} level, normal folic acid level, markedly increased LDH level, and absence of hydrochloric acid in the stomach support the diagnosis of pernicious anemia.
3. Many drugs can cause megaloblastic anemia by interfering with DNA synthesis, functioning as folic acid antagonists, or inhibiting purine and pyrimidine synthesis. Classic pernicious anemia is a chronic disease with a familial incidence, although no clear pattern of genetic transmission exists. Pernicious anemia usually becomes apparent in mid-life or later. The macrocytosis in pernicious anemia is the result of a defect in nuclear maturation or DNA impairment. Because RNA synthesis is normal, the normal nuclear-cytoplasmic ratio is maturationally asynchronous. The disease complex includes atrophy of the gastric mucosa and changes due to the deficiency of vitamin B_{12}. atrophic gastric mucosa secretes neither IF nor hydrochloric acid. A few patients have antibodies to IF in their gastric juice and serum. This antibody condition causes a failure in the absorption of vitamin B_{12} even if it is available.

✐ **Diagnosis: Megaloblastic anemia (pernicious anemia)**

BIBLIOGRAPHY

Harriman, G. R. et al. "Vitamin B_{12} Malabsorption in Patients With Acquired Immunodeficiency Syndrome." *Arch. Intern. Med.,* Vol. 149, September, 1989, pp. 2039–2041.
Hillman, R. S. and C. A. Finch. *Red Cell Manual* (7th ed.). Philadelphia: F. A. Davis, 1996.
Jandl, J. *Blood.* Boston: Little, Brown & Co., 1987, pp. 192–204.
Kapadia, C. and R. M. Donaldson. "Disorders of Cobalamin (Vitamin B_{12}) Absorption and Transport." *Ann. Rev. Med.,* Vol. 36, 1985, pp. 93–110.
Toh, Ban-Hock et al. "Pernicious Anemia." *N. Engl. J. Med.,* Vol 337, No. 20, November 13, 1997, pp. 1441–1448.
Turgeon, M. L. *Immunology and Serology in Laboratory Medicine* (2nd ed.). St. Louis: Mosby–Year Book, 1996.

REVIEW QUESTIONS

1. Megaloblastic anemias can be due to:

   A. Tapeworm infestation. C. Nutritional deficiency.
   B. Gastric resection. D. All of the above.

2. Megaloblastic anemia related to folic acid deficiency is associated with:

   A. Abnormal absorption. C. Nutritional deficiency.
   B. Increased utilization. D. All of the above.

3. The underlying gastritis that causes pernicious anemia is immunologically related to:

   A. Autoantibody to intrinsic factor.
   B. A serum inhibitor of intrinsic factor.
   C. Autoantibody to parietal cells.
   D. All of the above.

4. Cobalamin transport is mediated by:

   A. Intrinsic factor. C. R proteins.
   B. Transcobalamin II. D. All of the above.

5. In megaloblastic anemia, the typical erythrocytic indices are:

   A. MCV increased, MCH increased, and MCHC normal.
   B. MCV increased, MCH variable, and MCHC normal.
   C. MCV increased, MCH decreased, and MCHC normal.
   D. MCV normal, MCH increased, and MCHC normal.

6. The peripheral erythrocyte morphology in folate deficiency compares to that of pernicious anemia, the RBCs are:

   A. Small.
   B. Normal size.
   C. Large.

7. In a case of classic pernicious anemia, the patient has:

   A. Leukopenia.
   B. Hypersegmented neutrophils.
   C. Anemia.
   D. All of the above.

8. The reticulocyte count in a patient with untreated pernicious anemia is characteristically:

   A. 0%. C. Less than 1.0%.
   B. 0.3%. D. About 1.8%.

Questions 9 through 15: match the following clinical chemistry assays with their expected value in pernicious anemia:

9. ___ Serum haptoglobin-
    binding capacity.

10. ___ Serum B_{12}.

11. ___ Folate.

12. ___ Serum iron.

13. ___ Percent transferrin.

14. ___ Serum lactic dehydroge-
    nase (LDH).

15. ___ Unconjugated bilirubin.

A. Decreased.

B. Normal.

C. Increased.

D. Markedly increased.

Hemolytic Anemias

OBJECTIVES

Hemolytic anemia
- Define the term **hemolytic anemia.**
- Name two categories of inherited hemolytic disorders.
- Explain the basis of structural membrane defects.
- Name and discuss five types or varieties of membrane defects.
- Explain the nature of erythrocytic enzyme defects.
- Name and briefly explain three categories of acquired hemolytic anemia.
- Name three types of autoimmune hemolytic anemia.
- Give an example of isoimmune hemolytic anemia.
- Name four mechanisms of drug-induced hemolytic anemia.

- Describe the physiology of hemolytic anemia.
- Explain typical laboratory findings in hemolytic anemia.

Paroxysmal nocturnal hemoglobinemia (PNH)
- Characterize the etiology of PNH.
- Explain the physiology of PNH.
- Describe the clinical signs and symptoms of PNH.
- Discuss the laboratory findings in PNH.
- Briefly describe the treatment protocol of PNH.

Case studies
- Apply knowledge of characteristics, physiology, clinical signs and symptoms, laboratory findings, and treatment to the presented case studies.

HEMOLYTIC ANEMIAS

The common denominator in hemolytic anemia is an increase in red cell destruction initiated primarily by trapping of cells in sinuses of the spleen or liver and producing a decrease in the normal average life span of the erythrocyte. Increased bone marrow activity may compensate temporarily for this reduction. However, when the bone marrow fails to increase the production of erythrocytes to offset the loss of cells due to hemolysis, an anemia develops. Most anemias have a hemolytic component—even in the anemias of marrow failure, the red cell is somewhat defective. This is particularly evident in the case of dyserythropoietic syndromes, megaloblastic anemias, and thalassemias (Chapter 13).

Hemolytic disruption of the red cell involves an alteration in the erythrocytic membrane. The causes of this membrane alteration can be divided into inherited hemolytic disorders, an **intrinsic hemolytic anemia;** and acquired hemolytic disorders where a factor outside of the red blood cell acts on it, an **extrinsic hemolytic anemia**. Further subdivisions within each classification are based on the causative mechanism. The terms **intravascular** and **extravascular hemolysis** refer to the site of destruction of the red blood cell, within the circulating blood or outside of it, respectively.

Inherited Hemolytic Anemia

Etiology

Inherited hemolytic disorders may affect the basic membrane structure, the erythrocytic enzymes, or the hemoglobin molecules within the red cell. Table 12.1 outlines selected examples of the genetically based hemolytic anemias.

Structural Membrane Defects

Primary defects of the red cell membrane head the list as a matter of taxonomy, not of prevalence. Most membrane defects result from genetic aberrations of cytoskeletal components, some represent rare disorders of cation permeability, and others arise from abnormalities of the lipid bilayer or integral membrane proteins. Genetic aberrations of nearly half of these skeletal and integral proteins are associated with hereditary hemolytic anemias. Inherited abnormalities in the skeletal protein network of the red cell membrane can produce decreased membrane stability, decreased cell flexibility, and deviations from the normal discoid shape. Loss of membrane is another related disturbance. Membrane defects are commonly related to structural or quantitative defects in the skeletal protein, spectrin, or to abnormalities in the membrane's association with the other skeletal proteins. Cell membrane instability and decreased flexibility cause red cells to be removed from the circulation by the spleen. If the rate of hemolysis exceeds the erythropoietic compensatory mechanism of the bone marrow, anemia can result.

Examples of disorders in which skeletal protein defects have been described include hereditary spherocytosis and a variant, hereditary pyropoikilocytosis; hereditary elliptocytosis; and hereditary stomatocytosis. Another disorder in this grouping is hereditary xerocytosis.

Hereditary spherocytosis (HS) is transmitted in the majority of cases as an autosomal dominant trait; it is the most common prevalent hereditary hemolytic anemia among people of Northern European descent, although it is not restricted to any single race. Manifestations of the disorder range from almost-normal carriers of the trait to cases of severe hemolytic anemia. Anemia may manifest itself anytime, from early infancy to later life.

The underlying defect in HS is intrinsic to the red cell. Hemolysis is extravascular, occurring only in the presence of the spleen. In HS, secondary to membrane loss, the cell has a decreased surface-area-to-volume ratio, which changes the shape of the cell from discoid to spherocyte. Spherocytes have reduced cellular flexibility. The underlying mechanism of hemolysis is probably due to physical fragmentation of the membrane, however, contraction of the membrane surface by another mechanism is a possibility. A deficiency of spectrin and defective binding of spectrin to band 4.1 or some other cytoskeletal abnormality may be present. Spherocytic cells demonstrate an abnormal permeability to sodium ion (Na^+), causing an influx of sodium at 10 times the normal rate.

Some patients have compensated hemolytic disease, no anemia, little or no jaundice, and slight splenomegaly. Other patients may be severely anemic. Hemoglobin concentration can range from normal to decreased. Peripheral blood smears demonstrate spherocytes. The mean corpuscular volume (MCV) is normal or slightly decreased. The mean corpuscular hemoglobin (MCH) is normal but the mean corpuscular hemoglobin concentration (MCHC) is generally greater than 36%. Spherocytes are responsible for an increased MCHC. The osmotic fragility test is useful in diagnosis of this disorder.

Splenectomy corrects the anemia and hemolysis in severely afflicted patients but the basic membrane defect remains. Spherocytes can still be found. Some asplenic persons are at increased risk for life-threatening and fatal bacterial infections. Splenectomy carries a substantial risk for sepsis in children and adults (2.2% mortality).

TABLE 12.1 **Examples of Inherited Hemolytic Anemias**

Structural Membrane Defects
Acanthocytosis
Hereditary spherocytosis
Hereditary elliptocytosis
Hereditary stomatocytosis
Hereditary xerocytosis
Rh_{null} disease

Erythrocytic Enzyme Defects
Glucose-6-phosphate dehydrogenase (G6PD) deficiency
Glutathione reductase
Hexokinase
Pyruvate kinase

Defects of the Hemoglobin Molecule
Hb C disorder
Hb S-C disorder
Hb S-S disorder (sickle cell anemia)
Thalassemia

Hereditary elliptocytosis (HE) represents a comparatively common heterogeneous group of inborn disorders characterized by an overabundance of red blood cells and in some by a hemolytic process. HE and a closely related subtype of HE, hereditary pyropoikilocytosis (HPP), are caused by defects in the membrane skeleton.

HE is usually transmitted by a single (dominant) autosomal gene. In its homozygous form it may produce a severe hemolytic anemia in infancy. The heterozygous form may or may not show hemolysis.

Nine clinical variants of HE have been delineated, but these have been consolidated into three major categories based on the grounds of clinical severity and red cell morphology: common HE, spherocytic elliptocytosis, and stomatocytic elliptocytosis.

Spherocytic HE is a unique subset of elliptocytosis caused by dual inheritance of two nonallelic genes: one for mild HE and one for mild HS. This phenotypic hybrid is responsible for about 15% to 20% of HE cases in white families of European origin. The clinical course mimics that of conventional HS.

Stomatocytic HE is a unique variant peculiar to Melanesia and neighboring island groups. The red cells are only moderately oblong, and many of them display a transverse bridge of hemoglobin that connects with the opposite rim to create two central areas of pallor. Hemolysis is mild or absent.

The most prominent peripheral blood smear finding in HE is an increase in oval and elongated red cells (elliptocytes) to greater than 25% of the red blood cell population. A defect of the membrane cytoskeleton causes the elliptical red cell form and it is acquired in the circulation. In addition, the membrane may fragment under the stresses of circulation. Moderate weakening causes elliptocytosis, but severe weakening causes membrane fragmentation and elliptocytosis.

Several different membrane molecular defects are suspected as causes. Of the known mutations, the most common is a functional defect of tetramer assembly of varying degrees due to decreased association of spectrin dimers and tetramers, caused by defective spectrin chains. Other abnormalities may include a deficiency in band 4.1, which binds spectrin to actin, and various abnormal interactions among several membrane proteins, including defective binding of ankyrin of integral protein.

Cells have a nearly normal life span. A very small proportion (10%) of patients with common HE have significant chronic hemolytic anemia. If membrane fragmentation exists, the life span is shortened. In addition, red cells are abnormally permeable to sodium ion (Na^+).

Most patients show little or no hemolysis. No anemia exists if the hemolysis is compensated for by erythropoiesis. However, a variant in black infants is associated with moderately severe anemia at birth and neonatal jaundice.

In symptomatic patients, splenectomy may be indicated. This will prevent hemolysis and protect the patient from chronic hemolysis, but the elliptocytes will remain.

Hereditary pyropoikilocytosis (HPP) is a rare autosomal recessive disorder, representing a subset of common HE, seen primarily in blacks. It is manifested in infancy or early childhood as a severe hemolytic anemia with marked poikilocytosis. As the name of the disorder implies, bizarre red cell shapes are evident when a peripheral blood smear is examined. MCV values range from 55–74 fL because of the prevalence of microspherocytes and red blood cell fragments. This multiformity of the poikilocytosis is unmatched in any other hemolytic disease.

Hereditary stomatocytosis can be seen in the genetic hemoglobin defect, thalassemia, and in lead poisoning, hereditary spherocytosis, and alcoholic cirrhosis. The cellular appearance stems from a cation abnormality, because the erythrocytes contain increased sodium (Na^+) and decreased potassium (K^+). The specific membrane abnormality has not been identified, but abnormal membrane permeability has been implicated in the pathogenesis of hereditary stomatocytosis. Because the intracellular osmolality is exceeded and the intracellular concentration of cations increases, water enters the cell and overhydrated red cells take on the appearance of stomatocytes or red cells with a slit, mouthlike opening. The cells are uniconcave. The MCHC is usually decreased and the MCV may be increased.

Anemia is usually mild to moderate. Bilirubin is increased and reticulocytosis is moderate. Peripheral blood smears have 10% to 50% stomatocytes. Osmotic fragility and autohemolysis are increased. Autohemolysis is partially corrected with glucose and ATP. Splenectomy yields variable responses.

In addition, Rh null disease is also associated with the presence of stomatocytes. The lack of the Rh complex and stomatocytic membrane abnormality has not been explained.

Hereditary xerocytosis is a permeability disorder. In vitro, the thermal instability of spectrin suggests a defect in qualitative spectrin abnormality. The net loss of intracellular K^+ exceeds the passive Na^+ influx, yielding a net Na^+ gain. This causes the red cell to dehydrate. The MCHC increases and the red cell appears contracted and spiculated. When the MCHC increases beyond 37%, cytoplasmic viscosity increases and cellular deformability decreases. Rigid red cells are trapped in the spleen and removed from the circulation.

Peripheral blood smears demonstrate budding, fragments, microspherocytes, and bizarre red cell fragments. The osmotic fragility test is abnormal, especially after incubation. Autohemolysis is increased and the hemolysis is not corrected with glucose.

Rh$_{null}$ Disease

Rh$_{null}$ disease, or Rh deficiency syndrome is a rare hereditary disorder causing mild, compensated chronic hemolytic anemia. This disorder is associated with stomatocytosis, spherocytosis, and the deletion of all Rh-Hr determinants including the Landsteiner-Weiner (LW) antigen from the red blood cells. Rh$_{null}$ cells are abnormally permeable to K^+ and partly compensate for this leakiness and the resultant cation deficiency by reinforcing the number and activity of Na-K-ATPase pumps. The abnormal red cell morphology may be related to the increased K^+ leak rate. The resulting anemia is mild but variable. Typically the hemoglobin concentration is between 11 and 13 gm/dL and reticulocytes are moderately increased. Many of the red blood cells are spheroidal or stomatocytic. Hemoglobin F are often elevated.

Acanthocytosis

Acanthocytes are dense contracted or spheroidal red blood cells with multiple thorny projections or spicules. Acanthocytes are prevalent in two very different constitutional disorders: a betalipoproteinemia and spur cell anemia. A betalipoproteinemia is a rare derangement of lipid metabolism resulting from a genetic inability to synthesize apolipoprotein B (apoB), the protein that coats chylomicrons. Most red cell membrane lipids are in exchange equilibrium with the corresponding plasma lipoprotein lipids. Acanthocytes are a manifestation of the profound disturbances in plasma lipoprotein levels found in this disorder.

Young children may develop a moderate anemia but adults suffer from only a mild anemia. The MCV, MCH, MCHC, and osmotic fragility are normal.

Spur Cell Hemolytic Anemia

This form of acanthocyte-associated hemolytic anemia is seen in patients with established alcoholic cirrhosis. Approximately 5–10% of patients will develop a fatal hemolytic process. Hemolysis usually becomes severe and may necessitate maintenance transfusions. In most patients the hemoglobin concentrations level off at 5–7 gm/dL. Reticulocyte counts fluctuate between 10 and 20% and ^{51}Cr-labeled red cell half-life survival may be as short as 5 to 6 days. Maintenance blood transfusions are common therapy.

Other causes of acanthocytosis can include neonatal hepatitis, infantile pyknocytosis, the McLeod blood group, and severe malnutrition, e.g., anorexia nervosa.

Erythrocytic Enzyme Defects

Like the structural membrane defects, erythrocytic enzyme defects are inherited. The clinical effects of these enzymopathies vary widely. Some individuals manifest no hematological abnormalities, but the erythrocytes share the abnormality that produces a malfunction in other tissues. Certain inborn or genetic errors may produce hematological disorders other than hemolytic anemia. In a number of erythrocytic enzyme defects, such as deficiencies in hexokinase, glucose-phosphate isomerase, and pyruvate kinase, the sole clinical manifestation is hemolytic anemia. Many genetic enzyme errors cause multisystem disease with a hemolytic syndrome as one component.

The hemolytic anemia, glucose-6-phosphate dehydrogenase (G6PD) deficiency, is related to drug intake or oxidant stress in some individuals with this defect. Drugs such as primaquine can induce a hemolytic episode in about 10% of American black males, while the drugs chloramphenicol, quinine, and quinidine and the legume fava beans can precipitate a hemolytic incident in nonblacks.

All of the enzyme defects in this category are inherited. Some of them, such as G6PD deficiency, are sex-linked. G6PD is regulated by a mutant gene on the X chromosome and is inherited as an incomplete dominant trait. Full expression of the trait is seen in homozygous males. In females, full expression of the disorder occurs when two mutant genes are inherited. If only one mutant gene is inherited by a female (heterozygous), two populations of red blood cells exist. One population of red blood cells has a normal enzyme content; the other red blood cells are G6PD-deficient.

The erythrocyte, unlike other body cells, cannot compensate for an unstable enzyme. The absence of organelles to carry out oxidative phosphorylation on a compensatory basis creates unique problems for the red cells. The enzyme G6PD catalyzes this reaction:

$$\text{Glucose-6-phosphate} + \text{NADP} \xrightarrow{\text{G-6-PD}}$$
$$\text{6-phosphogluconate} + \text{NADPH}$$

This is the first step in the pentose-phosphate pathway (aerobic-glycolytic pathway). NADPH (nicotinamide-adenine dinucleotide phosphate) produced by this reaction is an important intracellular reducing agent. An excess intermediate product, oxidized glutathione, accumulates in the red cell because of the absence of NADPH and forms insoluble complexes with hemoglobin that result in Heinz body formation.

Laboratory findings in this disorder include a quantitatively decreased level of G6PD, a positive autohemolysis test result, and the presence of Heinz bodies on peripheral blood smears prepared for Heinz body screening. Heinz bodies are not visible on routinely stained, Wright stain preparations.

Acquired Hemolytic Anemia

Etiology

The acquired hemolytic anemias can be classified according to the agent or condition responsible for inducing the hemolysis. Selected examples of agents and conditions associated with acquired hemolytic anemias are presented in Table 12.2.

A major distinction exists between acute hemolysis of red cells, which result from damage done directly to the cell membrane, and hemolytic anemias caused by immunologic responses.

Chemicals, Drugs, and Venoms

Intravascular hemolysis can result from exposure to environmental agents and conditions. Fortunately, the destruction of red cells usually ceases when the conditions no longer exist. This is in contrast to congenital membrane defects, which are continuous. Lead from gasoline, paint, or other industrial products directly interferes with ATP production and inhibits heme synthesis.

Quinine sensitivity is a new, unusual cause of hemolytic uremic syndrome. Adult hemolytic uremic syndrome of acute onset with accompanying microangiopathic hemolytic anemia, thrombocytopenia, renal failure, neutropenia, and low-grade disseminated intravascular coagulation has been observed. Quinine, in one case in tonic water, was implicated by the finding of quinine-dependent antibodies reactive with platelets, granulocytes, and erythrocytes in patient serum.

This recently described syndrome can occur with or without associated disseminated intravascular coagulation or granulocytopenia. Only a small percentage of patients taking quinidine and quinine have this sensitivity (quinine and quinidine appear to do so more often than other agents). Platelets are the preferred target for drug-induced antibodies but granulocytes, erythrocytes, and probably other tissues are sometimes affected. Patients usually recover spontaneously when the provoking drug is withdrawn. The mechanism by which drugs promote selective binding of these immunoglobulins to target glycoproteins is not fully understood, but evidence suggests that the inciting medications bind reversibly to specific protein domains to form complexes or to induce conformational changes (neoantigens) for which the antibodies are specific. Deposition of fibrin in glomeruli and renal failure are characteristic features of the hemolytic uremic syndrome. Plasminogen-activator inhibitor type 1 (PAI-1) is believed to be the circulating inhibitor of fibrinolysis in the hemolytic uremic syndrome.

TABLE 12.2 Examples of Agents and Conditions Associated With Acquired Hemolytic Anemias

Chemicals, Drugs, Venoms
Aniline

Copper (Wilson's disease)

Lead from gasoline or paint

Naphthalene (found in moth balls)

Nitrobenzene

Phenacetin

Phenol derivatives

Resorcinol

Sulfonamides

Infectious Microorganisms
Bacteria: *Clostridium* sp., cholera, *E. coli* 0157:H7, typhoid fever

Protozoa: *Leishmania,* malaria (*Plasmodium* sp.), toxoplasmosis

Immune Mechanisms (Antibodies)
Autoimmune anemia due to cold-reactive antibodies
   Cold hemagglutinin disease
      Idiopathic or secondary
   Paroxysmal cold hemoglobinuria

Autoimmune anemia due to warm-reactive antibodies
   Drug-induced
   Idiopathic
   Secondary
      Lymphoproliferative disorders (chronic lymphocytic leukemia, malignancies, systemic lupus erythematosus, viruses)

Hemolytic disease of the newborn

Incompatible blood transfusion

Paroxysmal nocturnal hemoglobinuria

Physical Agents
Severe burns

Traumatic and Microangiopathic Hemolytic Anemias
Disseminated intravascular coagulation (DIC)

E. coli 0157:H7

Hemolytic-uremic syndrome

Prosthetic cardiac valves

Thrombotic thrombocytopenia purpura

Venoms from some types of snakes contain hemolysins that can produce intravascular hemolysis and also initiate disseminated intravascular coagulation.

Infectious Microorganisms

Several mechanisms of infectious organisms cause destruction of red cells. The intraerythrocytic protozoa, for example, malaria, rupture red cells. In some cases, such as *Clostridium perfringens,* hemolytic toxin is released from bacteria. In other cases, extravascular hemolysis can be caused by infectious agents such as *Bartonella.*

A significant infectious cause of hemolytic-uremic syndrome was discovered a decade ago. *Escherichia coli O157:H7* has emerged as a major cause of both sporadic cases and outbreaks of diarrhea in North America. The first report was associated with consumption of undercooked ground beef from a chain of fast-food restaurants. Little was known about the pathophysiology, epidemiology, or clinical sequelae of infection with *E. coli O157:H7*. Several studies have shown that infection with *E. coli O157:H7* is responsible for most cases of the hemolytic-uremic syndrome, which is a major cause of acute renal failure in children. This microorganism is estimated to cause more than 20,000 infections and as many as 250 deaths each year. Shiga toxins 1, 2, or both cause microangiopathic hemolytic anemia as a result of endothelial cell injury.

Immune Mechanisms (Antibodies)

A wide variety of disorders of acquired hemolytic anemia result from immune mechanisms. In these disorders, red blood cell survival is reduced because of the deposition of immunoglobulin or complement, or both, on the red blood cell membrane. The immune hemolytic anemias can be grouped according to the presence of autoantibodies, isoantibodies, or drug-related antibodies (Table 12.3).

Autoimmune anemias can be due to cold-reactive or warm-reactive antibodies. Other types of disorders in this category include hemolytic disease of the newborn, incompatible blood transfusion, and paroxysmal nocturnal hemoglobinuria.

Autoimmune Hemolytic Anemias (AIHA)

The AIHAs are caused by an altered immune response resulting in production of antibody against the patient's own red blood cells, with subsequent hemolysis. The cause of autoantibody production is unknown. Suggested mechanisms include infectious agents, e.g., *Mycoplasma pneumoniae,* or anti-i in the serum of patients with infectious mononucleosis. Development of AIHA in patients with lymphoproliferative or autoimmune disorders may be related to some abnormality with B cells, T cells, macrophages, or the interaction between these cells.

Warm-Type Autoimmune Hemolytic Anemia

In warm-type AIHA, there is IgG coating of red blood cells with or without complement fixation. Autoantibodies are usually directed at Rh antigens but also can be anti-U, anti-LW, anti-Kell, and Jk^a or Fy^a.

TABLE 12.3 Classification of Immune Hemolytic Anemia

Autoimmune hemolytic anemias
Associated with warm-type antibodies

Associated with cold-type antibodies

Both warm- and cold-type antibodies

Isoimmune Hemolytic Anemias
Hemolytic disease of the newborn
   Rh incompatibility
   ABO incompatibility

Drug-Induced Hemolytic Anemia
Adsorption of immune complexes to red cell membrane

Adsorption of drug to red cell membrane

Induction of autoantibody to drugs

Nonimmunologic adsorption of immunoglobulin to red blood cell membrane

Clearance of the red blood cell occurs mostly in the spleen. In the absence of complement fixation, it appears that the Fc portion of the IgG immunoglobulin bound to the red blood cell interacts with the Fc receptor present on the membrane of splenic macrophages. Therefore, sensitized red blood cells are retained, phagocytosed, or fragmented by splenic macrophages during their passage through the spleen.

A moderate to severe anemia can result. Peripheral blood smears frequently exhibit spherocytosis, schistocytes, polychromasia, and nucleated red blood cells. The percentage of reticulocytes is high in approximately half of affected patients.

The clinical course of patients with warm-type AIHA is characterized by periods of remissions and relapse. In secondary AIHA, the course and prognosis are related to the nature of the underlying disease. In idiopathic AIHA, the complications can be severe and fatal.

Cold-Type Autoimmune Hemolytic Anemia

In AIHA associated with cold-type autoantibody, e.g., cold hemagglutinin disease, the red blood cells are usually coated with IgM immunoglobulin. The antibody is usually anti-I. Complement fixation occurs frequently. If the entire complement system is activated, intravascular hemolysis can occur. Extravascular hemolysis can occur if complement activation is incomplete and no lysis of the red blood cells occurs.

IgG immunoglobulin can be a cause in cases of paroxysmal cold hemoglobinuria.

Warm-and-Cold-Type Autoimmune Hemolytic Anemia

AIHA associated with both warm and cold autoantibodies is mediated by IgG warm antibodies and complement as well as IgM cold hemagglutinins. A high percentage of patients also suffer from systemic lupus erythematosus.

Isoimmune Hemolytic Anemia

This form of anemia usually occurs in newborn infants because of transplacental passage of maternal antibodies directed toward antigens of the baby's cells. Isoimmune hemolytic anemia is most commonly the result of ABO incompatibility between mother and baby, e.g., the mother is group O whereas the baby is group A.

Drug-Induced Immune Hemolytic Anemia

Immune hemolytic anemia may occur following the administration of drugs, e.g., insulin, antihistamines, and sulfonamides. The drug-induced antibody is usually IgM and usually fixes complement which results in hemolysis.

Physical Agents

Hemolysis occurs within 24 hours of suffering severe burns. Because the red cells become fragile after exposure to heat, they form fragments and microspheres. These structures are removed by the spleen, with a subsequent rapid drop in the circulating red cell volume.

Trauma

Disseminated intravascular coagulation (DIC) is an example of a traumatic or microangiopathic hemolytic anemia. DIC is a consumptive coagulopathy that involves depositions of microthrombi in the blood vessels. These depositions form surfaces that damage circulating red cells. Traumatic injury due to repeated impact of the capillary bed produces red cell damage in **march anemia,** a condition diagnosed in soldiers after intense marches. Damage to capillary beds can also be seen in long-distance runners and individuals who perform high-impact sports.

Physiology

The normal erythrocyte has an average life span of 120 days. As the red cell becomes older, membrane changes occur and the cell is phagocytized. Most red cell destruction (80% to 90%) is presumed to be extravascular, within macrophages of the mononuclear phagocyte system of the liver and spleen. The red cell membrane and hemoglobin become separated. The red cell membrane remnants are phagocytized and eventually leave the body.

Hemoglobin is then further reduced into its two major components: heme and globin. The globin portion is further reduced to its constituent amino acids. Although some of the amino acids are further catabolized, most of the amino acids become part of the circulating amino acid pool and are reused in the synthesis of new proteins. The heme portion is broken down into iron, carbon monoxide, and biliverdin. Most of the iron will be recycled into new molecules of hemoglobin. Biliverdin will be converted to bilirubin. After entry into the plasma portion of the circulating blood as unconjugated bilirubin, being bound to albumin, and being transported to the liver where it is converted to conjugated bilirubin, it is finally excreted into the biliary system.

When red blood cell destruction is increased, the formation of unconjugated bilirubin exceeds the ability of the liver to conjugate it. This condition will produce elevated levels of unconjugated bilirubin in the blood plasma, and jaundice may result.

Some normal erythrocyte catabolism occurs intravascularly. In this situation, free hemoglobin is released into the blood plasma and is rapidly bound to the glycoprotein haptoglobin. This large molecular complex of hemoglobin and haptoglobin cannot pass through the renal glomeruli. Most of the molecular complex is taken up by the liver, whereas some is taken by the bone marrow.

If the amount of intravascular hemoglobin increases, all of the available haptoglobin will become saturated. Remaining free hemoglobin continues to circulate in the plasma and may dissociate into smaller components capable of passing through the glomeruli. If these smaller hemoglobin components are not reabsorbed by the proximal tubular cells of the kidney, the hemoglobin will be excreted in the urine (hemoglobinuria).

Laboratory Findings

The patient with hemolytic anemia will have a decreased hemoglobin, Hct, and red blood cell count. Blood smear examination will typically reveal the presence of many spherocytic erythrocytes (see Plate 15). Other red cell abnormalities may include acanthocytes, schistocytes, stomatocytes, polychromatophilia, target cells, and early erythroid forms such as metarubricytes.

TABLE 12.4 Typical Profile of Quantitative Laboratory Findings in the Hemolytic Anemias

Test	Result
Hemoglobin, hematocrit, RBC count	Decreased
Serum haptoglobin	Decreased
RBC survival (^{51}Cr)	Decreased
Lactic dehydrogenase (LDH) isoenzymes (LD$_1$ and LD$_2$)	Increased
Bilirubin (total)	Usually increased
Antiglobulin test	Positive or negative

RBC = red blood cell.

Other hematological tests can include a reticulocyte count, which is usually increased unless hematopoiesis is suppressed, and an osmotic fragility test, which will show increased fragility as a result of the presence of spherocytes.

Supporting laboratory tests can include:

The antiglobulin (AHG) (direct and indirect) test
Occult blood screening (to rule out bleeding)
Measurement of total serum haptoglobin level—decreased in hemolysis
Serum bilirubin determination
Measurements of serum LDH levels (LD isoenzymes)—increased LD$_1$ and LD$_2$
Chromium 51 red cell survival studies
Bone marrow studies
Determinations of G6PD values
Heinz body preparation

Tables 12.4 and 12.5 give, respectively, the typical laboratory findings in a hemolytic anemia and the supplementary tests that may be needed to establish a differential diagnosis.

PAROXYSMAL NOCTURNAL HEMOGLOBINURIA

Etiology

Paroxysmal nocturnal hemoglobinuria (PNH) is an acquired intravascular hemolytic disorder characterized by intermittent (paroxysmal) sleep-associated (nocturnal) blood in the urine (hemoglobinuria). PNH is a very complex disease that is more common than originally thought. It is an acquired clonal disorder associated with a somatic mutation in a pluri-

TABLE 12.5 Differential Testing in the Hemolytic Anemias

Antibody or drug identification, if direct antiglobulin test is positive
Bone marrow examination
Coagulation profile
Glucose-6-phosphate dehydrogenase (G6PD) screening
Major organ evaluations (renal or hepatic)
Lipoprotein electrophoresis

potent hematopoietic stem cell. Erythroid, myeloid, megakaryocytic, and some lymphoid lineage is involved in PNH.

This disorder is sometimes classified as a chronic myeloproliferative syndrome because of its potential to transform into acute leukemia or one of the myelodysplastic syndromes. But clinically, the disorder manifests itself and is sometimes classified as a chronic hemolytic anemia.

In this rare disorder, a red cell defect renders one population of red cells markedly sensitive to complement. Some patients with PNH suffer from chronic hemolysis that is not associated with sleep, and manifest no obvious hemoglobinuria.

In this disorder, mutations in a gene termed PIG-A result in the failure to present a large class of proteins on the hematopoietic cell surface. These proteins share a unique linkage to the surface membrane through a glycolipid structure called the glycosylphosphatidylinositol anchor. Some glycosylphosphatidylinositol-linked proteins inactivate complement on the red cell surface. This explains the characteristic intravascular hemolysis in the syndrome, but the biochemical basis of marrow failure in patients with PNH is unknown. Some observations have suggested that clones emerge because they are favored by certain extrinsic conditions. Patients may harbor clones with different PIG-A gene mutations, a finding consistent with the independent proliferation of genetically altered hematopoietic stem cells under some selective pressure.

Epidemiology

Twenty-five percent of cases will evolve into or from aplastic anemia. Approximately 5% to 10% of patients will have terminal acute myelogenous leukemia.

The median age of patients at diagnosis is 42 years (range 16 to 75 years). Median survival after diagnosis is 10 years. Spontaneous long-term remission can occur.

Physiology

The red cell defect is an intrinsic defect that is probably related to structural or biochemical defects of the cell membrane. The degree of hemolysis varies as a consequence of the proportion of abnormal stem cells.

PNH begins insidiously in patients between the age of 30 and 60 years. Irregular episodes of hemoglobinuria associated with sleep are a startling manifestation of this disorder.

Clinical Signs and Symptoms

Clinical manifestations include chronic hemolysis, thrombosis, recurrent infections, and a tendency toward bone marrow aplasia.

The leading cause of death in PNH is thrombosis, but related late-developing bacterial and fungal infections can also be life-threatening events.

Laboratory Findings

Most patients suffer from a severe anemia with hemoglobin concentrations below 6 gm/dL. Peripheral blood smears may reveal hypochromic, microcytic red cells if an iron deficiency state has developed owing to cell lysis. Autohemolysis is increased after 48 hours and hemolysis may increase with the addition of glucose to the test. Both the sucrose hemolysis (sugar-water) and Ham test (acid-serum lysis) are useful diagnostic procedures (see Chapter 24). Hemosiderinuria, the excretion of an iron-containing pigment derived from hemoglobin on disintegration of red cells, is a classic manifestation of chronic intravascular hemolysis.

Treatment

Patients have an average life expectancy of more than 10 years. Treatment includes blood transfusion therapy, antibiotics, and anticoagulants. If an induced marrow aplasia exists and the patient is younger than 50 years of age, bone marrow transplantation may be considered.

SUMMARY

The common denominator in hemolytic anemia is an increase in red cell destruction and a decrease in the normal average life span of the erythrocyte. Increased bone marrow activity may compensate temporarily for this reduction. However, when the bone marrow fails to increase the production of erythrocytes to offset the loss of cells due to hemolysis, an anemia develops.

Hemolytic disruption of the red cell always involves an alteration in the erythrocytic membrane. The causes of this membrane alteration can be divided into inherited hemolytic disorders (an **intrinsic hemolytic anemia**) and acquired hemolytic disorders where a factor outside of the red blood cell acts on it (an **extrinsic hemolytic anemia**). Further subdivisions within each classification are based on the causative mechanism. The terms **intravascular** and **extravascular hemolysis** refer to the site of destruction of the red blood cell, within the circulating blood or outside of it, respectively.

Inherited hemolytic disorders may affect the basic membrane structure, the erythrocytic enzymes, or the hemoglobin molecules within the red cell.

A variety of membrane defects are inherited. These include **hereditary spherocytosis**, **hereditary elliptocytosis**, **hereditary stomatocytosis**, **hereditary pyropoikilocytosis**, and **hereditary xerocytosis.**

Like the structural membrane defects, erythrocytic enzyme defects are inherited. The clinical effects of these enzymopathies vary widely. In a number of erythrocytic enzyme defects, such as deficiencies in hexokinase, glucose-phosphate isomerase, and pyruvate kinase, the sole clinical manifestation is hemolytic anemia.

The acquired hemolytic anemias can be classified according to the agent or condition responsible for inducing the hemolysis. These categories include chemicals, drugs, and venoms; infectious organisms; immune or antibody causes; physical agents; and trauma.

Autoimmune anemias can be due to cold-reactive or warm-reactive antibodies. Other types of disorders in this category include hemolytic disease of the newborn, incompatible blood transfusion, and paroxysmal nocturnal hemoglobinuria (PNH).

Patients with hemolytic anemia will have a decreased hemoglobin, Hct, and red blood cell count. Blood smear examination will typically reveal the presence of many spherocytic erythrocytes. Other red cell abnormalities may include acanthocytes, schistocytes, stomatocytes, polychromatophilia, target cells, and early erythroid forms such as metarubricytes.

Paroxysmal nocturnal hemoglobinuria (PNH) is an acquired intravascular hemolytic disorder characterized by intermittent (paroxysmal) sleep-associated (nocturnal) blood in the urine (hemoglobinuria). PNH is a very complex disease that is more common than originally thought. This disorder is sometimes classified as a chronic myeloproliferative syndrome because of its potential to transform into acute leukemia or one of the myelodysplastic syndomes. But clinically, the disorder manifests itself and is sometimes classified as a chronic hemolytic anemia.

Most patients suffer from a severe anemia with hemoglobin concentrations below 6 gm/dL. Peripheral blood smears may reveal hypochromic, microcytic red cells if an iron deficiency state has developed due to cell lysis. Autohemolysis is increased after 48 hours and hemolysis may increase with the addition of glucose to the test. Both the sucrose hemolysis (sugar-water) and Ham test (acid-serum lysis) are useful diagnostic procedures.

C A S E   S T U D I E S

CASE 1   A 5-year-old white boy was admitted with the diagnosis of a fractured tibia following a playground accident. A CBC was ordered on admission.

Laboratory Data
The results of the admission CBC were as follows:

Hemoglobin 10.2 gm/dL
Hct 0.27 L/L
RBC 3.6×10^{12}/L
WBC 12.5×10^{9}/L

The RBC indices were as follows:

MCV 96.4 fL
MCH 28.3 pg
MCHC 38%

The peripheral blood smear revealed anisocytosis, some spherocytosis, and polychromatophilia. Platelet distribution was normal on the smear.

Following receipt of the CBC results, the boy's physician ordered a serum bilirubin, a direct and indirect AHG test, reticulocyte count, and an osmotic fragility test. The findings of these tests were as follows:

Total serum bilirubin 2.4 mg/dL
Reticulocyte count 2.0%
Negative findings on direct and indirect AHG test
Increased osmotic fragility

Questions
1. What category of anemia is suggested by the laboratory findings?
2. What is the most probable etiology of this patient's anemia?
3. Describe the mechanism responsible for the increased bilirubin result.

(continued)

Discussion

1. When the spherocytes in the peripheral blood film are coupled with the laboratory results of an increased reticulocyte count, increased bilirubin, decreased haptoglobin, and a negative direct AHG test, a diagnosis of chronic hemolytic anemia is suggested. The increased osmotic fragility further demonstrates that the RBCs have a decreased surface-area-to-volume ratio or spherocytic shape. These findings are reflective of most cases of chronic hemolytic anemia; however, in about 20 to 25% of patients, spherocytes are not evident.

2. The laboratory findings of anemia and spherocytosis, and the inability to demonstrate antibodies either in the circulating blood or adhering to the RBCs in vivo, coupled with the associated clinical findings of jaundice, splenomegaly, and skeletal changes in this child, suggest a congenital membrane defect. In this case, the diagnosis of hereditary spherocytosis, which occurs in at a frequency of 1 in 5000, was made.

3. This disorder is usually an autosomal dominant trait with a variable hemolytic process. Although the condition is usually corrected by splenectomy, the spherocytosis remains. Physiologically, a decrease in the lipid content of the RBC membrane has been described as the source of the spherocytes. A membrane lipid alteration affects the permeability of the cell membrane to sodium ion (Na^+). As a result of the lack of permeability, the sodium increases within the cell and, in turn, demands greater glycolytic enzyme adenosine triphosphatase (ATPase) activity. Adenosine triphosphate (ATP) is needed to help maintain the normal, discoid erythrocytic shape. If ATP depletion occurs, the stability of the membrane will be altered, and result in the formation of spherocytes. The spleen adversely affects RBCs. The erythrocytes must pass through the splenic cords, where the Hct is increased, and blood flow is slow. The amount of available glucose diminishes, and blood pH is lowered. These conditions place a metabolic stress on the RBC, which depletes ATP. In stressed cells, such as in hereditary spherocytosis, the membrane becomes more unstable and is lost more readily than normally.

✎ Diagnosis: Hereditary spherocytosis

CASE 2   A 44-year-old white woman was seen in the emergency room. She complained of fatigue and weakness. Over the last 2 weeks, she had noticed that the whites of her eyes and her skin were becoming yellowish-looking. On physical examination, the spleen was palpable. The emergency room physician ordered a CBC, serum bilirubin, and urinalysis.

Laboratory Data
The test findings were as follows:

Hemoglobin 8.5 gm/dL
Hct 0.27 L/L
RBC 3.0×10^{12}/L

The RBC indices were as follows:

MCV 90 fL
MCH 28.3 pg
MCHC 32%

The WBC count was 9.0×10^9/L. The peripheral blood smear was essentially normochromic and normocytic; however, moderate polychromatophilia, spherocytes, rare basophilic stippling, 2 metrubricytes/100 WBC, and rouleaux formation were noted. The distribution of platelets on the peripheral smear was normal. The total serum bilirubin was 4.2 mg/dL, and the patient's urine was pinkish-red.

The patient was admitted to the hospital. The following tests were ordered by her attending physician: reticulocyte count, direct and indirect AHG, and serum haptoglobin. These test results were as follows:

Reticulocyte count 13%
Direct AHG 3+
Indirect AHG 2+
Serum haptoglobin decreased

The blood bank subsequently identified the serum antibody as a cold agglutinin. An elution (removal of antibodies from the RBCs that they are coating) demonstrated that the same cold agglutinin was responsible for the positive direct AHG test result.

Questions
1. Which category and specific type of anemia are presented in this case?
2. What is the etiology of this anemia?
3. What mechanism produced this patient's spherocytosis?

Discussion
1. The laboratory findings of a decreased hemoglobin, Hct, RBC count, and spherocytes on the peripheral blood smear coupled with an increased reticulocyte count, decreased haptoglobin, elevated bilirubin, and hemoglobinuria are typical findings in a patient who is suffering from increased RBC destruction. Supplementary laboratory testing in this case assisted in establishing a differential diagnosis. The positive direct and indirect AHG test results demonstrated that the hemolytic process was being caused by a circulating antibody. Further blood bank results established that the antibody was a cold-type antibody rather than a warm-type antibody or a complement-related problem. This information is needed in order to differentiate this type of spherocytic-hemolytic anemia from other, similar anemias. In addition to the test data, the patient's medical history indicated no history of a recent blood transfusion to account for the presence of these circulating antibodies. Therefore, the diagnosis of autoimmune hemolytic anemia was established.

2. Autoimmune hemolytic anemia occurs in 1 out of 75 persons annually. Of these cases, 70% are of the warm antibody type, and 16% are cold-reacting antibodies. The antibodies of the cold type are usually immunoglobulin M (IgM). Patients afflicted with this disorder suffer either acute life-threatening hemolysis or a chronic hemolytic anemia. Half of the cases of autoimmune hemolytic anemia of either the warm or the cold variety are secondary to an underlying disease such as a lymphoproliferative disorder or viral infection. The remaining cases have an unknown etiology and are classified as idiopathic.

3. Spherocytes are often formed in autoimmune hemolytic anemia as the cell membrane of antibody-coated RBCs is lost following interaction of the RBCs with splenic macrophages. RBCs coated with IgG or complement are partially phagocytized and bind to the macrophages. The macro-

(continued)

CASE STUDIES (continued)

phage subsequently removes portions of the RBC membrane, and releases the RBC in its spherocytic form with a typically decreased surface-area-to-volume ratio. In autoimmune hemolytic anemia, the slow flow of blood through the spleen provides an ample opportunity for the macrophages to come in contact with coated RBCs. This loss of membrane decreases the ability of RBCs to pass through the sinuses. Thus, the cells become trapped within the splenic cords. These events produce a cell that is highly vulnerable to hemolysis.

✏️ Diagnosis: Autoimmune hemolytic anemia due to cold antibody

CASE 3 A newborn girl, who was well hydrated, began developing jaundice at 24 hours of age. The mother's prenatal information sheet noted that she was O-negative, and had received immunoglobulin D after the delivery of her first two children. No irregular antibodies were present during her initial prenatal blood screening during the first trimester of pregnancy.

The neonatologist ordered the following tests on the neonate: CBC, serum bilirubin, blood type and Rh, and direct AHG test.

Laboratory Data
The results of the tests were as follows:

Hemoglobin 15.6 gm/dL
Hct 0.50 L/L
RBC 4.71 × 10^{12}/L
MCV 106.2 fL
MCH 33.1 pg
MCHC 31%

The peripheral smear revealed anisocytosis, macrocytosis, slight spherocytosis, 3+ polychromatophilia, and 3 metarubricytes/100 WBCs. The total serum bilirubin was 10.5 mg/dL. The infant was type O-positive. The result of the AHG test was positive (2+).

Following receipt of these laboratory findings, the physician ordered blood type and Rh determinations for both the mother and the baby, a direct AHG test on the routinely collected cord blood sample, and an irregular antibody screen on the mother. These tests revealed that the mother was type O-negative. Her irregular antibody screening was positive. The antibody was identified as anti-c̄. A further antibody elution study of the neonate's cells revealed the presence of anti-c̄. The mother's full genotype was determined as being D-negative, C-positive, c̄-negative, E-positive, e-positive. The neonate's genotype was D-positive, C-negative, c̄-positive, E-positive, e-positive.

Questions
1. Is this an inherited or acquired anemia?
2. Which category of anemias does this case represent?
3. What is the cause of the baby's increased red cell destruction?

Discussion
1. The neonate's decreased hemoglobin, Hct, and RBC count; elevated bilirubin; and positive direct AHG on both the cord blood specimen and the blood sample suggest an ac-

quired anemia. The presence of the antibody anti-c̄ in the mother's serum postpartum and the identification of the antibody adhering to the baby's RBCs as anti-c̄ confirmed that the baby has an acquired anemia. This type of acquired, hemolytic anemia in the newborn is referred to as hemolytic disease of the newborn, formerly called erythroblastosis fetalis.
2. An increased bilirubin and decreased RBC count with both spherocytes and immature RBCs (metarubricytes) indicate that a hemolytic process is taking place. The identification of antibody in the mother's serum and on the neonate's cells confirmed that this hemolytic anemia was acquired.
3. Although an incompatibility in the ABO blood group system between mother and neonate is the most frequent type of hemolytic disease of the newborn, in this case both the mother and the baby were type O. In ABO incompatibility, the most frequent cases occur when the mother is type O and the baby is type A. The neonate's direct AHG test result in ABO incompatibility is frequently negative or only slightly positive. In this case, no atypical or irregular antibodies had been detected during prenatal testing during the first trimester of the mother's pregnancy. However, the antibody did exist postpartum. Although the mother was Rh-negative, she did not exhibit the presence of anti-D. The mother's medical history indicated that she had delivered two Rh-positive babies in the past, but had been given an immunoglobulin D substance postpartum as a preventive measure. However, she had apparently been sensitized to the c̄ antigen during a previous pregnancy. When pregnant with this child, she built c̄ antibodies that crossed the placental barrier, and attached themselves to the c̄ antigen on the baby's RBCs. The anti-c̄ antibody is a warm-reacting, IgG-type antibody that is small enough to pass through the placental barrier and cause hemolytic disease. The antibody attaches itself if the specific c̄ antigen is present on the fetal cells. This coating of fetal cells with antibody makes the RBC membrane vulnerable to hemolysis, which subsequently leads to increased erythrocyte destruction. In this case, it was important to identify the disorder not only for the newborn's sake, but for the mother's sake as well. Because the mother did not demonstrate anti-D in her circulation, and met the other necessary criteria, she was again eligible to receive immunoglobulin D in order to protect any further babies against hemolytic disease of the newborn caused by the anti-D antibody.

✏️ Diagnosis: Hemolytic disease of the newborn

BIBLIOGRAPHY

Agre, P. "Hereditary Spherocytosis." *JAMA,* Vol. 262, No. 20, November 24, 1989, pp. 2887–2890.

Alter, P. B. "Advances in the Prenatal Diagnosis of Hematological Disease." *Blood,* Vol. 64, No. 2, August, 1984, pp. 329–340.

Aster, R. H. "Quinine Sensitivity: A New Cause of the Hemolytic Uremic Syndrome." *Annals of Internal Medicine,* Vol. 119, No. 3, Aug. 1, 1993, pp. 243, 244.

Bell, B. P. et al. "A Multistate Outbreak of *Escherichia coli* O157:H7-Associated Bloody Diarrhea and Hemolytic Uremic Syndrome From Hamburgers." *JAMA*, Vol. 272, No. 17, November 2, 1994, pp. 1349–1353.

Bergstein, J. M., M. Riley, and N. U. Bang. "Role of Plasminogen-Activator Inhibitor Type 1 in the Pathogenesis and Outcome of the Hemolytic Uremic Syndrome." *N. Engl. J. Med.*, Vol. 327, No. 11, September 10, 1992, pp. 755–759.

Bick, R. L. "Paroxysmal Nocturnal Hemoglobinuria." *Laboratory Medicine*, Vol. 25, No. 3, March, 1994, pp. 148–151.

Boyce, T., D. L. Swerdlow, and P. M. Griffin. "*Escherichia coli* O157:H7 and the Hemolytic-Uremic Syndrome." *N. Engl. J. Med.*, Vol. 333, No. 6, August 10, 1995, pp. 362–363.

Costa, F. F. et al. "Linkage of Dominant Hereditary Spherocytosis to the Gene for the Erythrocyte Membrane-Skeleton Protein Ankyrin." *N. Engl. J. Med.*, Vol. 323, No. 15, October 11, 1990, p. 1046.

Drozda, E. A., Jr. and R. Ciotola. "Unexpected Hemolytic Diseases of the Newborn." *Lab. Med.*, Vol. 15, No. 5, July, 1984, pp. 486–487.

Hillmen, P. et al. "Natural History of Paroxysmal Nocturnal Hemoglobinuria." *N. Engl. J. Med.*, Vol. 333, No. 19, Nov. 9, 1995, pp. 1253–1258.

Leach, A. P. and H. R. Gaumer. "Diagnosis and Detection of PNH Using GPI Anchored Proteins." *Clinical Laboratory Science*, Vol. 9, No. 4, July/August, 1996, pp. 191–197.

Marchand, A. "Immune Hemolytic Anemia." *Diagn. Med.*, Vol. 7, No. 10, November-December, 1984, pp. 51–64.

Scamurra, D. and F. R. Davey. "Anemias Associated With Spherocytic Erythrocytes." *Lab. Med.*, Vol. 16, No. 2, February, 1985, pp. 83–88.

Schilling, R. F. "Estimating the Risk for Sepsis After Splenectomy in Hereditary Spherocytosis." *Annals of Internal Medicine*, Vol. 122, No. 3, February 1, 1995, pp. 187–188.

Schwartz, R. S. "PIG-4—The Target Gene in Paroxysmal Nocturnal Hemoglobinuria." *N. Engl. J. Med.*, Vol. 330, No. 4, January 27, 1994, pp. 283–284.

Tarr, P. I. et al. "Hemolytic-Uremic Syndrome in a Six-Year-Old Girl after a Urinary Tract Infection with Shiga-Toxin-Producing *Escherichia coli* O103:H2." *N. Engl. J. Med.*, Vol. 335, No. 9, August 29, 1996, pp. 635–638.

REVIEW QUESTIONS

1. Hemolytic disruption of the erythrocyte involves:

   A. An alteration in the erythrocyte membrane.
   B. A defect of the hemoglobin molecule.
   C. An antibody coating the erythrocyte.
   D. Physical trauma.

Questions 2 and 3: match the following.

2. ___ Intravascular hemolysis.

3. ___ Extravascular hemolysis.

   A. Destruction of RBCs outside of the circulatory blood.
   B. Destruction of RBCs within the circulatory blood.

Questions 4 through 7: match the following disorders with the appropriate category of defect. An answer may be used more than once.

4. ___ G6PD deficiency.

5. ___ Hereditary spherocytosis.

6. ___ Thalassemia.

7. ___ Pyruvate kinase deficiency.

   A. Structural membrane defect.
   B. Erythrocytic enzyme defect.
   C. Defect of the hemoglobin molecule.

Questions 8 through 12: match the following (use an answer only once):

8. ___ Hereditary spherocytosis

9. ___ Hereditary elliptocytosis

10. ___ Hereditary pyropoikilocytosis

11. ___ Hereditary stomatocytosis

12. ___ Hereditary xerocytosis

   A. An overabundance of elliptic red cells.
   B. A permeability disorder.
   C. The most common prevalent hereditary hemolytic anemia among people of Northern European descent.
   D. Can be seen in the genetic hemoglobin defect, thalassemia.
   E. A subgroup of common hereditary elliptocytosis.

13. Heinz bodies are associated with the congenital hemolytic anemia:

   A. G6PD deficiency.
   B. Abetalipoproteinemia.
   C. Hereditary spherocytosis.
   D. Hemolytic anemias.

14. A hemolytic crisis may be precipitated in 10% of American black males by the drug G6PD deficiency by:

   A. Fava beans.   C. Quinine.
   B. Primaquine.   D. Quinidine.

15. Acquired hemolytic anemia can be caused by:

   A. Chemicals or drugs.   C. Antibody reactions.
   B. Infectious organisms.   D. All of the above.

16. The infectious microorganism directly associated with homolytic uremic syndrome is:

   A. *Pasturella tularensis.*   C. *Staphylococcus aureus.*
   B. *E. coli* O157-H7.   D. *Clostridia batulinum.*

Questions 17 through 19: match the following immune mediated acquired hemolytic anemias with their respective answers (use an answer only once):

17. ___ Warm-type autoimmune hemolytic anemia.

18. ___ Cold-type autoimmune hemolytic anemia.

19. ___ Isoimmune hemolytic anemia.

   A. IgM, usually anti-I.
   B. Rh antibodies are the most frequent cause.
   C. Usually occurs in newborn infants.

20. The erythrocyte alteration characteristically associated with hemolytic anemias is:

   A. Hypochromia.   C. Spherocytosis.
   B. Macrocytosis.   D. Burr cells.

21. What laboratory procedures would reflect a typical hemolytic anemia?
    A. Increased osmotic fragility.
    B. Increased total serum bilirubin.
    C. Increased reticulocyte count, unless hematopoiesis is suppressed.
    D. All of the above.

22. Which of the following is *not* associated with hemolytic anemia?
    A. Decreased hemoglobin and packed cell volume.
    B. Increased reticulocyte count.
    C. Increased haptoglobins.
    D. Decreased erythrocyte survival.

23. Paroxysmal nocturnal hemoglobinuria (PNH) exhibits sensitivity of one population of red blood cells to:
    A. Warm antibodies.   C. Complement.
    B. Cold antibodies.   D. Either A or B.

24. PNH episodes are usually associated with:
    A. Cold temperatures.
    B. Hot temperatures.
    C. Sleep.
    D. Certain foods or drugs.

25. The defect in PNH is a ___ associated defect of the red cell.
    A. Membrane.   C. Enzyme.
    B. Hemoglobin.   D. Either B or C.

CHAPTER 13

The Hemoglobinopathies

Hemoglobin defects
Sickle cell disease
Etiology
Epidemiology
Pathophysiology
Clinical signs and
   symptoms
General signs and
   symptoms
Laboratory testing
Special laboratory testing
Management of sickle
   cell disease

Sickle cell syndromes:
   Pathogenesis and new
   approaches
Sickle-beta thalassemia
Sickle-C disease
Sickle cell trait
Thalassemia
Etiology
Physiology
Alpha-thalassemia
Beta-thalassemia
Persistence of fetal
   hemoglobin

Laboratory findings
Other hemoglobinopathies
Hemoglobin C disease
Hemoglobin SC disease
Hemoglobin D disease
Hemoglobin E disease
Hemoglobin H disease
Methemoglobinemia
Unstable hemoglobins
Summary
Case studies
Bibliography
Review questions

OBJECTIVES

Hemoglobin defects
- Describe the common denominator in hemoglobinopathies.
- Name the three major categories of classification of hemoglobin defects.
- List the components and percentage of normal adult hemoglobin.
- Compare the disease state and trait condition of a hemoglobinopathy.

Sickle cell disease
- Describe the etiology of sickle cell disease.
- Explain the epidemiology of sickle cell disease.
- Describe the clinical signs and symptoms of sickle cell disease.
- Briefly explain the symptoms of sickle cell disease in children.
- Describe the symptoms of sickle cell disease associated with pregnancy.
- Discuss the clinical manifestations of sickle cell disease in adults.
- Characterize the general signs and symptoms in the categories of pain, pulmonary complications, and stroke associated with sickle cell disease.
- Outline laboratory findings that are typical of sickle cell disease.

- Briefly describe the value of the techniques of hemoglobin electrophoresis and DNA analysis.
- Explain the process of prenatal diagnosis of sickle cell disease.
- Delineate the general management of sickle cell disease.

Sickle cell syndromes
- Describe the conditions of sickle-beta thalassemia, sickle-C, and sickle cell trait.

Thalassemia
- Compare the conditions of alpha- and beta-thalassemia.
- Outline the laboratory findings in thalassemia.

Other hemoglobinopathies
- Describe the general characteristics of hemoglobin C disease, hemoglobin SC disease, hemoglobin D disease, hemoglobin E disease, hemoglobin H disease, methemoglobinemia, and unstable hemoglobins.

Case studies
- Apply knowledge of etiology, epidemiology, pathophysiology, clinical signs and symptoms, laboratory findings, and treatment to the presented case studies.

HEMOGLOBIN DEFECTS

As discussed in the preceding chapter, the hemolytic anemias are characterized by decreased red cell survival due to inherited or acquired mechanisms. In this chapter, a particularly unique type of genetic defect, the hemoglobinopathy, is presented. Hemoglobinopathies may or may not have a hemolytic manifestation. About 25% of all hemoglobinopathies demonstrate the decreased red cell survival that characterizes hemolytic disease.

The common denominator in the hemoglobinopathies is that all represent an inherited or genetic defect related to hemoglobin. This defect may result in an abnormal structure of the hemoglobin molecule or a deficiency in the synthesis of normal adult hemoglobin.

The hemoglobinopathies can be classified into three major categories:

1. Abnormal molecular structure of one or more of the polypeptide chains of globulin in the hemoglobin molecule
2. A defect in the rate of synthesis of one or more of the polypeptide chains of globulin in the hemoglobin molecule
3. Disorders that are a combination of abnormal molecular structure with a synthesis defect

Several hundred abnormal hemoglobins have been described in the literature. Selected examples of hemoglobinopathies within each of the three major categories are listed in Table 13.1.

Normal adult hemoglobin contains the following components: Hb A (95% to 98%), Hb A_2 (2% to 3%), Hb A_1 (3% to 6%), and Hb F (less than 1%). The major fraction is Hb A. Typically, the individual with a hemoglobinopathy will demonstrate an alteration in this pattern.

The hemoglobinopathies are inherited diseases. Some of these disorders are caused by the inheritance of an autosomal dominant gene that will produce hemolytic disease in its heterozygous state. Others are autosomal recessive genes and need to be in the homozygous state to produce the disease.

In the hemoglobinopathies, the distinction between the disease state and the trait condition is made. A disease is defined as either the homozygous occurrence of the gene for the abnormality or the possession of a heterozygous,

dominant gene that produces a hemolytic condition. In the case of sickle cell anemia, the trait must be inherited from both parents. A trait is described as the heterozygous and normally asymptomatic state. A review of inheritance and the synthesis of hemoglobin can be found in Chapter 5.

The major hemoglobinopathies have been identified as originating as mutations in Africa, Asia, and Europe. Two frequent hemoglobinopathies are sickle cell anemia/sickle cell trait and thalassemia. The sickle mutant has the highest frequency of occurrence in Central Africa. Thalassemia major can be traced back to the Mediterranean. The Middle East, South Asia, and the Orient have alpha thalassemia as a prevalent hemoglobinopathy. Because these anemias are among the most common hemoglobinopathies, they will be described in more detail.

SICKLE CELL DISEASE

Disorders of hemoglobin structure and synthesis constitute the most common group of genetic disorders in the world. Sickle cell disease is a general term for abnormalities of hemoglobin structure and function, hemoglobinopathies, in which the sickle gene is inherited from at least one parent. These genetic disorders are characterized by the production of hemoglobin S (Hb S), anemia, and acute and chronic tissue damage secondary to the blockage of blood flow produced by abnormally shaped red blood cells.

Sickle cell anemia (Hb SS), the most common form of hemoglobinopathy, is an expression of the inheritance of a sickle gene from both parents (see Chapter 3). Other sickle cell disorders result from the coinheritance of the sickle gene. Common variants include hemoglobin SC disease (Hb SC) and beta-thalassemia (SB-thalassemia).

Patients with this disease are living longer, new treatments are becoming available for adults as well as children, and early detection does matter. Almost every state in the United States screens the blood of all newborns for sickle cell disease.

Etiology

The sickle cell gene must be inherited from both parents. Hemoglobin S is different from hemoglobin A because of a single nucleotide change (GAT to GTT) that results in the substitution of valine for glutamic acid at the sixth position on the beta chain of the hemoglobin molecule. This results in abnormalities in polymerization (or gelation), with deoxygenation that leads to sickling. The end result of the polymerization is a permanently altered membrane protein. Two thirds of the RBCs are removed by extravascular mechanisms.

Epidemiology

Sickle cell disease is found most commonly in persons of African ancestry, but it also affects persons of Mediterranean, Caribbean, South and Central American, Arab, and East Indian ancestry. The sickle cell carrier state confers a selective advantage to *Plasmodium falciparum* malaria, because of preferential sickling of only the parasitized cells. The prevalence of the disease in some regions reflects this selective

---

TABLE 13.1 Examples of Selected Hemoglobinopathies

Abnormal Molecular Structure
Hb SS (sickle cell anemia)
Hb SA (sickle cell trait)
Hb C disease or trait

Rate of Synthesis
Beta-thalassemia
Alpha-thalassemia

Combination of Two Molecular Alterations or a Molecular Abnormality and Synthesis Defect
Hb S–C
Hb S–beta thalassemia

advantage. In the United States, an estimated 8% of the African-American population carries the trait, and approximately one in 375 African-American newborns are born with sickle cell anemia.

Hemoglobin SC disease (Hb SC) affects an estimated 1 in 835 African-American births, and sickle cell-beta thalassemia (Sβ-thalassemia) affects one in 1667 African-American live births. As a result, it is one of the most common genetic diseases in the United States.

Sickle cell anemia, the homozygous form of sickle cell disease, is the most common inherited hematologic disease affecting humans. More than 50,000 Americans suffer from sickle cell anemia.

The life expectancy of patients with sickle cell disease has improved considerably since 1960. The median age at death for individuals with sickle cell anemia, the most common form of the disease, is 42 years for men and 48 years for women, considerably younger than the general African-American population. For hemoglobin SC disease, the median age at death is 60 years for men and 68 years for women.

Pathophysiology

When Hb S is deoxygenated, it becomes polymerized and produces sickling. Subsequent hemolysis is probably a result of the extent of the red cell's capacity to sickle. The erythrocytic membrane in sickle cell anemia possesses significant membrane abnormalities, with an excessive increase in ionized calcium in the cell playing a role in the produced abnormality. Ionized calcium in the hemoglobin S-S cell is twice normal, with the most dense cells having four times the normal amount of ionized calcium.

Polymerization of Hb S occurs under conditions of extremely reduced oxygen and increased acidity in the blood. Sickling is promoted by low oxygen tension, low pH, increased 2,3-diphosphoglycerate, high cellular concentration of hemoglobins, loss of cell water, hemoglobin C, and HbO-ARAB. Sickling is retarded by hemoglobin A, hemoglobin F (at least 30%), hemoglobin J, and alpha-thalassemia.

When sickling occurs, it subsequently leads to an increased MCHC in proportion to the number of molecules in the deoxygenated state. Deoxyhemoglobin S is less soluble than deoxyhemoglobin A or oxyhemoglobin S.

Recently the understanding of the molecular basis of sickle cell disease has progressed rapidly. It is now possible to describe the structure of the gel of polymerized deoxyhemoglobin S, and to begin to understand the mechanism of the formation of this gelatinous hemoglobin solution in red cells. Initially, it is believed that with deoxygenation a continuum of cellular changes begins.

The first stage progresses from the formation of small amounts of polymer to larger amounts of highly ordered polymer as the result of severe and prolonged deoxygenation. This polymerization produces the resultant sickling. The red cell flexibility, which is governed by the amount and alignment of this intracellular polymer, is the principal determinant of the flow of sickled red cells.

Because cells that have large amounts of ordered polymer may be caught in the capillaries and venules, some cells at relatively high oxygen saturation with polymer but no deformability may have difficulty traversing the constriction of the precapillary arterioles. When the sickled cells attempt to travel through these small vessels, they become stuck, and the vessels become obstructed. This initiates a pattern of blood not flowing properly to the tissue and creating a lack of oxygen. The lack of oxygen causes more sickling and more deprivation of oxygen to the tissues. This process can cause intense pain.

When sickled cells receive oxygen, they return to their normal shape. Repeated cycles of sickling and unsickling lead to the red blood cell becoming permanently damaged. This process ends in hemolysis which leads to anemia. In addition, repeated episodes of this type lead to the necrosis of body tissues.

Clinical Signs and Symptoms

Acute crises are due to recurrent obstruction of the microcirculation by intravascular sickling. Aside from the painful crisis, sickling takes its toll on the body in other ways. Through the years, the cumulative damage from vascular occlusion can lead to organ and tissue failure. Other complications may include an enlarged heart, progressive loss of pulmonary or renal function, stroke, arthritis, liver damage, and other complications. There is significant activation of coagulation with consequent increase in fibrinolysis during both the sickle cell crisis and in the steady state.

There is variation in the severity of sickle cell disease. Many patients are reasonably well and have relatively few complications. However, 5% to 10% of patients account for 40% to 50% of hospital visits.

Symptoms in Children

In sickle cell anemia, splenic dysfunction is a potentially life-threatening complication that develops during infancy. The red blood cells become trapped in the spleen, leaving the infant vulnerable to shock and infection from encapsulated bacteria, particularly members of the *Streptococcus pneumoniae* and *Haemophilus influenzae* species. Infectious crises are the most frequent cause of death in patients younger than 5 years (Table 13.2).

Symptoms are not present unless the patient is older than 6 months. Vaso-occlusive disease develops between the ages of 12 months and 6 years. Chronic manifestations in children include a progressive lag in growth and development after the first decade of life and chronic destruction of bone and joints, with ischemia and infarction of the spongiosa.

TABLE 13.2 **Causes of Death Among Children With Sickle Cell Disease**

Cause	Percent of Total Deaths
Infection	44
Splenic sequestration	16
Sudden, unexpected death	14
Cerebrovascular accident	12
Congestive heart failure	7
Miscellaneous	7

Symptoms Associated With Pregnancy

In pregnancy, there is no increase in disease manifestation, but there is an increase in maternal mortality of 20% and fetal mortality of 20%.

Clinical Manifestations in Adults

SS homozygotes have a severe hemolytic anemia, with hematocrit values ranging between 15 and 30. Red cells with relatively low hemoglobin F levels are likely to become sickled cells and, therefore, have short life spans. In cases where erythropoiesis is also suppressed, anemia becomes increasingly severe. The two main causes of erythropoietic suppression are aplastic crises and megaloblastic erythropoiesis. Aplastic crises result from infection, particularly with parvovirus, whereas megaloblastic erythropoiesis occasionally occurs owing to the induction of folic acid deficiency by the increased requirements of the hyperplastic marrow. The hematocrit can plummet rapidly as a result of combined impairment in red cell production and ongoing hemolysis.

Acute chest syndrome is a significant cause of death in patients of all ages who have sickle cell anemia. Higher blood viscosity leads to several complications, including complications in the shoulders and hips, multiorgan dysfunction, and possibly some of the pain associated with the disease. There is an increased incidence of pigmented gallstones in 30% to 60% of adults, with symptoms in 10% to 15%. Renal manifestations include papillary necrosis. Leg ulcers may occur.

Fifty percent of patients with sickle cell anemia survive beyond the fifth decade. A large proportion of those who die have had no overt chronic organ failure but die during an acute episode of pain, chest syndrome, or stroke.

Patients with more symptomatic disease are at higher risk of early death. Risk of early death is inversely associated with the level of fetal hemoglobin. Patients with sickle cell anemia who had hemoglobin values below 7.1 gm and elevated white blood counts (>15.0) have a slightly higher risk.

General Signs and Symptoms

Pain

Painful sickle cell crisis is the hallmark of sickle cell anemia and is the most common complaint of patients with this disease. Acute painful episodes, often called vaso-occlusive crises, are the most frequent complication of sickle cell disease and are a common reason for visits to the emergency room and admission to the hospital. High-dose methylprednisolone decreases the duration of pain in children and adolescents with sickle cell disease, but they have more rebound attacks after therapy is discontinued.

Pulmonary Complications

Thoracic bone infarction is common in patients with sickle cell disease who are hospitalized with acute chest pain. Incentive spirometry can prevent the pulmonary complications (atelectasis and infiltrates) associated with the acute chest syndrome in patients with sickle cell diseases who are hospitalized with chest or back pain above the diaphragm. The cause of acute chest syndrome is uncertain.

Stroke

Because hemoglobin S tends to form intracellular polymers that distort the red cell, the disease is characterized clinically by chronic hemolytic anemia, recurrent bouts of pain, and organ infarction, including stroke. Cerebral infarction in sickle cell disease is associated with an occlusive vasculopathy involving the distal intracranial segments of the internal carotid artery, and the proximal middle and anterior cerebral arteries. Transcranial ultrasonography can identify children with sickle cell disease who are at highest risk for cerebral infarction. Periodic ultrasound examinations and the selective use of transfusion therapy could make the primary prevention of stroke an achievable goal.

Laboratory Testing

In addition to decreased hemoglobin (5 to 9.5 gm), hematocrit, and red blood cell count, a persistent increase in the WBC count of 12,000 to 15,000 $\times$ 10^9/L is common. The red cell morphology on peripheral blood smear can include moderate to marked anisocytosis, poikilocytosis, and hypochromia. Red cell abnormalities may include target cells, microcytes, polychromatophilia, and basophilic stippling. Howell-Jolly bodies may be present if hyposplenism is present. If the patient is in an acute crisis state, sickled red cells (drepanocytes) may be seen on peripheral smears (Table 13.3).

Other diagnostic laboratory tests (see Chapter 24) can include sickle cell screening tests, hemoglobin electrophoresis, the alkali denaturation test, an acid elution test, and determination of the osmotic fragility of erythrocytes.

Laboratory features of this chronic hemolytic state include reticulocytosis (8% to 12%), which may increase the MCV to levels up to 100 fL; elevated serum; unconjugated bilirubin and methemalbumin; decreased serum haptoglobin and hemopexin; increased serum lactate dehydrogenase (LDH); mildly increased aspartate transaminase (AST); and increased urine urobilinogen.

Special Laboratory Testing

Hemoglobin Electrophoresis

As early as 1949, Linus Pauling ascribed the altered electrophoretic mobility of the hemoglobin in patients with sickle cell anemia to a change in the hemoglobin. This cemented the fact that there was a direct link between defective hemo-

---

TABLE 13.3 Common Laboratory Signs of Hemolysis in Sickle Cell Disease

---

1. Reticulocytosis (polychromasia)
2. Unconjugated hyperbilirubinemia
3. Increased fecal and urine urobilinogen
4. Decreased serum haptoglobin
5. Decreased serum hemopexin
6. Increased serum methemalbumin
7. Elevated lactic dehydrogenase (LDH)
8. Mild elevation in aspartate transaminase (AST)

---

globin molecules and their pathological consequences, setting the groundwork for the concept of molecular disease.

In the laboratory, there is no single best screening method: hemoglobin electrophoresis, isoelectric focusing (IEF), and high-performance liquid chromatography are all acceptable, reliable, and accurate. Globin DNA analysis is also advocated as an alternative method, although the procedure is costly and limited in the number of genotypes it can identify. Electrophoresis is the most commonly used first step to characterize hemoglobin. Cellulose acetate and IEF are the most commonly used electrophoretic methods. Definitive diagnosis includes reassessment of the hemoglobin phenotype, measurement of hemoglobin concentration and red cell indices, inspection of red cell morphology, and correlation with the clinical history. In sickle cell disease, hemoglobin electrophoresis shows 80% to 95% hemoglobin S, 0 to 20% hemoglobin F, and a normal amount of hemoglobin A_2.

DNA Analysis

With the discovery of reverse transcriptase, and the cloning of the human globin genes, it became possible to probe specifically for the globin genes in the human genome. The hemoglobin disorders represent the first groups of disease where DNA analysis was applied.

This analysis has led to better understanding of the basic mechanism of diseases, clinical application, and in some countries, control of the diseases. Virtually all cases of sickle cell disease and most cases of thalassemia can be diagnosed by direct DNA analysis with polymerase chain reaction (PCR).

Prenatal and Neonatal Diagnosis

Prenatal diagnosis of abnormal hemoglobin is important because of the high frequency of sickle cell disease. As DNA from the fetus is available in the amniocytes, fetal diagnosis can be made by amniocentesis at about the 14th week of gestation. The current widespread use of chorionic villus biopsy allows DNA diagnosis to be performed at the 7th to 10th week of gestation.

The principal hemoglobin in the newborn is fetal hemoglobin (HbF). The distribution is 80% HbF and 20% HbA in a normal term infant. HbF is composed of two alpha and two gamma globulins. During the last trimester, there is a progressive increase in B globin synthesis and a decrease in gamma chain synthesis.

In a normal term infant, about 80% of the nonalpha globulin is gamma globin and 20% is beta globin. Because an infant with sickle cell trait has both a normal beta gene and a beta S gene, the infant will have a predominance of HbF and both HbA and HbS. There always will be more HbA than HbS in these infants because alpha chains preferentially pair with normal beta chains.

Screening of newborn infants is an important step in disease control. Although universal newborn screening can reliably identify all infants with sickle cell hemoglobinopathies, the initial screening result must not be considered the definitive diagnosis. Hemoglobin concentrations having a mean erythrocyte volume (MCV) that is higher or lower than expected should suggest concurrent beta-thalassemia.

Collection on the first day of life poses no problem for hemoglobin screening, provided the infant has not received a blood transfusion. A cord blood sample can be used, but it has the potential of being contaminated with blood from the mother. However, blood collected from a heel stick is the method of choice because it is easy to obtain and it is the same method used for other newborn screening, e.g., phenylketonuria (PKU), hypothyroiditis, and galactosemia. Samples collected onto filter paper from a heel stick remain stable for at least 1 week at room temperature.

The most popular procedure for screening infants is electrophoresis at alkaline pH on cellulose acetate followed by further examination of abnormal samples by electrophoresis at an acid pH on citrate agar (two-tiered approach). Electrophoresis separates hemoglobins by electrical charge. Hemoglobins with similar charges have similar migration patterns during electrophoresis. Several hemoglobins have similar motility on cellulose acetate. Hemoglobins D and G have migration patterns similar to hemoglobin S. Hemoglobin F migrates between hemoglobins A and S on cellulose acetate at alkaline pH.

In the newborn with a large amount of hemoglobin F, it is particularly important to detect small amounts of hemoglobin A and S reliably. Citrate agar electrophoresis clearly separates hemoglobins F, A, S, and C. Agar electrophoresis distinguishes HbS from hemoglobins C and D, and hemoglobin C from hemoglobins E and O. This method is rarely used as the primary electrophoretic method for screening, but it is used by many laboratories to confirm the presence of abnormal hemoglobins found by another technique. Advantages of the two-tiered approach include simplicity, low cost, and standardization. Disadvantages include the need for two different electrophoretic procedures to ensure accurate results and limited resolution of other abnormal hemoglobins.

Some newborn screening programs use thin-layer isoelectric focusing, an acceptable alternate method that provides better resolution of hemoglobins A, S, and C from hemoglobin F and detection of other abnormal hemoglobins by a single procedure. Other newborn screening programs use high-pressure liquid chromatography.

Metabisulfite sickle cell preparations and solubility testing are not acceptable screening methods for newborns or HbS confirmation in early infancy.

Management of Sickle Cell Disease

The management of sickle cell disease consists of:

1. Monitoring the severity of the anemia and transfusing blood only when necessary
2. Treating acute and chronic pain according to a rational guideline
3. Diagnosing organ failure and administering appropriate therapy. Over time, recurrent vaso-occlusion and its associated vasculopathy result in significant progressive organ failure.

Treatment

Conventional management of sickle cell anemia is primarily supportive. It is important to detect infections early and treat them with antibiotics, as these infections may trigger painful and aplastic crises. General supportive care includes daily oral folate supplementation, penicillin prophylaxis in childhood, Pneumovax, *Haemophilus influenzae* vaccine, meningococcal vaccine, a yearly flu shot, a yearly eye exam, prompt treatment of infections, and avoidance of dehydration. Treatment of pain crises includes hydration, adequate analgesia, and adequate oxygenation. Exchange transfusions may play a limited role in treatment, but possible reasons for their use include prevention of stroke recurrence, acute chest syndrome, in preparation for elective surgery, refractory priapism, refractory pain crises, and splenic sequestration crises.

Experimental treatment approaches include chemical inhibition of hemoglobin S polymerization, reduction of intracellular hemoglobin concentration, and pharmacological induction of hemoglobin F production.

Infectious Diseases. The primary treatment is prevention of infectious diseases. Vaccination including pneumococcal, influenza A, and *Haemophilus influenzae* immunizations are indicated. In addition, splenectomy is recommended for children who survive the initial splenic sequestration crisis.

Blood Transfusion. Blood transfusion and exchange transfusion are means of treatment of anemia. The major indications for blood transfusion in sickle cell disease are:

- To improve oxygen-carrying capacity and transport
- To dilute circulating sickle red blood cells in order to improve microvascular perfusion

Transfusion should be considered in a patient with:

1. Hemoglobin <5.0 gm/dL and significant signs and symptoms of anemia associated with erythroid aplasia or hypoplasia (aplastic crisis)
2. Angina or high output failure
3. Acute hemorrhage
4. Acute central nervous system complications
5. Acute chest syndrome with hypoxia
6. Sequestration crisis
7. Preoperative preparation (general anesthesia)

Exchange transfusion may be considered in patients with cerebrovascular accident, fat embolism, acute chest syndrome, eye surgery, unresponsive acute priapism, and leg ulcers, and before injection of contrast material. Prolonged hypertransfusion or an exchange transfusion regimen will result in iron overload and the consequent need for iron chelation therapy.

Drug Therapy

Drug therapy consisting of erythropoietin injection and the drug hydroxyurea are two treatment protocols. Hydroxyurea stimulates the production of fetal hemoglobin but suppresses bone marrow production. Hydroxyurea therapy can ameliorate the clinical course of sickle cell anemia in some adults with three or more painful crises per year. The beneficial effects of hydroxyurea do not become manifest for several months, and its use must be carefully monitored. Because of the effect of bone marrow suppression, patients must be monitored every two weeks to ensure that a life-threatening decrease in the number of hematopoietic cells does not occur. In addition, the long-term safety of hydroxyurea in patients with sickle cell anemia is uncertain.

Hydroxyurea alone can reduce symptoms of anemia that require some patients to undergo frequent transfusions. However, by combining hydroxyurea and recombinant erythropoietin, and adding iron supplements to the treatment, patients reportedly manifest increased levels of the protein fetal hemoglobin in their blood. By increasing the production of red blood cells containing the protein, the effect of the drug is to interfere with the process that makes hemoglobin abnormal in those who suffer from the disease.

Prevention

Genetic counseling may be useful in the prevention of sickle cell anemia. When the parents are both SA heterozygotes, antenatal diagnosis can be performed during the 18th to the 20th weeks of pregnancy by analyzing DNA from amniotic fluid.

SICKLE CELL SYNDROMES: PATHOGENESIS AND NEW APPROACHES

Sickle cell anemia was the first molecular disease to be recognized. The severity of illness in sickle cell disease differs with the quantity of hemoglobin S in the erythrocytes. The various states associated with the presence of hemoglobin S are listed in Table 13.4 in order of clinical severity.

Sickle-Beta Thalassemia

The inheritance of the sickle gene from one parent and a beta-thalassemia gene from the other results in the compound heterozygous state: sickle-beta thalassemia. This disorder is variable in its clinical manifestations, but tends to be milder in blacks than in Mediterranean people. Patients have mod-

TABLE 13.4 Various States Associated With the Presence of Hemoglobin S

Genotype	Percent Hb S	Percent Non-S Hb	Clinical Severity (Scale 0–4)	Other Clinical Features
SS	80–98	2–15 (fetal)	3–4	10–20% retics; rare splenomegaly
S-beta thalassemia	60–90	10–30	1–3	Splenomegaly; microcytosis; 4+ target cells
SC	50	50 (hgb C)	1–3	Splenomegaly, 4+ target cells
AS Sickle trait	30–40	60–70 (hgb A)	0	Normal morphology; no splenomegaly

erately severe hemolytic anemia. Splenomegaly occurs in 70% of the cases.

Patients who are unable to produce any Hb A (S-beta^0 thalassemia) have disease as severe as that of SS patients. Those with S-beta$^+$ thalassemia can make a small amount of hemoglobin A and have less extensive hemolysis and vaso-occlusive phenomena.

S-beta thalassemia can be diagnosed by examining the blood film and through hemoglobin electrophoresis. The blood film reveals hypochromic, microcytic red cells with polychromatophilia, target cells, stippling, and, rarely, sickled cells. Hemoglobin electrophoresis reveals that 60% to 90% of the hemoglobin is S and 10% to 30% is fetal (F). The therapy is the same as for SS disease. Splenectomy may be beneficial if the spleen is sequestering red cells in significant amounts.

Sickle-C Disease

The compound heterozygous state sickle-C (SC) disease is almost as common among adults as SS disease, even though the gene frequency for hemoglobin C is a quarter of that for hemoglobin S. The clinical manifestations in SC disease are highly variable. There are two reasons why SC is a disease whereas AS (i.e., sickle cell trait) is benign. First, in SC red cells, the intracellular hemoglobin concentration is significantly elevated because of the presence of Hb C. Second, SC red cells have at least a 10% higher level of hemoglobin S than SA red cells. Patients with sickle-C disease experience a mild to moderate hemolytic anemia and usually have splenomegaly. Target cell and occasional plump sickle forms are noted in the blood film. Complications commonly include retinopathy, hematuria from medullary infarcts, and aseptic necrosis of the femoral head (Table 13.5).

Sickle Cell Trait

About 8% of black Americans are heterozygous for hemoglobin S. Thus, their red cells contain hemoglobin S and A. The gene has persisted because heterozygotes are slightly protected against falciparum malaria. Life expectancy and morbidity of individuals with sickle trait (AS) resemble those

TABLE 13.5 Abnormalities Reported With Sickle Cell Trait

1. Associations with sickle cell trait very likely
   Splenic infarction at high altitude
   Hyposthenuria
   Hematuria
   Bacteriuria and pyelonephritis in pregnancy
2. Association with sickle cell trait possible
   Pulmonary embolism
   Complications induced by prolonged use of tourniquet
   Renal papillary necrosis
   Proliferative retinopathy
   Avascular necrosis of bone
   Intravascular sickling with strenuous exertion (especially in untrained subjects)

of a comparable group with hemoglobin A. AS red cells sickle far less readily than SS red cells. Accordingly, AS heterozygotes develop sickling crises rarely and only when severely hypoxic.

There are no manifestations of anemia, red blood cell abnormalities, increased risk of infection, or increased mortality associated with sickle cell trait. Electrophoresis of whole blood does reveal that 35% to 45% of hemoglobin in patients with sickle cell trait is hemoglobin S. Clinical signs and symptoms associated with sickle cell trait include hematuria, splenic infarction at high altitude (over 10,000), hyposthenuria, bacteriuria, pyelonephritis in pregnancy, and reduced mortality from *Plasmodium falciparum* infection.

In hemoglobin SC disease, the patients have only hemoglobin S and C, with an absence of hemoglobin A and normal or increased levels of hemoglobin F. The complications associated with this disorder are less severe than sickle cell disease with three exceptions: proliferative retinopathy, aseptic necrosis of femoral heads, and acute chest syndrome secondary to fat emboli in the final months of pregnancy. Mild anemia occurs in 10% of patients with the hemoglobin being less than 10 gm/dL. Sickle cells are rarely seen on a peripheral blood smear, but about 50% of red blood cells on a peripheral blood smear are target cells. The spleen remains functional.

Hemoglobin S/B-thalassemia is less severe than sickle cell disease. The spleen remains functional, but retinopathy is more common.

THALASSEMIA

Etiology

The thalassemia syndromes are among the most common genetic diseases in humans. The thalassemias are common in southern China, with the highest prevalence in areas where malaria has been or remains endemic. In Southeast Asia, with a population of approximately 450 million people, the burdens of inherited globin gene disorders in many regions are of such magnitude that they represent a public health concern.

These syndromes are caused by an abnormality in the rate of synthesis of the globin chains. This is in contrast to the true hemoglobinopathies (for example, Hb S and Hb C) that result from an inherited structural defect in one of the globin chains that produces hemoglobin with abnormal physical or functional characteristics.

Inheritance of thalassemia is autosomal; whether it is autosomal dominant or recessive is questionable because heterozygotes are not always symptomatic. Globin structural genes are found on chromosomes 11 and 16. The alpha chain and its embryonic counterpart, the zeta chain, are located on chromosome 16. Two genes on each homologous chromosome, four per diploid cell, specify the alpha-globin sequence. Only one gene per chromosome, two per diploid cell, specifies most of the nonalpha chain on chromosome 11. The gamma chain is also represented by two sites per chromosome. In terms of the genetic basis of alpha- and beta-thalassemia, this represents an important difference.

All thalassemia genes that have been studied to date have

been found to contain mutations that directly alter gene structure and subsequently gene function. One of five processes is now believed to be responsible for the genetic defect in thalassemia. These processes are:

1. A nonsense mutation leading to early termination of the globin chain synthesis
2. A mutation in one of the noncoding intervening sequences of the original globin chain gene, which causes inefficient splicing to mRNA
3. A mutation in the promoter area that decreases the rate of gene expression
4. A mutation at the termination of the gene that leads to lengthening of the globin chain with additional amino acids; the mRNA becomes unstable and causes a reduction in globin synthesis
5. A total or partial depletion of a globin gene, probably as the result of unequal chromosomes crossing over

Classical thalassemia has two main variants: major and minor (Table 13.6). These descriptions, however, usually reflect the clinical severity of the hemoglobinopathy. Thalassemia major is usually equivalent to beta-thalassemia in a homozygous form and is sometimes called **Cooley's anemia.** A third type of thalassemia, delta-thalassemia, occurs rarely but it is not clinically significant because the delta chain is a component of the minor hemoglobin, Hb A_2.

Physiology

Thalassemias are characterized by the absence or decrease in the synthesis of one of the two constituent globin subunits of a normal hemoglobin molecule. In alpha-thalassemia, decreased synthesis of alpha globulin results in accelerated red cell destruction because of the formation of insoluble Hb H inclusion in the mature erythrocyte. The more severe beta-thalassemia reflects the extreme insolubility of alpha globin, which is present in excess in the red cell because of decreased beta globin synthesis. Studies of RNA metabolism in erythroid cells have suggested that many patients with beta-thalassemia have a defect in RNA processing. This defect affects efficient RNA splicing during protein globin synthesis.

TABLE 13.6 Thalassemia Types

Phenotype	Clinical Descriptions
Thal "minor"	Mild anemia, microcytosis, abnormal erythrocyte morphology, splenomegaly
Thal "intermedia"	Moderate anemia and ineffective erythropoiesis, microcytosis, abnormal erythrocyte morphology, splenomegaly, iron overload, not transfusion dependent
Thal "major" (Cooley's anemia)	Severe anemia due to ineffective erythropoiesis, transfusion dependent, organ damage (heart, liver, etc.) secondary to iron overload, extra-medullary erythropoiesis, hepatosplenomegaly

Alpha-Thalassemia

Alpha-thalassemia is a group of disorders characterized by decreased synthesis of alpha chains. Alpha-thalassemias can be classified into four types on the basis of genotype and the total number of abnormal genes that result.

In thalassemia minor (silent carrier), patients are missing only one functioning alpha gene. The three remaining alpha genes direct the synthesis of an adequate number of alpha chains for normal hemoglobin synthesis; therefore, patients have no clinical manifestation of the hemoglobinopathy. Hemoglobin electrophoresis, red blood cell measurements, and peripheral blood smears are essentially normal.

Hemoglobin constant spring has one deletion and represents an mRNA termination defect. It is a hemoglobin formed from the combination of two structurally abnormal alpha chains, each elongated by 31 amino acids at the carboxy-terminal end, and two normal beta chains. The homozygous state is phenotypically similar to mild alpha-thalassemia.

Patients with alpha-thalassemia trait have two missing alpha genes. The imbalance of alpha- and beta-chain synthesis creates an excess in beta chains, which join in tetrads to form hemoglobin H. Manifestations of alpha-thalassemia are usually mild to moderate in nature. The most noticeable abnormality is the presence of a microcytic, hypochromic anemia.

Three deletions are present in patients with thalassemia major, Hb H disease. Hb H, formed from tetrads of beta chains, is unstable and has a high affinity for molecular oxygen ($10\times$ the affinity of Hb A). Erythrocytes containing Hb H produce precipitated Hb H when incubated with brilliant cresyl blue. These erythrocytes have a decreased life span because of the damage to the cell membrane by the precipitated Hb H and the poor handling of inclusions by the normal pitting function of the spleen. Hb H disease is a chronic, moderately severe hemolytic anemia that occurs most frequently in individuals from Southeast Asia. A slight variation in the degree of anemia exists. Conditions such as pregnancy, infection, or the consumption of oxidant drugs worsen the condition. Hemoglobin levels usually range from 8 to 10 gm/dL. Red cell indices (MCV, MCH, MCHC) are decreased. The reticulocyte count is increased from 5% to 10%. Hemoglobin electrophoresis demonstrates HB H (4% to 30%), small amounts of Hb Bart, and a normal or decreased amount of Hb A_2.

Hydrops fetalis represents a state of four deletions. This lack of alpha-chain production is incompatible with life. Affected fetuses die either in utero or shortly after birth.

Beta-Thalassemia

Beta-thalassemia is one of the most common single-gene disorders. More than 100 mutations in or around the β-globin gene are known to cause decreased production of β-globin, which in turn leads to the excess accumulation of unstable (gamma)-globin chains, ineffective erythropoiesis, and shortened red cell survival. Although the clinical severity of beta-thalassemia varies considerably, most patients who are homozygous for beta-thalassemia become dependent on transfusions and develop transfusion-related complications of iron overload, alloimmunization, and potential viral infection.

Prevention. Careful counseling and prenatal diagnosis in Sardinia reduced the incidence of homozygous beta-thalassemia by more than 90%.

Treatment. Bone marrow transplantation from HLA-identical related donors is an accepted treatment for patients with homozygous beta-thalassemia.

Any combination of normal beta genes and beta-thalassemia genes is possible, producing a wide variety of phenotypes. In the production of normal hemoglobin, equal quantities of alpha and beta chains are synthesized, which results in a 1:1 alpha-beta-chain ratio. In beta-thalassemia, synthesis of beta chains is decreased or absent; therefore, an excess of alpha chains results.

This underproduction of beta chains contributes to a decrease in the total erythrocyte hemoglobin production, ineffective erythropoiesis, and a chronic hemolytic process. The excess free alpha chains are unstable and precipitate within the cell, causing membrane damage. Marrow macrophages destroy precipitate-filled erythrocytes in the bone marrow, which results in ineffective erythropoiesis. Precipitate-filled circulating erythrocytes are destroyed prematurely in the spleen. This also contributes to the anemia of thalassemia.

In homozygous beta-thalassemia, symptoms are usually manifested in early life after hemoglobin synthesis switches from gamma-chain to beta-chain synthesis several months after birth. Infants fail to grow, and splenomegaly is common. Severe anemia is the most outstanding feature of the disorder and is responsible for many related problems. Regular transfusions are required to prevent death; however, the accumulation of iron from transfused blood is a problem.

Persistence of Fetal Hemoglobin

Hereditary persistence of fetal hemoglobin (HPFH) is a group of conditions characterized by the persistence of total hemoglobin synthesis in adult life. The distribution of fetal hemoglobin in red cells (see Chapter 24) determines the classification of this disorder. Heterocellular HPFH is found in a small percentage of cells. In contrast, the pancellular form displays a uniform distribution of hemoglobin F among the red cells. Heterocellular HPFH appears to be inherited. The number of fetal hemoglobin-containing cells is increased but no abnormalities in delta and beta chain production are evident. The common type of pancellular HPFH appears to be a form of delta-beta-thalassemia in which the gamma genes are not switched off and are able to compensate fully for the lack of delta and beta chain production.

Laboratory Findings

In beta-thalassemia, hematological findings include decreased hemoglobin, Hct, and red cell count. The hemoglobin concentration can be as low as 2 or 3 gm/dL in homozygous patients. Peripheral blood smears reveal anisocytosis, poikilocytosis, hypochromia, target cells, polychromatophilia, and few to many nucleated red cells. Erythrocytes are mark-

TABLE 13.7 Summary of Selected Laboratory Findings in the Hemoglobinopathies

Disorder	Test	Result
Sickle cell disease	Hemoglobin	Decreased
	PCV	Decreased
	Erythrocyte count	Decreased
	Hb S	Markedly increased
	Hb A	Decreased
	Hb F	Increased
Sickle cell trait	Hemoglobin	Normal
	PCV	Normal
	Erythrocyte count	Normal
	Hb S	Increased
	Hb A	Slightly decreased
	Hb F	Normal or slightly increased
Homozygous beta-thalassemia	Hemoglobin	Decreased
	PCV	Decreased
	Erythrocyte count	Decreased
	Hb S	Negative
	Hb A	Markedly decreased
	Hb F	Increased

PCV = packed cell volume.

edly microcytic and hypochromic. The red cell indices (MCV, MCH, MCHC) are markedly reduced. In addition, the red cell distribution width (RDW) is increased because of the anisocytosis. Other laboratory findings include increased reticulocyte formation (5 to 10%), decreased osmotic fragility, moderately increased bilirubin, increased serum iron, and saturated total iron-binding capacity. Hemoglobin electrophoresis reveals increased Hb F and decreased Hb A. A variable form of homozygous beta-thalassemia demonstrates no Hb A, increased Hb A_2, and decreased Hb F. The absence of Hb A is due to the absence of beta chain synthesis.

Heterozygous beta-thalassemia could be mistaken for a mild iron deficiency anemia on a peripheral blood smear. Other laboratory findings include decreased MCV, increased Hb A_2 on electrophoresis, and decreased osmotic fragility. Table 13.7 summarizes the significant test results in sickle cell anemia, sickle cell trait, and thalassemia.

Early treatment with deferoxamine in patients with thalassemia major (beta-thal) can improve survival and reduce the prevalence of major complications of iron overload such as cardiac impairment.

OTHER HEMOGLOBINOPATHIES

Hemoglobin C Disease

This hemoglobinopathy is prevalent in the same geographic area as Hb S (sickle cell) disease. Hemoglobin C differs from Hb A by the substitution of a single amino acid residual, lysine, for glutamic acid in the sixth position from the amino (NH_2) terminal end of the β chain. This is the exact point of substitution of Hb S; however, the amino acid is different.

Deoxyhemoglobin C has decreased solubility and forms intracellular crystals (see Plate 20). Erythrocyte morphology is usually normochromic and normocytic, with more than 50% target cells on peripheral blood smear examination. Clinical manifestations include mild, chronic hemolytic anemia with associated splenomegaly. Hemoglobin C trait is symptomless. Laboratory findings include target cells and possibly mild hypochromia.

Hemoglobin SC Disease

This disorder results from the inheritance of one gene for Hb S from one parent and one gene for Hb C from the other parent. The course of this disease is generally milder than sickle cell disease, although Hb C tends to aggregate and potentiate the sickling of Hb S.

Clinical signs and symptoms are similar to mild sickle cell anemia. Laboratory examination of a peripheral blood smear usually reveals target cells, folded erythrocytes, and occasionally, intracellular crystals.

Hemoglobin D Disease

Hemoglobin D has several variants. Patients who are homozygous or heterozygous are asymptomatic. Some target cells may be seen on examination of a peripheral blood smear. Hemoglobin D migrates to the same position as Hb S and Hb G at an alkaline pH but migrates with Hb A at an acid pH.

Hemoglobin E Disease

This hemoglobinopathy occurs with the greatest frequency in Southeast Asia. In some areas of Thailand, the frequency of the Hb E trait is almost 50%. Hemoglobin E results from the substitution of lysine for glutamic acid in the beta chain of hemoglobin. In the homozygous state, patients suffer from a mild microcytic anemia with decreased erythrocyte survival. Target cells are visible on peripheral blood smears. Hemoglobin E is slightly unstable and there is an associated thalassemic component. The presence of Hb E may have a protective effect against malaria.

Hemoglobin H disease is a mild to severe chronic hemolytic anemia. The disease most frequently results from an absence of three of the four alpha-globin genes.

This hemoglobin variant primarily affects individuals throughout Southeast Asia, the Mediterranean islands, and parts of the Middle East. Because of the large influx of immigrants from Southeast Asia in the last 20 to 30 years, the prevalence of hemoglobin H disease in the United States has increased significantly.

Hemoglobin H migrates at a fast rate at an alkaline pH during hemoglobin electrophoresis. The complete blood count may give important clues to the presence of hemoglobin H disease. All patients exhibit markedly abnormal findings. The results are similar to those in iron deficiency anemia, except that in hemoglobin H disease, the red blood cell count and RDW are usually greater, and the MCV is usually lower. A peripheral blood smear exhibits more target cells, anisocytosis, poikilocytosis, and polychromasia than do patients with iron deficiency. The reticulocyte count is generally between 5 and 10%, but it may be within the normal range. Serum ferritin can be normal or elevated.

Methemoglobinemia

Methemoglobinemia is a disorder associated with elevated methemoglobin levels (>2%) in the circulating blood. Causes of methemoglobinemia include acquired toxic substances, Hb M variants, and NADH-diaphorase deficiency.

Hemoglobin M has five variant forms. It displays a dominant inheritance resulting from a single substitution of an amino acid in the globin chain that stabilizes iron in the ferric form. NADH diaphorase is the enzyme that reduces cytochrome b5, which converts naturally occurring ferric iron back to the ferrous state.

Patients with congenital methemoglobinemia tolerate baseline methemoglobin levels of up to 40% without symptoms other than cyanosis. Patients with acquired methemoglobinemia caused by foreign oxidants begin to develop symptoms of hypoxia at methemoglobin levels of 20% to 40%. The symptoms produced by methemoglobinemia do not respond to oxygen therapy. Initial therapy consists of removal of any toxin which may be causing the accelerated hemoglobin oxidation. Except in cases of Hb M disease and in patients with G6PD deficiency, methylene blue effectively treats methemoglobinemia by quickly reducing the ferric heme iron to its useful ferrous state. If life-threatening levels of methemoglobin are present, exchange transfusion may be the therapy of choice.

Unstable Hemoglobins

Unstable hemoglobins are hemoglobin variants in which amino acid substitutions or deletions weaken the binding forces that maintain the internal portion of the globin chains of the hemoglobin molecule. Most unstable hemoglobins are inherited as autosomal dominant disorders.

Instability may cause abnormal hemoglobin to denature and precipitate in erythrocytes such as Heinz bodies. As a result, red blood cells become rigid, membrane damage occurs, and hemolysis results. Hemolysis is usually associated with a change in the normal environment such as the presence of an oxidizing drug or an infection. Heinz bodies are associated with alpha- or beta-chain abnormalities. Tetramers of normal chains, such as Hb Bart and Hb H, appear in thalassemias.

SUMMARY
Hemoglobin Defects

The hemolytic anemias are characterized by decreased red cell survival due to inherited or acquired mechanisms. Hemoglobinopathies may or may not have a hemolytic manifestation. About 25% of all hemoglobinopathies demonstrate the decreased red cell survival that characterizes hemolytic disease.

The common denominator in the hemoglobinopathies is that all represent an inherited or genetic defect related to hemoglobin. This defect may result in an abnormal structure of the hemoglobin molecule or a deficiency in the synthesis of normal adult hemoglobin. Hemoglobinopathies can be classified into abnormal molecular structure of one or more of the polypeptide chains of globulin in the hemoglobin molecule; a defect in the rate of synthesis of one or more of the polypeptide chains of globulin in the hemoglobin molecule; and a combination of abnormal molecular structure with a synthesis defect.

Normal adult hemoglobin contains the following components: Hb A (95% to 98%), Hb A_2 (2% to 3%), Hb A_1 (3% to 6%), and Hb F (less than 1%). The major fraction is Hb A. Typically, the individual with a hemoglobinopathy will demonstrate an alteration in this pattern.

The hemoglobinopathies are inherited diseases. Some of these disorders are caused by the inheritance of an autosomal dominant gene that will produce hemolytic disease in its heterozygous state. Others are autosomal recessive genes and need to be in the homozygous state to produce the disease.

In the hemoglobinopathies, the distinction between the disease state and the trait condition is made. A disease is defined as either the homozygous occurrence of the gene for the abnormality or the possession of a heterozygous, dominant gene that produces a hemolytic condition. A trait is described as the heterozygous and normally asymptomatic state.

Sickle Cell Disease

Sickle cell disease is a general term for abnormalities of hemoglobin structure and function, hemoglobinopathies, in which the sickle gene is inherited from at least one parent. These genetic disorders are characterized by the production of hemoglobin S (Hb S), anemia, and acute and chronic tissue damage secondary to the blockage of blood flow produced by abnormally shaped red blood cells.

Sickle cell anemia (Hb SS), the most common form of hemoglobinopathy, is an expression of the inheritance of a sickle gene from both parents. Other sickle cell disorders result from the coinheritance of the sickle gene. Common variants include hemoglobin SC disease (Hb SC) and beta-thalassemia (Sβ-thalassemia).

Sickle cell disease is found most commonly in persons of African ancestry, but it also affects persons of Mediterranean, Caribbean, South and Central American, Arab, and East Indian ancestry. The high prevalence in some regions is due to a selective advantage of the carrier state to malaria infection.

In the United States, an estimated 8% of the African-American population carries the trait, and approximately one in 375 African-American newborns are born with sickle cell anemia.

Hemoglobin SC disease (Hb SC) affects an estimated one in 835 African-American births and sickle cell beta-thalassemia (Sβ-thalassemia) affects one in 1667 African-American live births. As a result, it is one of the most common genetic diseases in the United States.

When Hb S is deoxygenated, it becomes polymerized and produces sickling. Subsequent hemolysis is probably a result of the extent of the red cell's capacity to sickle. Acute crises are due to recurrent obstruction of the microcirculation by intravascular sickling. Aside from the painful crisis, sickling takes its toll on the body in other ways. Through the years, the cumulative damage from vascular occlusion can lead to organ and tissue failure. Other complications may include an enlarged heart, progressive loss of pulmonary or renal function, stroke, arthritis, and liver damage.

In addition to decreased hemoglobin, hematocrit, and red blood cell count, a persistent increase in the WBC count is common. The red cell morphology on peripheral blood smear can include moderate to marked anisocytosis, poikilocytosis, and hypochromia. Red cell abnormalities may include target cells, microcytes, polychromatophilia, and basophilic stippling. Howell-Jolly bodies may be present if hyposplenism is present. If the patient is in an acute crisis state, sickled red cells (drepanocytes) may be seen on peripheral smears.

Other diagnostic laboratory tests can include sickle cell screening tests, hemoglobin electrophoresis, the alkali denaturation test, an acid elution test, and determination of the osmotic fragility of erythrocytes.

Conventional management of sickle cell anemia is primarily supportive. It is important to detect infections early and treat them with antibiotics, as these infections may trigger painful and aplastic crises. Drug therapy consisting of erythropoietin injection and the drug hydroxyurea are two treatment protocols.

Genetic counseling may be useful in the prevention of sickle cell anemia when the parents are both SA heterozygotes.

Sickle cell anemia was the first molecular disease to be recognized. The severity of illness in sickle cell disease differs with the quantity of hemoglobin S in the erythrocytes. The various states associated with the presence of hemoglobin S are sickle-beta thalassemia and sickle-C (SC) disease.

Thalassemia

The thalassemia syndromes are among the most common genetic diseases in humans. These syndromes are caused by an abnormality in the rate of synthesis of the globin chains. This is in contrast to the true hemoglobinopathies (for example, Hb S and Hb C) that result from an inherited structural defect in one of the globin chains that produces hemoglobin with abnormal physical or functional characteristics.

One of five processes is now believed to be responsible for the genetic defect in thalassemia. These processes are mutations of various types leading to early termination of globin chain synthesis, inefficient splicing of mRNA, a decrease in the rate of gene expression, a reduction in globin synthesis, or a total or partial depletion of a globin.

Classical thalassemia has two main variants: major and minor. These descriptions, however, usually reflect the clinical severity of the hemoglobinopathy. Thalassemia major is usually equivalent to beta-thalassemia in a homozygous form and is sometimes called **Cooley's anemia.** A third type of thalassemia, delta-thalassemia, occurs rarely but it is not clinically significant because the delta chain is a component of the minor hemoglobin, Hb A_2.

Alpha-thalassemia is a group of disorders characterized by decreased synthesis of alpha chains. Alpha-thalassemias can be classified into four types on the basis of genotype and the total number of abnormal genes that result.

Beta-thalassemia is one of the most common single-gene disorders. More than 100 mutations in or around the β-globin gene are known to cause decreased production of β-globin, which in turn leads to the excess accumulation of unstable (gamma)-globin chains, ineffective erythropoiesis, and shortened red-cell survival.

Hereditary persistence of fetal hemoglobin (HPFH) is a group of conditions characterized by the persistence of total hemoglobin synthesis in adult life.

In beta-thalassemia, hematological findings include decreased hemoglobin, Hct, and red cell count. The hemoglobin concentration can be as low as 2 or 3 gm/dL in homozygous patients. In contrast, heterozygous beta-thalassemia could be mistaken for a mild iron deficiency anemia on a peripheral blood smear. Other laboratory findings include decreased MCV, increased Hb A_2 on electrophoresis, and decreased osmotic fragility.

Other Hemoglobinopathies

Hemoglobin C disease is prevalent in the same geographic area as Hb S (sickle cell) disease. Hemoglobin C differs from Hb A by the substitution of a single amino acid residual, lysine, for glutamic acid in the sixth position from the amino (NH_2) terminal end of the β chain. This is the exact point of substitution of Hb S; however, the amino acid is different.

Hemoglobin E disease occurs with the greatest frequency in Southeast Asia. In some areas of Thailand, the frequency of the Hb E trait is almost 50%. Hemoglobin E results from the substitution of lysine for glutamic acid in the beta chain of hemoglobin.

Hemoglobin H disease is a mild to severe chronic hemolytic anemia. The disease most frequently results from an absence of three of the four alpha-globin genes.

Methemoglobinemia is a disorder associated with elevated methemoglobin levels (>2%) in the circulating blood. Causes of methemoglobinemia include acquired toxic substances, Hb M variants, and NADH-diaphorase deficiency.

Unstable hemoglobins are hemoglobin variants in which amino acid substitutions or deletions weaken the binding forces that maintain the internal portion of the globin chains of the hemoglobin molecule. Most unstable hemoglobins are inherited as autosomal dominant disorders.

CASE STUDIES

CASE 1 An 18-year-old black woman was admitted for elective surgery. She had a routine preoperative CBC and urinalysis.

Laboratory Data
The results of these tests were as follows:

Hemoglobin 13.0 gm/dL
Hct 0.40 L/L
RBC 4.35 × 10^{12}/L
WBC 7.3 × 10^9/L

The RBC indices were as follows:

MCV 92 fL
MCH 29.9 pg
MCHC 33%

The patient's peripheral blood smear revealed a normochromic, normocytic pattern; however, a moderate number of target cells (codocytes) were noted throughout the smear.

A repeat blood smear obtained from fingertip blood again had a moderate number of target cells (codocytes) present. The urinalysis revealed no abnormalities. A hematology technician notified the surgeon and anesthetist of the abnormal RBC morphology.

On receipt of these results, the patient's anesthetist postponed surgery and ordered a sickle cell preparation, sickle cell screening test, and hemoglobin electrophoresis. The results were:

Sickle cell preparation positive
Hb S screening test positive
Hb electrophoresis: Hb A 63%, Hb F 3%, and Hb S 34%

Questions
1. Why was it important to establish a diagnosis in this patient's asymptomatic state?
2. What kind of disorder did this patient suffer from?
3. What is the etiology of this patient's condition?

Discussion
1. This patient had sickle cell trait, which, under ordinary conditions, is usually asymptomatic except for the presence of codocytes on a peripheral blood smear. However, the fact that the patient was to undergo elective surgery made it important for the anesthetist to be aware of the patient's condition in order to carefully monitor the patient to prevent hypoxia.
2. The presence of a great number of true codocytes on a peripheral film is highly suggestive of a hemoglobinopathy. Because the codocytes (target cells) persisted on repeated smears, the possibility that the targeting was an artifact was eliminated. Supplementary laboratory assays provided the differential information needed to establish the diagnosis of sickle cell trait. The profile of this patient is typical of sickle cell trait. She is a heterozygous Hb A-Hb S. Both the sickle cell preparation, which exposed the cells to reduced oxygen levels, and the Hb S screening test confirmed the electrophoresis findings of the presence of the abnormal type S hemoglobin.
3. This patient suffered from a hemoglobinopathy, which is a genetically inherited trait. In her case, she received only one gene for S-type hemoglobin, and was fortunate to have received a normal gene for A-type hemoglobin. About 10% of American blacks possess the sickle cell trait. Identifying its existence in an individual is important for two reasons. Exposure to reduced oxygen levels will cause some of the cells of the individual to sickle, and the genetic consequences to future offspring are an important aspect of prenatal counseling in both men and women who possess the trait.

📖 **Diagnosis: Sickle cell trait**

(continued)

CASE 2 The 5-year-old son of a Liberian exchange student was hospitalized because of severe diarrhea, abdominal distention, and splenomegaly. The child had been previously diagnosed in Europe as suffering from sickle cell anemia, and had experienced several episodes of sickle cell crisis.

On admission, the following tests were ordered: CBC, platelet count, bilirubin determination, hemoglobin electrophoresis, Hb S screening test, electrolyte studies, urinalysis, and stool culture.

Laboratory Data
The results of the tests were as follows:

Hemoglobin 5.8 gm/dL
Hct 0.19 L/L
RBC 2.0 × 10^{12}/L

The RBC indices were as follows:

MCV 96 fL
MCH 29 pg
MCHC 31%

The total WBC count was 8.7 × 10^9/L. The peripheral blood smear revealed moderate anisocytosis, macrocytosis, microcytosis, poikilocytosis, polychromatophilia, occasional Howell-Jolly bodies, moderate basophilic stippling, many sickled RBCs (drepanocytes), and 12 (nucleated RBCs) metarubricytes/100 WBCs. The distribution of platelets was normal on the blood smear, and the total platelet count was 0.42 × 10^{12}/L.

The patient's total serum bilirubin was 6.0 mg/dL. Hemoglobin electrophoresis demonstrated Hb S 78% and Hb F 22%. The Hb S screening test result was positive. A routine urinalysis was positive for occult blood, and the stool culture was normal. The patient had severely abnormal electrolytes.

Questions
1. What is the cause of this patient's condition?
2. What is the clinical course of this disease?
3. Explain the presence of the drepanocytes on the peripheral blood film.

Discussion
1. The patient had been previously diagnosed as suffering from sickle cell anemia. However, the current "crisis" was undoubtedly precipitated by the dehydration caused by severe diarrhea. Although the exact trigger mechanism is not really known, events such as dehydration, fatigue, and emotional stress can trigger a crisis episode in patients with sickle cell anemia.
2. Sickle cell anemia takes a chronic clinical course. The course of the disease is characterized by hemolytic episodes, severe organ damage, and painful, acute episodes involving both bones and muscles. Painful crises are a feature of this disease. The crises correspond to obstruction of the microcirculation by the sickled cells, followed by ischemia which produces the associated pain and sometimes consequent necrosis of tissues.
3. Congestion in the microcirculation, tissue hypoxia, and the lowering of blood pH are all factors that promote the gelation of Hb S. With this gelation, the sickle cell assumes its characteristic shape. Many of these cells will assume a discoid shape following reoxygenation; however, dense sickle cells are irreversibly sickled. These cells have

a distinctive boat shape and will not resume the normal discoid shape after reoxygenation.

 Diagnosis: Sickle cell anemia

CASE 3 A 21-year-old white female college student of Greek ethnicity visited her gynecologist in San Francisco. She appeared to be healthy, and was 3 months pregnant. She was concerned about her future child, because she had been diagnosed as a child as having heterozygous beta-thalassemia. However, she had never had any "blood problems," but knew that her disorder had been inherited.

The following tests were ordered: CBC, urinalysis, and hemoglobin electrophoresis.

Laboratory Data
The results of these tests were as follows:

Hemoglobin 11.1 gm/dL
Hct 0.29 L/L
RBC 4.2 × 10^{12}/L

Her WBC count was 5.8 × 10^9/L. The peripheral blood smear revealed the presence of marked microcytosis, 2+ hypochromia, and some codocytes (target cells). Her RBC indices were as follows:

MCV 69 fL
MCH 26.4 pg
MCHC 37%

The distribution of platelets was normal on the peripheral smear. The hemoglobin electrophoresis revealed a slight increase in the Hb A_2 fraction (patient 3.5%, normal 2 to 3%), and the F fraction (patient 2%, normal is less than 1%). The urinalysis was normal.

On receipt of these results the patient's physician referred her to a research laboratory for prenatal testing and counseling.

Questions
1. Explain the asymptomatic state and peripheral blood findings in this patient.
2. Why did the patient's physician refer her to a research clinic for further prenatal testing?
3. What kind of advanced prenatal testing can be performed?

Discussion
1. Patients with heterozygous beta-thalassemia are frequently asymptomatic. The expression of this disorder can range from an asymptomatic state, as in this patient, to a fairly severe anemia. Her peripheral blood film is typical of the heterozygous patient with microcytosis, hypochromia, and codocytes. This condition can be confused with iron deficiency anemia until further laboratory studies are conducted, such as serum iron and TIBC and hemoglobin electrophoresis.
2. Modern prenatal testing for hematological disease began in 1974. Prior to that time, chromosomal studies were performed on amniotic fluid in older women with a high risk of Down's syndrome, or in order to determine fetal sex if the patient was at risk for a sex-linked disorder. Methods for obtaining fetal blood in utero were established in 1974, and this led to the development of prenatal diagnosis of any blood disorder that expressed itself in utero.

(continued)

C A S E   S T U D I E S (*continued*)

The first disorders to be studied were the hemoglobinopathies, specifically thalassemia. Recently, a third technique that utilizes amniotic fluid was developed for use with DNA probes. Sampling of fetal blood remains the method of choice for the detection of hematological diseases for which DNA probes are not available.

During the midtrimester, blood is aspirated from the placenta. In order to determine the proportion of fetal blood in the sample, RBC size (MCV) is performed immediately on the specimen. Fetal erythrocytes have an average MCV of 140 fL, compared with adult or maternal RBCs which have an average MCV of 100 fL. The sample is then labeled with a radioactive substance and incubated to label newly synthesized globin chains. Mutant beta globins are detected with this technique because they separate from normal beta globin on chromatographic analysis. The diagnosis of alpha- or beta-thalassemia can be made based on either the absence of or the substantially reduced amount of globin in the sample. By this method, 25% of the samples lead to a diagnosis of thalassemia in cases where the fetus is at risk. This frequency is proportional to the expected frequency for autosomal recessive disorders.

If amniocentesis studies are done, the fluid is obtained at 16 to 20 weeks of gestation. The sample must contain enough fetal cells to provide DNA for study of the globin genes. Earlier studies may now be done using chorionic villi specimens. All of these procedures are aimed at the early diagnosis of hematological diseases of genetic origin.

✏️ **Diagnosis: Prenatal patient with thalassemia minor (heterozygous beta-thalassemia)**

CASE 4 A 23-year-old Italian woman is noted to be suffering from mild anemia in a preemployment physical examination. The patient denied any significant illness in the past. She has no history of joint or abdominal pain and she was not sickly as a child. She has been told on several occasions that she has anemia and was given medications containing iron. She has not noticed any unusual bleeding. Her menstrual periods are regular at monthly intervals and they last for about 3 days. She has never been pregnant. She has no history of excessive alcohol intake.

Physical examination revealed an enlarged spleen. She has no icterus, purpura, or lymphadenopathy. Her liver is not enlarged.

Laboratory Data
Hemoglobin 11.0 gm/dL
Hematocrit 35%
RBC 5.0 × 10^{12}/L
WBC 9500 × 10^9/L

The peripheral blood smear shows target cells, an occasional sickle-shaped cell, microcytes, and slight hypochromia. Reticulocyte count: 7.2%.

Questions
1. What is the differential diagnosis?
2. What test will aid in the differential diagnosis?

3. What is the probable diagnosis?
4. How do you account for this patient's benign course?
5. Why does the patient have disease, compared to AS individuals who are asymptomatic?
6. What complications might arise in the future?
7. The husband has normal (AA) hemoglobin. They are expecting a child. What are the odds that the baby will have a clinically serious hemoglobin disorder? What are the odds that the baby will have a normal genotype (AA)?

Discussion
1. Striking target cells are seen in liver disease and hemoglobinopathies. The fact that hemolysis is present and this patient lacks clinical evidence of liver disease both favor the latter alternative.
2. Hemoglobin electrophoresis, serum Fe/TIBC to rule out iron deficiency, liver function tests, solubility test for the presence of hemoglobin S. Liver function was normal. The hemoglobin electrophoresis on acrylamide gel was abnormal.
3. Sickle-beta$^+$ thalassemia
4. The extent of polymer formation is less in S-beta$^+$ thalassemia, owing primarily to lower MCHC and less crowding of hemoglobin molecules in the red cell. The ability to synthesize some hemoglobin A also reduces intracellular polymer formation.
5. Cells contain much more hemoglobin S and therefore will form more polymer.
6. Proliferative retinopathy and avascular necrosis of hip; these complications are particularly common in sickle-beta$^+$ thalassemia and in SC disease for unclear reasons.
7. Nil Pedigree:

$$B^s B^+ thal ------------- B^A B^A$$

$$B^S B^A \quad B^S B^A \quad\quad B^+ thal B^A \quad B^+ thal B^A$$

✏️ **Diagnosis: Sickle-beta$^+$ thalassemia**

B I B L I O G R A P H Y

Adams, R. et al. "The Use of Transcranial Ultrasonography to Predict Stroke in Sickle Cell Disease." *N. Engl. J. Med.*, Vol. 326, No. 9, February 27, 1992, pp. 605–610.

Armbruster, D. A. "Neonatal Hemoglobinopathy Screening." *Lab. Med.*, Vol. 21, No. 12, December, 1990, pp. 815–822.

Ballas, S. K. and R. J. R. Castillo. "Pain in Sickle Cell Disease." *N. Engl. J. Med.*, Vol. 325, No. 24, 1991, p. 1747.

Ballas, S. K. "Management of Sickle Cell Disease." *Hospital Physician*, Vol. 29, No. 7, July, 1993, pp. 12–15, 29–35.

Bellet, P. et al. "Incentive Spirometry to Prevent Acute Pulmonary Complications in Sickle Cell Diseases." *N. Engl. J. Med.*, Vol. 333, No. 11, September 14, 1995, pp. 699–703.

Beutler, E. "Problems in the Diagnosis of the Hemoglobinopathies of Polycythemia." *Mayo Clin. Proc.*, Vol. 66, January, 1991, pp. 102–104.

Borgna-Pignatti, C. "Marrow Transplantation for Thalassemia." *Annu. Rev. Med.*, Vol. 36, 1985, pp. 329–336.

Brittenham, G. M. et al. "Efficacy of Deferoxamine in Preventing Complications of Iron Overload in Patients With Thalassemia Major." Vol. 33, No. 9, September 1, 1994, pp. 567–578.

Cao, A., L. Saba, R. Galanello, M. C. Rosatelli. "Molecular Diagnosis and Carrier Screening for B Thalassemia." *JAMA*, Vol. 278, No. 15, October 15, 1997, pp. 1273–1277.

Charache, S. et al. "Effect of Hydrourea on the Frequency of Painful Crises in Sickle Cell Anemia." *N. Engl. J. Med.*, Vol. 332, No. 20, May 18, 1995, pp. 1317–1322.

Dover, G. J. and D. Valle. "Therapy for B-Thalassemia—A Paradigm for the Treatment of Genetic Disorders." *N. Engl. J. Med.*, Vol. 331, No. 9, September 1, 1994, p. 609.

Embury, S. H. "The Clinical Pathophysiology of Sickle Cell Disease." *Annu. Rev. Med.*, Vol. 37, 1986, pp. 361–376.

Fabry, M. E. et al. "Dense Cells in Sickle Cell Anemia: The Effects of Gene Interaction." *Blood*, Vol. 64, No. 5, November, 1984, pp. 1042–1046.

Fishleder, A. J. and G. C. Hoffman. "A Practical Approach to the Detection of Hemoglobinopathies: Part I. The Introduction and Thalassemia Syndromes." *Lab. Med.*, Vol. 18, No. 6, June, 1987, pp. 368–372.

Fishleder, A. J. and G. C. Hoffman. "A Practical Approach to the Detection of Hemoglobinopathies: Part II. The Sickle Cell Disorders." *Lab. Med.*, Vol. 18, No. 6, July, 1987, pp. 441–443.

Fishleder, A. J. and G. C. Hoffman. "A Practical Approach to the Detection of Hemoglobinopathies: Part III. Nonsickling Disorders and Cord Blood Screening." *Lab. Med.*, Vol. 18, No. 8, August, 1987, pp. 513–518.

Gill, F. M. et al. "Clinical Events in the First Decade in a Cohort of Infants With Sickle Cell Disease." *Blood*, Vol. 86, No. 2, July 15, 1995, pp. 776, 783.

Griffin, T. C., D. McIntire, and G. R. Buchanan. "High-Dose Intravenous Methylprednisolone Therapy for Pain in Children and Adolescents With Sickle Cell Disease." *N. Engl. J. Med.*, Vol. 330, No. 11, March 17, 1994, pp. 733–737.

Habermann, Thomas M. "Hematology" (Chapter 18), in U. Prakash (ed.), *Mayo Internal Medicine Board Review* (1994–1995). Rochester, MN: Mayo Foundation for Medical Education and Research, 1994, pp. 440–442.

Hagger, D., S. Wolff, J. Owen, and D. Samson. "Changes in Coagulation and Fibrinolysis in Patients With Sickle Cell Disease Compared With Healthy Black Controls." *Blood Coagulation Fibrinolysis*, Vol. 6, No. 2, April, 1995, pp. 93–99.

Hall, R. B. et al. "Optimizing the Detection of Hemoglobin H Disease." *Laboratory Medicine*, Vol. 26, No. 11, November, 1995, pp. 736–741.

Henry, J. B. (ed.). *Clinical Diagnosis and Management by Laboratory Methods.* Philadelphia: Saunders, 1991.

Heguy, A. et al., "Gene Expression as a Target for New Drug Discovery." *Gene Expression*, Vol. 4, No. 6, 1995, pp. 337–344.

Hillman, R. S. and C. A. Finch. *Red Cell Manual* (7th ed.). Philadelphia: Davis, 1996.

Hiruma, H. et al. "Sickle Cell Rheology Is Determined by Polymer Fraction-Not Cell Morphology." *Am. J. Hematol.*, Vol. 48, No. 1, 1995, pp. 19–28.

Hoffman, G. C. "The Sickling Disorders." *Lab. Med.*, Vol. 21, No. 12, December, 1990, pp. 797–807.

Honda, S. A. A. et al. "Hemoglobinopathies Detected by CBC Analysis and HPLC Hemoglobin A1c Analysis." *Lab. Med.*, Vol. 25, No. 3, March, 1994, pp. 176–181.

Horan, P. and R. J. Lenox. "Acquired and Congenital Methemoglobinemia." *Guthrie J.*, Vol. 61, No. 4, Fall 1992, pp. 161–164.

Itoh, T., S. Chien, and S. Usami. "Effects of Hemoglobin Concentration on Deformability of Individual Sickle Cells After Deoxygenation." *Blood*, Vol. 85, No. 8, April 15, 1995, pp. 2245–2253.

Jandl, J. *Blood.* Boston: Little, Brown & Co., 1996.

Kan, Y. W. "Development of DNA Analysis for Human Diseases." *JAMA*, Vol. 267, No. 11, March 18, 1992, pp. 1532–1536.

Kodish, E. et al. "Bone Marrow Transplantation for Sickle Cell Disease." *N. Engl. J. Med.*, Vol. 325, No. 19, November 7, 1991, pp. 1349–1352.

Lang, H. K. "Sickle Cell Testing of All Newborns Urged." *ADVANCE for Clinical Laboratory Science*, Vol. 24, No. 9, September, 1993, p. 5.

Lau, Y. et al. "Prevalence and Genotypes of Alpha and Beta-Thalassemia Carriers in Hong Kong—Implications for Population Screening." *N. Engl. J. Med.*, Vol. 336, No. 18, May 1, 1997, pp. 1298–1301.

Ley, T. J. and A. W. Nienhuis. "Induction of Hemoglobin F Synthesis in Patients With Beta Thalassemia." *Annu. Rev. Med.*, Vol. 36, 1985, pp. 485–498.

Lubin, B. "Sickle Cell Disease and the Endothelium." *N. Engl. J. Med.*, Vol. 337, No. 22, November 27, 1997, pp. 1623–1624.

Lucarelli, G. et al. "Marrow Transplantation in Patients With Thalassemia Responsive to Iron Chelation Therapy." *N. Engl. J. Med.*, Vol. 329, No. 12, September 16, 1992, pp. 840–844.

Michaels, V. V. "Genetics," in Hematology (Chapter 16), in U. Prakash (ed.), *Mayo Internal Medicine Board Review* (1994–1995). Rochester, MN: Mayo Foundation for Medical Education and Research, 1994, p. 410.

Milner, P. F. et al. "Sickle Cell Disease as a Cause of Osteonecrosis of the Femoral Head." *N. Engl. J. Med.*, Vol. 325, No. 21, November 21, 1991, pp. 1476–1481.

Nagle, R. L. et al. "New Insights on Sickle Cell Anemia." *Diagn. Med.*, Vol. 7, No. 5, May, 1984, pp. 26–33.

Natta, C., C. Luritz, and C. Navarro. "Compartmentalization of Iron in Sickle Cell Anemia—An Autopsy Study." *Am. J. Clin. Pathol.*, Vol. 178, No. 1, January, 1985, p. 76.

Nienhuis, A. W. et al. "Advances in Thalassemia Research." *Blood*, Vol. 63, No. 4, April, 1984, pp. 738–758.

Noguchi, C. T. and A. N. Schechter. "The Intra-cellular Polymerization of Sickle Hemoglobin and Its Relevance to Sickle Cell Disease." *Blood*, Vol. 58, No. 6, December, 1981, pp. 1057–1068.

Orkin, S. H. "Prenatal Diagnosis of Hemoglobin Disorders by DNA Analysis." *Blood*, Vol. 63, No. 2, February, 1984, pp. 249–253.

Pelehach, Laura. "Understanding Sickle Cell Disease." *Lab. Med.*, Vol. 26, No. 11, November, 1995, pp. 720–728.

Platt, O. S. et al. "Mortality in Sickle Cell Disease." *N. Engl. J. Med.*, Vol. 330, No. 23, 1993, pp. 1639–1644.

Platt, O. S. et al. "Pain in Sickle Cell Disease—Rates and Risk Factors." *N. Engl. J. Med.*, Vol. 325, No. 1, July 4, 1991, pp. 11–16.

Platt, O. S. and E. C. Guinan. "Bone Marrow Transplantation in Sickle Cell Anemia—The Dilemma of Choice." *N. Engl. J. Med.*, Vol. 335, No. 6, August 8, 1996, pp. 426–427.

Rodgers, G. P. "Recent Approaches to the Treatment of Sickle Cell Anemia." *JAMA*, Vol. 265, No. 16, April 24, 1991, pp. 2097–2101.

Rogers, Z. R. and G. R. Buchanan. "Bacteremia in Children With Sickle Hemoglobin C Disease and Sickle Beta(+) Thalassemia: Is Prophylactic Penicillin Necessary?" *J. Pediatrics*, Vol. 127, No. 3, September, 1995, pp. 348–354.

Schechter, A. N. and G. P. Rodgers. "Sickle Cell Anemia—Basic Research Reaches the Clinic." *N. Engl. J. Med.*, Vol. 332, No. 20, May 18, 1995, pp. 1372–1374.

Scully, R. E. et al. "Case Records of the Massachusetts General Hospital." *N. Engl. J. Med.*, Vol. 324, No. 3, January 17, 1991, pp. 180–188.

Scully, R. E. et al. "Case Records of the Massachusetts General Hospital." *N. Engl. J. Med.*, Vol. 337, No. 18, October 30, 1997, pp. 1293–1301.

Sergeant, G. R. "Clinical Judgment and Sickle Cell Disease." *N. Engl. J. Med.*, Vol. 329, No. 7, August 12, 1993, pp. 501–502.

Smolinski, P. A., M. K. Offermann, J. R. Eckman, and T. M. Wick. "Double-Stranded RNA Induces Sickle Erythrocyte Adherence to Endothelium: A Potential Role for Viral Infection in Vaso-occlusive Pain Episodes in Sickle Cell Anemia." *Blood*, Vol. 85, No. 10, May 15, 1995, pp. 2945–2950.

Solovey, A. et al. "Circulating Activated Endothelial Cells in Sickle Cell Anemia." *N. Engl. J. Med.*, Vol. 337, No. 22, November 27, 1997, pp. 1584–1590.

Soloway, H. B. and J. B. Peter. "Interpretation of Tests." *Diagn. Med.*, Vol. 8, No. 4, April, 1985, pp. 10–11.

Splendiani, G., C. Tozzo, V. Mazzarella, C. U. Casciani. "Deferoxamine in Thalassemia Major." *N. Engl. J. Med.*, Vol. 332, No. 4, January 26, 1995, pp. 270–271.

Steinberg, M. H. "Genetic Modulation of Sickle Cell Anemia." *Proc. Soc. Exp. Biol. Med.*, Vol. 209, No. 1, May, 1995, pp. 1–13.

Strickland, D. K., R. E. Ware, and T. R. Kinney. "Pitfalls in Newborn Hemoglobinopathy Screening: Failure to Detect Beta(+)-Thalassemia." *J. of Pediatrics*, Vol. 127, No. 2, August, 1995, pp. 304–308.

Turgeon, Mary L. *Clinical Hematology* (2nd ed.). Boston: Little, Brown, & Co., 1996.

U. S. Department of Health and Human Services. "Guideline: Laboratory Screening for Sickle Cell Disease." *Lab. Med.*, Vol. 24, No. 8, August, 1993, pp. 515–522.

Valentine, W. N. and D. E. Paglia. "Erythrocyte Enzymopathies, Hemolytic Anemia, and Multisystem Disease: An Annotated Review." *Blood*, Vol. 64, No. 3, September, 1984, pp. 583–591.

Voskaridou, E., V. Kalotychous, and D. Loukopoulos. "Clinical and

Laboratory Effects of Long-Term Administration of Hydroxyurea to Patients With Sick-Cell/Beta-Thalassaemia." *Br J. Haematol.*, Vol. 89, No. 3, 1995, pp. 479–484.

Wallach, J. *Interpretation of Diagnostic Tests* (5th ed.). Boston: Little, Brown & Co., 1992.

Walters, M. C. et al. "Bone Marrow Transplantation for Sickle Cell Disease." *N. Engl. J. Med.*, Vol. 335, No. 6, August 8, 1996, pp. 369–376.

Weatherall, D. J. *Thalassemias: Methods in Hematology*, Vol. 6. New York: Churchill-Livingstone, 1983.

Winter, W. P. "The Tertiary Diagnosis of Rare Hemoglobin Variants." *Mayo Clin. Proc.*, Vol. 65, June, 1990, pp. 889–891.

Wintrobe, M. M. et al. *Clinical Hematology* (9th ed.). Philadelphia: Lea & Febiger, 1982.

Witkowska, H. E. et al. "Sickle Cell Disease in a Patient With Sickle Cell Trait and Compound Heterozygosity for Hemoglobin S and Hemoglobin Quebec-Chori." *N. Engl. J. Med.*, Vol. 325, No. 16, October 17, 1991, pp. 1150–1154.

REVIEW QUESTIONS

1. The common denominator in the hemoglobinopathies is that all are:

   A. Structural defects in the erythrocyte membrane.
   B. Metabolic defects in the erythrocytic physiology.
   C. Inherited or genetic defects related to hemoglobin.
   D. Acquired defects related to hemoglobin.

2. Hemoglobinopathies can be classified as:

   A. Abnormal hemoglobin globulin structure.
   B. A defect of hemoglobin globulin synthesis.
   C. A combination of defects of both structure and synthesis.
   D. All of the above.

3. True or false:
   Normal adult hemoglobin contains the following components: HbA (95–98%), HbA_2 (2–3%), HbA_1 (3–6%), and HbF (less than 1%).

   A. True.   B. False.

4. In the hemoglobinopathies, a trait is described as:

   A. Heterozygous and asymptomatic.
   B. Heterozygous and symptomatic.
   C. Homozygous and asymptomatic.
   D. Homozygous and symptomatic.

5. In sickle cell anemia the cause is:

   A. A change of a single nucleotide (GAT to GTT).
   B. The substitution of valine for glutamic acid at the 6th position on the beta chain of the hemoglobin molecule.
   C. Not genetic.
   D. Both A and B.

6. In sickle cell disease the abnormality is related to:

   A. The rate of synthesis of hemoglobin.
   B. An abnormal molecular structure of hemoglobin.
   C. An acquired defect.
   D. A membrane dysfunction.

7. The most common inherited hematologic disease is:

   A. Sickle cell trait.
   B. Sickle cell anemia.
   C. Sickle-beta thalassemic.
   D. Hemoglobin SC disease.

8. If a patient with sickle cell anemia is in an acute crisis state, peripheral blood smears may exhibit:

   A. Leptocytes.   C. Ovalocytes.
   B. Drepanocytes.   D. Stomatocytes.

9. What percentage of black Americans are heterozygous for hemoglobin S?

   A. 4%.   C. 12%.
   B. 8%.   D. More than 25%.

10. Thalassemias are characterized by:

    A. Abnormal hemoglobin molecules.
    B. Defective alpha globulin structure.
    C. Abnormality in the rate of synthesis.
    D. Skeletal membrane defects.

11. Homozygous beta-thalassemia patients:

    A. Have no manifestations of anemia.
    B. Have only a mild anemia.
    C. Have a moderate anemia.
    D. Have a severe transfusion dependent anemia.

12. In alpha type thalassemia, which of the following is characteristic?

    A. Hb A_2.   C. Hb H.
    B. Hb A.   D. Hb F and A_2.

13. Deoxyhemoglobin C has:

    A. Decreased solubility.
    B. Increased solubility.
    C. The ability to form intracellular crystals.
    D. Both B and C.

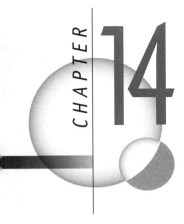

Leukocytes: The Granulocytic and Monocytic Series

The granulocytic series
Production of neutrophils, eosinophils, and basophils
Sites of development and maturation
Development and proliferation of neutrophils, eosinophils, and basophils
Distribution of neutrophils, eosinophils, and basophils
Normal maturational characteristics of neutrophils, eosinophils, and basophils

The monocytic-macrophage series
Production and development of monocytes and macrophages
Morphological characteristics
Normal values and functional properties of granulocytes and monocytes
Normal values
Phagocytosis
Specialized functions
Assessment methods
Total leukocyte count

Differential blood smear evaluation
Absolute cell counts
Erythrocyte sedimentation rate
Assessment of eosinophils and basophils
Leukocyte alkaline phosphatase test
Neutrophilic function
Summary
Bibliography
Review questions

OBJECTIVES

The granulocytic series
- Briefly explain the factors related to the development of multipotential progenitor cells into specific leukocyte cell lines.
- List each type of immature neutrophil found in the proliferative compartment of the bone marrow along with the percentage of each and the approximate time spent in each developmental stage.
- List each type of neutrophil found in the maturation-storage compartment of the bone marrow along with the percentage of each and the approximate time spent in this phase.
- Describe the chemical factors and cellular characteristics that permit neutrophils to leave the bone marrow and enter the peripheral circulation.
- Define the terms **marginating** and **circulating pools** and discuss the length of time the neutrophils, eosinophils, and basophils spend in each pool.
- Describe the nuclear and cytoplasmic characteristics of the neutrophils, eosinophils, and basophils throughout the maturation process.
- Explain the appearance and etiology of the various morphological abnormalities encountered in mature granulocytes.

- Describe the abnormalities associated with mature granulocytes in body fluids.

The monocytic-macrophage series
- Discuss the differentiation of monocytes and macrophages from the multipotential stem cell.
- Compare the bone marrow maturation of the monocyte with that of the neutrophil.
- Describe the nuclear and cytoplasmic characteristics of the monocyte as it develops.

Normal values and functional properties of granulocytes and macrophages
- List the normal values for neutrophils, eosinophils, basophils, and monocytes in normal peripheral blood.
- Describe the general characteristics and specific details of phagocytosis.
- Discuss the specialized functions of eosinophils, basophils, and monocytes.

Assessment methods
- Describe the rationale for each of the methods used in the assessment of inflammatory conditions.

The cellular elements of the blood are produced from a common, multipotential hematopoietic cell. This cell, the progenitor cell, undergoes mitotic division. Subsequent maturation of progenitor cells produces the major categories of the cellular elements of the circulating blood: the erythrocytes, leukocytes, and thrombocytes.

On the basis of function, leukocytes can be divided into the granulocytic, monocytic, and lymphoid series. In this chapter, the granulocytic leukocytes, which can be further subdivided on the basis of morphology into neutrophils, eosinophils, and basophils, and the monocytic-macrophage series are discussed.

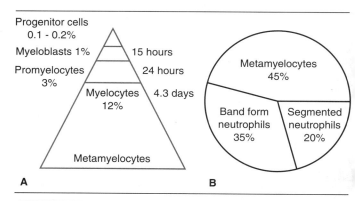

FIGURE 14.1 Bone marrow compartments. **A.** Proliferative. **B.** Maturation-storage.

THE GRANULOCYTIC SERIES

Production of Neutrophils, Eosinophils, and Basophils

Factors that regulate the commitment of a progenitor cell to a specific cell line, such as the granulocytic cell type, and their function are influenced by the hematopoietic growth factors, interleukins, and the microenvironment (see Chapter 4).

Cells that are committed to differentiation as granulocytes have been cloned in vitro and have produced a mixture of granulocytes and macrophage cells. Further growth of these cells is dependent on **colony-stimulating factor** (CSF) and interleukins. The presence of different CSFs favors interleukins, and the microenvironment of the progenitor cell favors differential development of either the granulocytic (**myeloid**) series or the macrophage-monocytic series. In addition to the differentiation of granulocytes and monocytes, different CSFs stimulate specific differentiation, such as the development of eosinophils.

Sites of Development and Maturation

The development, distribution, and destruction of neutrophils, eosinophils, and basophils are collectively referred to as **granulocytic kinetics.** The neutrophil, basophil, and eosinophil each begin as a multipotential cell in the bone marrow. Throughout the normal processes of differentiation, multiplication, and maturation, these cells remain in the bone marrow. After developing into either band or segmented forms, mature cells enter into the blood circulation.

Development and Proliferation of Neutrophils, Eosinophils, and Basophils

When the CFU-GEMM progenitor cell differentiates into the CFU-GM progenitor cell, the cell line becomes committed to developing into a myeloblast; the maturational development from the myeloblast through the myelocyte stage and mitotic division take place in what is referred to as the bone marrow's **proliferative compartment** (Fig. 14.1A). This is also called the **mitotic pool** and includes cells capable of DNA synthesis.

The **myeloblast** is the first identifiable cell in the granulocytic series. Myeloblasts constitute approximately 1% of the total nucleated bone marrow cells. This stage lasts approximately 15 hours. The next stage, the **promyelocyte,** constitutes approximately 3% of the nucleated bone marrow cells. This stage lasts about 24 hours. The **myelocyte** is the next maturational stage, with approximately 12% of the proliferative cells existing in this stage. The stage from myelocyte to **metamyelocyte** lasts an average of 4.3 days. Once the metamyelocyte stage has been reached, cells have undergone four or five cell divisions and the **proliferative phase** comes to an end.

Following the proliferative stage, granulocytes enter a **maturation-storage compartment** (see Fig. 14.1B). The metamyelocytes and most band forms mature into segmented granulocytes in this compartment of the bone marrow. The relative proportions of these cells are approximately 45%, 35%, and 20%, respectively. The segmented neutrophils in the maturation-storage compartment are frequently referred to as the **marrow reserve.** This reserve constitutes a 4- to 8-day supply of neutrophils. It is estimated that neutrophilic granulocytes normally remain in the maturation-storage phase for 7 to 10 days. Eosinophils remain for about 2.5 days, and basophils remain in this phase for the shortest period of time, approximately 12 hours.

Distribution of Neutrophils, Eosinophils, and Basophils

The release of neutrophils from the bone marrow into the circulatory system is a complex process. Certain characteristics (Fig. 14.2) and physiological regulators promote movement of the granulocytes through the sinusoid wall of the bone marrow, which is normally an anatomical barrier. Some of the factors that influence cellular release include the interleukins. Cellular characteristics include an overall reduction in cell size and a smaller nuclear-cytoplasmic ratio. The greater flexibility and mobility of mature cells enhance the migration of cells through the marrow sinusoids into the peripheral blood pool.

The peripheral blood circulation is subsequently divided into two pools of equal size: the **circulating** and the **margin-**

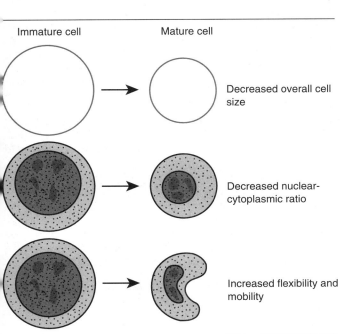

Immature cell   Mature cell

Decreased overall cell size

Decreased nuclear-cytoplasmic ratio

Increased flexibility and mobility

FIGURE 14.2 Comparative maturational characteristics. As cells mature, they are able to move through the sinusoids of the bone marrow because of a decreased overall cell size, a decreased nuclear-cytoplasmic ratio, and increased flexibility and mobility.

ating pools. The marginating granulocytes adhere to the endothelium of the blood vessels. Some granulocytes are additionally found in the spleen. Mature granulocytes in the peripheral blood are only in transit to their potential sites of action in the tissues. The movement of granulocytes from the circulating pool to the peripheral tissues occurs by a process called diapedesis. Once in the peripheral tissues, granulocytes, particularly the neutrophils, are able to carry out their function of **phagocytosis.**

The average life span of a segmented neutrophilic granulocyte in the circulating blood is approximately 7 to 10 hours.

Once mature cells have migrated into the tissues, their life span is considered to be several days, unless the cells encounter antigens, toxins, or microorganisms. Eosinophils are in the peripheral blood for a few hours and are believed to reside in the tissues for several days. Basophils have an average circulation time of about 8.5 hours. If excessive numbers of eosinophils are present because of a disease state, damaged or degenerated eosinophils give rise to **Charcot-Leyden crystals** found in body secretions, such as the sputum and stool. If cells are not prematurely destroyed while defending the body, they are sloughed off with various body secretions, such as the urine, saliva, or gastrointestinal secretions. An alternative route for the removal of granulocytes from the circulation is phagocytosis by the mononuclear phagocyte cells of the spleen.

Normal Maturational Characteristics of Neutrophils, Eosinophils, and Basophils

Myeloblast

In the maturational sequence (Table 14.1), the earliest morphologically identifiable granulocytic precursor is the **myeloblast** (Plate 27). This cell has an average overall diameter of 10 to 18 μm. The nuclear chromatin is finely reticular, with one to five light-staining nucleoli. The cytoplasm appears as a small rim of basophilic cytoplasm that lacks granules. **Auer rods,** which are aggregates of fused lysosomes, may appear as red, needlelike crystalline cytoplasmic inclusions. These inclusions may appear alone or in groups. Auer rods are pathological, not normal, inclusions.

Promyelocyte

The **promyelocyte** (Plate 28) represents the second maturational stage seen in granulocytes. The outstanding feature of this cell is the presence of prominent granulation that may actually obscure the other morphological features of the cell. These granules are primarily **azurophilic** granules and are rich in the enzymes myeloperoxidase and chloroac-

TABLE 14.1 Maturational Characteristics of Neutrophilic Granulocytes

	Myeloblast	Promyelocyte	Myelocyte	Metamyelocyte	Band	Segmented
Size (μm)	10–18	14–20	12–18	10–18	10–16	10–16
N:C	4:1	3:1	2:1–1:1	1:1	1:1	1:1
Nucleus						
Shape	Oval or round	Oval or round	Oval or indented	Indented	Elongated, curved	Distinct lobes (2–5)
Nucleoli	1–5	1–5	Variable	None	None	None
Chromatin	Reticular	Smooth	Slightly clumped	Clumped	Very clumped	Densely packed
Cytoplasm						
Inclusions	Auer rods	None	None	None	None	None
Granules	None	Heavy Nonspecific	Fine Specific	Fine Specific	Fine Specific	Fine Specific
Amount	Scanty	Slightly increased	Moderate	Moderate	Abundant	Abundant
Color	Medium blue	Moderate blue	Blue-pink	Pink	Pink	Pink

etate esterase. The promyelocyte is larger than the blast stage, with an average diameter of 14 to 20 μm. The N:C ratio is lower in the promyelocyte than in the myeloblast. The nuclear chromatin is more condensed than in the blast, and nucleoli are present. The cytoplasm is a pale grayish-blue.

Myelocyte

The **myelocyte** (Plate 29) is the third maturational stage. This cell is characterized by the recognizable appearance of secondary or specific cytoplasmic granulation. The separate cell types, neutrophils, eosinophils, and basophils, become visibly recognizable at this stage. Neutrophilic granules are fine and stain a blue-pink color with Wright stain. Eosinophilic granules are larger than neutrophilic granules. These round or oval-shaped granules are orange and have a glassy or semiopaque texture. Basophilic granules have a dark blue-black color and a dense appearance. The myelocyte has an average diameter of 12 to 18 μm. The N:C ratio continues to decrease. The nucleus has a more oval appearance than in previous stages, nucleoli are no longer visible, and the chromatin is much more clumped than in previous stages.

Metamyelocyte

The **metamyelocyte** (Plate 30) is the fourth maturational stage. Its most characteristic feature is that the nucleus begins to assume an indented or kidney-bean shape, which will continue to elongate as the cell matures through this phase. The chromatin continues to become more condensed or clumped. The color of the specific granulation continues to become a major distinguishing feature.

Mature Forms

Two stages of granulocytes are observed in the circulating blood: the **band form** and the **segmented form.** Both the band form of neutrophils (Plate 31), eosinophils, and basophils and, in the final stage of maturation, the segmented neutrophils (Plate 32), eosinophils (Plate 33), and basophils (Plate 34) are the cell forms normally found in the circulating blood. The band form has a typical elongated nucleus. The segmented neutrophil has a characteristic multilobed nucleus, whereas the eosinophil is normally bilobed. The separate lobes are attached to each other by a fine threadlike filament. The nucleus of the basophil is indented and is difficult to see because it is usually obscured by cytoplasmic granules.

Mast cells (tissue basophils) are not observed in the blood of normal persons. These cells have an appearance similar to that of the blood basophil. Mast cells have a round or oval nucleus. The granules of the mast cell do not overlie the nucleus as they do in basophils.

Granulation in Mature Forms

Although all granules are commonly produced by the rough endoplasmic reticulum and transported to the Golgi apparatus for packaging, the granules of each cell type stain differently because their contents vary. The characteristics of these granules are as follows.

The granules of **segmented neutrophils** are rich in various antibacterial substances, including lysosomal hydrolases, lysozyme, and myeloperoxidase. Some of these granules are typical lysosomes.

Eosinophilic granules differ from neutrophilic granules in that they lack lysozyme. These granules are of two types:

1. Smaller round granules, which have been identified as not containing crystalloids. These granules exist in small quantities in the mature eosinophil and are rich in acid phosphatase.
2. Larger crystalline granules, which are more numerous. These crystalline granules are elliptical, are larger than the granules of the neutrophil, and have an amorphous matrix surrounding an internal crystalline structure. The crystals are thought to represent the enzyme peroxidase (*not* the same as the myeloperoxidase found in neutrophils), and the matrix contains acid phosphatase.

Basophilic granules contain heparin and histamine. **Mast cells** have granules that have an enzyme content similar to those of the blood basophil.

THE MONOCYTIC-MACROPHAGE SERIES

Cells of the mononuclear phagocyte system include the monocytes and macrophages. Macrophages have a variety of names, including **histiocytes** in the loose connective tissues, **Kupffer cells** in the sinusoids of the liver, **osteoclasts** in bone, and **microglial cells** in the nervous system. The name of the cell changes with the location of the cell; however, mature macrophages are distributed throughout the body. These cells, along with the reticular cells of the spleen, thymus, and lymphoid tissues, are collectively referred to as the **mononuclear phagocyte system** or reticuloendothelial system (RES) (Fig. 14.3). The other major phagocytic cell, the segmented neutrophil, is confined to the circulating blood unless it is recruited into the tissues.

Production and Development of Monocytes and Macrophages

Cells of the macrophage system are formed from the progenitor cells in the bone marrow. These cells are derived from the CFU-GM, which can differentiate into either the CFU-M and develop into a monocyte or macrophage, or the CFU-G and develop into a segmented neutrophil. A monocyte is influenced by hematopoietic growth factors to transform into a macrophage in the tissues. Functionally, monocytes and macrophages have phagocytosis as their major role, although they also have regulatory and secretory functions.

In contrast to the granulocytic leukocytes, the promonocyte will undergo two or three mitotic divisions in approximately 2 to 2.5 days. Monocytes are released into the circulating blood within 12 to 24 hours after their precursors have completed their last mitotic division. Monocytes have no large reserve of cells in a maturation-storage pool as do the granulocytes. Once the monocytes have entered the circulation, cells may be located in a **circulating** or

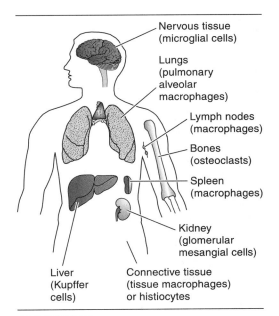

FIGURE 14.3 Mononuclear phagocyte system (reticuloendothelial system). Phagocytic cells are located in many body organs. In addition, the promonocyte precursors in the bone marrow develop into circulating monocytes in the peripheral blood. Monocytes ultimately become distributed throughout the body as macrophages. The other major phagocytic blood cells, the neutrophils, are located in the circulating blood, except when they enter the tissues during acute inflammation. (Adapted from I. Roitt, *Essential Immunology* [5th ed.]. Oxford, England: Blackwell Scientific, 1984, p. 183.)

marginating pool. The ratio of circulating to marginating cells is 1:3.5. Monocytes are estimated to have a circulatory half-life of approximately 8.5 hours. The life span of tissue monocytes is variable. However, cells in noninflammatory areas have been demonstrated to live for months to years.

Morphological Characteristics

Morphological identification of the monocyte is more difficult than that of the neutrophilic, eosinophilic, or basophilic granulocytes. Monoblasts, promonocytes (young monocytes), and monocytes vary greatly in their morphological appearance (Table 14.2). However, the monocytic series does have a characteristic nuclear chromatin pattern. The chromatin is clumped, although the clumps are smaller and more elongated than in neutrophils. This pattern can be described as lace-like. The shape of the nucleus of the monocyte may be round or oval, but it is frequently convoluted or twisted.

Mature monocytes (Plate 35) are the largest mature cells seen in peripheral blood. They may exhibit an irregular cytoplasmic outline. These cytoplasmic irregularities can include pseudopods. Vacuoles are also commonly observed. Classically, the cytoplasm is blue-gray in color, with fine granulation resembling ground glass.

NORMAL VALUES AND FUNCTIONAL PROPERTIES OF GRANULOCYTES AND MONOCYTES

Healthy adults and children have a relatively consistent number of each of the granulocytic and monocytic types of leukocytes. Normal variations occur along with daily rhythmic fluctuations; racial differences also occur.

The major function of the granulocytic leukocytes is **phagocytosis,** a body defense mechanism. Neutrophilic granulocytes are the major phagocytic cell of the circulating blood. Eosinophils and basophils are less effective as phagocytes but have additional specialized functions associated with body defense.

Normal Values

Each type of granulocyte and the monocytes have an established normal range (Table 14.3) and an average percentage

TABLE 14.2 Characteristics of Monocytes

	Monoblast	Promonocyte	Mature Monocyte
Size (μm)	12–20	12–20	12–18
N:C ratio	4:1	3:1–2:1	2:1–1:1
Nucleus			
Shape	Oval, folded	Elongated, folded	Horseshoe-shaped, folded
Nucleoli	1–2 or more	0–2	None
Chromatin	Fine	Lace-like	Lace-like
Cytoplasm			
Inclusions	Vacuoles variable	Vacuoles variable	Vacuoles common
Granules	None	None or fine	Fine, dispersed
Amount	Moderate	Abundant	Abundant
Color	Blue	Blue-gray	Blue-gray
Shape	Monocytes frequently demonstrate on irregular cytoplasmic shape with pseudopods		

TABLE 14.3 Normal Values of Granulocytes and Monocytes (Adults)

	Normal Range	Percentage Range
Neutrophils	$1.5–7.5 \times 10^9/L$	40–75
Eosinophils	$0.05–0.60 \times 10^9/L$	1–7
Basophils	$0.02–0.05 \times 10^9/L$	0–2
Monocytes	$0.0–0.80 \times 10^9/L$	1–10

Source: Modified from S. H. Robinson and P. R. Reich, *Hematology: Pathophysiologic Basis for Clinical Practice* (3rd ed.). Boston: Little, Brown & Co., 1993.

on a stained blood smear (refer to Chapters 3 and 24). Marked differences in the total leukocyte count do occur between black and white persons. Blacks have a lower total leukocyte count compared with whites, owing to a decreased number of neutrophils. Individual variations in the total leukocyte count occur, with a daily fluctuation of as much as 20%. Peak levels occur in the middle of the night and the early morning.

Variations may also occur with specific cells. For example, smoking causes a mild elevation of neutrophils. Monocytes have periodic oscillations of $0.2 \times 10^9/L$ every 3 to 6 days.

Eosinophils have a well-documented daily fluctuation, with a diurnal (time-related) variation in the number of circulating cells. The quantity of circulating eosinophils tends to be highest late at night during sleep, decreases during the morning, and begins to rise at midafternoon. This rhythmic variation in a person's eosinophil count is related to the fluctuation of the hormone adrenal glucocorticosteroid.

In women, the menstrual cycle affects the eosinophil count, with the number of circulating eosinophils dropping at the time of ovulation and rising during menstruation. The summer season may produce higher counts in a person without allergies. Exercise produces a brief rise in eosinophils, whereas stress can lower eosinophil counts.

Phagocytosis

Defense against infectious disease is the responsibility of both the phagocytic and the immune (antigen-antibody) systems in humans. The activities of these two systems are somewhat coordinated and interdependent. However, the granulocytic leukocytes constitute the body's initial defense against infectious agents and local noninfectious challenges that have penetrated the skin or mucous membranes. Phagocytosis is the process that enables particular cells to engulf and disable particles, such as bacteria.

General Characteristics

Although the major cells associated with phagocytosis are the neutrophilic leukocytes (neutrophils) and the monocytes-macrophages, the neutrophils are the principal leukocytes involved in a localized inflammatory response. The inflammatory exudate (pus), which develops rapidly in an inflammatory response, is primarily composed of neutrophils and monocytes.

Neutrophils are steadily lost to the respiratory system, the gastrointestinal system, and the urinary system, where

they participate in generalized phagocytic activities. Although the eosinophils and basophils are capable of participating in phagocytosis, they possess less phagocytic activity. Their ineffectiveness is due to both the small number of these cells in the circulating blood and the lack of powerful lytic enzymes. Eosinophils and basophils are functionally important in body defense in other ways.

The Role of Macrophages

Macrophages (Plate 36) participate in the phagocytic process and are particularly important in the processing of antigens as part of the immune response. Macrophages exist as either **fixed** or **wandering cells.** Fixed macrophages line the endothelium of capillaries and the sinuses of organs such as the bone marrow, spleen, and lymph nodes. Specialized macrophages, such as the **pulmonary alveolar macrophages,** are the dust phagocytes of the lung and function as the first line of defense against inhaled foreign particles and bacteria. Macrophages and their known precursor, monocytes, migrate freely into the tissues from the blood to replenish and reinforce the macrophage population. When there is tissue damage and inflammation, cellular activity increases with the release of substances that attract macrophages.

The Steps in Phagocytosis

Phagocytosis can be divided into three stages (Fig. 14.4). These stages are **movement of cells, engulfment,** and **digestion.** If microorganisms are not effectively immobilized, subsequent phagocytic activity may take place.

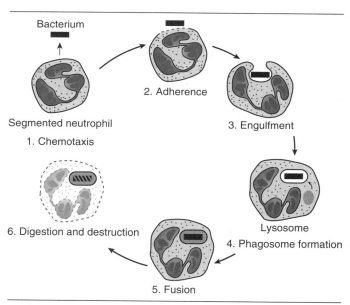

FIGURE 14.4 Phagocytosis. Step 1 depicts the movement of a segmented neutrophil toward the site of bacterial invasion, chemotaxis. Step 2 depicts the initiating event in engulfment, the adherence of the phagocytic membrane to the bacterial cell wall. This process can be enhanced by opsonization. If the surface tensions of the membranes are conducive to engulfment, the phagocytic cell membrane invaginates and engulfs the bacterium (step 3), and a phagosome is formed (step 4). The phagosome fuses with one or more lysosomal granules (step 5). Digestion of the bacterium occurs (step 6), and normally results in autolysis of the phagocyte. (Adapted from I. Roitt, *Essential Immunology* [5th ed.] Oxford, England: Blackwell Scientific, 1984, p. 186.)

Movement of Cells

Various phagocytic cells continually circulate throughout the blood, lymph, gastrointestinal system, and respiratory tract. The physical occurrence of damage to tissues, because of either trauma or microbial multiplication, releases substances that attract phagocytic cells.

Cells are guided to the site of injury by the concentration gradient of chemotactic substances. This event is termed **chemotaxis.** Actively motile segmented neutrophils are able to gather at the site of injury quickly, but monocytes are slower to arrive. Segmented neutrophils can be found in the beginning exudate in less than an hour. The marginating pool of neutrophils, adhering to the endothelial lining of nearby blood vessels, migrates through the vessel wall to the intestinal tissues. This amoeboid movement is called **diapedesis.**

Engulfment

After the phagocytic cells have arrived at the site of injury, the invading microorganisms or particles can be engulfed through active membrane invagination. It is important to realize that phagocytosis is an active process that requires a large expenditure of energy by the cells. The required energy is primarily provided by anaerobic **glycolysis.**

However, the principal factor in determining whether or not phagocytosis can occur is the physical nature of the surfaces of both the foreign particle and the phagocytic cell. Bacteria must be more hydrophobic than the phagocyte. Some bacteria, such as *Streptococcus pneumoniae,* possess a hydrophilic capsule and are not normally phagocytized. Most nonpathogenic bacteria are easily phagocytized because they are very hydrophobic.

Certain soluble factors, including complement (a plasma protein), coupled with antibodies, and substances such as acetylcholine, enhance the phagocytic process. Enhancement of phagocytosis through the process of **opsonization,** the coating of a particle with immunoglobulin and/or complement, speeds up the ingestion of particles. If the surface tensions are conducive to engulfment, the phagocytic cell membrane invaginates, a process that leads to the formation of an isolated vacuole, a **phagosome,** within the cell.

Digestion

Digestion follows ingestion of particles, the required energy being provided primarily by anaerobic glycolysis. The vacuole formed during the engulfment process fuses with one or more lysosomal granules that contain various lytic enzymes. The granules of neutrophils contain various antibacterial substances such as lysosomal hydrolases, lysozyme, and myeloperoxidase. The action of the oxygen-dependent myeloperoxidase-mediated system, hydrogen peroxide, and an oxidizable cofactor serve as major factors in the actual killing of bacteria within the vacuole. Other oxygen-independent systems, such as alterations in pH, lysozymes, lactoferrin, and the granular cationic proteins, also participate in the bactericidal process.

An energy-dependent respiratory burst accompanies phagocytosis. The respiratory burst generates oxidizing compounds through the hexose-monophosphate shunt. Oxidizing compounds produced from partial oxygen reduction are important in bacteriocidal activity. Utilization of NADPH or NADH as an electron donor subsequent to the activation of a membrane-bound oxidase produces superoxide (O_2^-) from oxygen. Hydrogen peroxide (H_2O_2) is either generated from superoxide spontaneously or is catalyzed by superoxide dismutase.

$$2 O_2 + NADPH \rightarrow 2 O_2^- + NADP^+ + H^+$$
$$2 O_2^- + 2 H^+ \rightarrow H_2O_2 + O_2$$

The killing effect of H_2O_2 is potentiated by the formation of peroxide-halide. This reaction requires the enzyme myeloperoxidase, found in the primary granules of neutrophilic granulocytes.

$$H_2O_2 + Cl^- \; myeloperoxidase \rightarrow HOCl + H_2O$$

Monocytes are particularly effective as phagocytic cells because of the large amounts of lipase in their cytoplasm. Lipase digests the lipid-rich cell wall of bacteria such as *Mycobacterium tuberculosis.* Monocytes are further able to bind and destroy cells coated with complement-fixing antibodies because of the presence of membrane receptors for specific components or types of immunoglobulin.

As the result of the release of lytic enzymes, the cytoplasmic membrane of the phagocytic cell is usually ruptured, and the engulfing cell itself is phagocytized by macrophages. Macrophage digestion proceeds without risk to the cell unless the ingested material is toxic. However, if the ingested material damages the lysomal membrane, the macrophage will also be destroyed because of the release of lysosomal enzymes.

Subsequent Phagocytic Activity

If invading microorganisms are not phagocytized at entry into the body, they may establish themselves in secondary sites, such as the lymph nodes or various body organs. Undigested bacteria produce a secondary inflammation, where neutrophils and macrophages again congregate. If bacteria escape from secondary tissue sites, **bacteremia** will develop. In patients who are unresponsive to antibiotic intervention, this situation can be fatal.

In cases of **acquired immunodeficiency syndrome (AIDS),** researchers at the National Cancer Institute have found evidence of the virus in mononuclear phagocytes. Infected phagocytes were found in brain and lung tissue specimens from AIDS patients, indicating that the brain infection might have been caused by the phagocytes. Phagocytes harboring AIDS virus were found to be more powerfully infective than T lymphocytes (discussed in Chapter 16). The infected phagocytes may be responsible for passing the virus back to the rest of the immune system, with other infected cells passing the virus back to healthy phagocytes.

Protozoan organisms, such as *Leishmania donovani* (popularly referred to as **kala-azar**), are cleared by the mononuclear phagocyte cells of the liver, spleen, and bone marrow. The **Leishman-Donovan bodies,** which are oblong or round, multiply in the phagocytic cells. Repeated multiplication produces extensive numbers of parasitized macrophages and monocytes (Plate 37). Infection with the pathogenic fungus *Histoplasma capsulatum,* which also infiltrates the mononuclear phagocytic system and appears within macrophages of the bone marrow, can mimic kala-azar.

Specialized Functions

Eosinophils

The eosinophil is considered to be a homeostatic regulator of inflammation that leaves the circulating blood when adrenal cortical hormone increases. Functionally, this means that the eosinophil attempts to suppress inflammatory tissue reactions in order to prevent the excessive spread of inflammation.

Eosinophils proliferate in response to antigenetic stimulation and contain substances that inactivate factors released by mast cells and basophils. The primary function of eosinophils appears to be their reactions with products from mast cells, lymphocytes, and other soluble substances in the blood, such as the coagulation factors, complement, and hormones.

Although eosinophils are ineffective in protecting the body against invading foreign particles, they do play a role in the body defense mechanism. Eosinophils have the ability to interact with the larval stages of some helminthic parasites and to damage them by means of oxidative mechanisms. Certain proteins released from eosinophilic granules are known to damage antibody-coated *Schistosoma* parasites.

Basophils

Basophils have high concentrations of **heparin** and **histamine** in their granules. Histamine plays an important role in acute, systemic allergic reactions. Degranulation (loss of granules) occurs when an antigen, such as pollen, binds to two adjacent immunoglobulin E (IgE)-type antibody molecules located on the surface of basophils. The release of the contents of these basophilic granules results in increased vascular permeability, smooth muscle spasm, and vasodilation. If this reaction is severe, it can result in **anaphylactic shock.**

A class of compounds, the **leukotrienes**, mediates the inflammatory functions of leukocytes. The observed systemic reactions that are related to these compounds were previously attributed to the slow-reacting substance of anaphylaxis (SRS-A).

Monocytes

In addition to phagocytosis, monocytes are able to synthesize various biologically important compounds, including transferrin, complement, interferon, and certain growth factors. In cellular immunity, monocytes assume a "killer role." In this role, they are activated by sensitized lymphocytes to phagocytize offending cells or antigen particles. This is important in fields such as tumor immunology.

ASSESSMENT METHODS

Inflammation almost always follows acute tissue damage. Diagnostic categories of acute inflammation can include bacterial causes and nonbacterial causes such as trauma, chronic inflammation, and viral disease. Among the many laboratory tests that have been advocated for the diagnosis of inflammation, the total leukocyte count, the percentage of band and segmented neutrophils determined by a differential leukocyte count, the absolute neutrophil cell count, and the erythrocyte sedimentation rate (ESR) are the most common.

Other tests include direct cell counts of eosinophils or basophils, the leukocyte alkaline phosphatase (LAP) cytochemical stain, and neutrophilic function tests.

Total Leukocyte Count

The total leukocyte count (refer to Chapters 24 and 25 for procedures) can be elevated above $10 \times 10^9/L$ in conditions such as pregnancy, strenuous exercise, and corticosteroid treatment. The total count may be depressed because of overwhelming bacterial infection (sepsis) or immunosuppressive agents. A diagnosis of acute inflammation is generally based on a total leukocyte count greater than $10.5 \times 10^9/L$ in combination with other factors.

Differential Blood Smear Evaluation

Although some authorities advocate doing away with the identification of band forms on the leukocyte differential procedure (see Chapter 24) because of individual variability in cell identification, the guidelines of the National Committee for Clinical Laboratory Standards (NCCLS) on leukocyte differential counting (H20-T) include bands as a routine category in the differential blood count. Patients with stress conditions can demonstrate an increase in the number of band forms in the presence of a normal total leukocyte count. The normal average for band neutrophils is considered to be 3% in adults, newborn infants having a somewhat higher normal average. A neutrophilic band count greater than 11% is considered to be consistent with an inflammatory condition. When the percentage of band forms and other immature neutrophils such as metamyelocytes and myelocytes increases, the condition is sometimes referred to as a "shift to the left." The normal average for segmented neutrophils is 56%, and for monocytes, approximately 4%.

Absolute Cell Counts

The absolute number of segmented neutrophils and bands is considered to be a less specific index of inflammation than other tests because the total leukocyte count drops in many patients with overwhelming infection. This condition results from the movement of circulating granulocytes into the tissue sites of infection. However, the absolute count may be of value in other cases of inflammation. An example of the method of calculating an absolute cell count is presented in Table 14.4.

Erythrocyte Sedimentation Rate

The ESR, or "sed rate," is a nonspecific indicator of disease with increased sedimentation of erythrocytes in acute and chronic inflammation and malignancies. Although this procedure is nonspecific, it is one of the most commonly performed laboratory tests.

Very few tests have as long a history as the ESR. A Swedish physician, Fahraeus, is credited with the discovery of this test in 1915. However, the sedimentation of blood was one of the principles on which ancient Greek medicine was based. The Greek philosophy of the four humors (fluids) in

TABLE 14.4 Absolute Cell Counts

Absolute count* = absolute cell value = total leukocyte count × percentage of cell type

Patient Data
Total leukocyte count: 15.0 × 10^9/L

Differential blood smear results: bands 12%, segmented neutrophils 80%, lymphocytes 8%

Sample Calculation
Absolute **segmented neutrophil** value = total leukocyte count × % of segmented neutrophils

Absolute value = 15.0 × 10^9/L × 0.80 = 12.0 × 10^9/L segmented neutrophils

---

*This formula can be used to determine the absolute value of any cell appearing on a leukocyte differential blood smear.

Normal absolute values include segmented neutrophils 1.5–6.0 × 10^9/L, bands 0.2–>1 × 10^9/L, monocytes 0.2–0.95 × 10^9/L.

the human body was established in the fifth century B.C. and further developed by Aristotle. This belief proposed that these fluids formed the body. On the basis of this philosophy, each person had a predisposition for a particular disease depending on the predominance of one of the four fluids, blood, phlegm, yellow bile, or black bile.

In 1836, Nasse recognized that a property of plasma, later identified as increased proteins, produced an increased sinking speed of erythrocytes in whole blood. The work of Nasse went unnoticed for nearly a century because medicine was undergoing a radical reform, moving away from the humoral philosophy of the Greeks toward the cellular pathology theories of Virchow (see Chapter 18). With the reestablishment by Fahraeus of the significance of the empirical basis of Greek medicine, Alf Westergren began working concurrently on refining the technique.

Except for some refinements, the ESR procedure continues to be an established parameter of inflammation in the modern clinical laboratory. Several ESR methods are in current use. They include the Westergren method, and the Wintrobe method (see Chapter 24). The Westergren method has been selected by the NCCLS as the standard method of choice.

Assessment of Eosinophils and Basophils

Examination of a peripheral blood smear normally demonstrates an average of approximately 4% eosinophils. Because this method of estimation is only semiquantitative, an absolute eosinophil count, either by manual chamber counting (see Chapter 24) or by the use of automated equipment, is preferred. This procedure is required only if an extreme increase in eosinophils is demonstrated on a peripheral blood smear or if clinical symptoms suggest an increase.

The basophil is the least numerous of the granulocytes. Normally, differential smears of normal blood have only one basophil, if any. If quantitative assays are needed, methods (see Chapter 24) similar to the eosinophil count are recommended. An increase in basophils is very significant

and is seen in conditions such as chronic myelogenous leukemia and polycythemia vera.

Leukocyte Alkaline Phosphatase Test

This procedure is discussed in detail in Chapters 21 and 24. The value of this cytochemical stain is in differentiating malignant disorders from leukemoid reactions.

Neutrophilic Function

A number of diseases are associated with leukocyte dysfunctions related to locomotion, chemotaxis (cell orientation along a concentration gradient), and the ability of cells to destroy infectious organisms. In vitro assays of the rate of cell movement and the directional orientation of the movement as well as the ability of granulocytes to destroy organisms have been in existence for more than 20 years.

A defect in cell adhesiveness can lead to decreased cell locomotion. The nylon fiber adherence test can be used to assess the adhesiveness of granulocytes. Patients who have consumed alcohol or are on medications such as salicylates or glucocorticoids can demonstrate inhibited granulocyte adherence. Cell migration can be assessed in a gradient of a chemotactic factor, such as the complement fraction C5a. Cell migration can be observed using a matrix, such as a Millipore filter or agarose gel, or a microscopic slide. A test that assesses the killing ability of granulocytes is the nitroblue tetrazolium (NBT) test. In the routine clinical laboratory, these procedures are infrequently performed.

SUMMARY

The following types of leukocytes are found in peripheral blood in this order of frequency: neutrophils, lymphocytes, monocytes, eosinophils, and basophils. The function of the entire leukocytic system is to defend the body against disease, with each type of leukocyte having a unique function.

The Granulocytic Series

The cellular elements of the blood are derived from a single, multipotential stem cell. This stem cell undergoes differentiation, multiplication, and maturation within the bone marrow. After a progenitor cell becomes committed to a specific cell line, mitosis and early development take place in the proliferative compartment of the bone marrow. A neutrophilic granulocyte matures in the following sequence: stem cell, myeloblast, promyelocyte, myelocyte, and metamyelocyte. Once the metamyelocyte stage has been reached, the proliferative phase comes to an end. In the next phase of bone marrow development, the maturation-storage compartment, metamyelocytes, and most band-type neutrophils mature into segmented granulocytes or polymorphonuclear neutrophils.

Release of granulocytes from the bone marrow is influenced by a variety of factors. These factors are chemical as well as physical. Chemical factors include neutrophil-releasing factor and leukocytosis-inducing factor. Physical factors include greater flexibility and mobility of cells, allowing the cells to pass through the sinusoid barrier of the bone marrow.

The earliest identifiable neutrophil-eosinophil-basophil precursor in the bone marrow is the myeloblast. This cell has a high N:C ratio and frequently contains Auer rods in the cytoplasm. The second stage of development is the promyelocyte, a heavily granulated cell, which may retain visible nucleoli in the nucleus. Following the promyelocyte, the myelocyte is the third stage. In this stage, granules that distinguish neutrophils, eosinophils, and basophils begin to become apparent. Myelocytes mature into metamyelocytes. The nucleus of the myelocyte progresses from an indented structure to an elongated structure as it matures. The last two maturational stages are the band and segmented forms. Band forms have a condensed chromatin pattern in the nucleus and a thin, elongated, curved nuclear shape. The segmented neutrophil is typified by the multiple segments of the nucleus that are attached to one another by fine filaments.

The Monocytic-Macrophage Series

Cells of the mononuclear phagocyte system include the monocytes and their bone marrow precursors, the macrophages. Macrophages have a variety of names, depending on their tissue location. Collectively, they are referred to as the mononuclear phagocyte system.

Morphological identification of monocytes is more difficult than granulocyte identification. A convoluted nuclear shape is typical of monocytes. The promonocyte, or young monocyte, has a greater N:C ratio than the mature monocyte. The cytoplasm is gray-blue, with fine granules that resemble ground glass. Vacuoles can frequently be observed.

Normal Values and Functional Properties of Granulocytes and Monocytes

Defense against infectious disease is the responsibility of both the phagocytic and immune (antigen-antibody) system. The neutrophils defend the body against infectious agents and local noninfectious challenges. Macrophages participate in the phagocytic process and are important in the processing of antigens as part of the immune system. Macrophages may be of either fixed or wandering types. Fixed types are located in the mononuclear phagocyte system.

Physical trauma initiates the events of phagocytosis. The attraction of phagocytic cells to the site of injury is termed **chemotaxis.** The neutrophils are the most abundant of the cells participating in phagocytosis and arrive at the site rapidly. Monocytes are slower in arriving. Engulfment of foreign particles, such as bacteria, is the next step. The physical nature of the membranes of both the bacteria and the phagocytic cell is the most important factor determining whether or not engulfment takes place. The presence of certain soluble substances, such as complement, enhances the process. If engulfment occurs, the phagocytic cell membrane invaginates to form an isolated vacuole, a phagosome, within the cell. Digestion of bacteria follows engulfment. Antibacterial enzymes contained in granules, and alterations within the

cell such as a change in pH, destroy the engulfed bacteria. Lytic enzymes disrupt the cellular membrane of the phagocytic cells, which are in turn phagocytized by macrophages. Macrophage digestion proceeds without risk to the cell unless the ingested material is toxic. If bacteria are not phagocytized or destroyed at entry, they may establish themselves at secondary sites, and bacteremia develops.

Both the eosinophils and basophils can participate in the phagocytic process, but they are relatively ineffective, for a variety of reasons. However, eosinophils and basophils have separate important and specialized functions. Eosinophils prevent the excessive spread of inflammation. Histamine found in basophils is important in acute allergic reactions, the most important being anaphylactic shock.

Assessment Methods

Several laboratory tests can be used to assess the inflammatory response. Two important indicators are the total leukocyte count and the differential count of leukocytes on a peripheral blood smear. Other assessments include the absolute cell count, erythrocyte sedimentation rate, absolute counts of eosinophils and basophils, the leukocyte alkaline phosphatase test, and neutrophilic function tests.

BIBLIOGRAPHY

Abrams, C. A. "Neutrophil Function Testing." *Advance for Medical Laboratory Professionals*, Vol. 7, No. 1, January 30, 1995, pp. 8–9, 32.

Abrams, C. A. "Neutrophil Function Testing." *Advance for Medical Laboratory Professionals*, Vol. 7, No. 2, January 16, 1995, pp. 17–19, 34.

Bass, David A. "Eosinophils," in *Fundamentals of Clinical Hematology*. Jerry L. Spivak (ed.). Hagerstown, MD: Harper & Row, 1975, pp. 119–135.

Bauer, John D. *Clinical Laboratory Methods* (9th ed.). St. Louis: Mosby, 1982, pp. 170–172.

Bentley, Stuart A. "An Overview of Granulopoiesis," in *Laboratory Hematology*, Vol. 1. John Koepke (ed.). Edinburgh: Churchill-Livingstone, 1984, pp. 143–152.

Boggs, Dane R. and Alan Winkelstein. *White Cell Manual* (4th ed.). Philadelphia: Davis, 1974, pp. 3–35.

Carpenter, Philip L. *Immunology and Serology*. Philadelphia: Saunders, 1975, pp. 8, 20–22, 38, 239–245.

Ciba. *The Cellular Elements of the Blood*. Summit, NJ: Ciba Pharmaceutical, 1962.

Dannenberg, Arthur M., Jr. "Macrophages and Monocytes," in *Fundamentals of Clinical Hematology*. Jerry L. Spivak (ed.). Hagerstown, MD: Harper & Row, 1980, pp. 137–153.

Dubost, J. J. et al. "From Sedimentation Rate to Inflammation Profile." *Rev. Med. Interne*, Vol. 15, No. 11, 1994, pp. 727–733.

Erslev, Allan J. and Thomas G. Gabuzda. "Phagocytes," in *Pathophysiology of Blood*. Philadelphia: Saunders, 1975, pp. 100–118.

Francis, G. E. et al. "DNA Strand Breakage and ADP-Ribosyl Transferase Mediated DNA Ligation During Stimulation of Human Bone Marrow Cells by Granulocyte-Macrophage Colony Stimulating Activity." *Leuk. Res.*, Vol. 8, No. 3, 1984, pp. 407–415.

Goldner, Morris et al. "Bacterial Phagocytosis Monitored by Fluorescence and Extracellular Quenching: Ingestion and Intracellular Killing." *Lab. Med.*, Vol. 14, No. 5, May, 1983, pp. 291–293.

Hellmann, Andrzej. "Production of Colony Stimulating Activity in Mixed Mononuclear Cell Culture." *Br. J. Haematol.*, Vol. 45, 1980, pp. 245–249.

Hicks, Roger G. and John M. Bennett. "An Improved Cytochemical Method for Nitroblue Tetrazolium Reduction by Neutrophils." *Am. J. Med. Technol.*, Vol. 37, No. 6, June, 1971, pp. 226–228.

Howard, John. "Myeloid Series Abnormalities: Neutrophilia." *Lab. Med.*, Vol. 14, No. 3, March, 1983, pp. 147–151.

Lopker, Anita et al. "Stereoselective Muscarinic Acetylcholine and Opiate Receptors in Human Phagocytic Leukocytes." *Biochem. Pharmacol.*, Vol. 29, 1980, pp. 1361–1365.

Luster, A. D. "Chemokines—Chemotactic Cytokines That Mediate Inflammation," *N. Engl. J. Med.*, Vol. 338, No. 7, February 12, 1998, pp. 436–444.

Marchand, Anthony. "How the Laboratory Can Monitor Acute Inflammation." *Diagn. Med.*, Vol. 7, No. 10, November/December, 1984, pp. 57–66.

Markell, Edward K. et al. *Medical Parasitology.* Philadelphia: Saunders, 1986, p. 314.

McCabe, Bennett H. "A Brief History of the Erythrocyte Sedimentation Rate." *Lab. Med.*, Vol. 16, No. 3, March, 1985, pp. 177–178.

O'Connor, Barbara H. *A Color Atlas and Instruction Manual of Peripheral Blood Morphology.* Baltimore: Williams & Wilkins, 1984.

Raphael, Stanley S. *Lynch's Medical Laboratory Technology* (4th ed.). Philadelphia: Saunders, 1983, pp. 653, 692.

Reference Procedure for the Human Erythrocyte Sedimentation Rate (ESR) Test. H2-T2. Villanova, PA: NCCLS, 1977.

Robinson, Stephen H. and Paul R. Reich. *Hematology: Pathophysiological Basis for Clinical Practice* (3rd ed.). Boston: Little, Brown & Co., 1993.

Statland, Bernard E. (ed.). "Normal Values for Bands." *Med. Lab. Observer.*, Vol. 17, No. 4, April, 1985, p. 12.

Tsan, Min-Fu. "Neutrophils," in *Fundamentals of Clinical Hematology.* Jerry L. Spivak (ed.). Hagerstown, MD: Harper & Row, 1980, pp. 109–117.

Wynn, Thomas E. Letters to the Editor. *Lab. Med.* Vol. 15, No. 4, April, 1984, pp. 276–277.

REVIEW QUESTIONS

1. The granulocyte cells that are believed to descend from a common multipotential stem cell in the bone marrow are:

   A. Neutrophils and eosinophils.
   B. Basophils and lymphocytes.
   C. Lymphocytes and monocytes.
   D. Both A & B

2. The types of granulocytic leukocytes found in the proliferative compartment of the bone marrow are:

   A. Myeloblasts, myelocytes, and metamyelocytes.
   B. Myeloblasts, promyelocytes, and myelocytes.
   C. Myeloblasts, promyelocytes, myelocytes, and metamyelocytes.
   D. Myeloblasts, promyelocytes, myelocytes, and metamyelocytes.

3. The types of granulocytic leukocytes found in the maturation-storage compartment of the bone marrow are:

   A. Metamyelocytes, band form neutrophils, segmented neutrophils, mature eosinophils, and mature basophils.
   B. Band form neutrophils, segmented neutrophils, mature eosinophils, and mature basophils.
   C. Metamyelocytes, band form neutrophils, segmented neutrophils, mature eosinophils, and mature basophils.
   D. Segmented neutrophils, immature and mature monocytes, and mature lymphocytes.

4. Release of neutrophils from the bone marrow is believed to be influenced by:

   A. Colony-stimulating factor (CSF).
   B. Interleukins.
   C. Interferon.
   D. All of the above.

5. The stages of neutrophilic granulocyte development are:

   A. Promyelocyte, myeloblast, myelocyte, metamyelocyte, and band and segmented neutrophils.
   B. Myeloblast, promyelocyte, myelocyte, metamyelocyte, and band and segmented neutrophils.
   C. Myelocyte, myeloblast, promyelocyte, metamyelocyte, and band and segmented neutrophils.
   D. Myeloblast, promyelocyte, metamyelocyte, myelocyte, and band and segmented neutrophils.

6. Marginating granulocytes in the peripheral blood can be found in:

   A. The circulating pool.
   B. The marginating pool.
   C. Adhering to the vascular endothelium.
   D. All of the above.

7. The *major* function of neutrophilic granulocytes is:

   A. Antibody production.
   B. Destruction of parasites.
   C. Phagocytosis.
   D. Suppression of inflammation.

8. The half-life of circulating granulocytes in normal blood is estimated to be:

   A. 2.5 to 5 hours.   C. More than 24 hours.
   B. 7 to 10 hours.   D. More than 2 days.

9. Identify the cell with these characteristics: prominent primary granules that are rich in myeloperoxidase and chloroacetate esterase and has a diameter of 14 to 20 μm.

   A. Myeloblast.   C. Myelocyte.
   B. Promyelocyte.   D. Promonocyte.

10. The earliest granulocytic maturational stage in which secondary or specific granules appear is:

    A. Myeloblast.   C. Promyelocyte.
    B. Monoblast.   D. Myelocyte.

11. The mature granulocytes seen in the peripheral blood of normal persons include:

    A. Band form and segmented neutrophils.
    B. Eosinophils and basophils.
    C. Lymphocytes and monocytes.
    D. Both A and B.

12. The granules of segmented neutrophils contain:

    A. Lysosomal hydrolases.   C. Myeloperoxidase.
    B. Lysozymes.   D. All of the above.

13. Which of the following are contents of basophilic granules?

    A. Heparin.   C. Myeloperoxidase.
    B. Histamine.   D. Both A and D.

14. The tissue basophil can be referred to as a:

    A. Mast cell.
    B. Macrophage.
    C. Mononuclear cell.
    D. Antibody-producing cell.

15. A leukocyte with the morphological characteristics of being the largest normal mature leukocyte in the peripheral blood and having a convoluted or twisted nucleus is the:

    A. Myelocyte.   C. Promonocyte.
    B. Metamyelocyte.   D. Monocyte.

16. The normal reference range of the total neutrophil count in adults is:

    A. 1 to 7.5 × 10^9/L.   C. 6.0 to 12 × 10^9/L.
    B. 4.5 to 11 × 10^9/L.   D. 10 to 15 × 10^9/L.

17. The principal leukocyte type involved in phagocytosis is the:

    A. Monocyte.   C. Eosinophil.
    B. Neutrophil.   D. Basophil.

18. The mononuclear phagocyte system consists of reticular cells. These cells can be found in the:

    A. Thymus.
    B. Spleen.
    C. Lymphoid tissues.
    D. All of the above.

19. The immediate precursor of the macrophage is the:

    A. Myeloblast.   C. Promonocyte.
    B. Monoblast.   D. Monocyte.

20. The correct sequence(s) of events in successful phagocytosis is (are):

    A. Chemotaxis, opsonization, phagosome formation, and the action of antibacterial substances.
    B. Opsonization, chemotaxis, phagosome formation, and the action of antibacterial substances.
    C. Engulfment, opsonization, digestion, and destruction of bacteria or particulate matter.
    D. Both A and C.

21. The *major* function of eosinophils is:

    A. Suppression of inflammatory reactions.
    B. Destruction of protozoa.
    C. Participation in anaphylaxis.
    D. Phagocytosis.

22. Monocytes are capable of:

    A. Phagocytosis.
    B. Synthesis of biologically important compounds.
    C. Assuming a "killer role."
    D. All of the above.

23. The hematology tests that are useful in the early diagnosis of acute inflammation are the:

    A. Total leukocyte count and total erythrocyte count.
    B. Total leukocyte count and white blood cell differential count.
    C. Erythrocyte sedimentation rate and absolute neutrophil cell count.
    D. Both B and C.

24. The total leukocyte count can be increased above normal in certain states. Select any of the following conditions that can belong in this category.

    A. Strenuous exercise.
    B. Overwhelming bacterial infection.
    C. Sepsis.
    D. Use of immunosuppressive agents.

25. Acute inflammation is characterized by:

    A. An increased total leukocyte count.
    B. Neutrophilic band count of less than 2%.
    C. Symptoms of long duration.
    D. An increase in lymphocytes.

26. On the basis of the following data, calculate the absolute value of the segmented neutrophils. Total leukocyte count = 12 × 10^9/L; percentage of segmented neutrophils on the differential count = 80%. The absolute segmented neutrophil value is:

    A. 2.5 × 10^9/L.   C. 6.5 × 10^9/L.
    B. 4.5 × 10^9/L.   D. 9.6 × 10^9/L.

27. An increase in metamyelocytes, myelocytes, and promyelocytes can be referred to as:

    A. Leukocytopenia.   C. A shift to the left.
    B. A shift to the right.   D. Pelger-Huet anomaly.

28. What is the normal range of the segmented neutrophil absolute value?

    A. 1.5 to 6 × 10^9/L.   C. 3.5 to 8 × 10^9/L.
    B. 2.5 to 6 × 10^9/L.   D. 5.5 to 10 × 10^9/L.

29. The absolute value of segmented neutrophils can be an unreliable indicator of overwhelming infection because:

    A. It drops in many patients because the circulating granulocytes are mobilized into the tissue site of infection.
    B. The bone marrow reserve becomes exhausted.
    C. The infection suppresses granulocytic production.
    D. All of the above.

30. The NCCLS-recommended method of choice for the erythrocyte sedimentation rate is the:

    A. Wintrobe method.   C. Duke.
    B. Westergren method.   D. Ivy.

CHAPTER 15

Leukocytes: Nonmalignant Disorders of Granulocytes and Monocytes

Quantitative disorders
Leukocytosis
Leukocytopenia
Morphological abnormalities of mature granulocytes
Toxic granulation
Döhle bodies
Hypersegmentation

Pelger-Huët anomaly
May-Hegglin anomaly
Chédiak-Higashi syndrome
Alder-Reilly inclusions
Abnormalities of mature granulocytes in body fluids
Qualitative disorders

Defective locomotion and chemotaxis
Defects in microbicidal activity
Monocyte-macrophage disorders
Summary
Case studies
Bibliography
Review questions

OBJECTIVES

Quantitative disorders
- Define the terms leukocytosis and leukocytopenia.
- List examples of common conditions that can cause leukocytosis or leukocytopenia.
- List at least one representative condition in which an increase or decrease in neutrophils, eosinophils, basophils, or monocytes can be found.

Morphological abnormalities of mature granulocytes
- Describe the appearance of cells when the following abnormalities are present: toxic granulation, Döhle bodies, hypersegmentation, Pelger-Huët anomaly, May-Hegglin anomaly, Chédiak-Higashi syndrome, Alder-Reilly inclusions, and abnormalities of mature granulocytes in body fluids.
- Briefly describe the conditions associated with the previously listed abnormalities of mature granulocytes.

Qualitative disorders
- Describe the consequences of defective locomotion and chemotaxis.

- Explain two defects in microbicidal activity.
- List and describe other functional anomalies of neutrophils.
- Compare defects found in monocytic-macrophage disorders, Gaucher's disease, and Niemann-Pick disease.

Case studies
- Apply laboratory data to the stated case studies and discuss the implications of these cases to the study of hematology.
- The diagnosis of nonmalignant disorders of granulocytes and monocytes is dependent on laboratory assays along with a patient's history and physical examination. Nonmalignant disorders of granulocytes range from general increases or decreases in the total leukocyte count to qualitative disorders, such as a defect in the killing ability of the leukocytes. A variety of laboratory tests are used to assess disorders related to the granulocytes and monocytes.

QUANTITATIVE DISORDERS

Quantitative disorders of leukocytes may reflect either a general increase (**leukocytosis**) or decrease (**leukocytopenia**) in the total leukocyte count, or a specific disorder (Table 15.1). Increases in neutrophils, eosinophils, and basophils are referred to as **neutrophilia, eosinophilia,** and **basophilia,** respectively. An increase in monocytes is called **monocytosis.** Decreases in these cellular elements are referred to as **neutropenia, eosinopenia, basopenia,** and **monocytopenia,** respectively.

Leukocytosis

Leukocytosis is an increase in the concentration or percentage of any of the leukocytes in the peripheral blood: neutrophils, eosinophils, basophils, monocytes, or lymphocytes.

TABLE 15.1 Leukocytic Increases or Decreases and Examples of Related Disorders	
Neutrophilia	Inflammatory conditions
	Infection
	Physical stimuli, e.g., heat or cold
	Surgery
	Burns
	Stress
	Some drugs and hormones
	Some types of leukemia
Eosinophilia	Active allergic disorders, e.g., asthma and hay fever
	Dermatoses
	Nonparasitic infections
	Some forms of leukemia
	Parasitic infections (nonprotozoan)
Basophilia	Ulcerative colitis
	Hyperlipidemia
	Smallpox and chickenpox
	Chronic sinusitis
	Chronic myelogenous leukemia
	Polycythemia vera
Monocytosis	Infections, e.g., tuberculosis and bacterial endocarditis
	Fever of unknown origin
	Inflammatory bowel disease
	Rheumatoid arthritis
	Hematological disorders, e.g., hemolytic anemia
Neutropenia	Bone marrow injury or infiltration
	Starvation
	Anorexia nervosa
	Cyclic neutropenia
	Increased destruction or utilization
	Entrapment in the spleen
Eosinopenia	Glucocorticosteroid hormones
	Acute bacterial or viral inflammation
Basopenia	Hormones, e.g., corticotropin and progesterone
	During ovulation in women
	Thyrotoxicosis
Monocytopenia	No known conditions

Although an increase in the total leukocyte count may be due to an increase in lymphocytes (see Chapter 16), an increase in neutrophils is the most frequent cause of nonmalignant increases in the total leukocyte count because of their proportionally higher concentrations in circulating blood.

Nonmalignant leukocytosis can be caused by various conditions in several general categories. These categories include:

1. Increased movement of immature cells out of the bone marrow's proliferative compartment
2. Increased mobilization of cells from the maturation-storage compartment of the bone marrow to the peripheral blood
3. Increased movement of mature cells from the marginating pool to the circulating pool
4. Decreased movement of mature cells from the circulation into the tissues

Neutrophilia

An increase in the number of neutrophils can be present in some forms of leukemia as well as nonmalignant conditions, such as inflammatory conditions or infection. Neutrophilia can also be caused by physical stimuli such as heat and cold, surgery, burns, stressful activities such as vigorous exercise, nausea, and vomiting. In addition, some drugs and hormones may produce neutrophilia.

Eosinophilia

Persistently and significantly increased numbers of eosinophils are most frequently observed in active allergic disorders, such as asthma and hay fever. Other causes of eosinophilia include dermatoses, nonparasitic infections, some forms of leukemia, and parasitic infections. Patients with significant eosinophilia usually demonstrate some abnormal morphology. Vacuolization and degranulation can be observed. Charcot-Leyden crystals can be found in the tissues, exudates, sputum, and stool of patients with active eosinophilic inflammation.

Eosinophilia is an index of host reaction to parasites and varies considerably from one patient to another. It is *not* characteristic of any of the protozoan infections. In general, tissue parasites provoke a higher eosinophilia than do parasites that live only in the lumen of the bowel. Marked eosinophilia (20% to 70% or higher) is most frequently seen in trichinosis, strongyloidiasis, hookworm infection, filariasis, schistosomiasis, and fasciolopsiasis. Moderate eosinophilia (6% to 20%) is related to trichuriasis, ascariasis, paragonimiasis, taeniasis, and eosinophilic meningitis.

Basophilia

The number of circulating basophils is not remarkably affected by factors such as time of day, age, and physical activity. Basophilia is considered to exist when the number of basophils exceeds 0.075×10^9/L. Hormones can cause an increase in basophils, and basophilia can be seen in many disorders, including ulcerative colitis, hyperlipidemia, smallpox, chickenpox, chronic sinusitis, chronic myelogenous leukemia, and polycythemia vera (P. vera).

Monocytosis

Because the normal value of circulating monocytes is not precisely defined, the association of monocytosis with disease may not be entirely accurate. Monocytosis is a significant absolute increase in circulating monocytes, which can represent a "reactive monocytosis" to many diseases. Some of the disorders commonly associated with monocytosis include infections (e.g., tuberculosis and bacterial endocarditis), fever of unknown origin, inflammatory bowel disease, rheumatoid arthritis, and various hematological disorders (e.g., hemolytic anemia). An increase in tissue macrophages may reflect a response to foreign antigens.

Leukocytopenia

The major leukocyte type associated with leukocytopenia or granulocytopenia is the segmented neutrophil.

Neutropenia

A reduction in the number of circulating neutrophils is referred to as **neutropenia.** Causes of neutropenia include underproduction of cells due to bone marrow injury or infiltration of the marrow by malignant cells, and nutritional deficiencies such as those caused by starvation or anorexia nervosa. Other causes can include cyclic neutropenia, a hereditary disorder; increased destruction or utilization of neutrophils; and entrapment in the spleen.

Most transient neutropenias in children are acquired disorders, and viral infections are a common cause. Congenital neutropenia can be caused by a variety of conditions. A rare congenital disorder of young children is congenital agranulocytosis of the Kostmann type. Another uncommon congenital disorder is **myelokathexis,** the inability to release mature granulocytes into the blood. Other rare causes of congenital neutropenia include reticular dysgenesis, type IB glycogen storage disease, and transcobalamin-II deficiency.

Eosinopenia

This is a rare, stress-related condition that may be due to several factors. Eosinopenia is frequently related to the action of glucocorticosteroid hormones or occurs as an aftermath of acute bacterial or viral inflammation.

Basopenia

This condition may be caused by hormones such as corticotropin and progesterone, or it may occur at the time of ovulation. Patients with thyrotoxicosis may also have basopenia.

Monocytopenia

No conditions are known to be related to a decrease in monocytes.

MORPHOLOGICAL ABNORMALITIES OF MATURE GRANULOCYTES

Abnormalities of mature granulocytes, particularly neutrophils, can be observed in stained smears of peripheral blood.

These conditions include the more frequently observed disorders of toxic granulation, Döhle bodies, and hypersegmentation as well as rarely observed disorders such as Pelger-Huët anomaly, May-Hegglin anomaly, Chédiak-Higashi syndrome, and Alder-Reilly inclusions.

Toxic Granulation

This is a condition in which prominent dark granulation, either fine or heavy, can be observed in band and segmented neutrophils or monocytes (Plate 38). Toxic granules are azurophilic (primary) granules that are peroxidase-positive. The granulation may represent the precipitation of ribosomal protein (RNA) caused by metabolic toxicity within the cells.

The extent of toxic granulation is usually graded on a scale of 1+ to 4+, with 4+ being the most severe. Grading of the granulation is dependent on the coarseness and amount of granulation within the cellular cytoplasm. This condition is most frequently associated with infectious states. It may be seen in conditions such as burns and malignant disorders, or as the result of drug therapy.

Döhle Bodies

These inclusion bodies are seen as single or multiple, light blue-staining inclusions on Wright-stained blood smears (Plate 39). They are usually seen near the periphery of the cytoplasm. These inclusions are predominantly seen in neutrophils, although they may be seen in monocytes or lymphocytes. Döhle bodies represent aggregates of rough endoplasmic reticulum (RNA) and may be associated with a variety of conditions such as viral infections, burns, or certain drugs. Döhle body-like inclusions may be seen in **May-Hegglin anomaly.**

Hypersegmentation

Hypersegmentation is most frequently seen in segmented neutrophils with more than five lobes or nuclear segments (Plate 40). This condition is frequently associated with deficiencies of vitamin B_{12} or folic acid and exists along with abnormally enlarged, oval-shaped erythrocytes. Pseudohypersegmentation may be seen in old segmented neutrophils.

Pelger-Huët Anomaly

This genetically acquired, autosomal dominant disorder produces **hyposegmentation** of many of the mature neutrophils (Plate 41). The nuclear shape may resemble a dumbbell or a pair of eyeglasses. Although the segments fail to lobulate normally, other characteristics, such as chromatin clumping and cytoplasmic maturation, are normal. Heavy chromatin clumping distinguishes Pelger-Huët anomaly from the "left shift" of infection. Abnormal nuclear maturation is presumed to be a reflection of abnormal nucleic acid metabolism, although the specific abnormality is unknown. A pseudoanomaly may be drug-induced or may occur in a maturational arrest associated with some acute infections. The function of the cell is considered to be normal despite the morphological abnormality. Therefore, it is considered to be a benign anomaly.

May-Hegglin Anomaly

This genetic condition is characterized by the presence of Döhle body-like inclusions in neutrophils, eosinophils, and monocytes (Plate 42). Abnormally large and poorly granulated platelets and thrombocytopenia (a decreased number of platelets) frequently coexist in this condition.

Although about 50% of patients have been reported as symptomless, others have manifested abnormal bleeding tendencies. The cause of the hemostatic defect is unclear, but it is proportionate to the degree of thrombocytopenia.

Chédiak-Higashi Syndrome

This rare disorder is a hereditary disease, an autosomal recessive trait. It is primarily seen in children and young adults and is characterized by very large granules (Plate 43). These gigantic, peroxidase-positive deposits represent abnormal lysosomal development in neutrophils and other leukocytes, such as monocytes and lymphocytes. Neutrophils display impaired chemotaxis and delayed killing of ingested bacteria. Patients with this disorder suffer from frequent infections, which suggests that neutrophils with this defect are not efficient bacteriocidal cells.

Alder-Reilly Inclusions

These purple-red particles are precipitated mucopolysaccharides seen primarily in neutrophils, eosinophils, and basophils (Plate 44). Occasionally, they are seen in monocytes and lymphocytes. These inclusions can resemble very coarse toxic granulation.

Alder-Reilly granules are most commonly seen in patients with Hurler, Hunter, and Maroteaux-Lamy types of genetic mucopolysaccharidosis. Most of these disorders are transmitted as autosomal recessive genes.

Abnormalities of Mature Granulocytes in Body Fluids

Certain abnormal inclusions can be seen in granulocytes obtained from body fluids. Examples of such inclusions are bacteria and *Histoplasma capsulatum.*

In Wright-stained sediments of body fluids, such as cerebrospinal fluid (refer to Chapter 23 for a complete discussion of the examination of body fluids) and pus from an abscess, engulfed bacteria can be observed as the result of phagocytosis. When this staining method is used, most bacteria appear as dark-blue, round or elongated structures in the cytoplasm.

H. capsulatum is a fungus. This organism lives intracellularly in cells of the mononuclear phagocyte system, cells of the bone marrow, or cells from sputum or effusion specimens. The fungus appears as a tiny oval body with a clear halo surrounding a small nucleus.

QUALITATIVE DISORDERS

Defective Locomotion and Chemotaxis

Defective locomotion and defects in chemotaxis represent qualitative defects. Leukocyte mobility may be impaired in diseases such as rheumatoid arthritis, cirrhosis of the liver, and chronic granulomatous disease (CGD). Defective locomotion or leukocyte immobility can be seen in patients receiving corticosteroids and in "lazy leukocyte syndrome." A marked defect in the cellular response to chemotaxis can be seen in patients suffering from diabetes mellitus, Chédiak-Higashi anomaly, and sepsis, and in patients with high levels of antibody IgE, such as those with Job's syndrome.

Defects in Microbicidal Activity

Neutrophils and monocytes possess oxidase systems capable of killing ingested microorganisms in the process of phagocytosis (see Chapter 14). These disorders include chronic granulomatous disease, myeloperoxidase deficiency, and other functional anomalies of neutrophils.

Chronic Granulomatous Disease

The most serious of disorders related to a defect in microbicidal activity is chronic granulomatous disease (CGD). CGD consists of a group of genetic disorders in which neutrophils and monocytes ingest, but cannot kill, catalase-positive microorganisms such as *Staphylococcus aureus,* gram-positive enteric bacteria, and various fungi, especially aspergilli. CGD is a rare disorder; the inability to kill microorganisms leads to recurrent life-threatening infections by catalase-positive organisms during the first year of life. In CGD, stimulated phagocytes do not generate O_2^-, produce H_2O_2, or consume O_2 at an accelerated rate via the hexose monophosphate (HMP) shunt; the respiratory burst is not activated, and free radical forms of reduced O_2 are not produced.

In many patients with CGD, the disease is X-linked, but in about one fourth of families the disease is transmitted by autosomal recessive genes. In most of these cases both parents have had normal neutrophil functions and their cytochrome b concentrations are normal, unlike the X-linked cases. However, abnormal oxidase activity is detectable by negative nitroblue tetrazolium (NBT) screening test, an indirect test for respiratory burst power. In addition to the two main categories of CGD, X-linked and the autosomal recessive forms, some cases do not conform to either classification. These cases are believed to be due to point mutations. Rare causes of CGD include severe deficiency or instability of leukocyte G6PD.

Myeloperoxidase Deficiency

Myeloperoxidase deficiency (Alius-Grignaschi anomaly) is a benign inherited disorder that is usually transmitted by autosomal recessive genes. This disorder is manifested by the absence of myeloperoxidase enzyme (MPO) from neutrophils and monocytes, but not eosinophils. A lack of MPO, which mediates oxidative destruction of microbes by H_2O_2, creates a microbicidal defect in phagocytes. The functional abnormality is not severe. Infections are not usually serious.

A partial deficiency of MPO has been observed in patients with acute and chronic leukemias, myelodysplastic syndromes, Hodgkin's disease, and carcinoma.

Other Functional Anomalies of Neutrophils

At least 15 hereditary defects and 30 additional disorders of neutrophil function have been described. A functional anomaly of neutrophils includes lactoferrin deficiency.

Lactoferrin deficiency is a rare disorder. In this disorder, specific granules are reduced in quantity and almost devoid of the specific granule protein, lactoferrin. This deficiency causes several dysfunctions including unresponsiveness to chemotactic signals and diminished adhesiveness to surfaces of particles. This deficiency leads to pyogenic infections, particularly deep-seated skin abscesses.

Monocyte-Macrophage Disorders

Qualitative disorders of monocytes-macrophages are manifested as lipid storage diseases, including several rare autosomal recessive disorders. The macrophages are particularly prone to accumulate undergraded lipid products, which subsequently leads to an expansion of the reticuloendothelial tissue. Monocytic disorders include Gaucher's disease and Niemann-Pick disease.

Gaucher's Disease

This inherited disease is caused by a disturbance in cellular lipid metabolism. Gaucher's disease is most frequently discovered in children, and the prognosis varies from patient to patient. If the disease is mild, the patient may live a relatively normal life; if it is severe, the patient may die prematurely.

The disorder represents a deficiency of beta-glucocerebrosidase, the enzyme that normally splits glucose from its parent sphingolipid, glucosylceramide. As the result of this enzyme deficiency, cerebroside accumulates in (macrophages) histiocytes (Plate 45). Gaucher's cells are rarely found in the circulating blood. The typical Gaucher's cell is large, with one to three eccentric nuclei and a characteristically wrinkled cytoplasm. These cells are found in the bone marrow, spleen, and other organs of the reticuloendothelial system. The production of erythrocytes and leukocytes decreases as these abnormal cells infiltrate into the bone marrow.

Niemann-Pick Disease

This disease is similar to Gaucher's disease because it is also an inherited abnormality of lipid metabolism. Niemann-Pick disease afflicts infants and children; the patient's average age at death is 5 years.

This disorder represents a deficiency of the enzyme that normally cleaves phosphoryl choline from its parent sphingolipid, sphingomyelin. Sphingomyelin accumulates in the tissue macrophages. The characteristic cell in this disorder, Pick's cell, is similar in appearance to the Gaucher's cell; however, the cytoplasm of the cell is foamy in appearance.

SUMMARY

Quantitative Disorders

Disorders of the quantitative type involve either an increase in leukocytes (leukocytosis) or a decrease (leukocytopenia). Any of the leukocyte types can be affected. A nonmalignant increase in specific granulocytes is referred to as neutrophilia, eosinophilia, or basophilia. An increase in monocytes is monocytosis. Neutrophils can be associated with physical stress, infection, inflammation, and drugs and hormones. Eosinophilia can be related to bronchial asthma, parasitic infections, and pulmonary and gastrointestinal disorders. Basophilia can be associated with asthma, smallpox, chickenpox, and drug therapy. Monocytosis is not a precisely defined state; however, tuberculosis, fever of unknown origin, and inflammatory bowel disease are a few of the disorders associated with an increase in circulating monocytes.

Decreases in leukocytes are caused primarily by either decreased production of normal granulocytes or increased destruction of circulating granulocytes. Neutropenia may be due to bone marrow injury or nutritional deficiencies, for example. Eosinopenia is rare and can be stress-related. Basopenia can be induced by the action of hormones, such as cortisone.

Qualitative Disorders

Qualitative abnormalities include defective locomotion and defective bacterial killing. Qualitative disorders of monocytes-macrophages include Gaucher's disease and Niemann-Pick disease. Both these disorders represent enzyme deficiencies that result in the accumulation of undegraded lipid products in macrophages.

CASE STUDIES

CASE 1 The 18-month-old son of a Nigerian exchange student was taken to his family doctor because he was losing weight and had been experiencing frequent fevers. The child had no history of disease or allergies. Physical examination revealed a well-nourished male infant. His rectal temperature was 101.8° F. The pediatrician ordered a complete blood count.

Laboratory Data
The patient had a slightly decreased hemoglobin and hematocrit. His total leukocyte count was $11.0 \times 10^9/L$. The total leukocyte differential count was as follows:

Neutrophilic bands 4%
Segmented neutrophils 35%
Lymphocytes 19%
Monocytes 2%
Eosinophils 40%

Additional Laboratory Tests
Allergy testing revealed no remarkable results. A stool examination was negative for ova and parasites.

Questions
1. What is the most probable cause of this child's eosinophilia?
2. Could pinworms (*Enterobius vermicularis*) be suspected?
3. What is the most probable source of this infection?

Discussion
1. In the absence of physical signs or symptoms such as asthma or other respiratory distress and with no history of allergies, the etiology of the eosinophilia must be considered to be systemic, that is, a condition throughout the body such as an invasive parasitic condition.

(continued)

CASE STUDIES (*continued*)

2. Children frequently suffer from pinworm infections. This parasitic infection is easily transmitted. However, the degree of eosinophilia is not usually as pronounced as in this case. In this case, a Scotch tape examination was subsequently performed and was negative for *E. vermicularis*.
3. A subsequent muscle biopsy revealed trichinosis. Trichinosis is contracted by eating pork that is infected with the parasite and improperly cooked. Because of laws that prohibit the marketing of hogs that have been fed garbage in the United States, trichinosis is uncommon today. However, in underdeveloped countries, improper swine management and improper food preparation can result in the transmission of this disease to humans.

> ### Diagnosis: Eosinophilia due to trichinosis

CASE 2 An 18-year-old female college freshman complaining of severe abdominal pain was brought to the emergency room by the college nurse. She had no history of prior illness but had begun having pain immediately after eating dinner.

Physical examination revealed tenderness in the lower right quadrant. No abdominal masses were noted. The patient had a temperature of 100° F. A complete blood count and urinalysis were ordered.

Laboratory Data
The hemoglobin and hematocrit values were within normal range. The total leukocyte count was 20×10^9/L. The leukocyte differential smear revealed the following:

Segmented neutrophils 72%
Band form neutrophils 16%
Lymphocytes 2%
Monocytes 6%
Eosinophils 4%

The result of urinalysis was essentially normal except for the presence of ketone bodies.

Questions
1. What general type of disorder is this patient suffering from?
2. What is the absolute segmented neutrophil value? Is it normal?
3. What is the probable diagnosis?

Discussion
1. The patient has symptoms and laboratory findings that support the classification of an acute inflammatory disorder.
2. The absolute value of segmented neutrophils = 20×10^9/L $\times 0.72 = 14.4 \times 10^9$/L. The patient's absolute segmented neutrophil value was above normal. The normal range for segmented neutrophils is 1.5 to 6.0×10^9/L.
3. The initial symptom of pain in the lower-right quadrant progressively became more severe, and the patient developed the classic rebound phenomenon found in acute appendicitis. The increased total leukocyte count and increased band form neutrophils supported the physical findings. Additionally, the presence of ketone bodies was consistent with acute appendicitis, although they may

also be found in other disorders such as starvation and diabetic ketosis.

> ### Diagnosis: Acute inflammation of the appendix (appendicitis)

CASE 3 A 45-year-old woman with a known diagnosis of diabetes mellitus visited her physician because of difficulty and pain on urination. Physical examination revealed that the patient had a slightly elevated temperature but no other abnormalities. A complete blood count, urinalysis, and urine culture were ordered.

Laboratory Data
The patient's hemiglobin and hematocrit were normal. However, the total leukocyte count was 28.5×10^9/L, with the following leukocyte differential results:

Segmented neutrophils 79%
Neutrophilic bands 10%
Eosinophils 2%
Lymphocytes 9%

Most of the segmented neutrophils displayed dark, coarse granulation. Many of the neutrophils were also vacuolated.

The patient's urine had an elevated concentration of protein, increased numbers of leukocytes, and many bacteria. The urine culture had a heavy growth of a gram-negative rod, *Pseudomonas* species.

Questions
1. What is the dark, coarse granulation in the neutrophils?
2. Does this condition alter the phagocytic effectiveness of the leukocytes?
3. What is the most probable explanation of the patient's elevated leukocyte count?

Discussion
1. The granulation observed is toxic granulation. This disorder is commonly seen in the hematology laboratory. However, care must be taken not to overlook the rarer finding of Chediak-Higashi syndrome. The inclusion granules in this disorder are gigantic.
2. No, toxic granulation is believed to represent the precipitation of ribosomal RNA due to metabolic toxicity occurring in the cell. This metabolic toxicity may shorten the life span of the cell, but the cell can remain fully functional until it dies.
3. Toxic granulation can be observed in granulocytes in a variety of conditions, including severe infections, burns, and drug therapy.

In this case, the combination of an elevated total leukocyte count, toxic granulation, and a positive urine culture with a gram-negative rod suggests that both the toxic granulation and the elevated leukocyte count were due to a severe urinary tract infection. Although the patient also had diabetes, that would not have directly affected the total leukocyte count. However, patients with diabetes tend to be more susceptible to bacterial infections than nondiabetic persons, due to circulatory problems and defective chemotaxis.

> ### Diagnosis: Toxic granulation due to bacterial infection

(*continued*)

CASE 4 A 6-month-old black child was admitted for repair of an inguinal hernia. Routine preoperative laboratory testing was ordered.

Laboratory Data
Hemoglobin and hematocrit were normal, and the total leukocyte count was 7.5 × 10⁹/L. The differential results revealed the following:

Band-type neutrophils 25%
Segmented neutrophils 10%
Lymphocytes 62%
Monocytes 2%
Eosinophils 1%

Questions
1. What is the condition most probably being observed in the neutrophils?
2. What is the etiology of this disorder?
3. Is it clinically significant?

Discussion
1. Further observation of the band-type neutrophils revealed that the nuclear chromatin was very coarsely clumped. The degree of clumping was much more than would normally be seen in bands and more consistent with the degree of chromatin clumping observed in segmented neutrophils. The cells classified as segmented neutrophils usually had only two lobes as compared with the multiple lobes seen in normal segmented neutrophils.

   Hypolobulation of neutrophils presents a peripheral blood picture that mimics an increase in neutrophilic bands. Because the total leukocyte count was within normal range, one would have expected the percentage of bands to be normal also. However, major discrepancies between these two measurements should alert the hematology technologist that an error has occurred. Repeated review of the peripheral smear confirmed that the band-type neutrophils were actually hypolobulated neutrophils. The condition was Pelger-Huët anomaly.
2. Pelger-Huët anomaly exists as a congenital disorder. This trait is inherited in an autosomal dominant manner. In persons who are heterozygous for this trait, more than three fourths of the mature neutrophils may be hypolobulated. Homozygous states for this trait are rare. A condition of pseudo-Pelger-Huët anomaly may be observed in leukemias, such as chronic granulocytic leukemia, or it may be induced by drugs such as the sulfa drugs or those used in chemotherapy.
3. Congenital Pelger-Huët anomaly has not been associated with any specific clinical disease. The abnormal nuclear maturation is presumed to be a reflection of abnormal nucleic acid metabolism, although the specific abnormality is unknown. Functionally, these leukocytes do not show any abnormality.

✐ **Diagnosis: Congenital Pelger-Huët anomaly**

CASE 5 A 31-year-old white male was admitted to the burn unit of a local hospital following an accident at a local foundry. Several stat laboratory blood tests were ordered, including a complete blood count.

Laboratory Data
The hemoglobin, hematocrit, and red blood cell count were all slightly elevated. The total leukocyte count was 15.8 × 10⁹/L. The differential count was as follows:

Band neutrophils 12%
Segmented neutrophils 65%
Lymphocytes 23%
Light blue-gray inclusions were observed in the cytoplasm of many of the bands and segmented neutrophils.

Questions
1. What is the etiology of the abnormal quantitative findings in this patient's complete blood count?
2. What are the blue-gray vacuoles in the cytoplasm of the leukocytes?
3. Is this abnormality diagnostically significant?

Discussion
1. The concentration of the red blood cells that produced the slightly elevated hemoglobin, hematocrit, and red blood cell count was undoubtedly due to the loss of fluids as the result of the serious burns. Elevation of the total leukocyte count is frequently seen as a response to stress, as in this type of trauma.
2. The blue-gray inclusions in the cytoplasm are Döhle bodies. However, care must be taken to distinguish these more common inclusions from May-Hegglin anomaly. The absence of unusual platelets and the admitting diagnosis would be helpful in not mistaking the more frequently encountered Döhle bodies from the May-Hegglin anomaly.
3. Döhle bodies are frequently seen in traumatic or toxic conditions such as severe burns. These leukocytic inclusions may also be seen in severe infections, during pregnancy, and as the result of cancer chemotherapy. Patients with viral infections, such as measles or hepatitis, may also have Döhle bodies. Although they are indicative of a metabolic abnormality, they are not specific for a particular disorder. However, it is diagnostically significant as a sign of abnormal stress on the bone marrow.

✐ **Diagnosis: Döhle inclusion bodies due to extensive burns**

BIBLIOGRAPHY

Bakken, J. S. et al. "Human Granulocytic Ehrlichiosis in the Upper Midwest United States." *JAMA,* Vol. 272, No. 3, July 20, 1994, pp. 212–218.

Barenfanger, J. et al. "Identifying Human Ehrlichiosis." *Lab. Med.,* Vol. 27, No. 6, June, 1996, pp. 372–374.

Beutler, E. "Gaucher's Disease." *N. Engl. J. Med.,* Vol. 325, No. 19, November 7, 1991, pp. 1354–1359.

Dannenberg, Arthur M., Jr. "Macrophages and Monocytes," in *Fundamentals of Clinical Hematology.* Jerry L. Spivak (ed.). Hagerstown, MD: Harper & Row, 1980, pp. 137–153.

Figueroa, M. L. et al. "A Less Costly Regimen of Alglucerase to Treat Gaucher's Disease." *N. Engl. J. Med.,* Vol. 327, No. 23, December 3, 1992, pp. 1632–1636.

Francis, G. E. et al. "DNA Strand Breakage and ADP-Ribosyl Transferase Mediated DNA Ligation During Stimulation of Human

Bone Marrow Cells by Granulocyte-Macrophage Colony Stimulating Activity.'' *Leuk. Res.,* Vol. 8, No. 3, 1984, pp. 407–415.

Grabowski, G. A. et al. ''Enzyme Therapy in Type I Gaucher Disease: Comparative Efficacy of Mannose-Terminated Glucocerebrosidase From Natural and Recombinant Sources.'' *Annals of Internal Med.,* Vol. 122, No. 1, January 1, 1995, pp. 33–39.

Hartmann, L. C. et al. ''Granulocyte Colony-Stimulating Factor in Severe Chemotherapy-Induced Afebrile Neutropenia.'' *N. Engl. J. Med.,* Vol. 336, No. 25, June 19, 1997, pp. 1776–1785.

Hellmann, Andrzej. ''Production of Colony Stimulating Activity in Mixed Mononuclear Cell Culture.'' *Br. J. Haematol.,* Vol. 45, 1980, pp. 245–249.

Henry, John B. *Clinical Laboratory Diagnosis and Management* (17th ed.). Philadelphia: Saunders, 1984, p. 638.

Howard, John. ''Myeloid Series Abnormalities: Neutrophilia.'' *Lab. Med.,* Vol. 14, No. 3, March, 1983, pp. 147–151.

Leukocyte Differential Counting, Tentative Standard H20-T. Villanova, PA: National Committee for Clinical Laboratory Standards (NCCLS), 1982.

Lopker, Anita et al. ''Stereoselective Muscarinic Acetylcholine and Opiate Receptors in Human Phagocytic Leukocytes.'' *Biochem. Pharmacol.,* Vol. 29, 1980, pp. 1361–1365.

Markell, Edward K. et al. *Medical Parasitology.* Philadelphia: Saunders, 1986, p. 314.

O'Connor, Barbara H. *A Color Atlas and Instruction Manual of Peripheral Blood Morphology.* Baltimore: Williams & Wilkins, 1984.

Raphael, Stanley S. *Lynch's Medical Laboratory Technology* (4th ed.). Philadelphia: Saunders, 1983, pp. 653, 692.

Robinson, Stephen H. and Paul R. Reich. *Hematology: Pathophysiological Basis for Clinical Practice* (3rd ed.). Boston: Little, Brown & Co., 1993.

Sidransky, E. and E. I. Ginns. ''Clinical Heterogeneity Among Patients With Gaucher's Disease.'' *JAMA,* Vol. 269, No. 9, March 3, 1993, pp. 1154–1157.

Stein, Robert B. ''Granulocytosis and Granulocytic Leukemoid Reactions,'' in *Laboratory Hematology.* John Koepke (ed.). Edinburgh: Churchill-Livingstone, 1984, pp. 153–187.

Tsan, Min-Fu. ''Neutrophils,'' in *Fundamentals of Clinical Hematology.* Jerry L. Spivak (ed.). Hagerstown, MD: Harper & Row, 1980, pp. 109–117.

Wynn, Thomas E. Letters to the Editor. *Lab. Med.,* Vol. 15, No. 4, April, 1984, pp. 276–277.

Zigmond, Sally H. and Douglas A. Lauffenburger. ''Assays of Leukocyte Chemotaxis.'' *Annu. Rev. Med.,* Vol. 37, 1986, pp. 149–155.

REVIEW QUESTIONS

1. Leukocytosis can be caused by:

   A. Increased proliferation of immature granulocytic cells.
   B. Increased mobilization of granulocytes from the maturation-storage compartment.
   C. Increased movement of granulocytes from the marginating pool to the circulating pool.
   D. All of the above.

2. Neutrophilia can be related to a variety of conditions or disorders. Select the appropriate conditions.

   A. Surgery. C. Stress.
   B. Burns. D. All of the above.

3. Charcot-Leyden crystals can be found in ___ of patients with active eosinophilic inflammation.

   A. Sputum. C. Stool.
   B. Tissues. D. All of the above.

4. Monocytosis can be observed in:

   A. Tuberculosis.
   B. Fever of unknown origin.
   C. Rheumatoid arthritis.
   D. All of the above.

5. Neutropenia can be observed in:

   A. Bone marrow injury.
   B. Nutritional deficiency.
   C. Increased destruction and utilization.
   D. All of the above.

Questions 6 through 9: match the following abnormalities with the appropriate characteristic.

6. ___ Alder-Reilly inclusions.
7. ___ Chédiak-Higashi syndrome.
8. ___ Döhle body inclusions.
9. ___ May-Hegglin anomaly.

A. Gigantic peroxidase positive deposits.
B. Precipitated mucopolysaccharides.
C. Döhle body-like inclusions.
D. Single or multiple pale-blue staining inclusions.

Questions 10 through 12: match the following abnormalities with the appropriate characteristic.

10. ___ Pelger-Huët anomaly.
11. ___ Toxic granulation.
12. ___ Hypersegmentation.

A. Dark blue-black precipitates of RNA.
B. Five or more nuclear segments.
C. Failure of the nucleus to segment.
D. Precipitated mucopolysaccharides.

Questions 13 through 16: match the following abnormalities with the appropriate condition.

13. ___ Chédiak-Higashi syndrome.

14. ___ Döhle bodies.

15. ___ Pelger-Huët anomaly.

16. ___ Hypersegmentation.

A. Associated with a deficiency of vitamin B_{12} or folic acid.

B. Associated with frequent infections in children or young adults.

C. May be related to a maturational arrest in some acute infections.

D. Associated with viral infections and burns.

Questions 17 through 21: select the appropriate cell type involved in the following disorders.

17. ___ Gaucher's disease.

18. ___ Niemann-Pick disease.

19. ___ Chédiak-Higashi syndrome.

20. ___ Chronic granulomatous disease.

21. ___ Lazy leukocyte syndrome.

A. Neutrophilic series.

B. Monocytic-macrophage series.

22. Gaucher cells have:

A. Wrinkled cytoplasm.
B. One to three nuclei.
C. A deficiency of betaglucocerebrosidase.
D. All of the above.

CHAPTER 16

Leukocytes: Lymphocytes and Plasma Cells

Anatomical origin and development of lymphocytes
The sites of lymphocytic development
Lymphocyte physiology
Normal values
Determining absolute lymphocyte values
Morphological characteristics of normal lymphocytes

Maturational stages
General variations in lymphocyte morphology
Specific lymphocyte morphological variations
The functions and membrane characteristics of lymphocytes
Major lymphocyte function
Major lymphocyte membrane characteristics and development

Lymphocyte subsets and function
Plasma cell development and maturation
Plasma cell development
Maturational morphology
Plasma cell disorders
Summary
Bibliography
Review questions

OBJECTIVES

Anatomical origin and development of lymphocytes
- Briefly describe the role of lymphocytes and plasma cells in the body defense mechanism against disease.
- Name and locate the two primary and three secondary lymphoid tissues.
- Identify the anatomical sites populated by T cells and B cells.
- Explain the importance of lymphocyte recirculation.
- Cite the percentage of T and B cells found in the peripheral circulation of adults.
- State the major type and percentage of leukocytes found in 6-month-old infants.
- Compare the normal percentages and quantities of lymphocytes in 6-month-old infants and adults.

Morphological characteristics of normal lymphocytes
- Compare the characteristics, such as chromatin patterns, of the three major developmental stages of lymphocyte maturation.
- Discuss the morphological abnormalities of variant lymphocytes.
- State at least three conditions associated with specific lymphocytic abnormalities that may be seen in peripheral blood.

The functions and membrane characteristics of lymphocytes
- Describe the major function of T, B, natural killer (NK), and K cells.
- Describe the major lymphocytic membrane characteristics.
- State the principles of the early tests that were used to distinguish T and B cells.
- Name several applications of lymphocyte subset testing.
- Briefly describe the production of monoclonal antibodies.
- Briefly describe membrane marker development in T cells.
- Explain the purpose of functional testing in lymphocytes.
- Name four cytokines.

Plasma cell development and maturation
- Describe the pathways of plasma cell development.
- Identify the maturational characteristics of plasma cells.
- Describe the appearance and cytoplasmic contents of Russell bodies, Mott cells, and flame cells.

ANATOMICAL ORIGIN AND DEVELOPMENT OF LYMPHOCYTES

In addition to the activities of the granulocytes, monocytes, and macrophages (discussed in Chapter 14), the lymphocytes and plasma cells cooperate in defending the body against disease through recognition of foreign **antigens** and **antibody** production.

The Sites of Lymphocytic Development

During embryonic development, lymphocytes arise from the pluripotent, precursor cells of the yolk sac and liver. Later in fetal development and throughout the life cycle, the bone marrow becomes the sole provider of hematopoietic stem cells. These cells, under the influence of hematopoietic growth factors IL-1 and IL-6, differentiate into the lymphoid stem cell. Continued cellular development of the lymphoid precursors and proliferation occur as the cells travel to specific microenvironments. Hematopoietic growth factors play an important role in differentiation into the pathway of the pre-B cell or prothymocyte. The majority of cells differentiate into either **T lymphocytes** or **B lymphocytes.** The plasma cell is the fully differentiated B cell.

Primary Lymphoid Tissue

In humans, both the bone marrow and the thymus are classified as primary or central lymphoid tissues (Fig. 16.1) and are active in lymphopoiesis. Stem cells that migrate to the thymus proliferate and differentiate under the influence of specific cytokines. These cells acquire thymus-dependent characteristics to become **immunocompetent** (able to function in the immune response) T lymphocytes. It is believed that the bone marrow functions as the bursal equivalent in humans. It is from the term **bursa** that the B lymphocytes derive their name. Most of the cells produced in the primary sites die before leaving; only a small percentage migrate to the secondary tissues.

Secondary Lymphoid Tissue

The secondary lymphoid tissues include the lymph nodes, spleen, and Peyer's patches in the intestine (see Fig. 16.1). Proliferation of the T and B lymphocytes in the secondary or peripheral lymphoid tissues is primarily dependent on antigenic stimulation. The T lymphocytes, or T cells (Fig. 16.2), populate these sites:

1. Perifollicular and paracortical regions of the lymph node
2. Medullary cords of the lymph nodes
3. Periarteriolar regions of the spleen
4. Thoracic duct of the circulatory system

The B lymphocytes, or B cells (see Fig. 16.2), multiply and populate these sites:

1. Follicular and medullary areas (germinal centers) of the lymph nodes
2. Primary follicles and red pulp of the spleen
3. Follicular regions of gut-associated lymphoid tissue (GALT)
4. Medullary cords of the lymph nodes

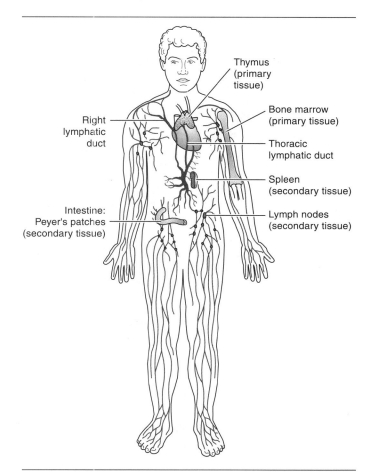

FIGURE 16.1 Primary and secondary lymphoid tissues and lymphatic system. The primary lymphoid tissues are the bone marrow and the thymus. The secondary tissues consist of the spleen, the lymph nodes, and the Peyer's patches of the small intestine. The lymphatic system consists of widely distributed lymph nodes and lymphatic vessels. The right lymphatic duct drains the heart, lungs, part of the diaphragm, and the right upper part of the body, the right side of the head and neck. The thoracic duct drains the rest of the body. Lymphatic fluid returns to the venous blood circulation. The principal return is into the left or right brachiocephalic vein or into one of the two veins that unite to form it, the left subclavian or left internal jugular vein.

Lymphocyte Physiology

The mature T lymphocyte survives for several months or years, whereas the average life span of the B lymphocytes is only a few days. Lymphocytes move freely between the blood and lymphoid tissues. This activity, referred to as **lymphocyte recirculation,** enables lymphocytes to come in contact with processed foreign antigens and to disseminate antigen-sensitized memory cells throughout the lymphoid system. Lymphocytes recirculate back to the blood via the major lymphatic ducts (see Fig. 16.1).

Lymphocytes enter the lymph node (Fig. 16.3) from the blood circulation via arterioles and capillaries to reach the specialized postcapillary venules. From the venule, the lymphocytes enter the node and either remain in the node or pass through the node and return to the circulating blood.

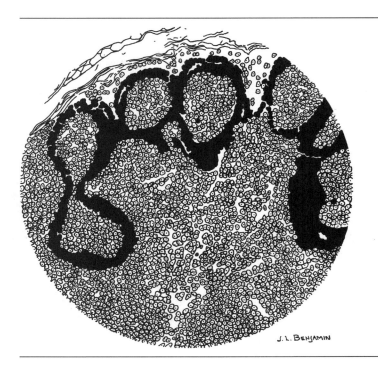

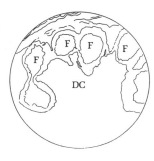

FIGURE 16.2 T and B cell areas in the lymph node. The lymphocytes of the outer cortex are mainly arranged in lymphoid follicles (F), which are the major sites of B lymphocyte localization and proliferation. The deep cortical zone (DC), or paracortex, is composed mainly of T lymphocytes that are *never* arranged in follicles. The number of cortical follicles and the depth of the deep cortical zone vary according to the immunological state of each lymph node and in each individual person.

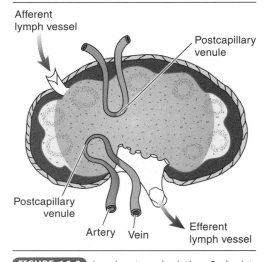

FIGURE 16.3 Lymphocyte recirculation. Recirculating lymphocytes, mostly T cells, pass from the blood circulation through the lymphoid system and back to the circulating blood. Lymphocytes enter the lymph node from the blood circulation via arterioles and capillaries to reach the specialized postcapillary venules. Both T- and B-type lymphocytes adhere to these large specialized venule walls and then move through the walls to enter the node. As the lymphocytes pass through the node, T lymphocytes circulate in close proximity to macrophages, B lymphocytes, and other T lymphocytes. This process allows for contact between lymphocytes and antigens processed by macrophages. Lymphatic fluid and lymphocytes enter the node through the afferent lymphatic duct and leave the node through the efferent duct. Valves are present in both the afferent and efferent ducts to prevent the backflow of lymphatic fluid. Fluid and lymphocytes leaving the node move into the medullary lymphatic sinuses and then to the efferent lymphatic duct, which in turn collects in the major lymphatic ducts (see Fig. 16.1).

Lymphatic fluid, lymphocytes, and antigens from certain body sites enter the lymph node through the afferent lymphatic duct and exit through the efferent lymphatic duct.

Normal Values

At any one time, approximately 5% of the total body lymphocyte mass is present in the circulating blood. Sixty to 80% of the blood lymphocyte pool in adults is composed of T lymphocytes and approximately 20% is composed of B lymphocytes. Total blood lymphocyte levels vary considerably with age (Table 16.1). Lymphocytes represent 31% of the total leukocytes present at birth; within a few days of birth, lymphocytes are the dominant type of leukocyte in the circulation. Most of the cells are T lymphocytes. In adults, lym-

TABLE 16.1 Average Lymphocyte Values in Peripheral Blood

Age	Total White Cell Count	Lymphocytes	
		absolute	percentage
Birth	18.1×10^9/L	5.5×10^9/L	31
6 months	11.9×10^9/L	7.3×10^9/L	61
2 years	10.6×10^9/L	6.3×10^9/L	59
12 years	8.0×10^9/L	3.0×10^9/L	38
21 years and over	7.4×10^9/L	2.5×10^9/L	34

Source: From P. L. Altman and D. S. Dittmer, *Blood and Other Body Fluids.* Bethesda, MD: Federation of American Societies for Experimental Biology, 1961, p. 125. With permission.

phocytes represent approximately 35% of the total circulation of leukocytes, or 2.5×10^9/L.

Determining Absolute Lymphocyte Values

The **absolute** number of lymphocytes is the total number of lymphocytes compared with the total number of leukocytes. The **relative** number of lymphocytes is the percentage of lymphocytes as determined by a differential blood smear enumeration of leukocytes (see Chapter 17).

MORPHOLOGICAL CHARACTERISTICS OF NORMAL LYMPHOCYTES

The stages of lymphocyte development are the **lymphoblast, prolymphocyte,** and mature **lymphocyte.** The morphological characteristics of these cells on a peripheral blood smear when stained with Wright stain are summarized in Table 16.2.

Under normal conditions, only mature lymphocytes are found in the peripheral blood. Mature cells can be classified as either large or small. Although T and B cells cannot be distinguished by routine Romanowsky-type staining of blood smears, most small lymphocytes are T cells and most large lymphocytes are B cells.

Maturational Stages

Lymphoblast

The lymphoblast (Plate 46) is the first morphologically identifiable cell of the lymphocytic maturational series in the bone marrow. The overall size ranges from 15 to 20 μm, with a nuclear-cytoplasmic (N:C) ratio of 4:1.

The nuclear shape is either round or oval. One or two nucleoli may be present. The chromatin pattern is delicate looking. The small amount of cytoplasm is medium blue and may have a darker-blue border. No granules are present.

Prolymphocyte

The second stage in the maturational development of the lymphocyte is the prolymphocyte (Plate 47). This cell may be seen in the bone marrow, thymus, and secondary lymphoid tissues. The overall size is usually about the same (15 to 18 μm) as the lymphoblast. The N:C ratio ranges from 4:1 to 3:1.

The nuclear shape is usually oval or slightly indented. The number of nucleoli varies from none to one. The chromatin pattern is slightly condensed. The small amount of cytoplasm is medium blue with a thin, darker-blue rim. A few azurophilic granules may be present.

Mature Lymphocyte

Mature lymphocytes (Plate 48) range in size from large (17 to 20 μm) in younger cells to small (6 to 9 μm) in older cells. The N:C ratio ranges from 2:1 in younger cells to 4:1 to 3:1 in older cells.

The nucleus is round or oval and may have an indentation (cleft). Nucleoli are not visible. The chromatin pattern is dense and appears clumped. The cytoplasm is light sky blue and very scanty. A few azurophilic granules may be present.

General Variations in Lymphocyte Morphology

Variant lymphocytes may be referred to by several names, including atypical lymphocytes, Downey cells, reactive or transformed lymphocytes, lymphocytoid or plasmacytoid lymphocytes, and virocytes. The National Committee for Clinical Laboratory Standards (NCCLS) has proposed that the term **variant lymphocyte** be included as one of the seven leukocyte types found in normal peripheral blood. This term denotes that a lymphocyte is not normal but does not further classify a lymphocyte. Normal persons may have up to 5% or 6% of variant lymphocytes. These represent morphological evidence of a normal immune mechanism. Variant lymphocytes can be found in increased numbers in disorders such as infectious mononucleosis, viral pneumonia, and viral hepatitis.

TABLE 16.2 Comparative Characteristics of Lymphocytes

	Lymphoblast	Prolymphocyte	Mature Lymphocyte
Size	15–20 μm	15–18 μm	Small 6–9 μm Large 17–20 μm
N:C ratio	4:1	4:1 to 3:1	Small 4:1 to 3:1 Large 2:1
Nucleus			
Nuclear shape	Round or oval	Oval, slightly indented	Round or oval; may have clefts
Nucleoli	1 or 2	0 or 1	Absent
Chromatin	Delicate	Slightly condensed	Dense and clumped
Cytoplasm			
Granules	None	May have a few azurophilic granules	Few azurophilic granules may be present
Amount	Small	Small	Very scanty
Color	Medium blue, may have a darker-blue border	Medium blue with a thin rim of darker blue	Light blue

The morphology of variant lymphocytes differs (Plate 49), and several distinct types have been described, including the classic grouping of lymphocytes seen in infectious mononucleosis, the Downey classification (see Table 16.3). Variant lymphocytes can embrace all transitional changes from mature unstimulated lymphocytes to immunoblasts to plasma cells (to be discussed later in this chapter). These lymphocytes represent stimulated lymphocytes that have increased DNA and RNA activity. Similarities between some variant lymphocytes and lymphoblasts can lead to difficulties in identification. The formation of distinctive nucleoli characterizes the immunoblast, the further transformation of which produces plasma cells or small sensitized committed lymphocytes called **memory cells.**

The general characteristics of **variant** lymphocytes include the following:

1. Usually the overall size is increased (16 to 30 μm).
2. The nucleus may be enlarged.
3. The nuclear shape may be lobulated or resemble the nucleus of a monocyte (**monocytoid**) with clefts or notching and may be folded.
4. Chromatin patterns vary from fine patterns to a coarsely granular appearance.
5. One to three nucleoli may be present.
6. The cytoplasm is frequently abundant and often foamy or vacuolated.
7. Cytoplasmic color may range from gray to light blue or intensely blue.
8. Granules may be present.

Specific Lymphocyte Morphological Variations

A variety of abnormal lymphocytes or lymphocyte-like cells are associated with specific disorders. They include the following.

Binucleated Lymphocytes

These cells can be seen in viral infections. If over 5% of the lymphocytes are binucleated, it is suggestive of either lymphocytic leukemia or leukosarcoma (the hematological spread of lymphosarcoma).

Rieder Cells

Rieder cells are similar to normal lymphocytes except that the nucleus is notched, lobulated, and cloverleaf-like. They occur in chronic lymphocytic leukemia (discussed in Chapter 20) or can be artificially produced through blood smear preparation.

Vacuolated Lymphocytes

Vacuolated lymphocytes (Plate 50) are frequently associated with Niemann-Pick disease, Tay-Sachs disease, Hurler's syndrome, and Burkitt's lymphoma. Vacuoles can also be seen in variant lymphocytes and as a reaction to viral infections, radiation, and chemotherapy.

Smudge Cells

Smudge cells (Plate 51) are a natural artifact produced in the preparation of a blood smear. They represent the bare nuclei of lymphocytes and neutrophils. Increased fragility of cells contributes to the increased percentage of smudge cells. Some laboratories enumerate smudge cells as a percentage of the total 100 leukocytes in a differential leukocyte count. Smudge cells are seen in increased proportions in lymphocytosis, particularly chronic lymphocytic leukemia.

THE FUNCTIONS AND MEMBRANE CHARACTERISTICS OF LYMPHOCYTES

Major Lymphocyte Function

Several major categories of lymphocytes are recognized as functionally active. These categories are the **T cells, B cells,** and the **natural killer (NK)** and **K-type** lymphocytes.

T Lymphocytes

T cells are responsible for cellular immune responses and are involved in the regulation of antibody reactions by either helping or suppressing the activation of B lymphocytes. Sensitized T lymphocytes protect humans against infection by mediating intracellular pathogens that are viral, bacterial, fungal, or protozoan. These cells are responsible for chronic rejection in organ transplantation.

B Lymphocytes

B cells serve as the primary source of cells responsible for humoral (antibody) responses. Participation of B cells in the humoral immune response is accomplished by their transformation into plasma cells, with subsequent synthesis and secretion of immune antibodies (immunoglobulins). Stimulation of B cells to produce antibodies is a complex process, usually requiring interactions between macrophages (that phagocytize, process, and present antigens to T cells), T cells, and B cells. B lymphocytes aid in body defense against encapsulated bacteria such as streptococci. The condition of hyperacute rejection of transplanted organs is mediated by the B cell.

Natural Killer and K-type Lymphocytes

A subpopulation of lymphocytes that lack most of the recognizable surface membrane markers of mature T or B cells includes the NK and K-type lymphocytes. The NK and K cells destroy target cells through an extracellular nonphagocytic mechanism, referred to as a **cytotoxic reaction.** NK cells are able to recognize, nonspecifically attach, and lyse a wide variety of target cells, including tumor cells, some cells of the embryo, cells of the normal bone marrow and thymus, and microbial agents. Increasing evidence suggests that a considerable number of NK cells may be present in other tissues, particularly in the lungs and liver, where they play important roles in inflammatory reactions and in host defense, including defense against certain viruses such as cytomegalovirus and hepatitis virus. NK cells are stimulated by **interferon** (an antiviral substance) released by an intracellular virus. These cells actively kill the virally infected target cell, and if this process is completed before the virus has time to replicate, it will combat viral infection.

NK cells are classified as a population of effector lymphocytes, which produce such mediators as **interferon** and **in-**

terleukin-2. Although these cells have long been classified as **null cells,** monoclonal antibodies demonstrate that NK cells share a variety of surface membrane markers with T cells as well as some surface membrane markers that are associated with monocytes, granulocytes, or B cells.

On a Wright-stained peripheral blood smear, NK cells vary morphologically from typical lymphocytes and appear as large lymphocytes with characteristic azurophilic granules in the cytoplasm. The term **large granular lymphocyte** (LGL) can synonymously refer to NK cells. Up to about 75% of LGLs function as NK cells, and LGLs appear to account fully for the NK activity in mixed cell populations. As a group, LGLs represent a small subpopulation in the blood and spleen (about 5% of mononuclear cells).

K-type cells have a different kind of cytotoxic mechanism than NK cells. The target cell must be coated with low concentrations of IgG antibody. This is referred to as an **antibody-dependent cell-mediated cytotoxicity reaction** (ADCC). An ADCC reaction may be shown by both K cells and phagocytic and nonphagocytic myelogenous-type leukocytes. K cells are capable of lysing tumor cells. Although the K cell is morphologically similar to a small lymphocyte, its precise lineage is uncertain.

Major Lymphocyte Membrane Characteristics and Development

Cells of the immune system have specialized receptors on their membrane surfaces for eliciting an immune response. Prior to 1979, human lymphocytes could be classified as B cells, which produce antibodies, and T cells, which regulate antibody production and directly kill certain cells (effector cells).

Several tests were used prior to the introduction of highly specific fluorescent monoclonal antibody tests to distinguish T and B cells (Table 16.3). T lymphocytes were defined by their ability to form rosettes with sheep erythrocytes and were further subclassified by their ability to form rosettes with bovine erythrocytes coated with immunoglobulin or **complement** (a soluble blood protein consisting of nine components, C1 through C9, which if activated can lead to rupture of the cellular membrane). This test demonstrated that the surface membrane of T cells had receptors for attachment to normal sheep erythrocytes. B cells had membrane-bound antibody and receptors, including the complement (C3) receptor. The presence of the C3 receptor could be demonstrated by the ability of B cells to bind erythrocytes with complement to form the erythrocyte-antibody-complement (EAC) rosettes. B lymphocytes were indisputably characterized by their surface membrane immunoglobulin markers. By use of these techniques, a population of non-B, non-T cells (atypical T cells) known as NK (null) cells could also be demonstrated.

B Cell Maturation

Certain immunologic characteristics are associated with B cell development (Table 16.4). The early pre-B cell is terminal deoxynucleotidyl transferase (TDT) positive and expresses HLA-DR, CD19, and usually CALLA (CD10) antigen. The first unique feature that identifies pre-B cells is the appearance of immunoglobulin chains in the cytoplasm. Immunoglobulins consist of light and heavy molecular weight chains. The heavy chain (μ) of IgM is synthesized first and characterizes the pre-B cell. Other markers include TDT, CD19, CD20, CALLA, and HLA-DR. In the next stage of maturation, the early or immature B cell has cytoplasmic (cIg) and surface immunoglobulin (sIg) in the form of complete heavy and light chain molecules of IgM. The surface-bound IgM is

TABLE 16.3 Techniques for Identification of Lymphocyte Types in Blood or Bone Marrow

Rosette Formation
Sheep erythrocytes incubated with lymphocytes for T cell identification

Bovine erythrocytes coated with antibody (IgG or IgM) or complement (C3) for the Fc portion of the IgG or IgM antibodies or complement (C3) receptor–bearing cells

Mouse erythrocytes for pre–B cell identification

Membrane Immunofluorescence
Manual methods of direct and indirect binding of fluorescent dyes coupled to antibodies for the detection of surface (antigen) markers

Laser flow cytometry methods

TABLE 16.4 B Cell Development Markers

Cell Type	Marker
Progenitor	Heavy chains = negative
	Light chains = negative
	TDT = positive
Early pre-B	
Early development	Heavy chains = positive
	Light chains = negative
	TDT = positive
	DR = positive
Latter development	Heavy chains = positive
	Light chains = negative
	TDT = positive
	DR = positive
	CD19 = positive
	CALLA (CD10) = positive
Pre-B	Heavy chains = positive
	Light chains = negative
	TDT = positive
	DR = positive
	CD19 = positive
	CALLA (CD10) = positive
	CD20 = positive
Mature B	Heavy chains = positive
	Light chains = negative
	DR = positive
	CD19 = positive
	CD20 = positive
	sIg = positive

TDT = Terminal deoxynucleotidyl transferase; CALLA = common ALL antigen; sIg = surface immunoglobulin; DR = HLA-DR.

structurally different from the IgM molecules that normally circulate in the plasma. Receptors for complement proteins and the Fc (*f*ragment, *c*rystallizable) portion of an immunoglobulin (IgG) also appear. All of this occurs while the cells reside in the bone marrow, prior to antigen stimulation.

The mature B cell produces two types of surface immunoglobulin, IgM and IgD. In addition, mature B cells possess CD19 and CD20 cell surface markers and HLA-DR. When activated, B cells undergo clonal expansion, producing daughter cells that retain the same antibody idiotype (antigen-binding region). Some daughter cells become memory cells and retain the small mature B cell morphology and phenotype; others continue development into a short-lived antibody secreting cell, the plasma cell.

The development of T and B lymphocytes is traditionally separated into sequential phases of antigen-independent and antigen-dependent maturational phases. Lymphocyte development in the thymus and bursal-equivalent are antigen-independent. Antigen-dependent maturation involves exposure of the T or B cell to a specific antigen, resulting in the expression of surface receptor molecules that can recognize the foreign antigen on representation. Lymphocytes in the peripheral lymphoid organs, including the lymph nodes, spleen, and other lymphoid tissues, remain in a resting state until they are stimulated to undergo antigen-dependent development.

T Cell Maturation

Maturation of T cells (Fig. 16.4) is recognized by the presence of surface membrane markers. Early T and B cells share the enzymes TDT, CD9, and CD10, which are lost during maturation. However, these markers, particularly CD9 and CD10, are used to identify the lineage of immature T cells.

Other surface markers are acquired during maturation. Some of these markers will be lost during maturation. The two characteristic markers of T lymphocytes, CD4 and CD8, are the hallmark markers of the mature lymphocyte subset.

Lymphocyte Subsets and Function

The introduction of monoclonal antibodies led to the present identification of surface membrane markers. In practical terms, surface markers are used to identify and enumerate various subclasses of T lymphocytes and other lymphocytes. Variations exist in the concentration of most marker antigens on the cell surface. The evaluation of surface membrane markers is useful in certain applications such as establishing lymphocyte maturity, identifying disorders of lymphocytes (e.g., acquired immunodeficiency syndrome [AIDS]), classification of leukemias (refer to Chapter 19), and monitoring patients receiving immunosuppressive therapy.

Monoclonal Antibodies

Monoclonal antibodies to cell surface antigens now provide a method of classifying and identifying specific cellular membrane characteristics. This technique is one application of laser technology (see Chapter 25). Monoclonal antibodies are produced by a complex process of fusing two cell types: a plasma cell derived from a malignant tumor and a lymphocyte activated by a specific antigen. The fusion products are incubated until enough cells exist to permit testing for antibody production. The resultant monoclonal reagent, an antibody specific for an activated lymphocyte, is finally tested for specificity. The process of producing monoclonal antibodies takes 3 to 6 months to complete.

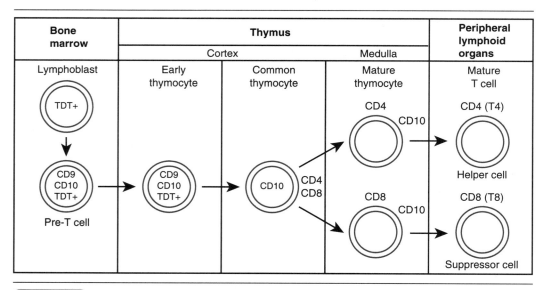

FIGURE 16.4 Examples of surface marker antigens present in T cell maturation. T cell development (antigen independent) in the thymus is divided into early thymocyte, common thymocyte, and mature thymocyte. Some of the surface membrane markers are depicted here. CD4 (T4) and CD8 (T8) are the hallmark markers of the lymphocyte subset.

Membrane Markers and Associated Function

T lymphocytes in the peripheral blood are divided into two subsets: the suppressor/cytotoxic subset and the helper/inducer subset. During T cell development, associated membrane antigens vary. Several monoclonal antibodies that distinguish functionally distinct subpopulations of lymphocytes have been developed. Among the commonly used surface markers are antibodies to CD4 and CD8. The naming of the surface membrane antigen varies with the monoclonal antibody used to identify it; each manufacturer of monoclonal antibodies has a separate nomenclature. The relationship between lymphocyte phenotype (expressed surface membrane marker) and the subset is presented in Table 16.5.

Identification of surface markers and the definition of cellular phenotypes are frequently associated with cellular function. However, an absolute correlation between phenotype and a particular function does *not* exist. Functionally, the helper/inducer subset cells signal B cells to generate antibodies, control production and switching of types of antibodies formed, and activate suppressor cells. The suppressor/cytotoxic lymphocytes control and inhibit antibody production either by suppressing helper cells or by turning off B cell differentiation. The normal ratio of helper cells and suppressor cells (approximately 2:1) can be reversed under certain conditions.

Monoclonal antibodies specific for B cells show patterns with less specificity than those for T cell markers. See Table 16.4 for the major surface markers for normal B cell differentiation. Surface immunoglobulins are usually determined in conjunction with monoclonal testing. Alterations in B cell surface markers are discussed in Chapter 20.

Functional Testing of Lymphocytes

In functional testing, phenotypes are enumerated in proportional relationship to one another. Functional assays evaluate the response of lymphocytes to nonspecific mitogens. In the case of T lymphocytes, mitogens such as pokeweed mitogen (PWM) and specific antigens such as purified protein derivative (PPD) are used. Functional testing of B lymphocytes is confined to determining the response to pure B cell mitogen such as *Staphylococcus aureus*—Cowan strain and antibody production. These substances provoke DNA synthesis and mitosis or production of antibodies that can determine which cells are functioning abnormally. A patient may have a normal proportion of phenotypically defined suppressor cells, but functional tests may show that those cells are impaired.

Other tests of T lymphocyte function measure mediator production. Soluble mediators (**cytokines**) are secreted by monocytes, lymphocytes, or neutrophils, providing the language for cell-to-cell communication. Important cytokines are as follows:

1. **Migration inhibition factor (MIF):** affects macrophage migration during delayed hypersensitivity reactions
2. **Interleukin-2 (T cell growth factor):** major factor stimulating T cell proliferation
3. **Chemotactic factor:** attracts granulocytes to affected areas
4. **Interleukin-1:** released by macrophages and activates helper T cells

PLASMA CELL DEVELOPMENT AND MATURATION

The function of plasma cells is the synthesis and excretion of immunoglobulins (antibodies). Plasma cells are not normally found in the circulating blood but are found in the bone marrow in concentrations that do not normally exceed 2%. Plasma cells arise as the end stage of B cell differentiation into a large activated plasma cell.

Plasma Cell Development

The pathway from the B lymphocyte to the antibody-synthesizing plasma cell (Fig. 16.5) occurs when the B cell is antigen-

TABLE 16.5 Examples of Normal T Lymphocyte Membrane Markers

Cell Type Detected	Designation	Monoclonal Antibody Source	Cells in Peripheral Blood (%)
All or most T lymphocytes	Leu-4	Becton-Dickinson	80–95
	OKT3	Ortho	95
	T11	Coulter	95
	Anti-CD5	Sigma	>90
T cell subsets			
Helper/inducer	Leu-3	Becton-Dickinson	40–60
	OKT4	Ortho	65
	T4	Coulter	60
	Anti-CD4	Sigma	30–50
Suppressor/cytotoxic	Leu-2	Becton-Dickinson	20–40
	OKT8	Ortho	35
	T8	Coulter	35
	Anti-CD8	Sigma	20–45

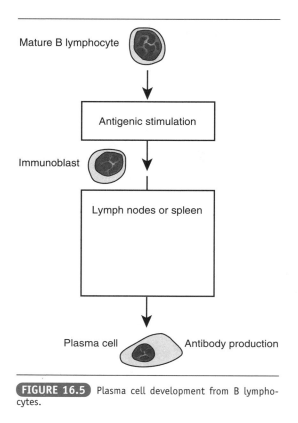

Mature B lymphocyte

↓

Antigenic stimulation

Immunoblast

↓

Lymph nodes or spleen

↓

Plasma cell   Antibody production

FIGURE 16.5 Plasma cell development from B lymphocytes.

ically stimulated and undergoes blast transformation. The immune antibody response begins when individual B lymphocytes encounter an antigen that binds to their specific immunoglobulin surface receptors. After receiving an appropriate "second signal" provided by interaction with helper T cells, these antigen-binding B cells undergo blast cell transformation and proliferation to generate a clone of mature plasma cells that secrete a specific type of antibody.

Maturational Morphology

Mature B Cell (After Blast Transformation)

The overall size is 8 to 20 μm. The nucleus may be round or oval and may be *eccentrically placed* (not in the middle of the cell). The chromatin may be arranged in a fine pattern. The cytoplasm is nongranular, is moderate in amount, and has a mottled blue color.

Plasmacytoid Lymphocytes

The overall size is 15 to 25 μm. The round or oval nucleus is eccentrically placed. The chromatin is coarse and irregularly spaced. Nucleoli may be visible. Usually, the cytoplasm is a distinctive dark blue with a lighter-staining area, the **hof,** next to the nucleus. The hof represents the area containing the Golgi apparatus.

Plasma Cell

The mature plasma cell (Plate 52) is not normally found in peripheral blood; however, 1% or 2% of plasma cell-like

lymphocytes may be encountered under stress conditions. The overall cell size is 14 to 20 μm. The nucleus is small and eccentrically located. More than one nucleus may be seen in a cell. The chromatin is condensed and has a cartwheel configuration.

Although the cytoplasm is dark blue, the hof area is usually visible. The cell has a well-developed, rough endoplasmic reticulum, which is characteristic of a cell producing proteins for export. The distinctive dark-blue cytoplasm is indicative of active synthesis and secretion of proteins (antibodies). The cytoplasm is oval in outline and abundant. Granules are absent, but vacuoles are common. Cytoplasmic inclusions can include Russell bodies, acidophilic refractile globules that represent gamma globulin (protein) secretions. Other forms of plasma cells, usually associated with abnormal conditions, are as follows:

1. **Grape** or **Mott cells,** in which the cytoplasm is completely filled with Russell bodies (Plate 53)
2. **Flame cells,** in which the cytoplasm stains a bright-red color and contains increased quantities of glycogen or intracellular deposits of amorphous matter

Plasma Cell Disorders

Although plasma cells are not normally found in the peripheral blood, an increase in these cells can be seen in a variety of nonmalignant disorders:

1. Viral disorders, for example, rubella, chickenpox, mumps, and infectious mononucleosis
2. Allergic conditions
3. Chronic infections
4. Collagen diseases

In plasma cell dyscrasias, the plasma cells may be greatly increased or may completely infiltrate the bone marrow, as in, for example, Waldenstrom's macroglobulinemia and multiple myeloma (discussed in Chapter 20).

SUMMARY

Anatomical Origin and Development of Lymphocytes

Lymphocytes and plasma cells represent the blood cells primarily concerned with antigen recognition and antibody production. Following embryonic and fetal development, the bone marrow becomes the sole provider of undifferentiated stem cells. Further development and proliferation of these cells continue in the primary tissues—the bone marrow and thymus—and the secondary tissues—the lymph nodes, spleen, and gut-associated lymphoid tissue. In the primary tissues, the lymphocytes differentiate into one of the major categories of lymphocytes: T cells or B cells.

Lymphocytes, mostly of the T type, move freely between the blood and lymphoid tissues. The process of recirculation is important in the dissemination of immunological information. At any one time, approximately 5% of the total body lymphocyte mass is present in the circulating blood. In newborn infants, lymphocytes, mostly T cells, represent

90% of the total peripheral leukocytes, whereas the adult has an average of 35% lymphocytes in the circulating blood, with a distribution of 60% to 80% T cells and 20% B cells.

Morphological Characteristics of Normal Lymphocytes

The stages of lymphocyte development are the lymphoblast, the prolymphocyte, and the mature lymphocyte. Mature lymphocytes can be classified as either large or small types. When lymphocytes are stained with Wright stain, their maturational characteristics are generally consistent with those seen in other leukocytes. However, in the lymphocyte, the N:C ratio does not decrease, nor does the cell develop specific granulation.

Lymphocytes can assume variant morphological features. Variant lymphocytes may be referred to as atypical, reactive, or Downey cells. As many as 5% to 6% of variant lymphocytes can be found in normal persons; however, an increase in these forms is associated with a variety of disorders. Some of the disorders that can produce an increase in variant lymphocytes are infectious mononucleosis, viral hepatitis, and viral pneumonia. The features of variant lymphocytes can include an increased amount of cytoplasm, cytoplasmic vacuolation, and a dark-blue cytoplasm. Nucleoli may be seen in the nucleus of some variant types.

Some morphologically abnormal lymphocytes or lymphocyte-like cells are associated with specific disorders. These abnormalities are binucleated lymphocytes, Rieder cells, vacuolated lymphocytes, and smudge cells.

The Functions and Membrane

Characteristics of Lymphocytes

The categories of lymphocytes that are recognized as functionally active are T cells, B cells, and NK and K-type cells. T lymphocytes are responsible for cellular immune responses and in either helping or suppressing the activation of B lymphocytes. B lymphocytes serve as the primary source of cells responsible for humoral immune (antibody) responses. NK and K-type lymphocytes lack the mature surface markers of T and B cells. These two types of cells destroy target cells through the nonphagocytic process referred to as a cytotoxic reaction.

All cells of the immune system have specialized receptors on their membrane surfaces. In the past, surface membranes could be studied only by use of the electron microscope or specialized agglutination tests. The introduction of monoclonal antibody tests allows for the identification of subpopulations of lymphocytes, such as the T-cell subsets of helper/inducer and suppressor/cytotoxic.

Functional testing may be used to evaluate the response of lymphocytes to mitogens.

Plasma Cell Development and Maturation

Plasma cells are not normally found in the circulating blood but can be seen in nonmalignant or malignant disorders. Plasma cells arise from stimulated B lymphocytes. Abnormal forms of the plasma cell include Russell body inclusions, grape cells, and flame cells.

A few plasma cells can be seen in the circulating blood in severe chronic infections or viral disorders. Increased numbers of plasma cells are associated with malignant conditions, such as **multiple myeloma.**

BIBLIOGRAPHY

Bauer, John D. *Clinical Laboratory Methods* (9th ed.). St. Louis: Mosby, 1982, pp. 163, 165, 166, 200, 201, 256, 257, 259.

Beck, J. Walter and John E. Davies. *Medical Parasitology* (2nd ed.). St. Louis: Mosby, 1976, pp. 58–61.

Fairbanks, Tod R. "Current Status of Lymphocyte Subpopulation Testing in Humans." *Am. J. Med. Technol.,* Vol. 46, No. 6, 1980, pp. 471–474.

Heberman, Ronald B. "Natural Killer Cells." *Annu Rev. Med.,* 1986, Vol. 37, pp. 347–352.

Henry, John B. *Clinical Diagnosis and Management* (17th ed.). Philadelphia: Saunders, 1984, pp. 824, 825, 827, 1049, 1286, 1290, 1291.

Hoffman, R. A. "Clinical Utility of Cell Surface Antigen Detection." *Am. Clin. Products Rev.,* April, 1985, pp. 16–31.

Kapff, Carola T. and James H. Jandl. *Blood: Atlas and Sourcebook of Hematology* (2nd ed.). Boston: Little, Brown & Co., 1991.

Keller, Robert H. et al. "Monoclonal Antibodies: Clinical Utility and the Misunderstood Epitope." *Lab. Med.,* Vol. 15, No. 12, December, 1984, pp. 795–802.

Leukocyte Differential Counting. Tentative Standard H2D-T Villanova, PA: National Committee for Clinical Laboratory Standards (NCCLS), 1982.

Monoclonal Antibodies. St. Louis: Sigma Diagnostics, 1985.

MMWR, Vol. 35, No. 20, May 23, 1986.

O'Connor, Barbara H. *A Color Atlas and Instruction Manual of Peripheral Blood Cell Morphology.* Baltimore: Williams & Wilkins, 1984, pp. 86–88.

Raphael, Stanley S. *Lynch's Medical Laboratory Technology* (4th ed.). Philadelphia: Saunders, 1983, pp. 478, 544, 655, 657, 658, 691.

Robinson, Stephen H. and Paul R. Reich. *Hematology: Physiopathologic Basis for Clinical Practice* (3rd ed.). Boston: Little, Brown & Co., 1993.

Roitt, Ivan. *Essential Immunology* (5th ed.). Oxford, England: Blackwell Scientific, 1984, pp. 76–85.

Wheater, Paul R. et al. *Functional Histology.* London: Churchill-Livingstone, 1979, pp. 31, 145–159.

Wolde-Mariam, Wondu and James B. Peter. "Recent Diagnostic Advances in Cellular Immunology." *Diagn. Med.,* Vol. 7, No. 3, March, 1984, pp. 25–30, 33, 34.

REVIEW QUESTIONS

Questions 1 through 6: match the following anatomical structures with the appropriate anatomical category.

1. ___ Lymph nodes.
2. ___ Liver.
3. ___ Spleen.
4. ___ Red bone marrow.
5. ___ Thymus.
6. ___ Peyer's patches of the intestine.

A. Primary lymphoid tissue.
B. Secondary lymphoid tissue.
C. Not a lymphoid tissue.

7. T cells are found in the:
   A. Perifollicular areas of the lymph nodes.
   B. Paracortical regions of the lymph nodes.
   C. Periarteriolar regions of the spleen.
   D. All of the above.

8. A major site of B lymphocyte localization and proliferation is:
   A. Lymphoid follicles.
   B. Deep cortical zone.
   C. Paracortex.
   D. All of the above.

9. The process of lymphocyte recirculation is important in:
   A. Antibody production.
   B. Lymphocyte proliferation.
   C. Dissemination of immunological information.
   D. Commitment of lymphocytes to T and B cells.
   E. Extending the life span of the lymphocytes.

10. T lymphocytes constitute ___% of the blood lymphocyte pool in adults.
    A. 0 to 20.
    B. 20 to 40.
    C. 40 to 60.
    D. 60 to 80.

11. Lymphocytes represent approximately ___% of the total circulating leukocytes in adults.
    A. 15.
    B. 35.
    C. 55.
    D. 75.

12. The percentage of lymphocytes as compared with the other types of leukocytes in the peripheral blood ___ as humans age.
    A. Increases.
    B. Decreases.
    C. Remains the same.

13. If a patient has a total leukocyte count of 20×10^9/L and a 50% lymphocyte count on the differential count, the **absolute** lymphocyte value is ___ $\times 10^9$/L.
    A. 1.
    B. 5.
    C. 10.
    D. 15.

Questions 14 through 18: complete the following statements with answers A, B, or C.

A. Increases.
B. Decreases.
C. Remains about the same.

14. As a lymphocyte matures, the nuclear-cytoplasmic ratio ___.
15. As a lymphocyte matures, the overall size ___.
16. As a lymphocyte matures, the number of nucleoli ___.
17. As a lymphocyte matures, the chromatin clumping ___.
18. As a lymphocyte matures, the quantity of cytoplasm ___.

19. The most characteristic morphological features of variant lymphocytes include:
    A. Increased overall size, possibly one to three nucleoli, and abundant cytoplasm.
    B. Increased overall size, round nucleus, and increased granulation in the cytoplasm.
    C. Segmented nucleus, light-blue cytoplasm, and no nucleoli.
    D. Enlarged nucleus, six to eight nucleoli, and dark-blue cytoplasm.

Questions 20 through 23: match the following using an answer only once.

20. ___ Rieder cells.
21. ___ Vacuolated lymphocytes.
22. ___ Crystalline inclusions.
23. ___ Smudge cells.

A. Niemann-Pick disease.
B. Chronic lymphocytic leukemia.
C. Leukosarcoma.
D. Natural artifact.

24. T cells are:
    A. Lymphocytes.
    B. Monocytes.
    C. Helper or suppressor types.
    D. Both A and C.

25. B cells are:
    A. Lymphocytes.
    B. Associated with antigen recognition.
    C. Found in the thymus and bone marrow.
    D. All of the above.

26. NK cells are classified as:
    A. Macrophages.
    B. Monocytes.
    C. Effector lymphocytes.
    D. K-type lymphocytes.

Questions 27 and 28: identification of membrane characteristics.

27. Which of the following statements are true of T cells?
    A. Responsible for humoral responses.
    B. Responsible for cellular immune responses.
    C. Responsible for chronic rejection in organ transplantation.
    D. Both B and C.

28. Which of the following statements is (are) true of B cells?
    A. Responsible for antibody responses.
    B. Protect against intracellular pathogens.
    C. Responsible for chronic rejection in transplantation.
    D. Both A and B.

29. An abnormal plasma cell with red-staining cytoplasm is a:
    A. Russell body.
    B. Mott cell.
    C. Grape cell.
    D. Flame cell.

17

Leukocytes: Nonmalignant Lymphocytic Disorders

Lymphocytosis
**Disorders associated with
  lymphocytosis**
Infectious mononucleosis
Cytomegalovirus infection
Toxoplasmosis
Infectious lymphocytosis

Bordetella pertussis
  (*Haemophilus pertussis*)
  infection
Lymphocytopenia
**Immune disorders
  associated with
  lymphocytopenia**

Acquired immunodeficiency
  syndrome
Systemic lupus erythematosus
Summary
Case studies
Bibliography
Review questions

OBJECTIVES

Lymphocytosis
- Define the term **lymphocytosis.**
- Name at least three disorders associated with lymphocytosis.

Disorders associated with lymphocytosis
- Describe the etiology, epidemiology, clinical signs and symptoms, and laboratory data for at least two disorders associated with lymphocytosis.

Lymphocytopenia
- Define the term **lymphocytopenia.**

- Name at least three disorders associated with lymphocytopenia.

Immune disorders associated with lymphocytopenia
- Describe the etiology, epidemiology, clinical signs and symptoms, and laboratory data for at least two disorders associated with lymphocytosis.

Case studies
- Apply the laboratory data to the stated case studies and discuss the implications of these cases to the study of hematology.

*T*he normal range for lymphocytes in an adult is 22% to 40%, with absolute values of 1.1 to 4.4 × 10⁹/L. The following is a sample calculation of the absolute lymphocyte count:

Absolute number = total leukocyte count × relative % of lymphocytes

Total leukocyte count = 25.0×10^9/L

Relative number of lymphocytes = 76%

Absolute number = 19.0×10^9/L

A value below the normal reference range is called **lymphocytopenia.** When the blood lymphocyte count increases above the upper limit of the reference range, the condition is referred to as **lymphocytosis.**

Disorders of lymphocytes (Table 17.1) are frequently encountered in the clinical laboratory. Many of these nonmalignant disorders result from viral or bacterial infections. Examples of viral diseases include infectious mononucleosis, cytomegalovirus (CMV) infection, and acquired immunodeficiency syndrome (AIDS). Bacterial diseases associated with lymphocytic disorders can include whooping cough. The parasitic infection toxoplasmosis, although rarer than viral and bacterial causes, can also display lymphocytic involvement. In addition, conditions such as drug-induced (immunological) hypersensitivity reactions elicit lymphocytic proliferative reactions that simulate or even surpass the lymphocytosis observed in infectious mononucleosis (Table 17.2).

LYMPHOCYTOSIS

Lymphocytosis is natural and normal in infants and children up to approximately 10 years old, with total lymphocyte counts as high as 9×10^9/L. This increase probably results from the limited production of adrenal corticosteroid hormones during this period of the life cycle. This limited production of hormones may underlie the lymphocytosis seen in later childhood in conditions such as malnutrition and scurvy.

Lymphocytosis is not a common nonspecific response to inflammation as is neutrophilia. In adolescence and adulthood, nonmalignant conditions associated with an absolute lymphocytosis include:

1. Acute viral infections (e.g., infectious mononucleosis, infectious hepatitis, posttransfusion syndrome, CMV infection, and infectious lymphocytosis)
2. Some bacterial infections (e.g., *Bordetella pertussis* infection [whooping cough] and brucellosis)
3. Parasitic infections (e.g., toxoplasmosis)

TABLE 17.1 Examples of Nonmalignant Disorders of Lymphocytes

Disorder	Etiology	Laboratory Data
Viral Disorders		
Infectious mononucleosis	Epstein-Barr virus	Lymphocytosis Variant lymphocytes Increased titer of heterophil antibodies
Infectious lymphocytosis	Coxsackie group	Lymphocytosis Negative for heterophil antibodies
CMV infection	Herpes group—CMV	Slight lymphocytosis Variant lymphocytes Negative for heterophil antibodies Positive for ANA, RA, and CMV nonspecific antibodies
Acquired immunodeficiency syndrome	HIV	Leukopenia Lymphocytopenia Abnormality of T cell subsets
Bacterial Disorders		
Whooping cough	*Bordetella pertussis*	Marked lymphocytosis Rare lymphoblasts All antibodies negative
Parasitic Disorders		
Toxoplasmosis	*Toxoplasma gondii*	Variant lymphocytes Negative for heterophil antibodies Positive for *Toxoplasma* antibodies
Autoimmune Disorders		
Systemic lupus erythematosus	Autoimmune	Positive LE cell preparation Positive for ANA antibodies Lymphocyte subset abnormalities

ANA = antinuclear antibodies; RA = rheumatoid factor antibodies; CMV = cytomegalovirus; HIV = human immunodeficiency virus.

TABLE 17.2 Causes of Lymphocytosis

Lymphocytosis Associated with Atypical Lymphocytes

percent of white cells that are atypical lymphocytes		uncommon causes	Lymphocytosis Associated with Small Mature Lymphocytes
>20	<20		
Infectious mononucleosis	Infections	Tertiary syphilis*	Infectious lymphocytosis
Infectious hepatitis	Mumps,* varicella,* rubeola, rubella, atypical pneumonia, herpes simplex, herpes zoster, roseola infantum, influenza,* other viral illnesses, tuberculosis,* rickettsialpox, brucellosis,* toxoplasmosis*	Congenital syphilis*	Pertussis
"Post-transfusion" syndrome		Smallpox	
Cytomegalovirus infection		Tetrachlorethane poisoning	
p-Aminosalicylic acid (PAS) hypersensitivity	Radiation	TNT poisoning	
Phenytoin (Dilantin) and mephenytoin (Mesantoin) hypersensitivity	Other	Organic arsenical hypersensitivity	
	Letterer-Siwe disease	Severe dermatitis herpetiformis	
	Agranulocytosis		
	Lead intoxication		
	Stress		
	Leukemia and lymphoma*		

*Higher counts of atypical lymphocytes are occasionally found.

Source: Modified from T. A. Wood and E. P. Frenkel. "The Atypical Lymphocyte." *Am. J. Med.,* Vol. 42, 1967, p. 923.

4. Drug reactions (e.g., *p*-aminosalicylic acid hypersensitivity and phenytoin hypersensitivity)
5. Uncommon causes (e.g., tertiary and congenital syphilis and smallpox)

Malignant conditions that produce lymphocytosis (discussed in Chapter 20) include:

1. Lymphocytic leukemia (acute and chronic forms)
2. The leukemic phase of lymphomas
3. Waldenstrom's macroglobulinemia
4. Cancer

DISORDERS ASSOCIATED WITH LYMPHOCYTOSIS

Infectious Mononucleosis

Infectious mononucleosis is usually an acute, benign, and self-limiting lymphoproliferative condition caused by Epstein-Barr virus (EBV). EBV is also the cause of Burkitt's lymphoma, a malignant tumor of the lymphoid tissue occurring mainly in African children; nasopharyngeal carcinoma; and neoplasms of the thymus, parotid gland, and supraglottic larynx.

Etiology

EBV was first discovered in 1964 as the cause of infectious mononucleosis. EBV is widely disseminated. It is estimated that 95% of the world's population is exposed to the virus, making it the most ubiquitous virus known.

EBV is a human herpes DNA virus. In infectious mononucleosis, the virus infects B lymphocytes but the variant lymphocytes produced in response to the virus and seen in microscopic examination of the peripheral blood have T cell characteristics. One of the habitats of the persisting viral genome in hosts with a latent infection is the B lymphocyte of the lymphoreticular system and the epithelial cell of the oropharynx.

Epidemiology

Although EBV appears to be transmitted primarily by close contact with infectious oro-pharyngeal secretions, the virus has been reported to be transmitted by blood transfusion and transplacental routes. Under ordinary conditions, transmission of EBV through transfusion or transplacental exposure is unlikely.

The frequency of **seronegativity** is nearly 100% in early infancy and declines with increasing age, more or less rapidly depending on socioeconomic conditions, to less than 10% in young adults. After primary exposure, a person is considered to be immune and generally no longer susceptible to overt reinfection. In western society, primary exposure to EBV occurs in two waves. Approximately half of the population is exposed to the virus before the age of 5 years; a second wave of seroconversion occurs during late adolescence (15 to 24 years old). Approximately 90% of adult patients demonstrate antibodies to the virus.

Individuals at risk include those who lack antibodies to the virus. EBV is only a minor problem for immunocompetent persons but it can become a major problem for immunologically compromised patients. In immunosuppressed patients the incidence of EBV infection ranges from 35% to 47%. Blood transfusion from an immune donor to a nonimmune recipient may produce a primary infection in the recipient known as infectious mononucleosis postperfusion syndrome. Infectious mononucleosis or infectious mononucleosis-like illness following blood transfusion may often be due to a concomitant CMV infection rather than the EBV.

A low percentage of patients experience symptomatic reactivation. Reactivation of latent infection has been implicated in a persistent illness referred to as the EBV-associated fatigue syndrome, but this phenomenon is not universally accepted.

In adolescents, clinically apparent infectious mononucleosis has an estimated frequency of 45/100,000. In immunosuppressed patients the incidence of EBV infection ranges from 35 to 47%. As occurs with other herpesviruses, there is a carrier state after primary infection.

Clinical Signs and Symptoms

The majority of individuals seroconvert without any signs and symptoms of disease. In children under 5 years old, infection is either asymptomatic or frequently characterized by mild, poorly defined signs and symptoms. Although anyone can suffer from this viral disorder, it is typically manifested in young adults.

The incubation period of infectious mononucleosis is from 10 to 50 days and once the disease is fully developed, it lasts for 1 to 4 weeks. Clinical manifestations include extreme fatigue, malaise, sore throat, fever, and cervical lymphadenopathy. Splenomegaly occurs in about 50% of patients, although the incidence of splenic rupture is low. When rupture occurs, however, mortality is significant. Jaundice is infrequent, although the most common complication is hepatitis. A smaller percentage of patients develop hepatomegaly or splenomegaly and hepatomegaly. Because abnormal liver function is more marked in EBV-induced infectious mononucleosis than in CMV-associated mononucleosis, EBV must be considered in the differential diagnosis of hepatitis. A significant number of patients with infectious mononucleosis do not manifest the classic signs and symptoms.

Laboratory Data

Laboratory testing is necessary to establish or confirm a diagnosis of infectious mononucleosis. Hematological studies reveal leukocyte counts ranging from 10 to 20 × 10⁹/L in about two thirds of patients; about 10% of the patients with this disorder demonstrate **leukopenia.** A differential leukocyte count may initially disclose neutrophilia, although mononuclear cells usually predominate as the disorder develops. Typical relative lymphocyte counts range from 60% to 90%, with 5% to 30% variant lymphocytes. These variant lymphocytes (Table 17.3) exhibit diverse morphological features and persist for 1 to 2 months in some patients and as long as 4 to 6 months in others.

If the classic signs and symptoms of infectious mononucleosis are absent, a diagnosis of infectious mononucleosis is more difficult to make. The diagnosis may be established by antibody testing. The antibodies present in patients with infectious mononucleosis are heterophil and EBV antibodies. Heterophil antibodies comprise a broad class of antibody. They are defined as antibodies that are stimulated by one antigen and react with an entirely unrelated surface antigen present on cells from different mammalian species. Heterophil antibodies may be present in normal individuals in low concentrations (titers), but a titer of 1:56 or greater is clinically significant in patients suspected to have infectious mononucleosis. Rapid slide tests (see Chapter 24) that use the princi-

TABLE 17.3 Descriptive Features of the Classic Downey Classification of Lymphocytes Seen in Infectious Mononucleosis	
Type I	
Nucleus	May be irregularly shaped
Cytoplasm	Usually many cytoplasmic vacuoles
	Dark blue (basophilic)
Type II	
Nucleus	Chromatin is coarse and clumped
Cytoplasm	Increased amount
	Dark blue (basophilic) around the periphery or in a radial pattern
	A few cytoplasmic vacuoles
*Type III**	
Nucleus	Nucleoli usually visible
	Enlarged in size
Cytoplasm	Dark blue (basophilic)

*This cell resembles an immature lymphocyte.

ple of agglutination of horse erythrocytes are available. The use of horse erythrocytes appears to increase the sensitivity of the test.

Within the adult population, 10% to 20% of individuals with acute infectious mononucleosis do not produce the associated heterophil antibody. The pediatric population is of particular concern because more than 50% of children under 4 years old with infectious mononucleosis are heterophil-negative.

For patients with diagnostically inconclusive infectious mononucleosis, a more definitive assessment of immune status may be obtained through an EBV serological panel. Candidates for EBV serology include those who do not exhibit the classic symptoms, those who are heterophil-negative, and those who are immunosuppressed.

EBV-infected B lymphocytes express a variety of "new" antigens encoded by the virus. Infection with EBV results in the expression of viral capsid antigen (VCA), early antigen (EA), and nuclear antigen (NA), with corresponding antibody responses. Assays for immunoglobulin M (IgM) and G (IgG) antibodies to these EBV antigens are available. EBV-specific serological studies (Table 17.4) are beneficial in defining immune status, and the time of antibody appearance may be indicative of the stage of disease (Fig. 17.1). This can provide important information for both the diagnosis and the management of EBV-associated disease.

Anti-i can be a clinically significant antibody in infectious mononucleosis. This antibody can be the cause of hemolytic anemia.

Cytomegalovirus Infection

Etiology

The first descriptive report of histological changes characteristic of the changes now associated with CMV infection was originally published in 1904. In 1956 and 1957, CMV was isolated in the laboratory. In 1966, actual isolation of the virus following a blood transfusion was noted.

Human CMV is classified as a member of the herpes family of viruses. There are presently five recognized human

TABLE 17.4 Characteristic Antibody Formation in Infectious Mononucleosis

	VCA IgM	VCA IgG	EA-D	EA-R	EBNA IgG	Heterophil
No previous exposure	−	−	−	−	−	−
Recent (acute) infection	+	+	+/−	−	−	+
Past infection (convalescent) period	−	+	−	−	+	−
Reactivation of latent infection	+/−	+	+/−	+/−	+	+/−

VCA = viral capsid antigen; EA-D = early antigen (diffuse); EA-R = early antigen (restricted); EBNA = Epstein-Barr nuclear antigen.

herpesviruses: herpes simplex I, herpes simplex II, varicella-zoster virus, EBV, and CMV. All of the herpesviruses are relatively large, enveloped DNA viruses that undergo a replicative cycle involving DNA expression and nucleocapsid assembly within the nucleus. The viral structure gains an envelope when the virus buds through the nuclear membrane that is altered to contain specific viral proteins.

Although the herpes family produces diverse clinical diseases, the viruses share the basic characteristic of being cell-associated. The requirements for cell association vary, but all five viruses may spread from cell to cell presumably via intercellular bridges, and in the presence of antibody in the extracellular phase. This common characteristic may play a role in the ability of the virus to produce subclinical infections that can be reactivated under appropriate stimuli.

Epidemiology

CMV is a ubiquitous human viral pathogen and is endemic worldwide. Dissemination of the virus can occur by oral, respiratory, and venereal routes. It can also be transmitted parenterally by organ transplantation or via the transfusion of fresh blood. Transmission of CMV appears to require close intimate contact with secretions or excretions (primarily urine, respiratory secretions, tears, feces, and genital secretions) of infected persons. The most likely mode of acquisition is via a venereal route through contact with infectious virus in body secretions.

The virus can be present in blood, urine, and breast milk. For more than 15 years, it has been recognized that transfusion of blood from healthy asymptomatic blood donors is occasionally followed by active CMV infection in the recipient. There is strong evidence to incriminate peripheral blood leukocytes and transplanted tissues as sources of CMV.

Although fatal infections have been reported in children with leukemia and premature infants with a birth weight of less than 1200 gm, the incidence of primary infections during childhood is low. The rate of exposure to the virus, however, may be accelerated during the first years of life in toddlers and children in day care centers. During adolescence the infection rate rises significantly. By adulthood, most individuals have experienced asymptomatic contact with CMV. Because CMV can persist latently, active infections may develop under a variety of conditions such as pregnancy and immunosuppression, and subsequent to organ or bone marrow transplantation. Active CMV infection is a major cause of morbidity and often mortality in patients with AIDS.

CMV can exist as a latent infection and is characterized by periods of reactivation. In addition, CMV is one of the most important causes of congenital viral infections in the United States. Primary as well as recurrent maternal CMV infection can be transmitted in utero.

Health care professionals are one of the groups becoming increasingly concerned about the risks associated with exposure to CMV. Nosocomial transmission from patients to

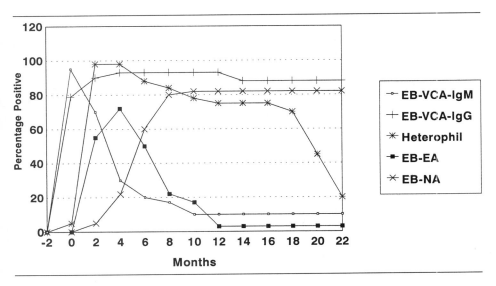

FIGURE 17.1 Percent of persons with positive antibody responses at specified time intervals. EBV = Epstein-Barr virus; VCA = virus capsid antigen (Ortho Diagnostic Systems, Raritan, NJ); EA = early antigen; NA = nuclear antigen. (Modified from Davey and Kurec, "Infectious Mononucleosis." *ASCP Hematology Check Sample*, Vol. 30, 1988.)

health care workers has not been documented, but observance of good personal hygiene and handwashing offer the best measures for preventing transmission.

Clinical Signs and Symptoms

Acquired CMV infection is usually asymptomatic and can persist in the host as a chronic or latent infection. In the majority of patients, CMV infection is asymptomatic. Occasionally, a self-limited, heterophil-negative, mononucleosis-like syndrome results. The symptoms include a sore throat and fever, chills, profound malaise, and myalgia. Lymphadenopathy and splenomegaly may be observed. Infections occurring in healthy immunocompetent individuals usually result in seroconversion. Virus may be excreted in the urine during both primary and recurrent CMV infection; it can persist sporadically for months or years.

Persons experiencing acquired infection, reinfection with the same or different strains of CMV, or reactivation of a latent infection can excrete the virus in titers as high as 10^6 infective units/mL in the urine and/or saliva for weeks or months.

Normal adults and children usually experience CMV infection without serious complications. Infrequent complications of CMV infection in previously healthy individuals, however, include interstitial pneumonitis, hepatitis, Guillain-Barré syndrome, meningoencephalitis, myocarditis, thrombocytopenia, and hemolytic anemia.

CMV infection, however, can be life-threatening in immunosuppressed patients. Infections in these patients may result in disseminated multisystem involvement including pneumonitis, hepatitis, gastrointestinal ulceration, arthralgias, meningoencephalitis, and retinitis. Interstitial pneumonitis, frequently associated with CMV infection, is a major cause of death following allogeneic bone marrow transplantation. In premature infants, acquired CMV infection can result in atypical lymphocytosis, hepatosplenomegaly, pneumonia, or death.

Transfusion-acquired CMV infections may cause not only mononucleosis-like syndrome but also hepatitis and an increased risk of rejection of transplanted organs.

The classic congenital CMV syndrome is manifested by a high incidence of neurological symptoms as well as neuromuscular disorders, jaundice, hepatomegaly, and splenomegaly. Congenitally infected newborns, especially those who acquire CMV during a maternal primary infection, are more prone to develop severe cytomegalic inclusion disease (CID).

Laboratory Data

In patients with CMV infection, hematological examination of the blood usually reveals a characteristic leukocytosis. A slight lymphocytosis with over 20% variant lymphocytes is common. Clinical chemistry assays may demonstrate abnormal liver function. Another assessment of the presence of infection is the demonstration of inclusion bodies in leukocytes in urinary sediment.

The incidence of viral exposure and subsequent antibody formation (seropositivity) varies greatly, depending on the socioeconomic status and living conditions of the population surveyed. The prevalence of CMV antibody varies with age and geographical location but ranges from 40% to 100%.

A definitive diagnosis, however, can only be made by isolating the virus from urine or blood samples or the demonstration of CMV-specific IgM or increasing CMV-specific IgG antibody titers. Serological methods to detect the presence of IgM antibodies can aid in the diagnosis of primary infection. Detection of CMV-specific IgM can represent primary infection or rare reactivation of infection. False-positive results, however, can occur because of the presence of other antibodies such as rheumatoid factor. Although results of tests for heterophil, EBV, and *Toxoplasma* antibodies are generally negative, elevated concentrations (titers) of several antibodies may occur. These include antinuclear antibody (ANA), rheumatoid factor antibody (RA), and nonspecific cold agglutinins.

Toxoplasmosis

Etiology

The microorganism *Toxoplasma gondii* causes toxoplasmosis. Toxoplasma was recently recognized as a tissue Coccidia.

Epidemiology

Toxoplasmosis is a widespread disease that occurs in humans and animals. *T. gondii* was first discovered in a North African rodent and has been observed in numerous birds and mammals around the world, including humans. It is a parasite of cosmopolitan distribution that is able to develop in a wide variety of vertebrate hosts. Human infections are common in many parts of the world. The incidence rates vary from place to place, for unknown reasons. The highest recorded rate (93%) occurs in Parisian women who prefer undercooked or raw meat, and there is a 50% rate of occurrence in their children.

The definitive host is the house cat and certain other *Felidae*. Domestic cats as a source of the disease produce oocysts that are present in their feces. Accidental ingestion of oocysts by humans and animals, including the cat, produces a proliferative infection in the body tissues. Feces-contaminated food, water, and hands, inadequately cooked infected meat, and raw milk can be important sources of human infection.

The hazard of transfusion-transmitted toxoplasmosis has been recently recognized in connection with the transfusion of leukocyte concentrates. Patients at risk are those who are receiving immunosuppressive agents or corticosteroids.

All mammals, including humans, can transmit the infection transplacentally. Transplacental transmission usually takes place in the course of an acute but inapparent or undiagnosed maternal infection. New evidence indicates that the number of infants born in the United States each year with congenital *T. gondii* infection is considerably higher than the 3000 previously estimated. It is estimated that 6 of every 1000 pregnant women in the United States will acquire primary infection with *Toxoplasma* during a 9-month gestation. Approximately 45% of the women who acquire the infection for the first time and who are not treated will give birth to congenitally infected infants. Consequently, the expected incidence of congenital toxoplasmosis is 2.7/1000 live births.

Clinical Signs and Symptoms

In adults and children other than newborn babies, the disease is usually asymptomatic. A generalized infection probably occurs. Although spontaneous recovery follows acute febrile disease, the organism can localize and multiply in any organ of the body or the circulatory system.

In acquired infection, symptoms are frequently mild if they are observable at all. The disease may resemble infectious mononucleosis, with chills, fever, headache, lymphadenopathy, and extreme fatigue. A chronic form of toxoplasmic lymphadenopathy has been described. *T. gondii* presents a special problem in immunosuppressed or otherwise compromised hosts, who can develop reactivation of a latent toxoplasmosis. This has been observed in patients with either Hodgkin's or non-Hodgkin's lymphomas as well as in recipients of organ transplants. Reactivation of cerebral toxoplasmosis is not uncommon in patients with AIDS. Primary infection may be promoted by immunosuppression.

Congenital toxoplasmosis infection can result in central nervous system malformation or prenatal mortality. Many infants who are serologically positive at birth fail to display neurological, ophthalmic, or generalized illness at birth. In as many as 75% of the congenitally infected newborns who are not serologically diagnosed at birth, the disease remains dormant, only to be discovered when other symptoms such as chorioretinitis, unilateral blindness, and severe neurological sequelae become apparent.

Laboratory Data

Both clinical and laboratory findings in this disease resemble infectious mononucleosis. An increased number of variant lymphocytes can be seen on a peripheral blood smear. The diagnosis is established by serologically demonstrating marked elevations of *Toxoplasma* antibodies. Antibodies are demonstrable within the first 2 weeks after infection, rise to high levels early in the infection, and fall slightly but persist at an elevated level for many months before declining to low levels after many years.

Because *T. gondii* is difficult to culture, diagnosis must be supported by serological methods. Diagnosis can be established by biopsy, necropsy, or intraperitoneal inoculation into mice.

Infectious Lymphocytosis

Acute infectious lymphocytosis is a poorly defined benign condition.

Etiology

Infectious lymphocytosis is caused by a virus, probably a member of the Coxsackie group.

Epidemiology

Infectious lymphocytosis is usually a mild disorder occurring in epidemics. Children are the most common victims.

A chronic form of infectious lymphocytosis has also been observed in children.

Clinical Signs and Symptoms

An incubation period of 10 to 21 days is typical. Symptoms can include vomiting, fever, abdominal discomfort, central nervous system involvement, rashes, upper respiratory distress, and diarrhea. Some patients may be asymptomatic or have symptoms that mimic infectious mononucleosis. The spleen and liver are rarely enlarged. Lymphadenopathy is also rare or minimal, if present.

Children with the chronic form of infectious lymphocytosis usually have a history of recurrent upper respiratory tract infections. In addition, enlargement of the tonsils, lymph nodes, and spleen is usually manifested.

Laboratory Data

Leukocytosis with lymphocytosis characterizes this disease. It may precede clinical manifestations of the disease with leukocyte counts of 20 to 50×10^9/L. Differential peripheral blood counts reveal up to 95% small, mature, normal-appearing lymphoctyes. These lymphocytes are probably of T cell origin. No lymphoblasts are present. An increase in eosinophils may be noted. Results of heterophil and EBV antibody tests are negative.

The illness and leukocytosis usually subside within 3 to 5 weeks. A moderate lymphocytosis, however, may persist for as long as 3 months.

In children with the chronic form of infectious lymphocytosis, the leukocyte count ranges from 10 to 25×10^9/L, with a predominance of normal-appearing lymphocytes. Other leukocytic alterations are minimal.

Bordetella Pertussis (*Haemophilus Pertussis*) Infection

Etiology

Whooping cough is caused by *B. pertussis*, a bacterial organism that produces inflammation of the entire respiratory tract.

Epidemiology

This illness occurs primarily in unimmunized children.

Clinical Signs and Symptoms

Following an incubation period of 2 weeks, symptoms become evident. Characteristically, symptoms include a cough and cold accompanied by pain in the neck and chest. A sputum-producing cough with pain over the trachea and bronchi characteristically emerges.

Laboratory Data

The total leukocyte count can be increased to as high as 100×10^9/L, with an absolute lymphocyte value of as high as 50×10^9/L. The absolute lymphocyte value is usually 15 to 40×10^9/L. These leukocyte and lymphocyte values are major laboratory findings and may be present if the characteristic cough has not yet developed or is mild enough to be missed during physical examination.

Lymphocytosis is most evident during the first 3 weeks of illness and then decreases. Lymphocytosis is caused by the release of lymphocytosis-promoting factor (LPF) from *B. pertussis*. This factor causes an increased mobilization of lymphocytes from lymphoid organs, followed by inhibition of recirculation of lymphocytes from blood into the lymph flow.

On a peripheral blood smear, the lymphocytes are small and mature, with only a rare occurrence of lymphoblasts. A definitive diagnosis can be made on isolation of the bacteria.

LYMPHOCYTOPENIA

Lymphocytopenia is generally defined as less than $3.0 \times 10^9/L$ lymphocytes in adults or less than $1.5 \times 10^9/L$ lymphocytes in children. A decrease in lymphocytes is a common response to stress and to the administration of corticosteroids, or it may be seen in normal persons with no apparent cause. Transient relative lymphocytopenia is generally associated with conditions resulting in granulocytosis. Pathological conditions that exhibit absolute lymphocytopenia are related to decreased production, mechanical loss, increased destruction, and various functional abnormalities. These conditions may be due to immune deficiency disorders, physical agents (e.g., radiation exposure), or cytotoxic drugs.

IMMUNE DISORDERS ASSOCIATED WITH LYMPHOCYTOPENIA

Immune disorders may be caused by defects in the numbers or functional properties of lymphocytes and may be congenital or acquired. These conditions are usually classified as either T cell or B cell disorders. Some of the less common disorders involve both T and B cells.

A number of T and B cell defects involve the alteration of some lymphocyte subpopulations. Patients with **DiGeorge's syndrome** exhibit a decrease in total T lymphocytes coupled with an increased ratio of helper to suppressor cells. In AIDS, a reversed phenotypic helper-to-suppressor ratio due to a decrease in helper cells is observed. A decrease in total T cells and a lack of, or reduced, suppressor cell population are among the immunological changes observed in active systemic lupus erythematosus (SLE).

Acquired Immunodeficiency Syndrome

The human T lymphotropic virus type III (HTLV-III) is also referred to as lymphadenopathy-associated virus (LAV) and most recently the human immunodeficiency virus (HIV). HIV type 1 (HIV-1) is the predominant virus responsible for AIDS. Although HIV was recently recognized, it is tentatively concluded that HIV-1 has infected humans for more than 20 but less than 100 years.

Etiology

At the beginning of the 1980s, no infectious retroviruses had been found in humans and many believed that no human retroviruses would be found. In spite of this skepticism,

however, the first human retrovirus, human T lymphotropic virus type I (HTLV-I), was isolated in 1980 and HTLV-II was isolated in 1982.

In 1983, researchers at the Pasteur Institute in Paris isolated a retrovirus from a homosexual man with lymphadenopathy. The virus was named the lymphadenopathy-associated virus, but the researchers were unable to prove that this agent caused AIDS. The American research team headed by Dr. Robert Gallo also isolated the same class of virus, which they labeled HTLV-III. In 1984, the Gallo team was able to demonstrate conclusively through virological and epidemiological evidence that it was the cause of AIDS. When it was demonstrated that LAV and HTLV-III were the same virus, an international commission changed the name of the virus to HIV, to eliminate confusion caused by two names for the same entity and to acknowledge that the virus does cause AIDS.

In addition to the original HIV-1, a second AIDS-causing virus, HIV type 2 (HIV-2), was identified in 1985. In evolutionary terms, the two viruses are related and have a similar overall structure. The pathogenic potential of HIV-2, however, is not as well established as that of HIV-1.

HIV has a marked preference for the helper/inducer subset of T lymphocytes. These cells, however, are not the only cells that have CD4 antigen embedded in their membrane. Macrophages; as many as 40% of the peripheral blood monocytes; and cells in the lymph nodes, skin, and other organs also express measurable amounts of CD4 and can be infected by HIV. In addition, about 5% of the B lymphocytes may express CD4 and be susceptible to HIV infection.

Although some cells do not produce detectable amounts of CD4, they do contain low levels of messenger RNA encoding the CD4 protein, which indicates that they do produce some CD4. These cell types include certain cells of the brain, **glial cells,** a variety of malignant brain tumor cells, and some cells derived from cancers of the bowel. In addition, cells of the gastrointestinal system do not produce appreciable amounts of CD4, but gut cells, called **chromaffin cells,** do sometimes appear to be infected by HIV in vivo. This suggests that gastrointestinal infection may be what leads to the AIDS-associated weight loss and emaciation known in Africa as slim disease.

Epidemiology

AIDS has become a major cause of morbidity and mortality in the United States. Through December 1997, 641,086 persons with AIDS have been reported to the Centers for Disease Control and Prevention (CDC). From 1995 to 1996, for the first time in the epidemic, the occurrence of AIDS-defined opportunistic infections among infected persons and deaths among persons reported with AIDS decreased 7% and 25% respectively. These declines are largely due to the increasing use of combination retroviral therapy including protease inhibitors. Perinatally acquired AIDS has also declined in incidence. The majority of all adults with AIDS continues to be gay men who have sex with men (47%) and intravenous drug abusers (21%). Heterosexual contact accounted for 57,360 (9%) of cases. A significant proportion are black or Hispanic. Other identifiable groups that have demonstrated the signs and symptoms of AIDS include sex partners of intravenous drug users and children below the age of 13 (pediatric AIDS), primarily infants and toddlers and recipients of unscreened blood or blood products (e.g., hemophiliacs). Of these cases of pediatric AIDS, most occur in children under 3 years old and the majority of these children are born to parents practicing high-risk behaviors or with AIDS.

In addition, a small number of health care workers who had accidentally punctured their skin with HIV-contaminated needles have developed HIV infection. At the present time, the interval between the time of diagnosis of AIDS to death varies greatly; in developed countries, 50% of untreated patients die within 18 months of diagnosis and 80% die within 36 months.

Three infection patterns of HIV have been traced worldwide. Pattern I is found in North and South America, western Europe, Scandinavia, Australia, and New Zealand. In these countries, it is primarily a disease of gay men and intravenous drug abusers. The male-female ratio of reported AIDS cases in pattern I areas ranges from 10:1 to 15:1. Pattern II is found in Africa, the Caribbean, and some areas of South America. In the pattern II areas, AIDS is primarily a heterosexual disease and the number of infected females and males is approximately equal. Pattern III is typically demonstrated in eastern Europe, North Africa, the Middle East, Asia, and the Pacific, excluding Australia and New Zealand. In the pattern III areas, relatively few cases of AIDS have been identified and most of them have had contact with people from pattern I or pattern II countries.

Clinical Signs and Symptoms

Early Stages

The early phase of the natural history of HIV-1 infection may last from many months to many years after the initiation of infection. Typically, patients in the early stages of HIV-1 infection either are completely asymptomatic or show mild, chronic lymphadenopathy.

An unknown number of infected patients experience a brief, infectious mononucleosis-like or flu-like illness with fever, malaise, and possibly a skin rash. Neurological complaints may also be reported. These symptoms parallel the first wave of HIV replications and develop at about the time antibodies produced by the body against HIV-1 can first be detected. This is usually between 2 weeks and 3 months after acquiring the infection, rarely later.

Following the early phase of HIV infection and any clinically manifested signs and symptoms, a person may remain symptom-free for years.

Late Phase

Untreated HIV causes a predictable, progressive derangement of immune function, and AIDS is just one late manifestation of that process. From 2 to 10 years after acquiring HIV-1 infection, replication of the virus flares again and the infection enters its final stage. An average of 8 or 9 years may pass before AIDS is fully developed. The virus behaves differently, depending on the kind of host cell and the cell's own level of mitotic activity. In T cells, however, the virus can lie dormant indefinitely but it can destroy the host cell in a burst of replication. HIV grows continuously but slowly

in macrophages/monocytes. This saves the cell from destruction but probably alters its function.

Clinical symptoms of the later phase of HIV-1 infection include extreme weight loss, fever, and multiple secondary infections. The end stage of AIDS is characterized by the occurrence of neoplasms and opportunistic infections. Lethal *Pneumocystis carinii* pneumonia has been a hallmark of AIDS. Other opportunistic infections, however, are frequent and may exist concurrently. Cryptosporidiosis and *Histoplasma capsulatum* infection are being recognized with increasing frequency. The most frequent malignancy observed is an aggressive, invasive variant of **Kaposi's sarcoma,** discovered in many patients at autopsy. Malignant B cell lymphomas are also being more commonly recognized in patients with AIDS or at high risk for AIDS. Because certain lymphomas can develop quite early, it is hypothesized that B cell hyperactivity plays a role in their development. Lymphomas and other cancers that appear late in HIV-1 disease could also stem from the failure of the compromised immune system to recognize and destroy cancer cells.

Disease Progression

Although a large enough dose of the right strain of HIV can cause AIDS on its own, cofactors can influence the progression of untreated disease. One is debilitation; for example, patients weakened by a medical condition existing before HIV infection occurred may progress toward AIDS more quickly than others. Stimulation of the immune system in response to later infections may also hasten disease progression. Other pathogenic microorganisms such as a herpesvirus called human B cell lymphotropic virus (HBLV) or human herpesvirus 6 (HHV-6) can interact with HIV-1 in a way that may increase the severity of HIV infection. HHV-6 is usually easily controlled by the immune system. If HIV compromises the immune system, however, HHV-6 may replicate more freely and become a health threat.

Laboratory Data

Laboratory evaluation of HIV-1-infected patients consists of an assessment of cellular and humoral components. Screening of blood donors and patients at risk is usually by serological methods. In patients who have developed the signs and symptoms of AIDS, assessment of the number of lymphocytes and their function becomes important.

Both a leukopenia and lymphocytopenia exist in AIDS patients. The number of circulating lymphocytes is severely decreased. The common denominator of the disease is a deficiency of a specific subset of thymus-derived (T4$^+$) lymphocytes. This abnormality (reversal of the ratio of helper-to-suppressor lymphocytes [i.e., T4$^+$:T8$^+$ cells]) has become synonymous with AIDS. Normally, this ratio is 2:1 in heterosexuals and 1.5:1 in homosexuals. In patients with AIDS, it is less than 0.5:1. T lymphocyte subset distribution is altered, with a decrease in the helper/inducer T cells and increase in suppressor/cytotoxic T cells. The absolute decrease in T4$^+$ cells, however, does not result from an absolute increase in T8$^+$ cells. This abnormality exists in the lymph nodes as well as in circulating T lymphocytes. Although characteristic, a diminished T4:T8 ratio is not diagnostic of AIDS because it can be observed in patients with other types of acute viral infections. In non-AIDS patients, the lymphocyte ratio reverts to normal after recovery from the viral infection.

The progressive decline of T4+ cells leads to a general decline in immune function. It is the primary underlying factor in determining the clinical progression of AIDS. The main host of HHV-6 is the B cell but this virus can also infect T4+ cells. If these lymphocytes are simultaneously infected by HIV-1, HHV-6 can stimulate the virus, which further impairs the immune system and promotes disease progression.

Total leukocyte and absolute lymphocyte concentrations need to be periodically assessed. Enumeration of lymphocyte subsets is usually performed by flow-cell cytometry (see Chapter 25). A decreased lymphocyte proliferative response to soluble antigens and mitogens, such as a diminished response to pokeweed mitogen (PWM), exists in this disorder.

Serological Markers

Detection of Viral Antigen. Following initial infection, the body mounts a vigorous immune response against viremia. Immunological activities include the production of different types of antibodies against HIV. Some antibodies neutralize it, others prevent it from binding to cells, and others stimulate cytotoxic cells to attack HIV-infected cells.

The time and sequence of the appearance and disappearance of antibodies specific for the serologically important antigen of HIV-1 during the course of infection is variable. A "window" of seronegativity exists from the time of initial infection until 6 or 12 weeks or longer thereafter. With enzyme immunoassay methods based on defined HIV-1 proteins produced by recombinant DNA methods, antibodies specific for glycoprotein (gp) 41 are detectable for weeks or months before assays specific for protein (p) 24 can detect antibodies. The appearance of antibodies specific for p24, however, has been shown in several studies to precede that of anti-gp41 when serum specimens are tested by Western blot analysis. This discrepancy in the sequence of antibody appearance is believed to be due to the greater sensitivity of the Western blot technique compared to viral lysate-based enzyme immunoassays used for the detection of anti-p24. Antibodies to gp41 persist throughout the course of infection. Antibodies specific for p24 not only rise to detectable levels after gp41 is detectable but also can disappear unpredictably and abruptly in a short period of time.

Increased production of core antigen is believed to be associated with a burst of viral replication and host cell lysis. The disappearance of antibody directed against p24 has been demonstrated to occur concomitantly with an increase in the concentration of core antigen in the serum. This parallel activity may be due to the sequestration of antibody in immune complexes, and the sudden decrease in anti-p24 is considered to be a grave prognostic sign in HIV-1-infected patients.

Antibodies to HIV-1. Antibodies to HIV-1 appear after a lag period of about 6 weeks between the time of infection and a detectable antibody response. Because of this, some virus-positive, antibody-negative individuals are undetected during initial screening assays.

In addition to positive test results for HIV antibody in 85% to 90% of patients, increased antibody titers to viruses such as CMV, EBV, hepatitis A and B, and *T. gondii*, and circulating immune (antigen-antibody) complexes can be found. At the present time, blood samples from donors that are initially reactive in HIV antibody testing are rechecked in duplicate in order to rule out technical errors. If on repeat testing, the result on one or more of the duplicate tests is positive, the specimen is considered "repeatably reactive." If the specimen is from a unit of blood, it is not used for transfusion. In order to rule out false-positive results, it is necessary to confirm repeatably reactive test results by an alternate protocol.

Other Immune Changes. A variety of other immune changes occur. These ancillary findings include polyclonal hypergammaglobulinemia and elevated levels of interferon alpha, alpha-1 thymosin, and beta microglobulin. Reduced levels of interleukin-1 or interleukin-2 have also been noted.

Systemic Lupus Erythematosus

Etiology, Signs, and Symptoms

This disease is a classic model of autoimmune disease that can affect practically every organ of the body. The name **systemic rheumatic disorders** is the one most commonly used for the disorders of the joints, connective tissues, and collagen-vascular disorders. SLE occurs primarily in adolescent and young adult females and may be present for years before a diagnosis is made. This disorder is eight times more common in female than in male patients.

Clinical symptoms can include fever, weight loss, malaise, arthralgia (joint pain), and arthritis (inflammation of the joints), and the characteristic erythematosus (butterfly) rash over the bridge of the nose. Drugs can produce an SLE-like syndrome. Those that have been implicated include hydralazine, procainamide, and isoniazid. In rare cases, drugs such as contraceptives, anticonvulsants, and phenothiazines have been suspected of producing symptoms.

Deterioration of the renal system is a usual consequence of the high levels of immune complexes in the blood that are deposited in tissues such as the kidneys. As the kidneys degenerate, the urinary sediment is typical of **acute nephritis** and later **chronic glomerulonephritis.** Although the disease can be rapidly fatal, it usually follows a chronic and irregular course, with periods of remission.

Laboratory Data

The laboratory findings in SLE are numerous. These tests include the classic LE cell preparation, testing for circulating antibodies, various antibody tests, and tests for lymphocyte subset abnormalities.

LE Cell Preparation

The classic but now outdated test for lupus is the LE cell test. An LE cell is either a normal segmented neutrophil or another phagocytic cell with the engulfed homogeneous and swollen nucleus of either a neutrophil or a lymphocyte.

Antibody Tests

Antibodies to DNA commonly occur in the systemic rheumatic disorders. The ANA procedure is a valuable screening tool for SLE and has virtually replaced the LE cell test because of its wider range of reactivity with nuclear antigens, greater sensitivity, and quality control characteristics. ANA refers to many different antibodies produced against a variety of antigens within the cell nucleus. These antigens are present on nucleic acid molecules (DNA and RNA) or proteins (histones and nonhistones) and on determinants consisting of both nucleic acid and protein molecules.

Some of these antibodies are directed against the double-stranded helical DNA (native DNA or DS-DNA). High titers of DS-DNA are seen primarily in SLE and parallel disease activity closely. Some antibodies are directed at the determinants of single-stranded DNA (SS-DNA). ANA testing may be by fluorescent antibody technique or by radioimmunoassay (RIA). In the fluorescent technique, a substrate that contains only DS-DNA is used. Antibody titers are frequently performed. Titers of 1:32 or greater indicate a substantial amount of antibody in an autoimmune response.

A positive ANA test result may be found in diseases other than SLE, in normal persons, in the elderly, in those with other chronic diseases, and in some patients receiving specific drug therapy. A negative ANA test result virtually eliminates SLE as a possible diagnosis if the patient is not being treated. Other antibodies, such as anti-Sm, are present in only 25 to 30% of all patients with SLE but are considered a marker for SLE. Patients with drug-induced SLE have a high incidence of antibodies to histones.

Lymphocytotoxic antibodies with predominant specificity for T lymphocytes may also be detected. These antibodies are able to lyse T lymphocytes in the presence of complement and antibodies coating the peripheral blood T cells. This can interfere with certain functional activities of T lymphocytes.

Lymphocyte Subsets

Disturbances of the lymphocyte subsets are major immunological features of SLE. Among the T cell subsets, a lack of, or reduced, generalized suppressor T cell function or hyperproduction of helper T cells occurs. Among the B cells, hyperactivity with corresponding enhancement of serum antibodies and autoantibodies, particularly IgG, and subsequent formation of pathogenic circulating immune complexes that lead to renal disease takes place.

SUMMARY

The normal range for lymphocytes in an adult is 22% to 40%, with absolute values of 1.1 to 4.4 $\times$ 10^9/L. When there is an increase in the blood lymphocyte concentration above the upper normal limit, the condition is referred to as **lymphocytosis.** A decrease below the normal limit is called **lymphocytopenia.**

Lymphocytosis

Lymphocytosis is natural and normal in infants and children up to approximately 10 years old, with total lymphocyte counts as high as 9.0 $\times$ 10^9/L. In adolescence and adulthood, nonmalignant conditions associated with an absolute lymphocytosis include acute viral infections (e.g., infectious mononucleosis) and some bacterial infections (e.g., whooping cough and brucellosis). Malignant conditions that pro-

duce lymphocytosis include cancer, lymphocytic leukemia (acute and chronic forms), the leukemic phase of lymphomas, and Waldenstrom's macroglobulinemia.

Disorders Associated With Lymphocytosis

Infectious mononucleosis is caused by EBV. This same virus is associated with Burkitt's lymphoma, a malignant tumor of the lymphoid tissue occurring mainly in African children. EBV is a human herpesvirus that has been isolated with increasing regularity.

Acute infectious lymphocytosis is a poorly defined benign condition caused by a virus, probably a member of the Coxsackie group. This is usually a mild disorder occurring in epidemics, with children being the most common victims.

CMV, a herpes family virus, can cause congenital infections in the newborn. The clinical syndrome resembles infectious mononucleosis.

Whooping cough is an infection caused by *B. pertussis,* a bacterial organism that produces inflammation of the entire respiratory tract. This is an illness that occurs primarily in children who have not been immunized.

Toxoplasmosis is an infection produced by the protozoa *T. gondii.* Both the clinical and the laboratory findings resemble those of infectious mononucleosis.

Lymphocytopenia

Lymphocytopenia is generally defined as less than 3.0 $\times$ 10^9/L lymphocytes in adults or less than 1.5 $\times$ 10^9/L lymphocytes in children. A decrease in lymphocytes is a common response to stress and to the administration of corticosteroids or may be seen in normal persons with no apparent cause. Specific categories of lymphocyte disturbances include immune deficiency disorders.

Immune Disorders Associated With Lymphocytopenia

Immune deficiency disorders may be caused by defects in the quality (defects) or quantity (deficiencies) of lymphocytes and may be congenital or acquired. These conditions are usually classified as either T cell or B cell disorders. Some of the less common disorders involve both T and B cells.

AIDS is a contemporary example of a leukopenia and lymphocytopenia. The number of circulating T lymphocytes is severely decreased. A decreased lymphocyte proliferative response to soluble antigens and mitogens exists in this disorder. This condition additionally demonstrates defective natural killer cell activity. T lymphocyte subset distribution is also altered, with a decrease in the helper/inducer T cells and an increase in the number of suppressor/cytotoxic T cells.

SLE is a collagen-vascular disorder. It occurs most frequently in young adult females. A characteristic manifestation of SLE is a "butterfly rash" over the bridge of the nose. The renal system usually deteriorates because of high levels of immune complexes in the blood. Testing for antinuclear antibody is the most significant screening in SLE.

CASE STUDIES

CASE 1 A college freshman woman complaining of extreme fatigue, headaches, and a sore throat was seen by the college physician. A routine physical examination revealed that the patient had puffiness around the eyes, swollen lymph nodes (lymphadenopathy), slight splenomegaly, and pharyngitis. A complete blood count, urinalysis, and mononucleosis screening test were ordered.

Laboratory Data
The blood count demonstrated normal values for erythrocytes and hemoglobin; however, the total leukocyte count was 13.5×10^9/L. The percentage of lymphocytes on the differential smear was 56%. Many variant forms of lymphocytes (25%) were seen, including cells with convoluted nuclei and highly vacuolated cytoplasm. The result of urinalysis was normal. The result of mononucleosis screening test was negative.

The physician prescribed medication for the patient's headache, and bed rest. A follow-up appointment was scheduled for 10 days later.

Questions
1. What was this patient's absolute lymphocyte count? Is this considered normal?
2. What is the most probable diagnosis of this disorder?
3. If repeat testing were performed on the patient after 10 days, could any of the results vary?
4. Discuss the antibodies that could occur in this condition.
5. Why are increased variant lymphocytes produced in this disorder?

Discussion
1. The patient's absolute lymphocyte count is 7.83×10^9/L. This represents an increase; hence, a lymphocytosis is present.
2. The age and physical findings in this patient are highly suggestive of infectious mononucleosis. The laboratory findings of normal erythrocyte parameters and an increase in variant lymphocytes further support the diagnosis of mononucleosis. However, the absence of a positive heterophil screening test precludes a definitive diagnosis of infectious mononucleosis.
3. The heterophil antibody test usually becomes positive within 3 weeks after the initial symptoms.
4. Heterophil antibodies are the antibodies normally encountered in infectious mononucleosis. Rare cases of infectious mononucleosis have been described as heterophil-negative. The clinical manifestations of infectious mononucleosis are present in these patients, but the heterophil test result remains negative for weeks after the onset. An Epstein-Barr antibody test may be helpful in distinguishing these cases from syndromes caused by other agents such as CMV or *Toxoplasma*. Occasionally, unusual antibodies occur in cases of infectious mononucleosis. Some of them may produce false-positive results for ANA, rheumatoid factor, and syphilis. Anti-i can also be encountered in acquired hemolytic anemias subsequent to infectious mononucleosis.
5. Several types of nonneoplastic disorders, such as systemic infection, diffuse inflammation, virus infections, and autoimmune disease, can produce a transient lymphocytosis. This lymphocytosis results from either an increased production, a release of cells from peripheral lymphatic tissue, or both. If the normal proliferation and mobilization of lymphocytes from the lymph nodes and spleen is augmented by significant stimulation from other factors, increased numbers of variant lymphocytes can be seen in the peripheral blood. Lymphocytosis associated with infectious mononucleosis results from preferential infection of B cells by EBV. This infection results in a short burst of B cell proliferation and mobilization, which produces the transient rise in the number of B cells with the variant lymphocyte structure. The altered membrane of the B cells further induces a prolonged proliferation response in T cells.

Diagnosis: Infectious mononucleosis

CASE 2 A 6-year-old boy was taken to the emergency room by his parents. The child had been having extreme difficulty in breathing for the last several days and had been experiencing diarrhea for the past 24 hours. There was no history of illness or infections.

Physical examination revealed that the child was severely dehydrated, had an elevated temperature, and had swollen lymph nodes (lymphadenopathy). The physician on duty ordered a complete blood count, serum electrolyte determination, urinalysis, infectious mononucleosis screening test, and a chest radiograph.

Laboratory Data
The boy's blood count was normal, except for the leukocytes. The total leukocyte count was 28×10^9/L, with 78% of leukocytes being lymphocytes. Most of the lymphocytes were small and normal in appearance. The serum electrolytes were consistent with a mild state of dehydration. The urinalysis was normal, and the infectious mononucleosis screening test result was negative. The chest radiograph displayed mild congestion in the upper quadrant of the lungs.

Questions
1. What is the possible etiology of this disorder?
2. What other laboratory tests can assist in making a definitive diagnosis?
3. What mechanism is responsible for the lymphocytosis?
4. What is the expected duration of this condition?

Discussion
1. Pediatric patients with lymphocytosis, respiratory distress, and diarrhea are usually prime candidates for infectious lymphocytosis due to bacterial or viral agents. Leukocytosis with a concurrent lymphocytosis can be caused by alterations in lymphocyte recirculation or abnormalities in lymphocyte turnover. Disorders producing this type of abnormality can include *B. pertussis*, certain viral infections, systemic infection, diffuse inflammation, autoimmune disease, immunoproliferative disorders, and some medications.
2. Laboratory tests that can assist in making a definitive diagnosis include microbiological culture for *B. pertussis* or viral cultures. A culture was positive for *B. pertussis*.
3. In normal persons, the rate of the entry and exit of lymphocytes from the blood is relatively constant. This balance can be disrupted by bacterial or viral agents, such as *B. pertussis* and adenoviruses, or by medications such as heparin and dextran. If disruption of lymphocyte recirculation occurs because the lymphocytes are unable to recog-

(continued)

nize and attach to the endothelial venules in the lymph nodes, the number of lymphocytes in the blood circulation rapidly increases. However, the normal morphology of the lymphocytes is not altered.

4. In cases of acute infectious lymphocytosis, the elevated peripheral blood lymphocyte count may persist for 2 or 3 weeks and then begin to decline. Frequently, a transient eosinophilia is noted during the period of lymphocyte decline.

✏ Diagnosis: *B. pertussis* infection producing an infectious lymphocytosis

---

CASE 3 A 5-year-old girl was taken to the pediatrician by her mother because of recurrent high fevers over the past few days. Physical examination revealed a light-colored rash but no other abnormalities. The child was referred to the clinic for a complete blood count.

Laboratory Data

The complete blood count revealed normal erythrocyte parameters; however, the total leukocyte count was 4.0×10^9/L.

The differential count revealed a lymphocyte count of 40%; all of the lymphocytes were mature and small.

Questions

1. Are the leukocyte count and differential count normal?
2. What is the probable etiology of this disorder?
3. What is the mechanism of this disorder?

Discussion

1. The total leukocyte count and percentage of lymphocytes are slightly below normal for a child of this age.
2. Mild lymphopenias can occur in some types of viral diseases, such as measles, varicella, and polio. The most common worldwide cause of lymphopenia is malnutrition. Other congenital defects due to disturbed maturation of T or B cells are rare, and related disorders usually appear in early childhood.
3. Some severe viral infections produce a noticeable decrease in B cells. These alterations are due to the ability of the virus to infect and destroy B cells. Because B cells constitute only a small percentage of circulating lymphocytes in children, the decrease in circulating lymphocytes is not dramatic.

✏ Diagnosis: Measles

CASE 4 A 27-year-old white woman sought medical attention because of persisting pain in her wrists and ankles and an unexplained skin irritation of the face. On physical examination, swelling of the joints of the hands and ankles was evident, along with erythema of the skin over the bridge of the nose and the upper cheeks. The patient had a slightly elevated temperature. The following laboratory tests were ordered: a complete blood count, urinalysis, and rheumatoid arthritis screening test.

Laboratory Data

The hemoglobin and hematocrit were normal, with a total leukocyte count of 7.0×10^9/L. The differential count was as follows: segmented neutrophils 80%, bands 1%, lymphocytes 17%, monocytes 1%, and eosinophils 1%. The morphology of the erythrocytes, leukocytes, and platelets was nor-

mal. The gross and microscopic urinalysis results were normal. A positive result was obtained with the rheumatoid arthritis screening test.

An ANA screening test was ordered. The results were positive.

Questions

1. What is the most probable diagnosis in this case?
2. What is the principle of the ANA test?

Discussion

1. The patient's symptoms are all highly suggestive of a collagen-type disease, such as one of the rheumatoid disorders. However, both a positive LE test result and a positive ANA test result are highly suggestive of SLE.
2. Antibodies to DNA with high titers of DS-DNA are seen primarily in SLE. ANA testing may be by fluorescent antibody technique or by RIA. In the fluorescent technique, a substrate that contains only DS-DNA is used. Titers of 1:32 or greater indicate a substantial amount of antibody.

✏ Diagnosis: Systemic lupus erythematosus

BIBLIOGRAPHY

Angell, M. "A Dual Approach to the AIDS Epidemic." *N. Engl. J. Med.*, Vol. 324, No. 21, May, 1991, pp. 1498–1500.

Barbara, J. A. J. and R. S. Tedder. "Viral Infections Transmitted by Blood and Its Products." *Clin. Haematol.*, Vol. 13, No. 3, October, 1984, pp. 693–707.

Barman, M. R. "AIDS Precautions in Practice." *Med. Lab. Observer*, Vol. 10, No. 4, April, 1990, pp. 24–33.

Bowden, R. et al. "Cytomegalovirus Immune Globulin and Seronegative Blood Products to Prevent Primary Cytomegalovirus Infection After Marrow Transplantation." *N. Engl. J. Med.*, Vol. 314, 1986, pp. 1006–1010.

Brady, M. T. "Cytomegalovirus Infections: Occupational Risk for Health Professionals." *Am. J. Infect. Control*, Vol. 14, No. 5, October, 1986, pp. 197–203.

Breo, D. L. "Blood, Money, and Hemophiliacs—The Fatal Story of France's AIDSgate." *JAMA*, Vol. 266, No. 24, December 25, 1991, pp. 3477–3482.

Brown, J. W. "Lab-Related Findings from the Sixth International Conference on AIDS." *Med. Lab. Observer*, August, 1990, pp. 59–65.

Brown, J. W. "Laboratorians: On the Front Lines of Exposure." *Med. Lab. Observer*, Vol. 11, No. 8, August, 1991, pp. 54–60.

Brown, K. A. "Nonmalignant Disorders of Lymphocytes." *Clin. Lab. Sci.*, Vol. 10, No. 6, Dec, 1997, pp. 329–335.

Bruce-Chwatt, L. J. "Transfusion Associated Parasitic Infections," in *Infection, Immunity, and Blood Transfusion*. New York: Liss, 1985, pp. 101–125.

Centers for Disease Control and Prevention. *HIV/AIDS Surveillance Report*. Vol. 9, No. 2, 1997, pp. 1–43.

Chaisson, R. E. and D. E. Griffin. "Progressive Multifocal Leukoencephalopathy in AIDS." *JAMA*, Vol. 264, No. 1, July 4, 1990, pp. 79–82.

Chamberland, M. E. et al. "Health Care Workers with AIDS." *JAMA*, Vol. 266, No. 24, December 25, 1991, pp. 3459–3462.

de Smet, M. D. and R. B. Nussenbatt. "Ocular Manifestations of AIDS." *JAMA*, Vol. 266, No. 21, December 4, 1991, pp. 3019–3022.

Ellerbrock, T. V. et al. "Epidemiology of Women With AIDS in the United States, 1981 through 1990." *JAMA*, Vol. 265, No. 22, June 12, 1991, pp. 2971–2975.

Evans, A. S. and J. C. Niederman. "Epstein-Barr Virus," in *Viral Infections of Human Epidemiology and Control* (2nd ed.). A. S. Evans (ed.). New York: Plenum Medical, 1982, pp. 580–586.

Fleischer, G. R. "Epstein-Barr Virus," in *Textbook of Human Virology.* M Belshe (ed.). Littleton, MA: PSG Publishing, 1984, pp. 490–558.

Fleischer, G. R. et al. "Primary Epstein-Barr Virus Infection in Association With Reye Syndrome." *J. Pediatr.,* Vol. 97, 1980, pp. 935–937.

Fossel, E. T. "Correspondence: Importance of Age in Prognostic Staging System for AIDS." *N. Engl. J. Med.,* Vol. 321, No. 20, November, 1989, pp. 1408–1410.

Gallo, D. et al. "Comparison of Detection of Antibody to the Acquired Immune Deficiency Syndrome Virus by Enzyme Immunoassay, Immunofluorescence, and Western Blot Methods." *J. Clin. Microbiol.,* Vol. 23, 1986, pp. 1049–1051.

Gallo, D., K. H. Walen, and J. L. Riggs. "Improved Immunofluorescence Antigens for Detection of Immunoglobulin M Antibodies to Epstein-Barr Viral Capsid Antigen and Antibodies to Epstein-Barr Virus Nuclear Antigen." *J. Clin. Microbiol.,* Vol. 15, 1982, pp. 243–248.

Gallo, R. C. and L. Montagnier. "AIDS in 1988." *Sci. Am.,* Vol. 259, No. 4, October, 1988, pp. 40–51.

Geltosky, J. E. et al. "Use of a Synthetic Peptide-Based ELISA for the Diagnosis of Infectious Mononucleosis and Other Diseases." *J. Clin. Lab. Anal.,* Vol. 1, 1987, pp. 153–162.

Goudsmit, J. et al. "Intrathecal Synthesis of Antibodies to HTLV-III in Patients Without AIDS or AIDS Related Complex." *Br. Med. J.,* Vol. 292, 1986, pp. 1231–1234.

Hall, S. M. "The Diagnosis of Toxoplasmosis." *Br. Med. J.,* Vol. 289, 1984, pp. 570–571.

Haseltine, W. A. and F. Wong-Stall. "The Molecular Biology of the AIDS Virus." *Sci. Am.,* Vol. 259, No. 4, October, 1988, pp. 52–63.

Henle, W. et al. "Antibodies to Early Antigens Induced by Epstein Barr Virus in Infectious Mononucleosis." *J. Infect. Dis.,* Vol. 124, 1971, pp. 8–67.

Henle, W. and G. Henle. "Epstein-Barr Virus and Infectious Mononucleosis." *N. Engl. J. Med.,* Vol. 288, 1973, pp. 263–264.

Henle, W. and G. Henle. "Epstein-Barr Virus and Infectious Mononucleosis," in *Human Herpesvirus Infections: Clinical Aspects.* R. Glaser and T. Gotlieb-Stematsky (eds.). New York: Marcel Dekker, 1982, pp. 704–715.

Henle, W. and G. Henle. "Epstein-Barr Virus and Blood Transfusions," in *Infection, Immunity, and Blood Transfusion.* New York: Liss, 1985, pp. 201–209.

Heyward, W. L. and J. W. Curran. "The Epidemiology of AIDS in the U.S." *Sci. Am.,* Vol. 259, No. 4, October, 1988, pp. 72–81.

Horwitz, C. A. et al. "Heterophil-Negative Infectious Mononucleosis and Mononucleosis-like Illnesses: Laboratory Confirmation in 43 Cases." *Am. J. Med.,* Vol. 63, 1977, pp. 947–957.

Kinney, J. S. et al. "Cytomegaloviral Infection and Disease." *J. Infect. Dis.,* Vol. 151, 1985, pp. 772–774.

Konvolinka, C. W. and D. B. Wyatt. "Splenic Rupture and Infectious Mononucleosis." *J. Emerg. Med.,* Vol. 7, 1989, p. 471.

Krogstad, D. J. et al. "Blood and Tissue Protozoa," in *Manual of Clinical Microbiology* (4th ed.). E. H. Lennette et al. (eds.). Washington, DC: American Society of Microbiology, 1985, pp. 612–630.

Lamberson, H. V. "Cytomegalovirus (CMV): The Agent, Its Pathogenesis, and Its Epidemiology," *Infection, Immunity, and Blood Transfusion.* New York: Liss, 1985, pp. 149–173.

Lemp, G. F. et al. "Survival Trends for Patients With AIDS." *JAMA,* Vol. 263, No. 3, January 19, 1990, pp. 402–406.

Lennette, E. T. and W. Henle. "Epstein-Barr Virus Infections: Clinical and Serologic Features." *Lab. Management,* Vol. 25, 1987, pp. 23–28.

Leyvraz, S. et al. "Association of Epstein-Barr Virus With Thymic Carcinoma." *N. Engl. J. Med.,* Vol. 312, 1985, pp. 1296–1299.

Liskowsky, D. R. "Update: Acquired Immunodeficiency Syndrome—United States, 1981-1990." *JAMA,* Vol. 265, No. 24, June 26, 1991, p. 3226.

Mandell, G. E. (ed.). *Principles and Practices of Infectious Disease* (2nd ed.). New York: Wiley, 1985.

Mann, J. M. et al. "The International Epidemiology of AIDS." *Sci. Am.,* Vol. 259, No. 4, October, 1988, pp. 40–51.

Markell, E. K. et al. *Medical Parasitology* (6th ed.). Philadelphia: Saunders, 1986, pp. 112–117, 131–138.

Martin, W. J., II and T. F. Smith. "Rapid Detection of Cytomegalovirus in Bronchoalveolar Lavage Specimens by Monoclonal Antibody Method." *J. Clin. Microbiol.,* Vol. 23, 1986, pp. 1006–1008.

Mayer, K. H. et al. "Human T-Lymphotropic Virus Type III in High-Risk, Antibody-Negative Homosexual Men." *Ann. Intern. Med.,* Vol. 104, 1986, pp. 194–196.

McHugh, T. M. et al. "Comparison of Six Methods for the Detection of Antibody to Cytomegalovirus." *J. Clin. Microbiol.,* Vol. 22, 1985, pp. 1014–1019.

McKeating, J. A. et al. "Detection of Cytomegalovirus in Urine Samples by Enzyme-Linked Immunosorbent Assay." *J. Med. Virol.,* Vol. 16, 1985, pp. 367–373.

Moore, R. D. et al. "Zidovudine and the Natural History of the Acquired Immunodeficiency Syndrome." *N. Engl. J. Med.,* Vol. 324, No. 20, May 16, 1991, pp. 1412–1416.

Panjwani, D. D. et al. "Virological and Serological Diagnosis of Cytomegalovirus Infection in Bone Marrow Allograft Recipient." *J. Med. Virol.,* Vol. 16, 1985, pp. 357–365.

Paul, J. R. and W. W. Bunnell. "The Presence of Heterophil Antibodies in Infectious Mononucleosis." *Am. J. Med. Sci.,* Vol. 183, 1932, pp. 90–104.

"Percent Distribution of AIDS Cases, by Transmission Category and Year of Report, United States, 1981–1988." *MMWR,* Vol. 38, No. S-4, 1989.

Raub, W. "Possible AIDS Virus Subgroup Identified." *JAMA,* Vol. 263, No. 5, February 2, 1990, p. 628.

Ray, C. G., M. J. Hicks, and L. L. Minnich. "Viruses, Rickettsia, and Chlamydia," in *Clinical Diagnosis and Management by Laboratory Methods.* John B. Henry (ed.). Philadelphia: Saunders, 1984, pp. 1290–1291.

Redfield, R. R. and D. S. Burke. "HIV Infection: The Clinical Picture." *Sci. Am.,* Vol. 259, No. 4, 1988, pp. 90–98.

Saemundsen, A. K. et al. "Epstein-Barr Virus in Nasopharyngeal and Salivary Gland Carcinomas of Greenland Eskimoes." *Br. J. Cancer,* Vol. 46, 1982, pp. 721–728.

Schrier, R. D., J. A. Nelson, and M. B. Nelson. "Detection of Human Cytomegalovirus in Peripheral Blood Lymphocytes in a Natural Infection." *Science,* Vol. 230, 1985, pp. 1048–1051.

Schuster, V. et al. "Detection of Human Cytomegalovirus in Urine by DNA-DNA and RNA-DNA Hybridization." *J. Infect. Dis.,* Vol. 154, 1986, pp. 309–314.

Shuster, E. A. et al. "Monoclonal Antibody for Rapid Laboratory Detection of Cytomegalovirus Infections: Characterization and Diagnostic Application." *Mayo Clin. Proc.,* Vol. 60, 1985, pp. 577–585.

Smith, R. S. et al. "A Synthetic Peptide for Detecting Antibodies to Epstein-Barr Virus Nuclear Antigen in Sera from Patients with Infectious Mononucleosis." *J. Infect. Dis.,* Vol. 154, 1986, pp. 885–889.

Stagno, S. et al. "Congenital Cytomegalovirus Infection." *N. Engl. J. Med.,* Vol. 306, 1982, p. 945.

Stagno, S. and R. J. Whitley. "Herpesvirus Infections of Pregnancy. Part I: Cytomegalovirus and Epstein-Barr Virus Infections." *N. Engl. J. Med.,* Vol. 313, 1985, pp. 1270–1274.

Starr, S. E. and H. J. M. Friedman. "Human Cytomegalovirus," in *Manual of Clinical Microbiology* (4th ed.). E. H. Lennette et al. (eds.). Washington, DC: American Society of Microbiology, 1985, pp. 711–719.

Steel, E. and H. W. Haverkos. "Increasing Incidence of Reported Case of AIDS." *N. Engl. J. Med.,* Vol. 325, No. 1, July 4, 1991, pp. 65–66.

Sullivan, J. L. and J. B. Hanshaw. "Cytomegalovirus Infections," in *Human Herpesvirus Infections: Clinical Aspects.* R. Glaser and T. Gotlieb-Stematsky (eds.). New York: Marcel Dekker, 1982, pp. 57–83.

Sumaya, C. V. "Epstein-Barr Virus Serologic Testing: Diagnostic Indications and Interpretations." *Pediatr. Infect. Dis.,* Vol. 5, 1986, pp. 337–342.

Sumaya, C. V. "Infectious Mononucleosis and Other EBV Infections: Diagnostic Factors." *Lab. Management,* Vol. 24, 1986, pp. 37–45.

Sumaya, C. V. and Y. Ench. "Epstein-Barr Virus Infectious Mononucleosis in Children. I. Clinical and General Laboratory Findings." *Pediatrics,* Vol. 75, 1985, pp. 1003–1010.

Sumaya, C. V. and Y. Ench. "Epstein-Barr Virus Infectious Mononucleosis in Children. II. Heterophil Antibody and Viral-Specific Responses." *Pediatrics,* Vol. 75, 1985, pp. 1011–1019.

Taswell, H. F. et al. "Comparison of Three Methods for Detecting Antibody to Cytomegalovirus." *Transfusion,* Vol. 26, No. 3, 1986, pp. 285–289.

Tegtmeier, G. E. "Cytomegalovirus and Blood Transfusion," in *Infection, Immunity, and Blood Transfusion.* New York: Liss, 1985, pp. 175–199.

U.S. Department of Health and Human Services. "Human Immunodeficiency Virus Infection in the United States: A Review of Current Knowledge." *MMWR,* Vol. 36, December 18, 1987, pp. s-6, 1–48.

U.S. Department of Health and Human Services. "Update: Acquired Immunodeficiency Syndrome and HIV Infection Among Health Care Workers." *MMWR,* Vol. 37, April 22, 1988, p. 229.

Walls, K. W. "Serodiagnostic Tests for Parasitic Diseases," in *Manual of Clinical Microbiology* (4th ed.). E. H. Lennette et al. (eds.). Washington, DC: American Society of Microbiology, 1985, pp. 945–948.

Walls, K. W. and M. Wilson. "Immunoserology in Parasitic Infections," in *Immunodiagnostics.* New York: Liss, 1983, pp. 191–214.

Weiss, S. H. et al. "Screening Test for HTLV-III (AIDS Agent) Antibodies. Specificity, Sensitivity, and Applications." *JAMA,* Vol. 253, 1985, pp. 221–225.

Wilson, C. B. and J. J. Remington. "What Can Be Done to Prevent Toxoplasmosis?" *Am. J. Obstet. Gynecol.,* Vol. 138, 1980, pp. 357–363.

REVIEW QUESTIONS

1. Lymphocytopenia means:
   A. A total increase in leukocytes.
   B. A total increase in lymphocytes.
   C. A total increase in the absolute value or percentage of lymphocytes.
   D. A total decrease in lymphocytes.

2. The helper subset of T lymphocytes is ___ in AIDS.
   A. Increased. C. Not altered.
   B. Decreased.

Questions 3 through 8: match the following disorders with either the A or the B answer.

3. ___ Radiation exposure. A. Lymphocytosis.
4. ___ Infectious mononucleosis. B. Lymphocytopenia.
5. ___ Cytotoxic drugs.
6. ___ Whooping cough.
7. ___ Immune deficiency disorders.
8. ___ Toxoplasmosis.

9. Which of the following characterizes infectious mononucleosis?
   A. Etiology: Epstein-Barr virus.
   B. A T cell disorder.
   C. A greater incidence in Africa.
   D. Nonheterophil antibodies.

10. The laboratory findings in infectious mononucleosis are generally characterized by:
    A. An increase in variant lymphocytes.
    B. A heterophil titer of less than 1:56.
    C. No agglutination of the patient's serum with horse erythrocytes.
    D. All of the above.

11. Which of the following characterizes infectious lymphocytosis?
    A. An adult disorder.
    B. Leukocytopenia in the early stages.
    C. Lymphocyte differential counts of 60 to 95%.
    D. Lymphoblasts on the peripheral blood smear.

12. Which of the following are characteristics of cytomegalovirus infection?
    A. Etiology: a herpes family virus.
    B. Lymphocytopenia.
    C. A positive heterophil test result.
    D. Both A and B.

13. Acquired immunodeficiency syndrome (AIDS) is caused by:
    A. A herpes family virus. C. HIV-1.
    B. Cytomegalovirus. D. Epstein-Barr virus.

14. Which of the following generally characterize toxoplasmosis?
    A. Symptoms may resemble infectious mononucleosis.
    B. Occurrence in pregnant women who own cats.
    C. Etiology: parasitic.
    D. All of the above.

15. Which antibody test has replaced the LE cell preparation in the diagnosis of systemic lupus erythematosus?
    A. Rheumatoid arthritis factor.
    B. Antinuclear antibody test.
    C. Complement fixation test.
    D. Antibody Sm test.

16. Which of the following characteristics is associated with plasma cells?
    A. Arise from plasmablasts.
    B. Many are found in the bone marrow.
    C. Arise from stimulated T lymphocytes.
    D. Synthesize and excrete antibodies.

Characteristics of Leukemias and Lymphomas

OBJECTIVES

Comparison of leukemias and lymphomas
- Define and compare the terms **leukemia** and **lymphoma.**

Forms of leukemia
- Describe the terms **acute** and **chronic** leukemia.

Classification of leukemias
- List the traditional forms of the major types of leukemias.
- List the more uncommon forms of leukemias.

Prognosis and treatment
- Compare the early treatment of leukemias and lymphomas with current therapy.

Factors related to the occurrence of leukemia
- Describe the role of oncogenes in leukemias and lymphomas.
- Describe the effects of ionizing radiation on the incidence of leukemia.

- Name one chemical that is correlated with an increased incidence of leukemia.
- Name several occupations that are associated with a higher-than-normal risk of hematological malignancies.
- Name one genetic defect that is correlated with an increased incidence of leukemia.
- Explain the significance of the discovery of the HTLV family and describe the disorders associated with HTLV-I, HTLV-II, and HIV.

Demographic distribution of leukemia
- Describe the variations in the incidence of leukemia in different ethnic and racial groups.
- Correlate patient age to the overall incidence of various leukemias.
- Describe the overall differences between the incidence of leukemia in female and male patients.

Although the symptoms of leukemia had been reported since the time of Hippocrates, Virchow first recognized leukemia as a distinct clinical disorder between 1839 and 1845. He named this disorder **leukemia** because of the white appearance of the blood from patients with fever, weakness, and **lymphadenopathy.** Virchow originally divided the leukemias into two classes, those with and those without lymphadenopathy. Since that time, sophisticated classification systems of leukemias and lymphomas have been developed.

COMPARISON OF LEUKEMIAS AND LYMPHOMAS

Leukemias and lymphomas are both neoplastic proliferative diseases predominantly involving the leukocytes. Leukemias are characterized by an overproduction of various types of immature or mature leukocytes in the bone marrow and/or peripheral blood. Lymphomas are solid, malignant tumors of the lymph nodes and associated tissues; hence, the lymphocyte is the distinctive cell type. Another distinction between a leukemia and a lymphoma is that in the leukemias, malignant cells freely trespass the blood-tissue barrier, whereas in a lymphoma the malignant cells are initially confined to the organs containing mononuclear phagocyte cells such as the lymph nodes, spleen, liver, and bone marrow. Lymphomas can "spill over" into the circulating blood and present a leukemic-appearing picture on a peripheral blood smear.

FORMS OF LEUKEMIA

The clinical symptoms, maturity of the affected cells, and total leukocyte count determine whether a leukemia will be classified as **acute** or **chronic.** Acute leukemias are characterized by symptoms of short duration, many immature cell forms in the bone marrow and/or peripheral blood, and an elevated total leukocyte count. Chronic leukemias have symptoms of long duration, mostly mature cell forms in the bone marrow and/or peripheral blood, and total leukocyte counts that range from extremely elevated to lower than normal. The prognosis of survival in untreated acute forms is from several weeks to several months, compared with the untreated chronic forms, which can have a prognosis of survival ranging from months to many years after diagnosis.

CLASSIFICATION OF LEUKEMIAS

Although Virchow divided leukemias into two groups based on the presence of lymphadenopathy, today the different forms of leukemia are usually classified according to the predominant blood cell morphology, associated supplementary testing, and clinical criteria. On the basis of morphological and cytochemical results, the predominant type of proliferative cell can be determined in a specific patient.

In the commonly encountered cases, the leukemias are separable into three broad leukocyte groups: **myelogenous, monocytic,** and **lymphocytic.** When this information is coupled with the degree of cell maturity, the traditional classifi-cations of the major types of leukocytic leukemia are as follows:

1. Acute or chronic myelogenous
2. Acute or chronic monocytic
3. Acute or chronic myelomonocytic
4. Acute or chronic lymphocytic

More uncommon forms of leukocytic leukemia are these: acute undifferentiated (stem cell), eosinophilic, and basophilic. Overproliferation of the erythrocytic and megakaryocytic cell lines, either solely or in conjunction with abnormalities of the leukocytic line, also exist.

PROGNOSIS AND TREATMENT

Untreated leukemias and lymphomas are ultimately fatal. Radiation therapy in the 1920s provided the first type of curative intervention. The first effective drug therapy, adrenoglucocorticosteroids and antifolate agents, was discovered in the late 1940s. Modern drugs, which are more effective against malignant cells and less toxic to the patient, have had a significant impact on the longevity of patients with many forms of leukemia and lymphoma. However, effective treatment requires selecting the proper mode and method of treatment. The time of administration of treatment can also have an effect (refer to Chapter 25 for applications of flow-cell cytometry). Specific treatment requires accurate diagnosis and classification of the disorder by the clinical laboratory.

FACTORS RELATED TO THE OCCURRENCE OF LEUKEMIA

Leukemia is a clonal disease that develops subsequent to the malignant transformation of one or more normal hematopoietic progenitor cells. It appears likely that mutation and the altered expression of specific genes cause this transformation. Leukemic stem cells are capable of proliferation and self-renewal, which gives rise to one or more dominant clones of cells that eventually fill the bone marrow and suppress normal hematopoiesis.

Many agents or factors have been implicated in the occurrence of leukemias and lymphomas (Table 18.1). These factors include:

1. Oncogenes
2. Ionizing radiation
3. Chemical exposure
4. Genetic factors
5. Infectious agents

Oncogenes

A single oncogene produced through mutation in a target cell is not sufficient to convert these cells into full-blown cancer cells. Cancer cells typically carry multiple genetic changes that act together. Cancer-predisposing genes may act in several ways:

1. They may affect the rate at which exogenous precarcinogens are metabolized to actively carcinogenic forms that can damage the cellular genome directly.

TABLE 18.1   Known Environmental Factors Associated With Leukemias and Lymphomas

Factor	Type of Cancer
Benzene	Leukemia
Hydantoins	Lymphoma
Chloramphenicol, alkylating drugs	Leukemias, lymphomas
Ionizing radiation (fallout, industrial exposure)	Leukemias, thyroid tumors
Isotopes, radium	Osteogenic sarcoma
Therapeutic	Osteogenic sarcoma; fibrosarcoma; skin, breast, thyroid carcinoma
Infectious Agents	
Herpesvirus (Epstein-Barr virus)	Burkitt's lymphoma, nasopharyngeal carcinoma
Human immunodeficiency virus (HIV)	Kaposi's sarcoma, non-Hodgkin's lymphoma, primary lymphoma of the brain, bladder cancer

2. Some genes may affect a host's ability to repair resulting damage to DNA.
3. Predisposing genes may alter the immune system's ability to recognize and wipe out incipient tumors.
4. Some genes may affect the function of the apparatus responsible for the regulation of normal cell growth and associated proliferation of tissue.

Relatively few cancer-predisposing genes have been described. An absence of functional alleles at a specific loci, however, allows the genesis of a malignant process.

The Role of Oncogenes

Malignant proliferation of cells is related to genes. Cancer often begins when a carcinogenic agent such as a chemical or ionizing radiation damages the DNA of a critical gene in a cell. The mutant cell multiplies and the succeeding generations of cells aggregate to form a malignant tumor.

Proto-oncogenes act as central regulators of growth in normal cells and are antecedents of oncogenes. Not one of the proto-oncogenes, however, has yet been linked to genes that are thought to increase the risk of cancer. The rare involvement of these genes in the cancer process is a consequence of somatic mutations that take place in specific target tissues and convert these genes into oncogenic alleles. Because oncogenic alleles arise somatically, they cannot be used to explain genetic susceptibilities to cancer that exist at the moment of conception.

The genetic targets of carcinogens are known to be oncogenes. Oncogenes have been associated with various tumor types that stem in large part from preexisting genes present in the normal human genome. Therefore, oncogenes are considered to be altered versions of normal genes. In the course of a lifetime, a variety of mutations can convert a normal gene into a malignant oncogene. Once an oncogene is activated by mutation, it promotes excessive or inappropriate cell proliferation. Oncogenes have been detected in about 15% to 20% of a variety of human tumors and appear to be responsible for specifying many of the malignant traits of these cells. More than 30 distinct oncogenes, some of which are associated with specific tumor types, have been identified (Table 18.2). Each gene has the ability to evoke many of the phenotypes characteristic of cancer cells.

Tumor-Suppressing Genes

A very different class of cancer genes has been discovered recently. These tumor-suppressing genes appear to regulate the proliferation of cell growth in normal cells. When this type of gene is inactivated, a block to proliferation is removed and cells begin a program of deregulated growth, or the genetically depleted cell itself may proliferate uncontrollably. Thus, tumor-suppressing genes are referred to as "anti-oncogenes" and their discovery will in time lead to the reformulation of ideas about how the growth of normal cells is regulated.

There is much speculation as to how tumor-suppressing genes operate in normal tissue. It is known that normal cells exert a negative growth influence on each other within a tissue. Normal cells also secrete factors that are negative regulators of their own growth and that of adjacent cells. Diffusible factors may also be released by normal cells in order to induce the end-stage differentiation of other cells in the immediate environment. Examples of such factors include:

1. Beta-interferon
2. Tumor growth factor
3. Tumor necrosis factor

TABLE 18.2   Oncogenes Formed by Somatic Mutation of Normal Genetic Loci

Oncogene	Disorder
Abl	Chronic myelogenous leukemia
Myc	Burkitt's lymphoma
Ras type	Variety of tumors

Normal gene products appear to prevent malignant transformation in some way. It is speculated that normal cells have receptors able to detect the presence of these growth-inhibiting and differentiation-inducing factors, which allows the receptors to process the signals of negative growth and respond with appropriate modulation of growth. Genes may specify proteins that are necessary to detect and also respond to the negative regulators of growth. If this process becomes dysfunctional owing to inactivation or the absence of a critical component such as the loss of chromosomal loci, a cell may continue to respond to mitogenic stimulation but lose its ability to respond to negative feedback to cease proliferation.

Animal experiments suggest that humans carry a repertoire of genes, each of which is involved in the negative regulation of the growth of specific cell types. Somatic inactivation of these genes may be involved in the initiation of tumor-cell growth or the transformation of benign tumors into malignant ones. Therefore, the somatic inactivation of tumor-suppressing genes may be as important to carcinogenesis as the somatic activation of oncogenes.

Immunologic Surveillance

Clinical immunologists regard the immune response as a means of diagnosing and treating malignancy. Although no single satisfactory explanation exists to explain the success of tumors in escaping the immune rejection process, it is believed that early clones of neoplastic cells are eliminated by the immune response. Cells such as the large granular lymphocytes (LGLs), antibody-dependent cell-mediated cytotoxicity (ADCC) effector cells, and cytotoxic T cells dominate the rejection process that leads to the elimination of foreign tissue; therefore, cells rather than immunoglobulins are believed to dominate tumor immunity. The functions of normal antitumor mechanisms and the failure of these mechanisms in the pathogenesis of cancer are incompletely understood at the present time.

Ionizing Radiation

Ionizing radiation is associated with an increased incidence of leukemia. The acute and chronic forms of myelogenous leukemia are most frequently associated with radiation. Historically, Madame Curie and her daughter, Irene, both succumbed to leukemia, and the survivors of Hiroshima were found to have a dose-related increase in the incidence of leukemia. Prior to the use of protective measures, radiologists were found to suffer from leukemia 10 times more frequently than the general population.

Chemical Exposure

Occupational exposure to chemicals is also highly correlated with an increased incidence of acute and chronic myelogenous leukemia. Prolonged exposure to the chemical benzene is known to increase the probability of various forms of cancer, including leukemia. The occupations associated with job-related death due to a higher-than-average risk of malignancy in the hematopoietic system are presented in Table 18.3. All but one of these occupations (radiologist) is associated with chemical exposure.

TABLE 18.3 Occupations Related to a Higher-Than-Average Risk of Malignancy in Hematologically Related Sites

Occupation	Site
Chemist	Lymphatic system
Petrochemical worker	Blood
Painter	Blood
Radiologist	Bone marrow
Rubber industry worker	Blood
Woodworker	Lymphatic system

Source: Adapted from William F. Allman, "We Have Nothing to Fear." *Science '85*, October, 1985, p. 32.

Genetic Factors

Genetic factors have been correlated with the incidence of leukemia. In studies of twins, if one member develops leukemia, the other has one chance in five of developing leukemia. Children with Down's syndrome are 20 times more likely to develop acute leukemia than children without this genetic disorder. Cytogenetic abnormalities are now associated with many varieties of leukemia. The link between certain genetic abnormalities and leukemia is consistent with a germinal or somatic mutation in a stem cell line, and the increased incidence of lymphomas in congenital, acquired, and drug-induced immunosuppression is consistent with the failure of normal immune mechanisms or antigen overstimulation with a loss of normal feedback control. The incidence of cancers such as lymphoma is extremely increased (10,000 times greater than expected) in patients suffering from acquired immunodeficiency syndrome (AIDS).

Infectious Agents

In the last decade, specific viruses have been found to be associated with the development of several disorders, including leukemias and lymphomas. These viruses can be separated epidemiologically into two groups:

1. Those that are ubiquitous, such as the Epstein-Barr virus (EBV)
2. Those that have a higher incidence in certain populations, such as human immunodeficiency virus (HIV)

A variety of RNA and DNA viruses have been associated with human malignancies. Some viral agents have a clear causative role such as the Epstein-Barr virus (EBV) and certain papilloma viruses that are the etiologic agents in Burkitt's lymphoma and cervical carcinoma, respectively.

Viral oncogenes are carried by viruses into target cells, where they become firmly established. Clonal descendants then carry the viral genes that maintain the malignant phenotype of the cell clones.

The association of the DNA-related EBV with Burkitt's lymphoma was the first recognized link between a specific virus and a human malignant disease. Burkitt's lymphoma represents a well-characterized epidemiological entity in equatorial Africa and is found less frequently elsewhere. In nonendemic areas such as Europe and the United States, it has been shown that only 15% to 18% of the Burkitt's type of malignant lymphomas in children are associated with EBV. Among adolescents in western countries, EBV is the etiological agent in the nonmalignant disorder infectious mononucleosis.

Human T Cell Leukemia Viruses

The first member of the HTLV family of viruses was isolated in 1978. Since this discovery, an enormous amount of accumulated data has established this viral family as the etiological agent of unusually aggressive forms of adult T cell leukemia or lymphoma. HTLV is the first RNA tumor virus (retrovirus) known to occur in humans. The original isolates of HTLV were obtained from two adult patients from the United States who had aggressive T cell disorders. This historic discovery was made possible because of the availability of a protein called T cell growth factor (TCGF) or interleukin-2 (IL-2), which was discovered in 1976. This factor allows for the growth of mature human T cells in long-term cultures.

These original American isolates, as well as additional isolates from Japan and the Caribbean, were shown by core and envelope protein analysis serology and nucleic acid studies to be closely related to each other and were designated as HTLV-I. Subsequently, specimens from two patients were discovered to have a member of the HTLV family that was related to HTLV-I but was distinct from it. Core and envelope protein analysis and nucleic acid studies established these isolates to be HTLV-II and HTLV-III (now called HIV).

With the original American virus isolates in 1978 and subsequent Caribbean and Japanese isolates, researchers recognized that adult T cell leukemia (ATL) was a distinct clinical entity. Cases of ATL have since been recognized in the United States and patients with HTLV-associated lymphoma have been identified.

The prevalence of HTLV-I and HTLV-II varies widely among drug abusers in the United States according to geography, age, and race. In contrast, HTLV-I and HTLV-II are rare among drug abusers in the United Kingdom.

HTLV-I

HTLV-I was the first retrovirus to be isolated from patients suffering from aggressive T cell cancers with skin involvement. Although these patients were actually suffering from ATL, they were originally diagnosed as having mycosis fungoides or Sézary syndrome. ATL represents a high proportion of the lymphomas seen in part of the Caribbean. Although cases of ATL occur in the United States, they have been unusual. HTLV-I has also been associated with the rare tropical neurological illness acute spastic hemiplegia or paraplegia and perhaps other neurological problems. It has been suggested that other lymphoreticular malignancies may be directly or indirectly associated with HTLV-I, and that seropositive persons may be at increased risk for infections.

The features of ATL are clinical rather than histological and are characterized by onset in adulthood, dermal involvement, lymphadenopathy, and splenomegaly. Evidence of a disorder of calcium, including hypercalcemia and lytic bone lesions (nonmalignant), is common. Patients may have a circulating leukemia as well. The leukemic cells have mature T cell properties and morphologically distinctive features. Although the malignant ATL cells in some individuals have been shown to have suppressor function, they are T4+. Patients with ATL have a poor prognosis, often dying within a year of disease onset despite therapy. Subtypes of ATL may include subacute and chronic forms. Some overlap may exist with cutaneous T cell lymphomas and T cell chronic lymphocytic leukemias.

HTLV-I may be indirectly involved in some B cell leukemias in endemic areas, including Alaska, and among rural blacks residing in the southeastern portions of the United States and in the Caribbean islands. In general, the prevalence of antibodies against HTLV-I is high in southern Japan and the Caribbean, where approximately 5% to 10% of the population has antibody. In Africa, the results are inconsistent, ranging from 0 to 4%. The prevalence of antibodies in the United States is less than 1% but may be slightly higher in the southern states and among blacks. Prevalence increases with age and may be more common in older women than men.

HTLV-II

HTLV-II was isolated in 1981 and has only been marginally studied. The first isolate of HTLV-II, "mo," was isolated from a patient with hairy cell leukemia of a very rare T cell variety; infections are uncommon but increasing in frequency. HTLV-II has been isolated from a New York City drug abuser with *Pneumocystis carinii* pneumonia and a hemophilia A patient. In part, the disease association and natural history of HTLV-II remain difficult to establish because of the extensive serological cross-reactivities between this agent and the apparently more common HTLV-I. The two agents share about 60% homology, which accounts for the cross-reactivity.

HIV

HIV is the etiological agent in acquired immunodeficiency syndrome (see Chapter 17). This virus is now believed to be only distantly related to HTLV-I and HTLV-II and is recognized as the clinical entity characterized by helper T cell depletion and immunodeficiency.

HIV belongs to the retrovirus group, and since its discovery, much has been learned about the impact of the virus on human cells. Retroviruses carry a single, positive-stranded RNA and use a special enzyme, called **reverse transcriptase,** to convert viral RNA into DNA. This reverses the normal process of transcription where DNA is converted to RNA—hence, the term **retrovirus.**

DEMOGRAPHIC DISTRIBUTION OF LEUKEMIA

The number of new cases annually of all types of leukemia in the United States is approximately 68 per 1 million persons in the general population. The overall occurrence of leukemia can be correlated with a variety of factors, including ethnic origin, race, age, and gender.

Ethnic Origin and Race

Although leukemia occurs worldwide, the highest incidence is in the Scandinavian countries and Israel, whereas the lowest incidence is in Japan and Chile. In whites, chronic lymphocytic leukemia accounts for over 20% of the new cases of leukemia, but among Asians it is rare. Deaths due to leukemia are higher among the white American population than among American blacks.

Age

Age has a marked correlation with the various types of leukemia seen. Acute lymphoblastic leukemia ranks first among nonaccidental causes of death in children. Over 40% of cancers in American children under the age of 15 years are either acute lymphoblastic leukemia or lymphoma, although leukemia in very young infants (under 18 months old) is generally of a myelogenous nature. Persons over 60 years old are more likely to develop chronic lymphocytic leukemia than other types of leukemias. The myelogenous leukemias, both acute and chronic forms, have a peak incidence among young and middle-aged adults.

Gender

Most forms of leukemia are diagnosed more frequently in American males than in females regardless of race or age, except among children under 18 months old. The gender differences tend to be most dramatic in chronic lymphocytic leukemia, where the male:female ratio is 2:1.

SUMMARY
Comparison of Leukemias and Lymphomas

Leukemias are neoplastic proliferative diseases that are characterized by an overproduction of immature or mature cells of various leukocyte types in the bone marrow and/or blood. Lymphomas are similar to leukemias; however, lymphomas are solid tumors of lymph nodes and associated tissues or bone marrow.

Forms of Leukemia

The clinical symptoms, the maturity of the affected cells, and the total leukocyte count determine whether a leukemia will be classified as **acute** or **chronic.** Acute leukemias are characterized as having symptoms of short duration, many immature cell forms in the bone marrow and/or peripheral blood, and an elevated total leukocyte count. Chronic leukemias have symptoms of long duration, mostly mature cell forms in the bone marrow and/or peripheral blood, and total leukocyte counts that range from extremely elevated to less than normal. The prognosis of survival in untreated acute forms is from several weeks to several months, com-

pared with the untreated chronic forms, which can have a prognosis of survival ranging from months to many years after diagnosis.

Classification of Leukemias

The commonly encountered types of leukemia are separated into three broad groupings by cell type: **myelogenous, monocytic,** and **lymphocytic.** When cell type, degree of maturity, and clinical symptoms are considered, the most frequently encountered traditional forms of leukocytic leukemia are these:

1. Acute or chronic myelogenous
2. Acute or chronic monocytic
3. Acute or chronic myelomonocytic
4. Acute or chronic lymphocytic

More uncommon forms of leukemia are these: acute undifferentiated (stem cell), eosinophilic, and basophilic. Overproliferation of eythrocytic and megakaryocytic cells, either solely or in combination with a leukocytic cell type, may also occur.

Prognosis and Treatment

Untreated leukemias and lymphomas are ultimately fatal. Since the advent of radiation therapy in the 1920s, the treatment of these malignancies has become more effective and less toxic, thereby increasing patient's expected longevity. Effective treatment requires selection of the proper mode and method of treatment. The time of administration of treatment can also have an effect (refer to Chapter 25 for applications of flow-cell cytometry). Specific treatment requires accurate diagnosis and classification of the disorder by the clinical laboratory.

Factors Related to the Occurrence of Leukemia

The occurrence of leukemias and lymphomas has been related to a variety of factors. These factors include:

1. Oncogenes
2. Ionizing radiation
3. Chemical exposure
4. Genetic factors
5. Infectious agents

Viruses are now known to be the etiological factor in certain leukemias and lymphomas. Although EBV was the first virus directly associated with a human malignant disorder, Burkitt's lymphoma, the discovery of HTLV-I in 1978 initiated a new era in the study of leukemia. HTLV-I has been identified as the etiological agent in ATL; HTLV-II is associated with hairy cell leukemia; and HTLV-III is the virus associated with AIDS.

Demographic Distribution of Leukemia

The overall occurrence of leukemia can be correlated with a variety of factors: ethnic origin, race, age, and gender.

BIBLIOGRAPHY

Blattner, W. A. et al. "Epidemiology of Human Lymphotropic Retroviruses: An Overview." *Cancer Res. Suppl.*, Vol. 45, September, 1985, pp. 4598–4601.

Boice, J. D. et al. "Diagnostic X-ray Procedures and Risk of Leukemia, Lymphoma, and Multiple Myeloma." *JAMA,* Vol. 265, March 13, 1991, pp. 1290–1294.

Buckley, J. D. et al. "Occupational Exposures of Parents of Children with Acute Nonlymphocytic Leukemia: A Report from the Children's Cancer Study Group." *JAMA,* Vol. 263, January 5, 1990, p. 100.

"Current Trends, Childhood Cancers—New Jersey, 1979–1985." *MMWR,* Vol. 40, No. 33, 1991, pp. 572–574.

DeThe, G., L. Gazzolo, and A. Gessain. "Viruses as Risk Factors or Causes of Human Leukemias and Lymphomas?" *Leuk. Res.,* Vol. 9, No. 6, 1985, pp. 691–696.

Hardy, I. et al. "The Incidence of Zoster After Immunization With Live Attenuated Varicella Vaccine. A Study in Children with Leukemia." *N. Engl. J. Med.,* Vol. 325, No. 22, November 28, 1991, pp. 1545–1550.

Hershey, D. W. "Detection of Minimal Residual Diseases in Childhood Leukemia With the Polymerase Chain Reaction." *N. Engl. J. Med.,* Vol. 324, No. 11, March 14, 1991, pp. 772–773.

Kleiler, K. R. "Lymphocytic Leukemia: A Review of the Literature." *Am. J. Med. Technol.,* Vol. 45, No. 6, 1979, pp. 590–599.

Miller, R. W. "The Features in Common Among Persons at High Risk of Leukemia," in *Cancer Epidemiology in the USA and USSR.* David L. Levin (ed.). Bethesda, MD: National Cancer Institute, 1980, pp. 125–127.

Neri, G. "Some Questions on the Significance of Chromosome Alterations in Leukemias and Lymphomas: A Review." *Am. J. Med. Genet.,* Vol. 18, 1984, pp. 471–481.

Neugut, A. I. et al. "Poor Survival of Treatment-Related Acute Nonlymphocytic Leukemia." *JAMA,* Vol. 264, No. 8, August 22/29, 1990, pp. 1006–1008.

Powers, L. W. and M. K. Register. "Down Syndrome and Acute Leukemia: Epidemiological and Genetic Relationships." *Lab. Med.,* Vol. 22, No. 9, September, 1991, pp. 630–636.

Pui, C. H. et al. "Acute Myeloid Leukemia in Children Treated with Epipodophyllotoxins for Acute Lymphoblastic Leukemia." *N. Engl. J. Med.,* Vol. 325, No. 24, December 12, 1991, pp. 1682–1687.

Stevens, W. et al. "Leukemia in Utah and Radioactive Fallout From the Nevada Test Site. A Case-Control Study." *JAMA,* Vol. 264, No. 5, August, 1990, pp. 585–591.

Weiss, S. H. and R. J. Biggar. "The Epidemiology of Human Retrovirus-Associated Illnesses." *Mt. Sinai J. Med.,* Vol. 53, No. 8, December, 1986, pp. 579–587.

Windebank, K. P. et al. "Acute Megakaryocytic Leukemia (M7) in Children." *Mayo Clin. Proc.,* Vol. 64, November, 1989, pp. 1339–1351.

Wing, S. et al. "Mortality Among Workers at Oak Ridge National Laboratory." *JAMA,* Vol. 265, No. 11, March 10, 1991, pp. 1397–1408.

REVIEW QUESTIONS

1. A definition of a leukemia could include:

   A. An overproduction of leukocytes.
   B. Solid, malignant tumors of the lymph nodes.
   C. Trespassing the blood-tissue barrier.
   D. Both A and C.

2. Descriptive terms for most lymphomas can include:

   A. A nonneoplastic proliferative disease.
   B. A solid malignant tumor of the lymph nodes.
   C. A lymphocytopenia.
   D. Freely trespassing the blood-brain barrier.

3. An acute leukemia can be described as:

   A. Of short duration with many mature leukocyte forms in the peripheral blood.
   B. Of short duration with many immature leukocyte forms in the peripheral blood.
   C. Of short duration with little alteration of the leukocytes of the peripheral blood.
   D. Of long duration with many mature leukocyte forms in the peripheral blood.

4. The etiological agents of leukemias can include:

   A. Ionizing radiation.
   B. Certain infectious agents.
   C. Chemical exposure to benzene.
   D. All of the above.

5. HIV is associated with:

   A. Hairy cell leukemia.   C. AIDS.
   B. Sézary cell syndrome.   D. Lymphoma.

6. The incidence of leukemia is higher in:

   A. Scandinavian versus Japanese populations.
   B. American blacks versus white Americans.
   C. Chronic forms in children versus chronic forms in adults.
   D. Acute forms in older adults versus acute forms in children.

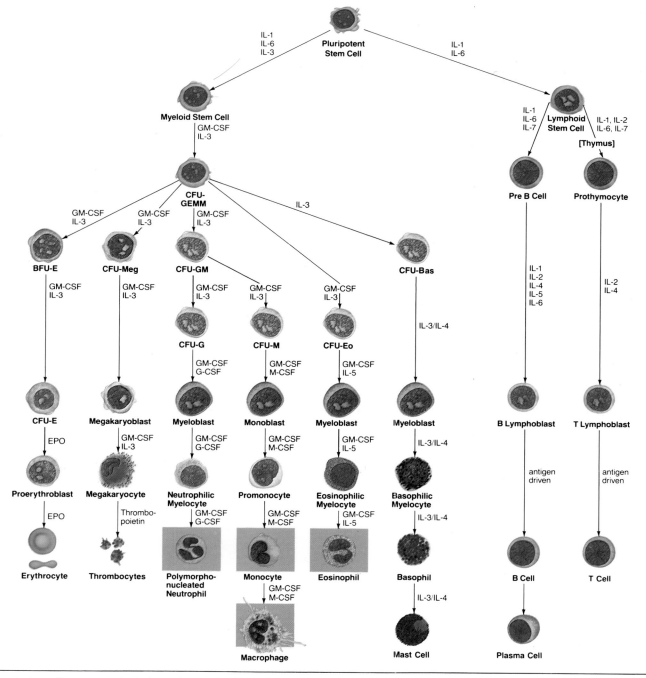

1. Regulation of hematopoiesis by colony stimulating factor.

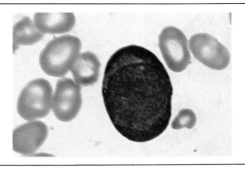

2. Rubriblast (pronormoblast).

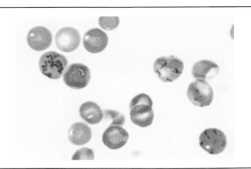

6. Reticulocyte.

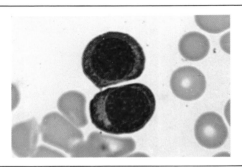

3. Prorubricyte (basophilic normoblast).

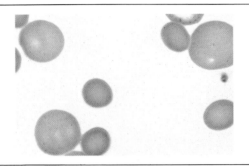

7. Polychromatophilia.

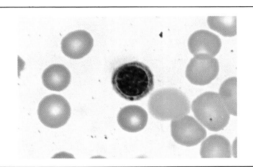

4. Rubricyte (polychromic normoblast).

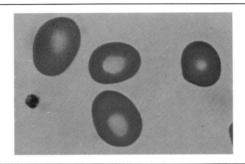

8. Macroovalocytes (oval macrocytes).

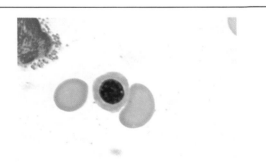

5. Metarubricyte (orthochromic normoblast).

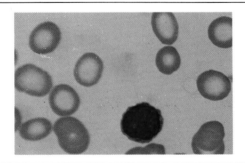

9. Microcytes.

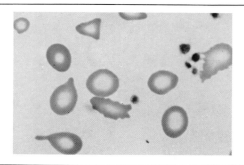

10. Poikilocytes.

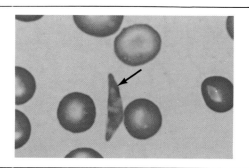

14. Sickle cell (*arrow*).

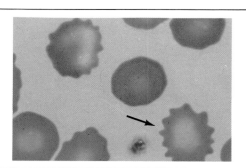

11. Burr cells. The *arrow* points to a typical Burr cell.

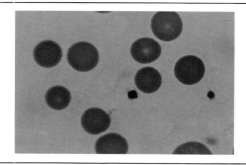

15. Spherocytes.

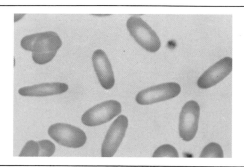

12. Elliptocytes.

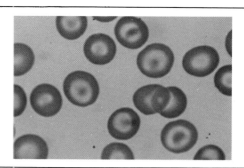

16. Target cells.

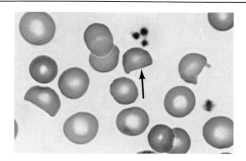

13. Helmet cells. The *arrow* points to one of several helmet cells present in this microscopic field.

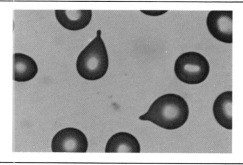

17. Teardrop cells.

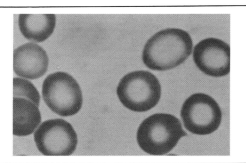

18. Hypochromia.

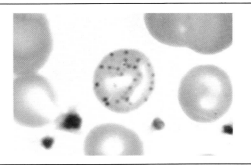

19. Basophilic stippling.

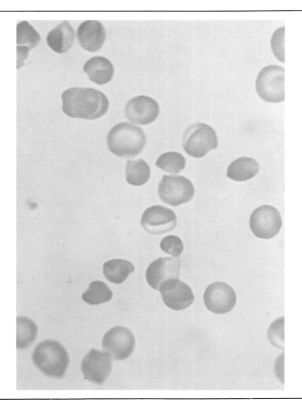

20. Hemoglobin C disease.

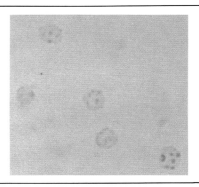

21. Heinz bodies (crystal violet stain).

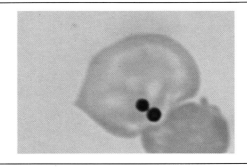

22. Howell-Jolly bodies.

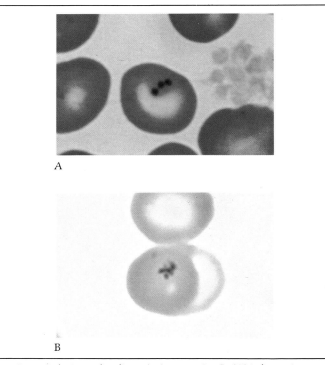

A

B

23. Pappenheimer bodies. A. Iron stain. B. Wright stain.

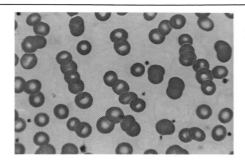
24. Rouleaux formation.

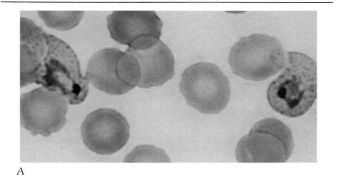

A

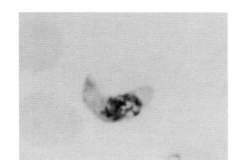

B

25. Malaria. A. *Plasmodium vivax.* B. *Plasmodium falciparum.*

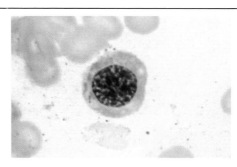

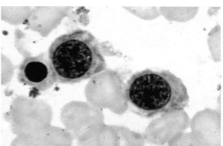

26. Megalocytes.

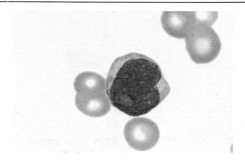

27. Myeloblast.

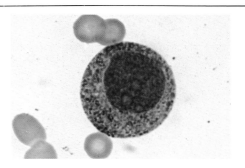

28. Promyelocyte.

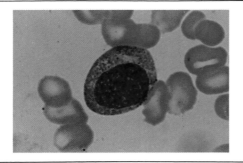

29. Myelocyte.

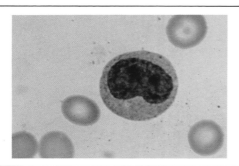

30. Metamyelocyte.

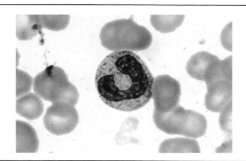

31. Band neutrophil.

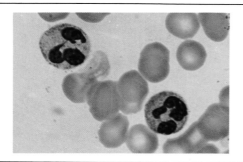

32. Segmented neutrophil.

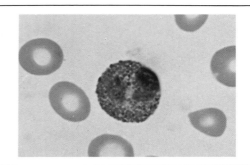

33. Eosinophil.

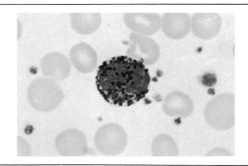

34. Basophil.

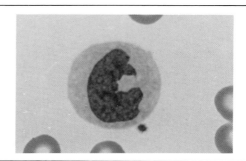

35. Monocyte.

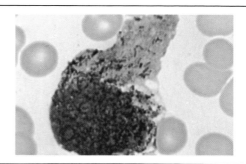

36. Macrophage (bone marrow).

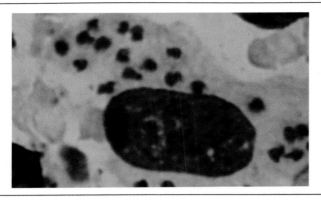

37. Leishmann-Donovan bodies.

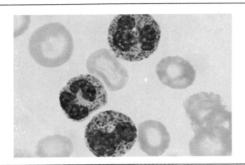

38. Toxic granulation.

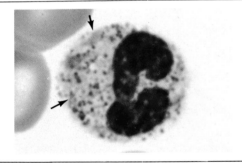

39. Döhle bodies (*arrows*) and toxic granulation in leukocytic cytoplasm.

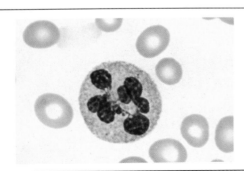

40. Hypersegmentation.

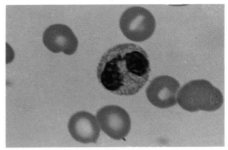

A

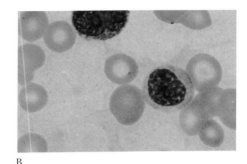

B

41. Pelger-Huët anomaly. A. Heterozygous. B. Homozygous.

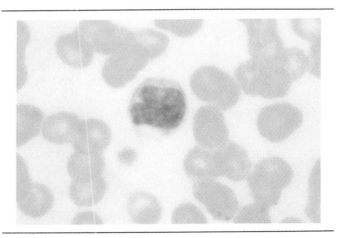

42. May-Hegglin anomaly.

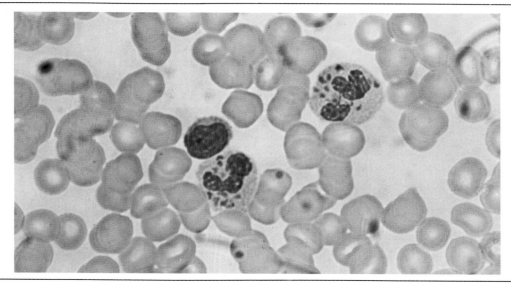

43. Chédiak-Higashi syndrome.

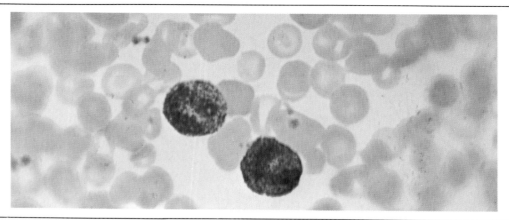

44. Alder-Reilly inclusions.

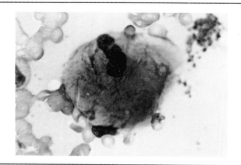

45. Gaucher's cell (histiocyte).

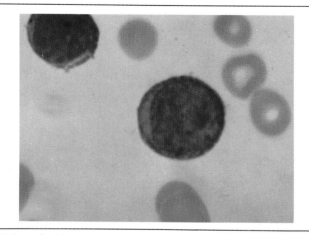

46. Lymphoblast.

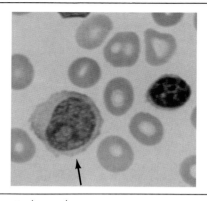

47. Prolymphocyte (*arrow*).

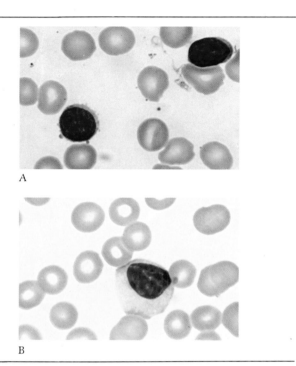

A

B

48. Mature lymphocytes. A. Small. B. Large.

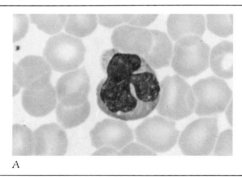

A

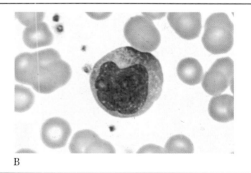

B

49. Variant lymphocytes. A. Monocytoid nucleus.
B. Nucleoli.

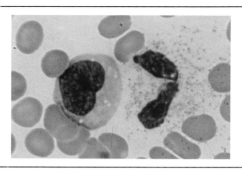

50. Vacuolated lymphocytes.

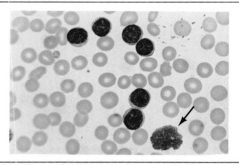

51. Smudge cell (*arrow*) and six mature lymphocytes in chronic lymphocytic leukemia (CLL).

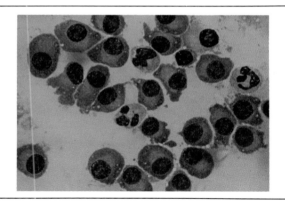

52. Plasma cells.

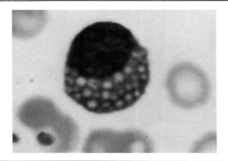

53. Mott cell (Russell bodies).

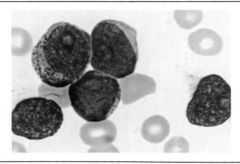

54. Acute myelogenous leukemia (FAB M1).

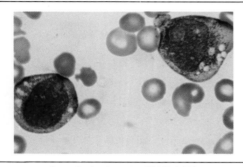

55. Acute promyelocytic leukemia (FAB M3).

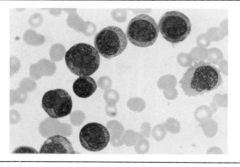

56. Acute myelomonocytic leukemia (FAB M4).

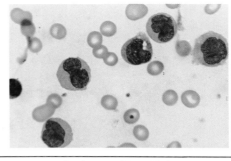

57. Acute monocytic leukemia (FAB M5).

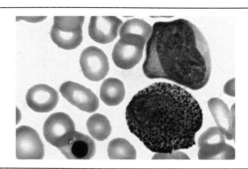

58. Erythroleukemia (FAB M6).

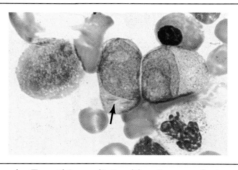

59. Auer rods. Two thin, splinter-like Auer rods (*arrow*) are present in the cytoplasm of this immature leukocyte.

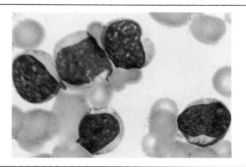

60. Acute lymphoblastic leukemia (ALL).

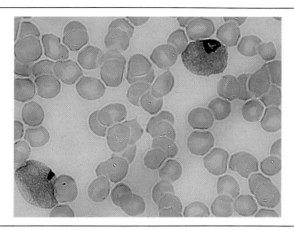

61. FAB M1 stained for Sudan black B. Note the similarity of structure to that seen in Plate 62.

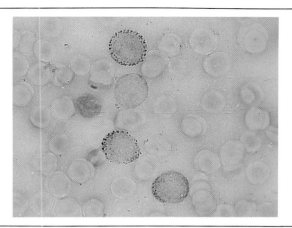

63. Periodic acid-Schiff (PAS) reactivity. The lymphoblasts demonstrate dots or blocks of PAS-reactive material circumscribing the cell.

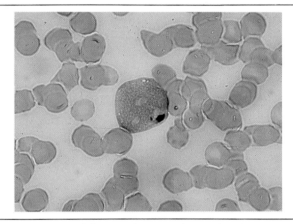

62. FAB M1 stained for myeloperoxidase. The distinctly stained structure is a so-called phi body, which may prove pathognomonic of acute myelogenous (granulocytic) leukemia.

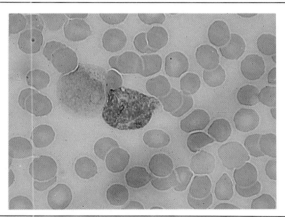

64. FAB M2 stained for naphthol AS-D chloracetate esterase. The more primitive cell is unstained.

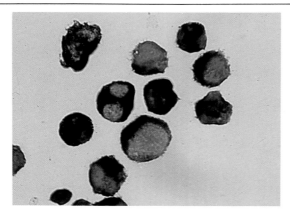

A

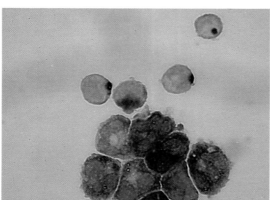

B

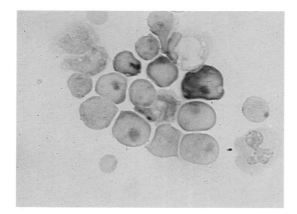

C

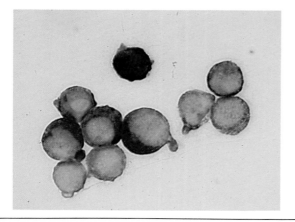

D

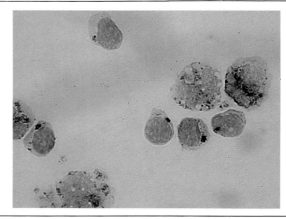

66. Cytospin preparation from normal individual stained for acid phosphatase. The lymphocytes displaying a single focal area of activity are T cells.

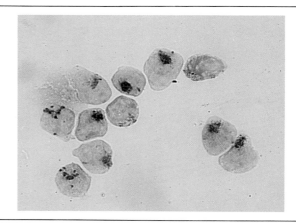

67. FAB L1 stained for acid phosphatase. Blasts demonstrate intense Golgi reactivity characteristic of T-cell disease.

65. A. FAB M5 stained for alpha-naphthyl acetate esterase. Cells of monocytic origin demonstrate an intense black granular stain. B. Cytospin preparation demonstrating alpha-naphthyl butyrate esterase from healthy individuals. Note the focal staining characteristic of T lymphocytes and the intense diffuse staining of monocytes. C. FAB L2 stained for alpha-naphthyl butyrate esterase. The focal stain is evident but of less intensity than seen in B. Cells arrested at an earlier stage of development do not stain. D. FAB M5 stained for alpha-naphthyl butyrate esterase showing an intense positive reaction indicative of a monocytic cell line.

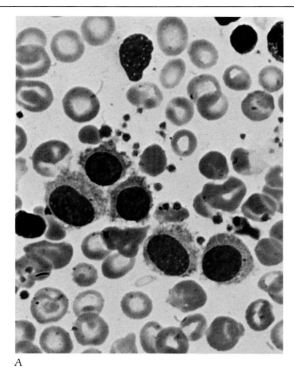

A

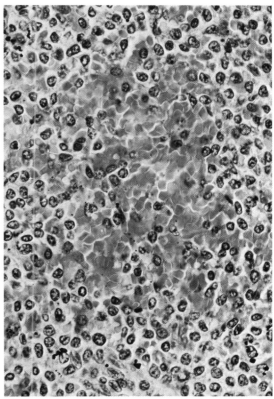

C

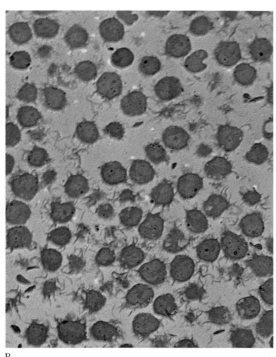

B

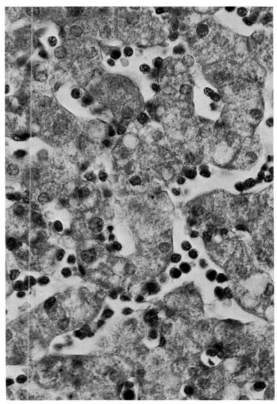

D

68. Morphology of hairy cell leukemia (HCL) cells. A. Romanovsky-stained blood smear. B. Thin section of hairy leukemic cells stained with toluidine blue; the characteristic "hairy" appearance of cells is seen. C. Spleen section in hairy cell leukemia showing a thick conglomerate of hairy cells and erythrocytes (pseudoinfarctual area). D. Liver section in HCL showing accumulation of leukemic cells in the liver sinusoids.

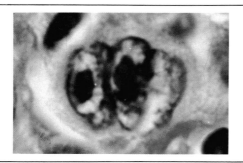

69. Reed-Sternberg cells.

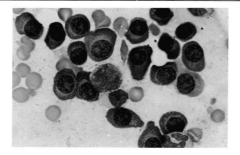

70. Plasma cells.

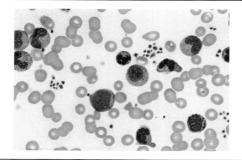

71. Chronic myelogenous leukemia (CML).

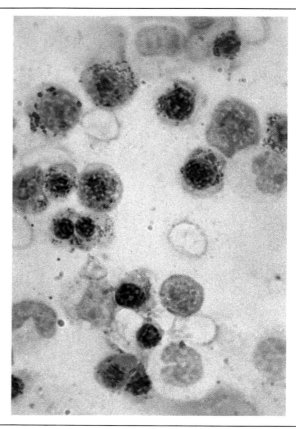

72. Prussian blue stain showing free iron granules distributed throughout the cytoplasm of most of the erythroblasts, either as confluent clumped masses or arranged as a ring around the nuclei ("ringed sideroblasts").

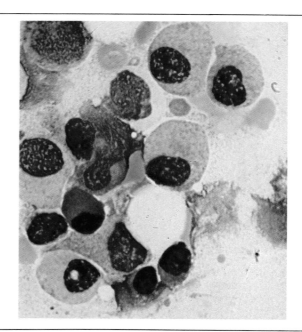

73. Myelodysplastic syndrome (refractory anemia with erythroblastopenia and excess blasts; RAEB). Myelocytes with very few granules and coarse nuclear chromatin are prominent.

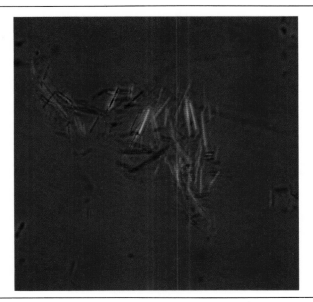

74. A group of negatively birefringent monosodium urate (MSU) crystals.

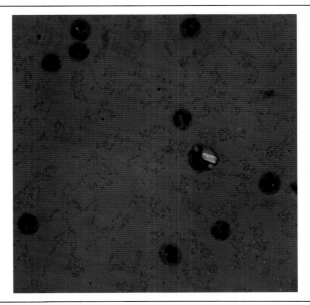

75. A phagocytosed calcium pyrophosphate dihydrate (CPPD) crystal in a synovial fluid leukocyte, seen on Wright's stained smear.

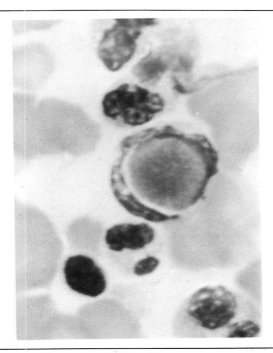

76. Lupus erythematosus (LE) cell.

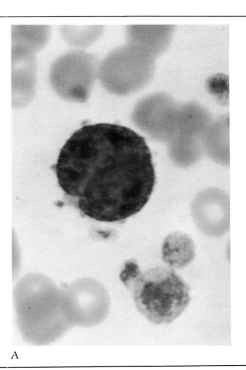

A

77. A. Megakaryoblast.

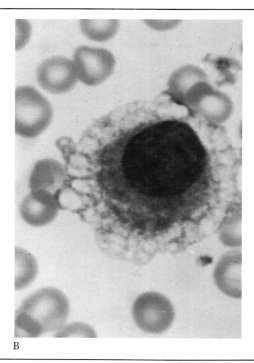

B

77. B. Promegakaryocyte.

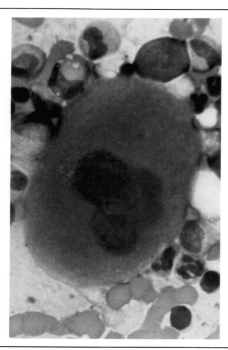

78. Megakaryocyte.

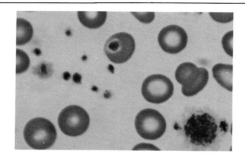

79. Platelets.

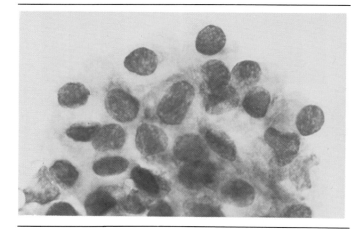

80. A cluster of ependymal cells in CSF.

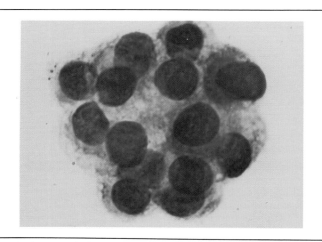

81. A cluster of choroid plexus cells in CSF.

Acute Leukemias

OBJECTIVES

General characteristics
- Describe the general characteristics of the acute leukemias.

Categories
- Name and briefly describe the classification of leukemias according to the French-American-British (FAB) system.

Acute nonlymphoblastic leukemias
- List and name the various types of acute leukemias, including the FAB nomenclature.
- Describe the clinical symptoms and laboratory findings, including peripheral blood morphology, of acute myelogenous, acute promyelocytic, acute myelomonocytic, and acute monocytic leukemia.
- Explain some of the general features of eosinophilic leukemia, basophilic leukemia, and erythroleukemia.

Acute lymphoblastic leukemia
- Describe the clinical symptoms, laboratory findings, and special identification techniques in acute lymphoblastic leukemia.

Electron microscope examination
- Describe the ultrastructure of myeloblasts, monoblasts, and lymphoblasts.

Cytogenetic analysis
- Explain the chromosomal alterations that may be observed in various myelogenous and lymphoblastic leukemias.

Chemical methods of cellular identification
- Explain the principle and purpose of the Sudan black B stain.
- Describe the location of myeloperoxidase in blood cells and explain the purpose of the test.
- State the biochemical class that the periodic acid–Schiff test detects, and describe the purpose of the test.
- Compare the two common esterase procedures in terms of their purposes.

Monoclonal antibodies
- Describe the utility of monoclonal antibodies in differentiating between various leukocytic disorders.

Case studies
- Apply the laboratory data to the stated case studies and discuss the implications of these cases to the study of hematology.

*E*ach type of leukemia, acute or chronic, has unique characteristics. The general characteristics, classification, clinical symptoms, and laboratory data of the various types of acute leukemias are presented in this chapter.

GENERAL CHARACTERISTICS

As a group, the acute leukemias are characterized by the presence of blasts and immature leukocytic forms in the peripheral blood and bone marrow. Anemia is usually present, caused by bleeding, possible secondary anemia, and the replacement of normal marrow elements by leukemic blasts. Although the total leukocyte count is usually elevated, some patients may demonstrate normal or decreased leukocyte counts. Thrombocytopenia is also usually present in the acute leukemias.

Nearly 70% of adult patients with acute leukemia ultimately die of infection. The median survival time for an untreated patient with acute leukemia is 3 months. Ninety percent of children and 70% of adults achieve at least one remission. Modern treatment methods have produced a high rate of survival in children.

The best time to achieve the longest remission and possible cure of acute leukemia via maximum cell kill is when the disease is first diagnosed. Because treatment regimens vary, accurate diagnosis of the acute types of leukemia is critically important.

CATEGORIES

The two major divisions of the acute leukemias are the acute nonlymphoblastic leukemias (ANLLs) and acute lymphoblastic leukemias (ALLs). In 1976, a group of seven French, American, and British hematologists proposed a system of nomenclature, the **French-American-British (FAB)** classification system. This FAB classification is based on the morphological characteristics of Wright-stained cells in periph-

eral blood or bone marrow. Special cytochemical stains are used as supplementary sources of information.

Since its introduction, the FAB classification (Table 19.1) has been widely accepted internationally. The system groups ANLL into seven categories (M1 through M7) and ALL into three categories (L1 through L3). In a revision of the original criteria, over 30% blasts in the marrow suffice for the diagnosis of acute leukemia in any of the six categories including M1 to M6.

The myelogenous subcategories (M1, M2, and M3) reflect three maturational phases of myelogenous leukemias. M4 represents a combination of myelogenous and monocytic leukemias. M5 is the designated category for monocytic leukemias with additional subcategories. The M6 category is reserved for erythroleukemias, an abnormality of both erythrocytic and myelogenous cell lines. M7 is the designation for megakaryocytic leukemias. The lymphoblastic types (L1 through L3) are classified according to cell size, nuclear chromatin patterns, nuclear shape, the presence of nucleoli, and the amount and coloration of the cytoplasm.

ACUTE NONLYMPHOBLASTIC LEUKEMIAS

Among the acute forms of myelogenous leukemia, some forms are more common than others. When a population of 358 untreated patients, children and adults, with acute myelogenous leukemia were classified, FAB M2 represented about 45% of the cases and FAB M4 represented 19% of the cases. Together these two types comprised the majority of the cases. The least common varieties were FAB M3 and FAB M5B.

Acute Myelogenous Leukemia (FAB M1)

This form of leukemia is the most common type of leukemia in the first few months of life; however, it typically occurs in middle-aged adults with a median age of 46 years. The typical male-female ratio of FAB M1 is 1:1. The median survival time is 3-1/2 months after diagnosis.

TABLE 19.1 **The FAB Classification System**

M1 myelogenous	Blasts and promyelocytes predominate without further maturation of myelogenous cells
M2 myelogenous	Myelogenous cells demonstrate maturation beyond the blast and promyelocyte stage
M3 promyelocytic	Promyelocytes predominate in the bone marrow
M4 myelomonocytic	Both myelogenous and monocytic cells are present to the extent of at least 20% of the total leukocytes
M5 monocytic	Most cells are monocytic; two subtypes are recognized, one characterized by large blasts in bone marrow and peripheral blood, the other (differentiated type) by monoblasts, promonocytes, and monocytes
M6 erythroleukemia	Known as Di Guglielmo syndrome; abnormal proliferation of both erythroid and granulocytic precursors; may include abnormal megakaryocytic and monocytic proliferations
M7 megakaryocytic	Large and small megakaryoblasts with a high nuclear-cytoplasmic ratio; pale, agranular cytoplasm
L1 homogeneous	One population of cells within the case. Small cells predominant; nuclear shape is regular with an occasional cleft; chromatin pattern is homogeneous and nucleoli are rarely visible; cytoplasm is moderately basophilic
L2 heterogeneous	Large cells with an irregular nuclear shape; clefts in the nucleus are common; one or more large nucleoli are visible; cytoplasm varies in color
L3 Burkitt's lymphoma type	Cells are large and homogeneous in size; nuclear shape is round or oval; one to three prominent nucleoli; cytoplasm is deeply basophilic with vacuoles often prominent

Clinical Signs and Symptoms

FAB M1 is characterized by either a rapid or gradual onset that may resemble an acute infection. The patient may have a history of fever, infections, fatigue, and bleeding episodes. Physical examination may reveal tenderness of the bones, particularly the ribs and sternum; ulcerated mucous membranes; petechiae; and purpura. Additional physical findings may include hepatomegaly, splenomegaly, and lymphadenopathy; however, about 50% of patients exhibit no organomegaly or lymphadenopathy.

Cellular infiltration of organs is less prominent in ANLL compared to ALL. Occasional localized tumor masses consisting of myeloblasts may arise in bone or soft tissues in patients with acute myelogenous leukemia. In these tumors, the presence of large quantities of the enzyme myeloperoxidase produces a green appearance if the tissue is cut. This type of tumor is referred to as a **chloroma.** In some cases, the appearance of these tumors is an early sign of acute myelogenous leukemia.

Laboratory Data

Anemia and thrombocytopenia are present in approximately 85% of all acute myelogenous leukemias. Leukocytosis is encountered in more than one third of patients, and the total leukocyte count is usually greater than 100×10^9/L.

The peripheral blood smear does not usually exhibit many immature erythrocytes, which are more common in other forms of acute leukemia. If severe disruption of erythrocyte development does occur and many immature forms are present, the leukemia is possibly an erythroleukemia (FAB M6).

The outstanding feature of the peripheral blood smear (Fig. 19.1 and Plate 54) and bone marrow is the predominance of myeloblasts. These blasts usually have a regular cytoplasmic outline and may contain slender, red-staining

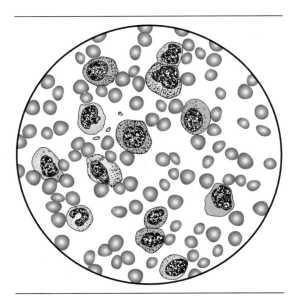

FIGURE 19.1 Acute myelogenous leukemia. Increased numbers of immature cells are seen in acute leukemias. The predominating cells in this peripheral blood smear are myeloblasts and promyelocytes. The number of platelets (thrombocytes) is severely decreased. (Simulates magnification ×1000.)

Auer rods in the cytoplasm. The nuclear chromatin is very fine and homogeneous. Three to five nucleoli are usually evident. Some differential development of the myeloid cell line may be noted. Depending on the type, some promyelocytes may be present. Agranular or hypogranular segmented neutrophils may be seen (acquired Pelger-Huët anomaly). Abnormal eosinophils may also be seen. Monocytes usually constitute less than 1% of the nucleated cells in the peripheral blood.

Acute Myelogenous Leukemia (FAB M2)

The FAB M2 form of leukemia typically occurs in middle-aged persons. The median age of occurrence is 48 years; however, about 40% of cases occur in individuals 60 years or older. The approximate male-female ratio is 1.6:1. The median survival time is 8-1/2 months.

Clinical Signs and Symptoms

Hemorrhagic manifestations such as easy bruising, epistaxis, gingival bleeding, and petechiae are common initial symptoms. Hepatomegaly, splenomegaly, and lymphadenopathy are seen infrequently.

Laboratory Data

Anemia and thrombocytopenia are present in most cases. Leukocytosis is commonly seen, with rare patients having total leukocyte counts exceeding 300×10^9/L.

Myeloblasts predominate on peripheral blood smears. The nuclei are usually round or oval with one or more prominent nucleoli and fine reticular chromatin. The cytoplasm is basophilic with a variable number of azurophilic granules. Auer rods are commonly seen. Maturation of the granulocytic cell line is also observed.

Acute Promyelocytic Leukemia (FAB M3)

In acute promyelocytic leukemia the median age of occurrence is 38 years, with a median survival of about 16 months. The approximate male-female ratio is 2:1.

Clinical Signs and Symptoms

Fatigue and symptoms of bleeding such as bruising, hematuria, and petechiae are common. Hepatomegaly, splenomegaly, and lymphadenopathy are seen infrequently.

Laboratory Data

Laboratory findings may be similar to those of the FAB M2 type. Anemia and thrombocytopenia are present in most cases. Total leukocyte counts range from conditions of leukopenia to leukocytosis. Leukopenia is seen frequently. Promyelocytes are the predominating cell type (Plate 55). The promyelocytes may be hypergranular, microgranular, or hypogranular variations. Coarsely granular promyelocytes with dumbbell-shaped or bilobed nuclei may be seen. The nuclear chromatin is finely reticular and the cells often lack nucleoli. Myeloblasts and cells at the myelocyte level of development may also be present and contain many small Auer rods. An increased incidence of disseminated intravascular coagulation (DIC) (see Chapter 27) is common.

Acute Myelomonocytic Leukemia (FAB M4)

This form of leukemia may also be referred to as **Naegeli-type** monocytic leukemia. Occurrence of this form of leukemia is uncommon in children and young adults. The highest frequency of occurrence is in adults over 50 years old. The average male-female ratio is 1.4:1. Most forms of myelomonocytic leukemia are of the acute form, with the average length of survival being about 8 months.

Clinical Signs and Symptoms

Symptoms of this form of leukemia are similar to those of other forms of acute leukemia. Fatigue, fever, and bleeding manifestations are common. Pharyngitis may be observed. Hepatomegaly and splenomegaly are seen in about one third of patients. Gingival hyperplasia due to leukemic infiltration may be noted.

Patients with FAB M4 or FAB M5 leukemia or ALL (predominantly of the T-cell type) with hyperleukocytosis (an excessive increase in the total leukocyte count) are at risk of developing leukostasis. **Leukostasis** refers to a pathological finding of slightly dilated, thin-walled vessels filled with leukemic cells. The brain and lungs are the most commonly involved organs. Symptoms of leukostasis are headache, visual impairment, and shortness of breath.

Laboratory Data

In FAB M4, proliferation of granulocytes and monocytes is characteristic. Anemia and thrombocytopenia are present. The total leukocyte count varies from leukopenia to leukocytosis. The total leukocyte count rarely exceeds $100 \times 10^9/L$. In many patients, the absolute monocyte count reaches or exceeds $5 \times 10^9/L$ in the peripheral blood.

On a peripheral blood smear (Plate 56), early myelogenous cells predominate, but approximately 20% of the cellular elements are monocytes. The blasts may have indented and convoluted nuclei as in monocytes. The number of nucleoli averages from three to five. Auer rods may be present. Promyelocytes are often present but do not predominate. Agranular and hypogranular neutrophils may be seen and acquired pseudo-Pelger-Huët anomaly may be noted. The number of platelets is usually reduced. Erythrocytic precursors are not usually seen. DIC can be observed.

Acute Monocytic Leukemia (FAB M5)

Pure monocytic leukemia is uncommon and comprises less than 15% of all leukemias. Two forms, FAB M5A and FAB M5B, have been distinguished. The FAB M5A form is most common in young adults (median age of 16 years); the FAB M5B form has a peak occurrence characteristically during middle age (median age of 49 years). The male-female ratio is about 0.7:1 in the M5A form; the male-female ratio is approximately 1.8:1 in the M5B form. Because this form of acute leukemia is very resistant to therapy, the life expectancy is short, ranging from 5 to 8 months depending on the type.

Clinical Signs and Symptoms

The onset of this form of leukemia is dramatic, headaches and fevers being the chief complaints. Typical symptoms of monocytic leukemia additionally include fatigue, weight loss, and bleeding from the mouth or nose. Physical examination frequently reveals gingival (mouth and gums) hyperplasia, as in myelomonocytic leukemia; pallor; and skin lesions. Enlargement of the lymph nodes and spleen is uncommon. Extramedullary masses may be seen in about one third of patients.

Laboratory Data

As in other forms of acute leukemia, anemia and thrombocytopenia are usually evident. The total leukocyte count ranges from 15 to $100 \times 10^9/L$. Peripheral blood smears (Plate 57) normally exhibit a high proportion of blast forms. Monocytes and promonocytes constitute 25% to 75% of the nucleated cells. Blasts frequently have a "muddy" or "smoggy" gray-blue cytoplasm containing tiny granules, and pseudopods are common. The nucleus has a reticular granular chromatin pattern and may contain from one to five large nucleoli. A few immature erythrocytes may be seen occasionally.

Erythroleukemia (FAB M6)

Erythroleukemia, also referred to as erythemic myelosis or Di Guglielmo leukemia, represents a proliferation of both immature granulocytic and erythrocytic cell types (Plate 58). This form of leukemia is usually acute. The median age of occurrence is 54 years; usually, more than half of patients are over 50 years old. The male-female ratio is 1.4:1. The average length of survival is 11 months.

Clinical Signs and Symptoms

A common presenting symptom is a bleeding manifestation. Hepatomegaly, splenomegaly, and lymphadenopathy are infrequently observed.

Laboratory Data

Blast cells of erythroid and myelogenous origin are found in both the bone marrow and the peripheral blood. Erythroblasts on blood smears typically have an irregular outline with a high nuclear-cytoplasmic ratio. Some of the blasts exhibit the intense blue color associated with rubriblasts. Blasts of myelogenous origin may have Auer rods (Plate 59). Promyelocytes may also be present as well as monocytes and promonocytes.

Selected Examples of Unusual Forms

Eosinophilic Leukemia

Eosinophilic leukemia is extremely rare, although it can be indistinguishable from reactive eosinophilia or chronic myelogenous leukemia. If eosinophilic leukemia is present, it is usually acute. Death generally occurs within a year. Tissue infiltration and cardiac failure have been described in this form of leukemia. Signs and symptoms include a chronic cough, pulmonary infiltration by leukocytes, and central nervous system involvement.

Twenty percent of patients demonstrate anemia and thrombocytopenia. Leukocytosis with total leukocyte counts of 50 to 200 $\times$ 10^9/L may exist. A few patients may have absolute eosinophil counts greater than 100 $\times$ 10^9/L. On peripheral blood smears, more than 60% of the leukocytes can be eosinophils. These cells are usually mature with segmented nuclei; however, the granules may not have the typical appearance of eosinophils. The granules may not stain uniformly, and some of the granules may appear empty. In the terminal phases of this leukemia, blasts may constitute 80% of the nucleated cells. Abnormal eosinophils are often present in small numbers in all leukemias.

Basophilic Leukemia

Basophilic leukemia (mast cell leukemia) is the rarest form of all leukemias. Frequently, an infiltration of mast cells in large numbers into affected skin is observed. Patients with this form of leukemia generally exhibit leukocytosis, with total leukocyte counts exceeding 30 $\times$ 10^9/L. Peripheral blood smears can demonstrate greater than 50% basophils in this disorder.

ACUTE LYMPHOBLASTIC LEUKEMIA

General Characteristics

The predominant type of leukemia in children 2 to 10 years old is lymphoblastic leukemia of the acute type. Ninety percent of childhood leukemias in western cultures are of the acute lymphoblastic variety. A second peak in the incidence of this form of leukemia occurs in adults later in life.

ALL is divided into FAB L1 (children), L2 (older children and adults), and L3 (patients with leukemia arising secondary to Burkitt's lymphoma).

Clinical Signs and Symptoms

The history of symptoms in ALL can vary from a few days to a few weeks. Symptoms can include fatigue, fever, infection, headache, nausea, and vomiting. Bone and joint pain related to the replacement of normal hematopoietic elements is common. Pain in the extremities, particularly the legs, is produced by an infiltration of leukemic cells into the tissues. Physical examination may reveal petechiae or other evidence of hemorrhage, and pallor. Gastrointestinal hemorrhage and hematuria are less common findings. Lymphadenopathy and hepatomegaly are present in 75% of patients. Leukemic meningitis and cranial nerve palsies due to nerve infiltration by leukemic blasts are quite common. Nephropathy may be present but is usually precipitated later by therapy that lyses the abundant leukocytes.

Laboratory Data

The total leukocyte count is elevated in 60% to 70% of patients, with total leukocyte counts ranging from 50 to 100 $\times$ 10^9/L. Less than 15% of patients have extreme leukocytosis with a total leukocyte count of over 100 $\times$ 10^9/L. In only about 25% of patients is a leukocytopenia present.

Peripheral blood smears (Fig. 19.2 and Plate 60) show a predominance of blast cells in about 50% of patients. In addition to blasts, the peripheral blood is usually composed of close to 100% lymphoblasts, lymphocytes, and smudge cells. The blast forms have one or two nucleoli in the nucleus, and Auer rods are absent from the cytoplasm. These blasts have a high nuclear-cytoplasmic ratio. The shape of the nucleus is usually round rather than indented or twisted. In addition, blood smears reveal a granulocytopenia, although some immature granulocytes are often seen in the blood as a response to leukemic replacement of the bone marrow. In the FAB L2 variety, the lymphoblasts may have indented nuclei and frequently show mature cells of the myelogenous type. Early forms of erythrocytes and megakaryocytes are absent in all forms of this type of leukemia. The presence of anemia, due to decreased red cell production and blood loss, and severe thrombocytopenia is remarkable on peripheral smears.

Patients may develop meningeal leukemia following prolonged remission without evidence of abnormalities in the peripheral blood or bone marrow. In adults, ALL is differentiated from lymphosarcoma by the presence of poorly differentiated lymphocytes, which may have prominent nucleoli.

Special Identification Techniques

Surface markers, proteins on the cell membrane that can be detected with immunologic reagents, are extremely helpful in differentiating ALL. Different proteins are expressed at different stages of maturation, which allows them to be used

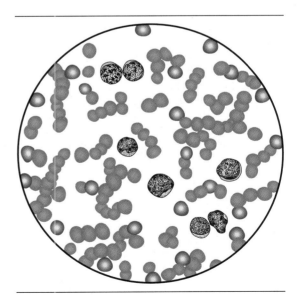

FIGURE 19.2 Acute lymphoblastic leukemia (ALL). Increased numbers of immature cells are seen in acute leukemias. The predominating cell in this peripheral blood smear is the lymphoblast. Blood platelets (thrombocytes) are completely absent from this field of the smear. (Simulates magnification $\times$1000.)

TABLE 19.2   Immunological Markers in Acute Lymphoblastic Leukemia

Type	FAB	TDT	CALLA	CD7	CD19	HLA-DR	Slg
Precursor B cell ALL	L1, L2	+	0	0	+	+	0
Common ALL	L1, L2	+	+	0	+	+	0
Pre-B cell ALL	L1, L2	+	+	0	+	+	0
B cell ALL	L3	0	0*	0	+	+	+
T cell ALL	L1, L2	+	0*	+	0	0	0
Null cell ALL	L1, L2	+	0	0	0	+	0

*Some cases are positive.

TDT = Terminal deoxynucleotidyl transferase; CD = cluster designation; CALLA = common ALL antigen; Slg = surface immunoglobulin; + = positive; 0 = negative.

as markers of both cell lineage and maturation (Table 19.2). Terminyl deoxynucleotidyl transferase (TDT) is an intracellular enzyme that catalyzes the nonspecific incorporation of nucleotides into DNA. TDT (+) lymphoblasts are found in the bone marrow and blood of the majority of patients with ALL of T and B cell lineage, except in some cases of B cell ALL, and are believed to occur in a small number of patients with ANLL. TDT is also present in most cases of lymphoblastic lymphoma and in about one third of patients with chronic myelogenous leukemia in blast crisis. In the latter patients, this surface marker is a predictor of favorable response to treatment.

The common ALL antigen (cALLA) is found on the surface of lymphoblasts from 70% of patients with ALL.

ELECTRON MICROSCOPE EXAMINATION

Laboratory investigation of leukemias begins with the careful examination of a peripheral blood smear and bone marrow stained with Wright stain. However, additional information regarding various leukemias can be gained through electron microscope observation, chromosome analysis, surface markers, and cytochemical staining.

Examination of the ultrastructure of leukemic blast cells is helpful in the classification of acute leukemias. Various morphological differences between myelobasts, monoblasts, and lymphoblasts as seen through the electron microscope can be a useful adjunct to light microscope examination. These differences are shown in Table 19.3 and discussed in more detail in the next few paragraphs.

Myeloblasts

Blast cells of this variety have an oval nucleus with a thin rim of heterochromatin. Euchromatin predominates in the nucleus. Nucleoli are prominent and are usually multiple. The cytoplasm may contain granules, scattered mitochondria, microfilaments in bundles, and polyribosomes. Rough endoplasmic reticulum is rare.

Monoblasts

The blasts seen in acute monocytic leukemia have a lobulated nucleus with a predominance of euchromatin. Usually one to three small nucleoli can be observed; however, one central macronucleolus may be seen in some cells. The cytoplasm is generally abundant, with numerous organelles. These organelles include lysosomes, microfilaments, and mitochondria. A well-developed Golgi complex is frequently encountered, although both smooth and rough endoplasmic reticula are scant. The cytoplasm may additionally contain lipid vacuoles and glycogen aggregates in greater concentration than in other blasts.

Lymphoblasts

Blasts of this variety usually have an irregular nucleus with a dense peripheral rim of heterochromatin. Some central euchromatin and a small, inconspicuous nucleolus may also be observed in the nucleus. The cytoplasm contains a few organelles. These organelles can include mitochondria, poly-

TABLE 19.3   Electron Photomicrograph Characteristics of Blast Cells

Cell Types	Nucleus	Cytoplasm
Myeloblasts	Euchromatin predominates; multiple nucleoli	Rough endoplasmic reticulum is rare
Monoblasts	Euchromatin predominates; one to three small nucleoli; may have one central macronucleus	Well-developed Golgi complex; lipid vacuoles; glycogen
Lymphoblasts	Dense rim of heterochromatin; central euchromatin; small nucleolus	Well-formed Golgi complex; glycogen

ribosomes, lysosomes, and diffusely distributed microfilaments. The Golgi complex is a well-formed cytoplasmic structure. Additionally, large glycogen deposits may be seen in the cytoplasm.

CYTOGENETIC ANALYSIS

The study of chromosomes, **cytogenetics,** and molecular pathology have become fields of major importance in the diagnosis and treatment of various types of malignancies, including leukemias. Approximately 50% of leukemia patients demonstrate some type of chromosomal abnormality; it has been shown that the karyotype of the leukemic cells provides diagnostic as well as prognostic information. A patient's response to therapy and survival can be correlated with the karyotype and gene rearrangement. Diagnosed patients can be monitored for remission and relapse using chromosomal and molecular analysis.

Since the initial observation of the Philadelphia chromosome, a number of other recurring chromosome abnormalities (such as gains and losses of entire chromosomes, deletions, translocations, and inversions) have been described in human leukemias and lymphomas, including ANLL, ALL, and non-Hodgkin's lymphomas. Analysis of chromosome morphology (karyotyping) and specific banding patterns of individual chromosomes (refer to Chapter 3 and Figs. 3.4 and 3.5) have been particularly useful in terms of the acute leukemias. The most consistent and specific chromosomal abnormalities that are found in human leukemia cells are translocations (Table 19.4). These alterations are found in leukocytes but not in other somatic (body) cells. Examples of chromosomal translocations and gene rearrangements consistently associated with specific hematologic malignancies are given in Table 19.5.

Because this is an area of active research interest, the list of chromosomal translocations and gene rearrangements is constantly being expanded. Gene rearrangement studies are excellent examples of molecular tests used for diagnosis, prognosis, and monitoring of patients with leukemia. Abnormal gene rearrangements result from chromosomal abnor-

malities that are usually the consequence of chromosomal translocations and involve cellular oncogenes. Activation of normal cellular oncogenes by translocation-induced gene rearrangement is an important part of the process of malignant transformation.

Cytogenetics in Acute Nonlymphoblastic Leukemia

Specific chromosomal alterations have been demonstrated in many of the acute leukemias. Although a translocation has been observed in acute myelogenous leukemia (FAB M1), it is not a specific marker. In erythroblastic leukemia (FAB M6), a specific marker has not yet been identified.

Acute Myelogenous Leukemia (FAB M2)

About 10% of patients with FAB M2 have a translocation between the long arms of chromosomes 8 and 21, t(8;21). This chromosome abnormality is generally associated with a good response to therapy and improved survival; however, if this translocation is coupled with the loss of one sex chromosome, the patient's prognosis is particularly grave. The t(8;21) abnormality is the most frequent chromosomal alteration in children with this type of leukemia. Although this abnormality is generally associated with the FAB M2 category, a few patients with this translocation who were included in the Fourth International Workshop on Chromosomes in Leukemia were classified as FAB M4.

TABLE 19.5 Examples of Chromosomal Translocations and Gene Rearrangements Consistently Associated With Hematologic Malignant Disease

Disorder	Translocation	Rearranged Genes
CML, ALL, AML	t(9;22) (q34;q11)	BCR, ABL*
AML (FAB M2)	t(8;21) (q22;q22)	Hu-ETS-2*
AML (FAB M3)	t(15;17) (q22;q21)	G-CSF, ERB-B-2/NEU, ERB A
Burkitt's lymphoma, ALL (FAB M3)	t(8;14) (q24;q32)	MYC*, IgH
	t(8;22) (q24;q11)	MYC*, Igλ
	t(2;8) (p11;q24)	MYC*, Igκ
Lymphoma (follicular)	t(14;18) (q32;q21)	IgH, BCL-2*
CLL, multiple myeloma	t(11;14) (q13;32)	BCL-1*, IgH
T cell leukemia/ lymphoma	t(8;14) (q24;q11)	MYC*, TCR α
	t(10;14) (q23;q11)	TCL-3*, TCR δ

*Denotes cellular oncogenes or putative oncogenes.

CML = chronic myelogenous leukemia; ALL = acute lymphoblastic leukemia; AML = acute myelogenous leukemia; FAB = French-American-British classification; CLL = chronic lymphocytic leukemia.

Source: D. Crisan and E. R. Carr, "BCR/*abl* Gene Rearrangement in Chronic Myelogenous Leukemia and Acute Leukemias." *Lab. Med.,* Vol. 23, No. 1, November, 1992.

TABLE 19.4 Example of Chromosomal Translocation: t(9q+;22q−)

Code	Meaning
t	The translocation of chromosomal material from one chromosome to another nonhomologous chromosome
9;22	The numbers of the 22 pairs of autosomal chromosomes or pair of sex chromosomes that are involved in the translocation
q	The lower portion (arm) of a chromosome involved in the translocation
p	The upper portion (arm) of a chromosome
+/−	The chromosome that *gained* the extra chromosomal material followed by the chromosome that lost the chromosomal material; these symbols may be absent

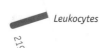
...yelocytic Leukemia (FAB M3)

...tients with acute promyelocytic leukemia (FAB ..., a reciprocal translocation of chromosomes 15 and 17 has been observed in bone marrow cells. This translocation of chromosome 17 to chromosome 15, t(15;17), is seen only in patients suffering from FAB M3.

Acute Myelomonocytic Leukemia (FAB M4)

An alteration of chromosome 16 has been detected in patients suffering from acute myelomonocytic leukemia (FAB M4). This alteration may be a deletion type of defect.

Acute Monoblastic Leukemia (FAB M5)

In this form of acute leukemia, translocations or deletions of the long arm of chromosome 11 are common. A rearrangement of the long arms of chromosome 11 is most frequently associated with either chromosome 9 or 19. Although the t(9;11) alteration has been demonstrated, no specific markers have yet been identified.

Cytogenetics in Acute Lymphoblastic Leukemia

About half of patients with lymphoblastic leukemia have abnormal karyotypes. Structural changes in ALL include t(9;22), t(4;11), t(8;14), t(8;22), t(2;8), and the Ph[1] chromosome. Gains in chromosome 21 and losses in chromosome 7, 9, or 20 have all been cited. Although no consistent markers have been associated with L1 and L2 types of ALL, the t(8;14) alteration is commonly seen in the L3 type of ALL with Burkitt's lymphoma morphology and other abnormalities of chromosome 14.

Patients with more than 50 chromosomes in their leukemic cells have the longest survival; patients with an abnormal karyotype have somewhat shorter survival times, and those with a t(4;11), t(9;22), or t(8;14) do relatively poorly.

CHEMICAL METHODS OF CELLULAR IDENTIFICATION

Principles of Special Cytochemical Stains

Special cytochemical stains are a frequently used supplementary source of information in the identification and differentiation of leukemias. Cytochemistry is the application of biochemical stains to blood and bone marrow cells. These stains reflect the chemical composition of cells through the use of color reactions, without damaging the cell to the point where the cell itself can no longer be recognized (see Table 19.9). Cytochemical stains include Sudan black B, myeloperoxidase, periodic acid–Schiff (PAS), naphthol AS-D chloroacetate (NASDCA) esterase, alpha-naphthyl acetate-butyrate esterase with fluoride inhibition, leukocyte alkaline phosphatase (LAP), and acid phosphatase with or without tartaric acid inhibition. In using various cytochemical stains, the resulting color will vary depending on the manufacturer of the reagents (refer to Chapter 24 for procedures).

Sudan Black B Stain

The Sudan stains, such as Sudan black B, are substances belonging to a series of lipid-soluble pigments that detect cellular lipids. Hematopoietic cells contain finely dispersed cytoplasmic lipids as well as complex lipids such as lipoproteins in the cell membrane and in the membranes of the mitochondria and other organelles. These lipids are not identifiable in Wright-stained smears. However, when lipid-containing blood or bone marrow cells are stained with a solution containing Sudan black B, this lipophilic dye leaves the solvent because the pigment is more soluble in the lipids than in the solvent. On microscopic examination, the concentrated pigment produces a black color in positive reactions.

Positive staining reactions are associated with the granulocytic leukocytes. The intensity of staining becomes more pronounced as the neutrophilic granulocytes mature. In this procedure, the monocytic cell line displays variable reactions, and the lymphocytic cell line is negative (Table 19.6).

This procedure (see Chapter 24) is very helpful in differentiating acute myelogenous leukemia from ALL (Plate 61). In the FAB M1 variant of acute leukemia, intensely positive groups of particles may be localized in the Golgi region of the cell. Auer rods also demonstrate a strong sudanophilic reaction. Acute monocytic leukemia cells may display scattered positive granulation, and lymphocytes and their precursors are usually negative.

Myeloperoxidase Stain

Peroxidase enzymes are relatively rare in animal tissues; however, they are very common in plant tissues. In humans, peroxidases are found in the microbodies of liver and kidney cells and in the granules of myeloid and monocytoid cells.

Myeloperoxidase is located in the primary, azurophilic granules. However, primitive blasts that are committed to the myeloid cell line demonstrate myeloperoxidase activity in areas such as the endoplasmic reticulum and the Golgi region. Positive peroxidase reactions produce a black precipitate, depending on the procedure.

A positive reaction pattern in early cells may appear as dots or rod-type structures, referred to as phi bodies (Plate 62). Cells of the myelogenous series exhibit positive reactions that intensify as the cells mature, whereas cells in the monocytic cell line display a less intense positive reaction that is characterized by fine granular deposits scattered throughout the cell. Other cell types demonstrate negative reactions. Myeloperoxidase reactions (Table 19.7) and Sudan black B reactions frequently parallel each other.

This procedure (see Chapter 24) is useful in differentiating acute myelogenous and acute monocytic leukemia from ALL. Although myeloperoxidase and Sudan black B reactions are usually parallel, rare cases can deviate from this pattern. Occasionally a myeloperoxidase-negative reaction may be associated with a Sudan black B-positive reaction, or a myeloperoxidase-positive reaction with a Sudan black B-negative reaction. Examples of exceptional reactions include negative evidence of myeloperoxidase in some persons who are in preleukemic states or suffering from severe infections, and cases of positive reaction of lymphocytes in persons

TABLE 19.6 Sudan Black B Reactions

Cell Type	Reaction
Positive Reactions	
Granulocytic cells (neutrophils and eosinophils)	Become increasingly positive (sudanophilic) as they mature
Myeloblasts	May have a few, small granules in the Golgi region
Promyelocyte	Increased granulation
Neutrophilic myelocytes	Granules concentrated near the nucleus or rim of cytoplasm
Metamyelocytes, bands, and segmented neutrophils	Strongly positive
Eosinophils at all stages	Granules react positively at the periphery of the granule
Monocytes and precursors	May have granules scattered over the entire cell
Variable Reactions	
Basophils	
Negative Reactions (Sudanophobic)	
Lymphocytes and lymphocytic precursors	
Megakaryocytes and thrombocytes (platelets)	
Erythrocytes	
Erythroblasts may display a few granules that represent mitochondrial phospholipid components	

with hairy cell leukemia (leukemic reticuloendotheliosis). A condition of hereditary decreases in myeloperoxidase also exists.

Periodic Acid–Schiff Stain

The PAS reaction is important in carbohydrate histochemistry. Positive staining reactions indicate the presence of glycogen, a polymer of glucose, and other 1,2-glycol-containing carbohydrates. Mature neutrophils contain high levels of cytoplasmic glycogen, which is physiologically related to the high energy needs of neutrophils in phagocytosis.

The PAS stain involves a two-step procedure. The first step is an oxidation reaction with periodic acid, in which hydroxy groups on adjacent carbon atoms are oxidized to aldehydes. The second step is the demonstration of the re-

sulting dialdehydes formed, using Schiff's reagent. A basic fuchsin dye in the Schiff's reagent produces a color ranging from magenta to purple, depending on the percentage of fuchsin dye in the solution. The color produced is at the site of the oxidizable carbohydrates. Several classes of carbohydrates produce positive reactions: monosaccharides, polysaccharides, glycoproteins, and mucoproteins.

The PAS reaction is strongly positive in neutrophilic granulocytes except blast forms, immature and mature platelets, and erythrocytes in erythroleukemia (FAB M6).

The usefulness of this procedure is in establishing the negative characteristics of myeloblastic and monoblastic leukemias from lymphoblastic leukemias (Table 19.8 and Plate 63).

Esterase Stains

Esterases are a very diverse group of enzymes. Perhaps the most significant property of these enzymes is that their natural substrates are esters of carboxylic acids. The esterase enzymes are capable of hydrolyzing aliphatic and aromatic ester bonds. Many esterases have a low substrate specificity and are referred to as nonspecific esterases. Those with high substrate specificity are given specific names, such as chloroacetate esterase. Several types of esterase enzyme reactions can be used in leukocytes to differentiate neutrophilic granulocytes and earlier forms from monocytic cell lines.

If a NASDCA substrate (see Chapter 24) is enzymatically hydrolyzed by a cell's specific chloroacetate esterase, a free naphthol compound is liberated. This compound is then coupled with a diazonium salt to form a highly colored deposit at the sites of enzyme activity. Positive reactions are observable in cells of granulocytic lineage (Plate 64). This enzyme has occasionally been observed in promonocytes and mature monocytes. Monoblasts are negative. The reac-

TABLE 19.7 Myeloperoxidase Reactions

Cell Type	Reaction
Positive Reactions	
Neutrophilic granulocytes except blast forms	Strongly positive
Eosinophils	Positive
Monocytes except blast forms	Positive, but reaction is faint with few granules
Negative Reactions	
Basophils	
Lymphocytic cell series	
Plasma cell series	
Erythrocytic cell series	

TABLE 19.8 Periodic Acid–Schiff (PAS) Reactions

Cell Type	Reaction
*Positive Reactions**	
Neutrophilic granulocytes except blast forms	Strongly positive
Megakaryoblasts in malignant or proliferative disease; both blasts and megakaryocytes are strongly positive	Strongly positive
Erythrocytes in erythroleukemia (FAB M6)	Strongly to moderately positive
Variable Reactions	
Eosinophils, basophils	Granules are negative; cytoplasm may contain faintly positive (PAS) granules
Monocytes	Faint pink cytoplasm, with or without granules
Lymphocytes	May contain a few pink or red granules
Thrombocytes	Intense pink or red
Megakaryocytes	Diffuse pink or red; may have coarse red granules
Lymphoblasts (leukemic)	30% to 40% may show strong coarse or block-like positivity
Negative Reactions	
Erythrocytic series	Negative
Myeloblasts and monoblasts	Faint diffuse reaction may be occasionally observed

*Appear as a diffuse pink or large red aggregates of particles.

tions with this enzymatic substrate, with the exception of the FAB M1 class of acute myelogenous leukemia which is invariably negative for NASDCA, are similar to those with both Sudan black B and myeloperoxidase stains but appear later in cellular development, usually at the differentiated myeloblast/progranulocyte stage (Table 19.9).

The nonspecific esterase enzymes alpha-naphthyl acetate and butyrate esterase (see Chapter 24) are used clinically to recognize cells of monocytic origin (Plate 65). If the enzyme is of monocytic origin, it is inhibited by sodium fluoride; however, no sodium fluoride inhibition of enzyme occurs if the enzyme is of granulocytic or lymphocytic origin. This reaction also liberates a free naphthol compound from alpha-naphthyl acetate substrate. The naphthol compound couples with a diazonium salt, as in the previous enzyme reaction, to form a black deposit at the sites of enzyme activity.

Alpha-naphthyl acetate esterase, unlike NASDCA esterase, is strongly positive for monocytes, weakly positive or negative for granulocytes, and positive for other cell types (see Table 19.9).

Phosphatase Stains

The phosphatase enzymes are widely distributed in mammalian tissue. As a group, these enzymes liberate orthophosphate from organic phosphates. The two major classifications, based on pH, are alkaline and acid phosphatase. Microscopic determinations of these enzymes are based on methods that produce a visible precipitate of the organic phosphates hydrolyzed by these enzymes.

Alkaline Phosphatase

Refer to Chapter 21, "Chronic Myeloproliferative Disorders," for a discussion of this cytochemical staining procedure and its clinical applications.

Acid Phosphatase

Acid phosphatase is one of many acid hydrolases that have been demonstrated in lysosomes. The acid phosphatases and other lysosomal enzymes appear to be formed in the endoplasmic reticulum of cells that are metabolically active. These enzymes are then packaged into primary lysosomes in the Golgi apparatus and later take part in intracellular digestive processes.

TABLE 19.9 Esterase Staining Reactions

Naphthol AS-D Chloroacetate Esterase
Positive reactions[a]
    Promyelocyte
    Myelocyte
    Metamyelocyte
    Bands and segmented neutrophils
Negative reactions
    Myeloblasts (variable)
    Monoblasts (uniformly negative)
    Promonocytes and monocytes[b]

Alpha-naphthyl Esterase (pH 7.6)
Positive reactions
    Monocytes
    Histiocytes
    Segmented neutrophils (rare)
    Mature lymphocytes (rare)
    Megakaryoblasts
    Erythroblasts
Negative reaction (with sodium fluoride incubation)
    Monocytes

[a]Reaction becomes more intense with maturation.

[b]Occasionally weakly positive.

TABLE 19.10 Cytochemical Reactions in Selected Leukemias

FAB Class	SB	MP	PAS	NASDCA	(α) NA (7.6)	Acid Phos
M1 myelogenous	+	+	−	−	−	−
M2 myelogenous	+ +	+ +	−	+	−	−
M4 myelomonocytic	+/−	+/−	−	+/−	+ +	−
M5 monocytic	+/−	+/−	−	−	+ +	−
M6 erythrocytic	−	−	+	+	+ + +	−
M7 megakaryocytic	−	(+)[a]	+	+	+ + +	−
L1 or L2 (TALL)	−	−	+/−	−	−	(+ +)[b]

[a]Test is performed on unfixed preparation.

[b]The reactivity must be focal or Golgi in nature.

SB = Sudan black B; MP = myeloperoxidase; NASDCA = naphthol AS-D chloroacetate esterase; (α) NA = alpha-naphthyl acetate esterase; Acid Phos = acid phosphatase; and PAS = periodic acid–Schiff.

Note: Negative reactions for all tests, except for the PAS, indicate common acute lymphoblastic leukemia, pre-B or B cell lymphoblastic leukemia, or unclassified acute lymphoblastic leukemia.

Source: Adapted from William H. Starkweather, Gloria J. Small, and Sandra K. Hill. "A Systematic Approach to the Cytochemical Classification of Acute Leukemia." *Lab. Perspect.*, No. 5, 1985, p. 3.

Using a naphthol AS-B1 phosphoric acid and fast garnet dye procedure (see Chapter 24), a maroon pigment is precipitated at the cellular sites of acid phosphatase activity. Most leukocytes exhibit a positive reaction in varying degrees (Table 19.10) to this test. However, monocytes demonstrate a more intense positive reaction than do neutrophils. Although lymphocytes display little activity, T cells do exhibit intense positivity in the Golgi region (Plate 66), whereas B cells may be positive or negative. For this reason, the procedure is useful in differentiating subgroups of ALL (Plate 67).

An additional tartaric acid inhibition study may be conducted. Most of the acid phosphatase isoenzyme is inhibited by L-tartaric acid. However, the cells in hairy cell leukemia (leukemic reticuloendotheliosis), Sézary syndrome, and some T cell ALLs are tartrate-resistant.

MONOCLONAL ANTIBODIES

In addition to the surface membrane markers discussed previously, it is important to realize the role of monoclonal antibodies in supplementary differential testing in the various leukemias and lymphomas (Table 19.11).

During the last decade, considerable progress has been made in the identification and characterization of surface membrane antigens that are expressed by human leukemic cells. The majority of patients with ALL express surface antigens characteristic of normal B lymphocyte lineage cells; smaller numbers express antigens of T cells. The use of immunological surface membrane markers has improved diagnostic accuracy. Rapid identification of the T cell leukemias is important clinically because the prognosis is generally worse and therapy is difficult. Surface marker analysis has become standard practice in ALL.

B Cell Markers

Early B cell maturation is divided into the early pre-B, pre-B, and mature B cell stages. The specific surface marker for

TABLE 19.11 Monoclonal Antibodies Used in Leukemia and Lymphoma Identification

Cluster	Common Name	Cell Type
CD1a	T6, Leu 6	T
CD2	T11, Leu 5	T
CD3	T3, Leu 4	T
CD4	T4, Leu 3	T
CD5	T1, Leu 1	T
CD7	Leu 9	T
CD8	T8, Leu 2	T
CD10	CALLA	B
CD11b	Leu 15	M/G
CD11c	Leu M5	M/G precursors
CD13	MY 7	G/M (most G, some M)
CD14	MY 4, Leu M3	M, some G
CD19	B4, Leu 12	B
CD20	B1, Leu 16	B
CD21	B2	B
CD22	Leu 14	B
CD25	IL-2R1, IL-2R	T
CD33	MY 9	G
CD41	J15	Megakaryocytes and platelets
CD42b	AN51	Megakaryocytes and platelets
CD45	HLE, LCA, T200	Various cells
	Ia, HLA-DR	Various cells

CD = cluster designation, M = monocytes, G = granulocytes, T = T lymphocyte, B = B lymphocyte.

early B cells is CD19. The mature B cell is identifiable by the presence of surface immunoglobulin (SIg). The immunologic classification of ALL is based on potentially identifying cells in one of the preceding stages. Before the availability of specific B cell monoclonal antisera against CD19 and CD20, many cases of ALL were incorrectly classified. The CD21 marker reacts with cells from patients suffering from B cell chronic lymphocytic leukemia (B-CLL), B cell lymphomas, B cell leukemias excluding ALL, T-CLL Sézary syndrome, acute myelogenous leukemia, and chronic myelogenous leukemia in blast crisis.

Other Surface Membrane Markers

Other surface membrane markers are widely distributed among plasma cells, some bone marrow cells, and some B cell malignancies. The HLA-DR surface marker is found in various cells. In addition, some surface markers such as CD11b, CD11c, CD13, and CD14 are unique to granulocytes and monocytes.

SUMMARY
General Characteristics

Acute leukemias are characterized by the presence of blast and immature cells in peripheral blood and bone marrow. The majority of adult patients will die of infection in a relatively short time after diagnosis. The best time to achieve the longest remission is when the disease is first diagnosed.

Categories

In addition to the traditional system of classification for leukemias, a new nomenclature for the acute leukemias has been proposed. This system, the French-American-British (FAB) system, classifies cells on the basis of their appearance and classifies the acute leukemias in ANLL and ALL types. The nonlymphoblastic types are categorized as M1 to M6, and the lymphoblastic types as L1 to L3.

Acute Nonlymphoblastic Leukemias

Some forms of myelogenous leukemia are more common than others. FAB M2 and M4 constitute the majority of cases. The least common varieties are FAB M3 and M5B. Each type has distinctive characteristics, clinical signs and symptoms, and laboratory features.

Acute Lymphoblastic Leukemia

This is the predominant type of leukemia in children 2 to 10 years old. ALL is divided into three FAB categories: FAB L1, FAB L2, and FAB L3. Cellular identification techniques include surface marker analysis. Terminyl deoxynucleotidyl transferase (TDT) is a surface marker found in the majority of patients with ALL.

Electron Microscope Examination

Examination of the ultrastructure of leukemic blast cells is helpful in the classification of acute leukemias. Electron mi-

croscope studies can be used as an adjunct to light microscope examination.

Cytogenetic Analysis

Demonstration of chromosomal alterations and molecular pathology can be valuable in the diagnosis and treatment of patients with leukemias. At least half of patients demonstrate some type of chromosomal abnormality. Certain chromosomal abnormalities and gene rearrangements are consistently associated with specific hematological malignancies.

Chemical Methods of Cellular Identification

Supplementary testing in the acute leukemias is important because they typically have more than 20% to 30% blast cells. Cytochemical staining of peripheral blood and bone marrow smears is the most common supplementary test. The cytochemical stains include Sudan black B, myeloperoxidase, periodic acid–Schiff (PAS), esterases, and phosphatases. Other testing may include electron microscope examination and chromosome and genetic analysis.

Monoclonal Antibodies

Monoclonal antibodies have become increasingly important in the study of leukemias and lymphomas. B cell markers are found in most cases of ALL and in 50% of patients with chronic myelogenous leukemia. The CD21 marker reacts with cells from patients with B cell chronic lymphocytic leukemia (B-CLL), B cell lymphomas, B cell leukemias excluding ALL, T-CLL Sézary syndrome, acute myelogenous leukemia, and chronic myelogenous leukemia in blast crisis.

Other surface membrane markers are widely distributed among plasma cells, some bone marrow cells, and some B cell malignancies.

CASE STUDIES

CASE 1 An 8-year-old white girl had been complaining of fatigue and had experienced night sweats for several weeks. Her mother took her to the pediatrician when she noticed that the child was beginning to look pale and had some unexplained large bruises.

Physical examination revealed that the mucous membranes were pale. Hepatomegaly was present, but lymphadenopathy was absent. The physician ordered a routine complete blood count (CBC) and urinalysis.

Laboratory Data
The erythrocytes and hemoglobin were severely decreased. The total leukocyte count was 110×10^9/L. The leukocyte distribution on the differential counts was as follows:

Blast cells 53%
Promyelocytes 12%
Myelocytes 8%

(continued)

Metamyelocytes 6%
Bands 4%
Segmented neutrophils 10%
Lymphocytes 7%

Auer rods were seen in many of the blast cells. The thrombocyte distribution was severely diminished on the peripheral blood smear. The result of urinalysis was normal.

Follow-up cytochemical staining demonstrated that the blast cells were positive for Sudan black B, with a variable number of moderate and coarse black granules. The PAS stain was negative. A bone marrow aspiration revealed hyperproliferation of the granulocytic precursors.

Questions
1. What is the most probable diagnosis in this case?
2. What types of supplementary testing could be done to establish the diagnosis?
3. What is the prognosis in such a case?

Discussion
1. Although children are more frequently afflicted with ALL, the presence of increased numbers of immature granulocytes on the peripheral blood smear in conjunction with the blast forms suggests a myelogenous leukemia. The absence of lymphadenopathy and the presence of hepatomegaly are consistent with the physical findings in acute myelogenous leukemia.
2. In addition to the Sudan black B and peroxidase cytochemical stains, which were positive, cytogenetic studies to determine any chromosomal translocations or alterations may be helpful in establishing a diagnosis. A translocation of a portion of the long arm of chromosome 8 to chromosome 21, t(8;21), is seen only in leukemia of the FAB M2 type. The t(8;21) alteration is the most frequent chromosomal alteration in children.
3. The complete chromosomal analysis on this patient demonstrated not only a t(8;21) alteration but also the loss of a sex chromosome. This karyotype is predictive of a grave prognosis.

✎ Diagnosis: Acute myelogenous (FAB M2) leukemia

CASE 2 A 12-year-old white boy had a sudden onset of fatigue, which increased. He had been diagnosed at birth as suffering from Down's syndrome and mental retardation.

Physical examination revealed that the patient had the physical abnormalities associated with Down's syndrome, pale mucous membranes, and slight splenomegaly. No lymphadenopathy or hepatomegaly was present. The physician ordered a CBC and urinalysis.

Laboratory Data
The erythrocytes and hemoglobin were severely decreased. The total leukocyte count was 255×10^9/L. Distribution of the leukocytes on differential smear was as follows:

Blast cells 82%
Promyelocytes 2%
Myelocytes 2%
Metamyelocytes 1%
Segmented neutrophils 7%
Lymphocytes 6%

The distribution of platelets was markedly decreased. Auer rods were noted in many of the blast forms. The urinalysis was normal.

Follow-up cytochemical staining revealed that some blasts were positive for Sudan black B, and for NASDCA esterase without inhibition by sodium fluoride. Negative results were obtained with alpha-naphthyl acetate esterase (monocytic esterase), PAS, and acid phosphatase.

Questions
1. What is the most probable diagnosis?
2. What supporting laboratory tests would be helpful?
3. Does this patient have any special circumstances that are often correlated with leukemia?

Discussion
1. The presence of a severe leukocytosis and blast cells with Auer rods is diagnostic of an acute myelogenous leukemia. However, additional testing of blood and bone marrow is needed to confirm a diagnosis.
2. In addition to the cytochemical stains that were ordered, a peroxidase stain could be performed. The results of a peroxidase staining procedure should roughly parallel the results of the Sudan black B stain. Cytogenetic analysis might be of additional value in differentiating between FAB M1 and M2 types.
3. The incidence of acute leukemias among persons with Down's syndrome is about 20 times that in the general population. Several other congenital disorders, such as Fanconi's anemia, are also known to be associated with a higher incidence of acute leukemia. Karyotypes of persons suffering from Down's syndrome and other congenital disorders show a high frequency of chromosome breaks that may be responsible for malignant transformations.

✎ Diagnosis: Acute myelogenous (FAB M1) leukemia

CASE 3 A 38-year-old white woman had been referred to her family physician after seeing her dentist. She had gone to the dentist because she had been suffering from swollen, bleeding gums for several weeks. Physical examination revealed that the patient was pale and febrile, and had hepatomegaly, splenomegaly, and lymphadenopathy. Her physician sent her to the clinic laboratory directly from his office for a CBC. On receipt of the results, the family physician admitted her to the hospital and requested a hematological consultation.

Laboratory Data
The CBC revealed a moderate decrease in erythrocytes and hemoglobin. The total leukocyte count was 32×10^9/L. The leukocyte distribution was as follows:

Blast forms 89%
Promonocytes 6%
Monocytes 4%
Lymphocytes 1%

The distribution of platelets was markedly decreased.

Subsequent hematological study showed a platelet count of 0.12×10^{12}/L. Bone marrow aspiration revealed a predominance of immature and abnormal monocytes. No increase in granulocyte precursors was noted. The cytochemical findings

(continued)

CASE STUDIES (*continued*)

were as follows: Sudan black B, slightly positive; NASDCA, blue granulation over the nucleus and cytoplasm of the majority of cells; alpha-naphthyl esterase, positive, but negative after incubation with sodium fluoride; and PAS reaction, negative.

Questions
1. What is the most probable type of leukemia in this case?
2. Would you expect the blasts to have any distinctive morphological features?
3. What are the cytogenetic findings in this type of leukemia?

Discussion
1. Pure monocytic leukemia is rare. Because this form of leukemia has a peak incidence after middle age, the patient's age is consistent with the peak incidence period. The rather abrupt physical finding of bleeding from the mouth and gums is also consistent with either acute monocytic or acute myelomonocytic leukemia.

   The supplementary cytochemical test results are consistent with a monocytic leukemia rather than a mixed myelomonocytic or other form of granulocytic leukemia. Additional analysis of the patient's karyotype might be of value.
2. Monoblasts can also have the Auer rods that are characteristic of myeloblasts. The nuclei of monoblasts are frequently convoluted and twisted rather than being evenly rounded, as in most other blast forms. The cytoplasm might additionally have a smoggy blue-gray appearance. The cytoplasmic membrane is fragile and can be slightly irregular in shape.
3. In the FAB M5 type of leukemia, a chromosomal alteration of t(9;11) has been demonstrated.

   ✏️ **Diagnosis: Acute monocytic (FAB M5) leukemia**

CASE 4 A 60-year-old white male bank manager saw his physician because he had been experiencing severe pain in his abdomen and back. He had also experienced frequent nausea for the last few weeks. These symptoms were very disturbing to the patient because he worked out regularly and was very health-conscious. He neither smoked nor consumed alcohol. Physical examination revealed no abnormalities.

The patient's physician ordered a CBC and urinalysis. A radiographic examination of the lower back was also ordered.

Laboratory Data
Both the erythrocytes and the hemoglobin were below normal limits. The total leukocyte count was 185 × 10⁹/L. Distribution of the leukocytes was as follows:

Blast cells 45%
Promyelocytes 4%
Myelocytes 10%
Metamyelocytes 3%
Bands 3%
Segmented neutrophils 5%
Monocytes 13%
Promonocytes 10%
Lymphocytes 7%

Platelet distribution was within the lower range of normal on the peripheral blood smear. The urinalysis revealed a small amount of protein.

Questions
1. On the basis of the peripheral blood smear, what is the probable diagnosis in this case?
2. What additional tests are needed to establish a diagnosis?
3. What type of leukemia is the patient suffering from, and what is the probable prognosis?

Discussion
1. The presence of granulocytic precursors and monocytic precursors along with blast forms is suggestive of a mixed myelocytic-monocytic leukemia.
2. Cytochemical staining is particularly helpful in establishing a diagnosis. In this case, it gave the following results: 98 blast cells were positive for Sudan black B stain, with few to many black granules; blast cells were negative for PAS; 73 blasts showed a few reddish granules (monocytic esterase) to the combined esterase test; 5 blasts had a few fine blue granules with the granulocytic esterase test; and 4 blasts with both red and blue granules appeared on the monocytic and granulocytic esterase tests.
3. On the basis of the peripheral blood smear morphological appearance and the cytochemical staining results, a diagnosis of acute myelomonocytic (FAB M4) leukemia was established. It is basically a granulocytic leukemia, which usually runs an acute, fulminant course and carries a life expectancy of less than a year.

   ✏️ **Diagnosis: Acute myelomonocytic (FAB M4) leukemia**

CASE 5 A 3-year-old black girl was taken to the emergency room by her mother because of an elevated temperature that could not be controlled by aspirin. The mother also reported that her daughter had been crying, pulling at her ear, and complaining of a sore throat for the last several days.

Physical examination revealed a well-nourished but listless child. The tympanic membrane was inflamed. The child had both lymphadenopathy and hepatosplenomegaly. The emergency room physician ordered a stat CBC.

Laboratory Data
The child's erythrocyte count and hemoglobin level were substantially below normal. The total leukocyte count was 66.0 × 10⁹/L. Leukocyte distribution on the differential smear was as follows:

Blast forms 76%
Prolymphocytes 12%
Lymphocytes 12%

The blast cells had one to two nucleoli and a high nuclear-cytoplasmic ratio. The nuclear shape of the blasts was round, and no Auer rods were seen in the cellular cytoplasm. The number of platelets (thrombocytes) was severely decreased.

Subsequent cytochemical examination revealed a strongly positive PAS reaction on the bone marrow lymphoblasts. The Sudan black B and esterase cytochemical stains were negative. Additional immunological testing revealed that the lymphoblasts exhibited a common ALL surface marker phenotype.

(*continued*)

Questions

1. What is the most probable diagnosis in this case?
2. What additional tests could be done?
3. What is the prognosis?

Discussion

1. The predominant type of leukemia in children from ages 2 to 10 years is lymphoblastic leukemia. Peripheral smears in these cases show a predominance of blasts. The morphological appearance of the blasts is consistent with lymphoblasts rather than other types of blasts. These findings are consistent with a probable diagnosis of ALL.
2. Common ALL antigen is found on the surface of lymphoblasts of 70% of patients with ALL. Cytogenetic analysis would be of little value in a case such as this. An additional PAS cytochemical stain may be of value because PAS-positive particles are frequently found in lymphoblasts, sometimes in large quantities. This feature is important in differentiating between lymphoblasts and myeloblasts or monoblasts.
3. Although meningeal leukemia is frequently encountered in childhood ALL, remission rates for children are high. About 90% of children achieve at least one remission. According to current statistics, about 50% of children with ALL will live at least 5 years.

✎ **Diagnosis: Acute lymphocytic (FAB L1) leukemia**

BIBLIOGRAPHY

Adamson, P. C. et al. "Pharmacokinetics of Mercaptopurine in Children With Acute Lymphocytic Leukemia." Letter to the Editor. *N. Engl. J. Med.*, Vol. 323, No. 22, November 29, 1990, pp. 1565–1566.

Bell, A., T. Hippel, and H. Goodman. "Use of Cytochemistry and FAB Classification in Leukemia and Other Pathological States." *Am. J. Med. Technol.*, Vol. 47, No. 6, June, 1981, pp. 437–470.

Berman, E. et al. "Reasons That Patients With Acute Myelogenous Leukemia Do Not Undergo Allogeneic Bone Marrow Transplantation." *N. Engl. J. Med.*, Vol. 326, No. 3, January 16, 1992, pp. 156–157.

Buckley, J. D. et al. "Occupational Exposures of Parents of Children With Acute Nonlymphocytic Leukemia: A Report From the Children's Cancer Study Group." *JAMA*, Vol. 263, No. 1, January 5, 1990, p. 100.

Carovsky, D., J. V. Melo, and E. Matutes. "Biological Markers in Lymphoproliferative Disorders," in *Chronic and Acute Leukemias in Adults.* C. D. Bloomfield (ed.). Boston: Martinus Nijhoff, 1985, pp. 69–101.

Cheson, B. D. et al. "Report of the National Cancer Institute-Sponsored Workshop on Definitions of Diagnosis and Response in Acute Myeloid Leukemia." *J. Clin. Oncol.*, Vol. 8, No. 1, May, 1990, pp. 813–819.

Cochran, D. L. "Unique Features of Acute Promyelocytic Leukemia." *Clin. Lab. Sci.*, Vol. 10, No. 6, November/December, 1997, pp. 315–319.

"Current Trends, Childhood Cancers—New Jersey, 1979–1985." *M.M.W.R.* Vol. 40, No. 33, pp. 572–574.

DeThe, G., L. Gazzolo, and A. Gessain. "Viruses as Risk Factors or Causes of Human Leukemias and Lymphomas?" *Leuk. Res.*, Vol. 9, No. 6, 1985, pp. 691–696.

Fenaux, P. and L. Degos. "Differentiation Therapy for Acute Promyelocytic Leukemia." *N. Engl. J. Med.*, Vol. 337, No. 15, Oct. 9, 1997, pp. 1076–1077.

Gallo, R. "Human T-Cell Leukemia (Lymphotropic) Retroviruses and Their Causative Role in T-Cell Malignancies and Acquired Immune Deficiency Syndrome." *Cancer*, Vol. 55, No. 10, May 15, 1985, pp. 2317–2323.

Gallo, R. C. "The Human T Cell Leukemia/Lymphotropic Retroviruses (HTLV) Family: Past, Present and Future." *Can. Res. Suppl.*, Vol. 45, September, 1985, pp. 4524–4533.

Griffin, J. D. "Surface Marker Analysis of Acute Myeloblastic Leukemia," in *Chronic and Acute Leukemias in Adults.* C. D. Bloomfield (ed.). Boston: Martinus Nijhoff, 1985, pp. 113–137.

Gupta, P. "Granulocyte Colony-Stimulating Factor in Children With Acute Lymphoblastic Leukemia." *N. Engl. J. Med.*, Vol. 337, No. 18, October 30, 1997, p. 1320.

Hanker, J. S. et al. "Facilitated Demonstration of Leukocyte Peroxidases: Importance in Leukemia Diagnosis and Classification." *Lab. Perspect.*, Issue 5, 1985, pp. 10–15.

Hardy, I. et al. "The Incidence of Zoster After Immunization With Live Attenuated Varicella Vaccine. A Study in Children With Leukemia." *N. Engl. J. Med.*, Vol. 325, No. 22, November 28, 1991, pp. 1545–1550.

Henry, J. B. *Clinical Diagnosis and Management* (19th ed.). Philadelphia: Saunders, 1991.

Hershey, D. W. "Detection of Minimal Residual Diseases in Childhood Leukemia With the Polymerase Chain Reaction." *N. Engl. J. Med.*, Vol. 324, No. 11, March 14, 1991, pp. 772–773.

Hirai, H. et al. "A Point Mutation at Codon 13 of the N-ras Oncogene in Myelodysplastic Syndrome." *Nature*, Vol. 372, June 4–10, 1987, pp. 430–432.

Howard, J. "Myeloid Series Abnormalities: Neutrophilia." *Lab. Med.*, Vol. 14, No. 3, March, 1983, pp. 147–152.

Kantarjian, H. M. "Adult Acute Lymphocytic Leukemia: Critical Review of Current Knowledge." *Am. J. Med.*, Vol. 97, Aug. 1994, pp. 176–184.

Keinanen, M. et al. "Clonal Chromosomal Abnormalities Showing Multiple-Cell-Lineage Involvement in Acute Myeloid Leukemia." *N. Engl. J. Med.*, Vol. 318, No. 18, May 5, 1988, pp. 1153–1156.

Kleiler, K. R. "Lymphocytic Leukemia: A Review of the Literature." *Am. J. Med. Technol.*, Vol. 45, No. 6, 1979, pp. 590–599.

Koepke, J. A. *Laboratory Hematology*, Vol. 1. Edinburgh: Churchill-Livingstone, 1984, pp. 251–357.

Leclair, S. J. "Case Studies Reveal Laboratory Characteristics of ALL." *Advance for Medical Laboratory Professionals*, Vol. 6, No. 14, May 2, 1994, pp. 8–9, 16.

Linet, M. S. et al. "Residential Exposure to Magnetic Fields and Acute Lymphoblastic Leukemia in Children." *N. Engl. J. Med.*, Vol. 337, No. 1, July 3, 1997, pp. 1–7.

Lowenberg, B. "Post-remission Treatment of Acute Myelogenous Leukemia," *N. Engl. J. Med.*, Vol. 332, No. 4, Jan. 26, 1995, pp. 260–262.

Lowenberg, B. "Autonomous Proliferation of Leukemic Cells in Vitro as a Determinant of Prognosis in Adult Acute Myeloid Leukemia." *N. Engl. J. Med.*, Vol. 328, No. 9, March 4, 1993, pp. 614–619.

McMillan, A. K. et al. "High-Dose Chemotherapy and Autologous Bone Marrow Transplantation in Acute Myeloid Leukemia." *Blood*, Vol. 76, No. 3, August 1, 1990, pp. 480–488.

Minowada, J. "Marker Utility in the Diagnosis and Management of Leukemias." *Lab. Med.*, Vol. 16, No. 5, May 1985, pp. 305–309.

Neugut, A. I. et al. "Poor Survival of Treatment-Related Acute Nonlymphocytic Leukemia." *JAMA*, Vol. 264, No. 8, August 1990, pp. 1006–1008.

Paietta, E. and P. H. Wiernik. "Acute Versus Chronic Leukemic Cells: Is Phenotyping a Good Prognostic Indicator." *Diagn. Med.*, November/December, 1984, pp. 20–34.

Pedraza, M. A. et al. "Acute Leukemias: Ultrastructural, Cytochemical, and Immunologic Diagnostic Approaches." *Lab. Med.,* Vol. 14, No. 1, January, 1983, pp. 45–49.

Penchansky, L. and J. R. Krause. "Flow Cytochemical Study of Acute Leukemia of Childhood With the Technicon H-1." *Lab. Med.,* Vol. 22, No. 3, March, 1991, pp. 184–190.

Pui, C. H. et al. "Human Granulocyte Colony-Stimulating Factor After Induction Chemotherapy in Children With Acute Lymphoblastic Leukemia." *N. Engl. J. Med.,* Vol. 336, No. 25, June 19, 1997, pp. 1781–1788.

Pui, C. H. et al. "Acute Myeloid Leukemia in Children Treated With Epipodophyllotoxins for Acute Lymphoblastic Leukemia." *N. Engl. J. Med.,* Vol. 325, No. 24, December 12, 1991, pp. 1682–1687.

Rebulla, P. et al. "The Threshold for Prophylactic Platelet Transfusions in Adults With Acute Myeloid Leukemia." *N. Engl. J. Med.,* Vol. 337, No. 26, December 25, 1997, pp. 1870–1875.

Reich, P. R. *Hematology* (2nd ed.). Boston: Little, Brown & Co., 1984, pp. 311, 314, 316, 322, 324, 328, 330, 375, 377.

Rowley, J. D. "Consistent Chromosome Abnormalities in Human Leukemia and Lymphoma." *Can. Invest.,* Vol. 1, No. 3, 1983, pp. 267–280.

Sachs, B. P. "Myeloid-Antigen Expression in Childhood Acute Lymphoblastic Leukemia." Letter to the Editor. *N. Engl. J. Med.,* Vol. 325, No. 19, November 7, 1991, pp. 1378–1379.

Shaw, G. M. and R. Broder. "Human T-Cell Leukemia Viruses: Its Discovery and Role in Leukemogenesis and Immunosuppression." *Adv. Intern. Med.,* Vol. 30, 1984, pp. 1–27.

Stanley, M. et al. "Classification of 358 Cases of Acute Myeloid Leukemia by FAB Criteria: Analysis of Clinical and Morphologic Features," in *Chronic and Acute Leukemias in Adults.* C. D. Bloomfield (ed.). Boston: Martinus Nijhoff, 1985, pp. 147–173.

Starkweather, W. and R. L. Searcy. "New Stabilized Staining Procedures for Classification of Specific Acute Leukemia Subgroups." *Am. Clin. Products Rev.,* February, 1987, pp. 8, 10–15.

Starkweather, W. H., G. J. Small, and S. K. Hill. "A Systemic Approach to the Cytochemical Classification of Acute Leukemia." *Lab. Perspect.,* Issue 5, 1985, pp. 2–7.

Stevens, W. et al. "Leukemia in Utah and Radioactive Fallout From the Nevada Test Site. A Case-Control Study." *JAMA,* Vol. 264, No. 5, August, 1990, pp. 585–591.

Tallman, M. S. et al. "All-*Trans*-Retinoic Acid in Acute Promyelocytic Leukemia." *N. Engl. J. Med.,* Vol. 337, No. 15, October 9, 1997, pp. 1021–1028.

Warrell, R. P. et al. "Differentiation Therapy of Acute Promyelocytic Leukemia With Tretinoin." *N. Engl. J. Med.,* Vol. 324, No. 20, May 16, 1991, pp. 1385–1393.

Welte, K. and H. Riehm. "Granulocyte Colony-Stimulating Factor in Children With Acute Lymphoblastic Leukemia." *N. Engl. J. Med.,* Vol. 337, No. 18, October 30, 1997, p. 1320.

Wiersma, S. R. et al. "Clinical Importance of Myeloid-Antigen Expression in Acute Lymphoblastic Leukemia of Childhood." *N. Engl. J. Med.,* Vol. 324, No. 12, March 21, 1991, pp. 800–808.

Windebank, K. P. et al. "Acute Megakaryocytic Leukemia (M7) in Children." *Mayo Clin. Proc.,* Vol. 64, November, 1989, pp. 1339–1351.

Wong-Staal, F. and R. Gallo. "The Family of Human T-Lymphotropic Leukemia Viruses: HTLV-I as the Cause of Adult T Cell Leukemia and HIV as the Cause of Acquired Immunodeficiency Syndrome." *Blood,* Vol. 5, No. 2, February, 1985, pp. 253–263.

Zittoun, R. A. et al. "Autologous or Allogeneic Bone Marrow Transplantation Compared With Intensive Chemotherapy in Acute Myelogenous Leukemia." *N. Engl. J. Med.,* Vol. 332, No. 4, January 26, 1995, pp. 217–223.

REVIEW QUESTIONS

1. Which of the following are typical characteristics of an acute leukemia?

   A. Replacement of normal marrow elements by leukocytic blasts and bleeding episodes.

   B. Blasts and immature leukocyte forms in the peripheral blood and anemia.

   C. Leukocytosis.

   D. All of the above.

Questions 2 through 5: match the following types of acute leukemia with their FAB classifications.

2. ___ Myelogenous and mono-cytic.

3. ___ Monocytic.

4. ___ Myelogenous without maturation.

5. ___ Lymphoblastic (one cell population).

A. M1.

B. M4.

C. M5.

D. L1.

6. Characteristics of FAB M1 include:

   A. Leukocytosis with maturation of the myelogenous cell line in the peripheral blood.

   B. Leukocytosis with maturation of the lymphocytic cell line in the peripheral blood.

   C. Leukocytosis without maturation of the myelogenous cell line in the peripheral blood.

   D. Leukocytosis with many mature leukocytes in the peripheral blood.

7. The incidence of FAB M1 is:

   A. High in children under 18 months old.

   B. High in children between 1½ and 12 years old.

   C. High in middle-aged adults.

   D. Both A and C.

Questions 8 through 12: match the following predominant peripheral blood cell morphological appearances with the FAB classifications.

8. ___ A mixture of myelogenous and monocytic blasts.

9. ___ Blasts of the monocytic type.

10. ___ Many coarsely granular promyelocytes with dumbbell-shaped or bilobed nuclei.

11. ___ Myeloblasts, promyelocytes, and myelocytes.

12. ___ Immature leukocytic and erythrocytic cell types.

A. FAB M2.
B. FAB M3.
C. FAB M4.
D. FAB M6.
E. FAB M5.

Questions 13 through 15: match the FAB classifications with the correct descriptive term.

13. ___ Leukemia secondary to Burkitt's lymphoma.

14. ___ Childhood lymphoblastic leukemia.

15. ___ Older children and adults.

A. FAB M1.
B. FAB L1.
C. FAB L2.
D. FAB L3.

16. Chloromas are associated with:
   A. FAB M1.
   B. FAB M3.
   C. FAB M4.
   D. FAB M5.

17. A common characteristic of acute lymphoblastic leukemia is:
   A. Bone and joint pain.
   B. Many blast cells with Auer rods.
   C. Leukocytopenia.
   D. A leukemia of older persons.

18. In electron microscopy comparisons of myeloblasts, monoblasts, and lymphoblasts, the myeloblasts have:
   A. Great amounts of rough endoplasmic reticulum.
   B. Multiple and prominent nucleoli.
   C. One to three nucleoli.
   D. An inconspicuous nucleolus.

Questions 19 through 21: match one of the following chromosomal alterations with the appropriate FAB type.

19. ___ t(15q+;17q-).
20. ___ t(8q-;21q+).
21. ___ t(9;11).

A. FAB M2.
B. FAB M3.
C. FAB M5.

Questions 22 through 24: match one of the following cytochemical stains with the appropriate constituent.

22. ___ Sudan black B.
23. ___ Myeloperoxidase.
24. ___ PAS.

A. Glycogen.
B. Enzymes.
C. Lipids.

25. The Sudan black B cytochemical stain differentiates:
   A. Acute myelogenous from acute lymphoblastic leukemia.
   B. Acute monocytic from acute myelogenous leukemia.
   C. Myelogenous leukemia from a leukemoid reaction.
   D. Acute myelogenous from acute myelomonocytic leukemia.

26. Myeloperoxidase differentiates:
   A. Acute myelogenous from chronic myelocytic leukemia.
   B. Acute myelogenous and acute monocytic from acute lymphoblastic leukemia.
   C. Acute myelomonocytic from acute monocytic leukemia.
   D. Acute lymphoblastic from acute monocytic leukemia.

27. The periodic acid–Schiff (PAS) reaction is:
   A. Positive in the normal erythrocytic maturational series.
   B. Positive in a block-like pattern in some lymphoblasts.
   C. Negative in megakaryoblasts.
   D. Negative in myelocytes.

28. Esterase (naphthol AS-D chloracetate) differentiates:
   A. Granulocytic (promyelocytic to segmented neutrophils) from the monocytic cell line.
   B. Promyelocytes from myelocytes.
   C. Monoblasts from myeloblasts.
   D. Metamyelocytes from myelocytes.

29. In the nonspecific esterase (alpha-naphthyl acetate or butyrate esterase) staining reaction, the cells of monocytic origin are:
   A. Positive.
   B. Positive initially and positive after sodium fluoride incubation.
   C. Positive initially and negative after sodium fluoride incubation.
   D. Negative.

30. The alpha-naphthyl acetate esterase cytochemical staining reaction is:
   A. Positive in lymphocytes.
   B. Commonly positive in segmented neutrophils.
   C. Strongly positive in monocytes.
   D. Negative in erythroblasts.

20 Malignant Lymphoid and Monocytic Disorders and Plasma Cell Dyscrasias

OBJECTIVES

Chronic leukemias
- Describe the general characteristics, including clinical symptoms and laboratory data, of monocytic leukemia and chronic lymphocytic leukemia.
- Explain the usefulness of electron microscopy and chromosome analysis in the diagnosis and prognosis of chronic lymphocytic leukemia.

Lymphomas
- Describe the relationship between leukemias and lymphomas.
- Explain the characteristics of lymphomas and their relationship to clinical hematology.

- Describe some of the characteristics of Hodgkin's disease.

Plasma cell dyscrasias
- Describe the general characteristics and laboratory data in multiple myeloma.
- Describe the general characteristics and laboratory data in Waldenstrom's macroglobulinemia.

Case studies
- Apply the laboratory data to the stated case studies and discuss the implications of these cases to the study of hematology.

CHRONIC LEUKEMIAS

Chronic leukemias are generally characterized by the presence of leukocytosis with an increased number of mature leukocytes on peripheral blood films. For example, malignant lymphoproliferative disorders (Table 20.1) are characterized by an accumulation of malignant lymphocytes; chronic monocytic leukemia is distinguished by an increased number of monocytes. Chronic lymphocytic leukemia (CLL) is the most common form of chronic leukemia.

Chronic Monocytic Leukemia

This form of leukemia is less common than other chronic forms. About 10% to 15% of all leukemias are classified as chronic monocytic leukemia. The occurrence of this variety is rare in young persons; it is characteristically seen after middle age. The overall prognosis for survival varies from 6 months to 5 years, with an average of 18 months.

The symptoms of this disorder are gradual and insidious. It is most often discovered in the course of investigating anemia. Physical examination usually reveals enlarged lymph nodes and spleen.

Many patients have a leukopenia. The total leukocyte count ranges from 3 to 70 × 10⁹/L. Peripheral blood smears are usually unremarkable on examination. However, the most frequent abnormal finding is an increase in large mature monocytes with convoluted, indented, or irregular nuclei and cytoplasmic pseudopods. Moderately decreased platelets may also be observed.

Chronic Lymphocytic Leukemia

General Characteristics

This form of leukemia is rare before age 20 and uncommon before age 50. The median age of onset is 68 years. Twice as many males as females are afflicted by the disorder. The

course of treatment is variable. The typical length of survival from the time of diagnosis is 2 to 10 years, although some patients survive more than 30 years. Prognosis is roughly related to the extent of organ infiltration at the time of diagnosis. The principal cause of death is usually infection, although 25% of CLL patients die of causes unrelated to the disorder because of older age. The high risk of infection in patients with CLL is the result of altered humoral (antibody) immunity caused by suppression of immunoglobulin synthesis that leads to hypogammaglobulinemia. Patients may also develop autoimmune disease; about one third of patients develop autoimmune hemolytic anemia.

Classic CLL is usually a B cell disease, as are most of the other CLL subtypes. Malignant proliferation of T lymphocytes (T-CLL) can occur.

More than 90% of cases of CLL represent clonal overgrowth of B-type cells and accumulation of malignant lymphocytes. CLL can resemble lymphoma. Clinically, CLL can be divided (staged) as a disease of progressive accumulation of nonfunctioning lymphocytes. The stages of reflecting accumulation of lymphocytes are as follows:

Stages of Chronic Lymphocytic Leukemia

0 Bone marrow and blood lymphocytosis

I Lymphocytosis with enlarged nodes
II Lymphocytosis with enlarged spleen or liver or both
III Lymphocytosis with anemia
IV Lymphocytosis with thrombocytopenia

Normal bone marrow elements get crowded out because of the excessive lymphoid production and packing of the marrow space by malignant lymphocytes. This infiltration by the leukemic clone results in anemia, thrombocytopenia, and neutropenia.

The median survival time (in months) decreases with each stage. The average survival times are related to each stage, as follows: 0, 150 months; I, 101 months; II, 71 months; III, 19 months; and IV, 19 months. Elderly patients, treated and untreated, survive from 3 to 5 years, on the average.

Clinical Signs and Symptoms

The onset of this disorder is insidious and is commonly discovered by chance. Twenty-five percent of patients are asymptomatic at diagnosis. Usually, the disease is suggested by abnormal findings discovered on a complete blood count for the evaluation of an unrelated illness. Common symptoms can include malaise, low-grade fever, and night sweats. Other symptoms may be weakness, fatigue, anorexia, and weight loss. Physical examination usually reveals cervical and supraclavicular adenopathy. Hepatosplenomegaly is also frequently present.

Laboratory Data

Although leukocytosis may be observed, it is less pronounced than in chronic myelogenous leukemia. Total leukocyte counts can range from 30 to 200 × 10⁹/L. In one third of patients, the total leukocyte count is greater than 100 × 10⁹/L. However, absolute lymphocytosis is a usual finding. Peripheral blood smears (Fig. 20.1; see also Plate 51) com-

---

TABLE 20.1 Classification of Lymphoproliferative Disorders

Type	Alternate Names
Acute lymphoblastic leukemia (ALL)	
Chronic lymphocytic leukemia (CLL)	
B cell	
T cell	
Prolymphocytic leukemia	
Hairy cell leukemia	Leukemic reticuloendotheliosis
Plasma cell leukemia	Leukemic phase of multiple myeloma
Sézary syndrome	Leukemic phase of mycosis fungoides
Non-Hodgkin's lymphoma	
Large granular lymphocytosis*	
Reactive lymphocytosis*	

*These disorders usually have a benign clinical course.

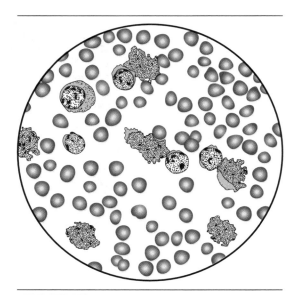

FIGURE 20.1　Chronic lymphocytic leukemia (CLL). Mature cells predominate in the chronic leukemias. In this blood smear, a typical increase in the number of smudge cells is seen. (Simulates magnification ×1000.)

monly exhibit up to 80% or 90% small lymphocytes. Many of these cells have an overmature look because of the hyper-condensed nuclear chromatin pattern. An occasional large lymphoblast may be noted. Smudge cells are highly characteristic. Both the granulocytes and the platelets are normal.

Other mild to severe immunological dysfunction typifies the disease. Serum electrophoresis studies usually show a hypogammaglobulinemia.

Electron Microscope Studies in Chronic Lymphocytic Leukemia

The study of cellular ultrastructure is less commonly performed in chronic leukemias than in acute leukemias because of the more apparent nature of the leukemia. However, investigators have studied some of the unique characteristics of the blood cells seen in chronic leukemias.

Scanning electron microscope studies that compared normal lymphocytes to the lymphocytes of patients with CLL have demonstrated that normal lymphocytes have a small or moderate number of finger-like projections, while the lymphocytes from CLL patients have a smooth, homogeneous surface. The CLL-associated lymphocytes had abundant amounts of cytoplasm that contained notable azurophilic granulation and bundles of parallel tubular arrays.

Transmission electron microscope studies do not usually demonstrate consistent differences between normal and CLL lymphocytes. However, occasionally the lymphocytes seen in CLL may have endoplasmic reticulum-associated structures that are globular, crystalline, or cylindrical. The unusual crystalline inclusions seen on some Wright-stained smears from CLL patients are within the endoplasmic reticulum. In addition, the Auer body-like inclusions seen in rare cases of CLL are Golgi-associated rather than endoplasmic-associated crystalline inclusions.

Cytogenetics in Chronic Lymphocytic Leukemia

In CLL, cytogenetic analysis has been hampered by the low mitotic index of typical CLL cells. However, cytogenetic studies after stimulation with B cell mitogens have shown clonal chromosome abnormalities in about 75% of patients with B cell CLL. The most consistent finding is an extra chromosome 12 (trisomy 12), which is present in about half of the patients. A translocation of chromosomes 8 and 14 is also associated with B cell CLL. Chromosome abnormalities can be found in TCLL and adult T cell leukemia. A variety of chromosomal abnormalities are found, the most consistent being trisomy 7. In non-T, non-B types, a translocation of chromosomes 9 and 22 may be observed. Immunologically, B cells display the classic SIg (surface immunoglobulin) marker. In addition, B cells can be identified by monoclonal antibodies as expressing CD19, CD20 or CD24, and CD5 markers. Other new techniques that can be of value in CLL include the polymerase chain reaction (PCR). This procedure reveals the nature of a lymphoid neoplasm and detects residual disease, which can lead to relapse of the disease. PCR produces multiple copies of a scarce sequence of DNA by using recombinant DNA methods.

Prolymphocytic Leukemia

Prolymphocytic leukemia is characterized by a large number of small lymphocytes with scant cytoplasm and the immature features of prolymphocytes in the peripheral blood. The leukocytosis can exceed $100 \times 10^9/L$. Most patients have a disease of B cell origin and demonstrate immunologic markers for CD19, CD20, CD24, or CD22. In addition, the cells display strong SIg. This disease progresses rapidly and does not respond well to chemotherapy.

Hairy Cell Leukemia

Hairy cell leukemia is another form of B lymphocyte-derived chronic leukemia. This form of leukemia was originally called leukemic reticuloendotheliosis. Epidemiologically it is much more common in males than females (7:1, respectively) and it has been suggested that a locus on the X chromosome might be involved in hairy cell leukemia.

Hairy cell leukemia is so named because of the fine, hair-like, irregular cytoplasmic projections that are characteristic of lymphocytes (Plate 68) in this disease. These cells are large lymphocytes with moderately large nuclei. Pancytopenia is common. The bone marrow may become fibrotic; therefore, bone marrow aspirates frequently are unsuccessful (a dry tap). Treatment with interferon may have a positive effect on bone marrow fibrosis.

The cytochemical features of hairy cell leukemia include a strong acid phosphatase reaction that is not inhibited by tartaric acid or tartrate-resistant acid phosphatase (TRAP) stain. The immunologic markers include CD19, CD20, CD22, CD24, and CD25 reactivity to the monoclonal antibody that recognizes the interleukin-2 (Tac) receptor. In addition, the cells display strong surface immunoglobulin (SIg).

The clinical course of hairy cell leukemia is more benign than many forms of leukemia. Patients frequently live more than a decade after diagnosis. The greatest risk of death is from infection.

LYMPHOMAS

Relationship Between Lymphomas and Leukemias

The term lymphoproliferative disorder includes the various forms of leukemias and malignant lymphomas that are of lymphoreticular origin. In the broadest sense, all neoplasms of lymphoid cells could be included, from immature lymphoblasts to mature-looking lymphocytes, even when they transform into immunoglobulin (Ig)-secreting cells or plasma cells, but clinically disorders such as acute lymphoblastic leukemia are considered as a separate group. The neoplastic cells of leukemia and lymphoma have an intimate relationship. Frequently, the neoplastic cells of these two disorders are identical (Table 20.2).

Characteristics

The lymphomas are a group of closely related disorders that are characterized by the overproliferation of one or more types of cells of the lymphoid system such as lymphoreticular stem cells, lymphocytes, reticulum cells, and histiocytes. During the progression of the disease, the malignant cells may spill into the blood circulation. This spillover may produce a leukemic phase of the disease. Such transitions to a leukemic phase are rare in disorders such as Hodgkin's disease but are common in the well-differentiated lymphocytic lymphomas.

Malignant lymphoma expresses itself as a disorder of the lymph nodes. It is characterized by the infiltration of abnormal lymphocytes and destruction of the normal architecture of the node. This results in the invasion and destruction of the lymph node capsule and subcapsular sinuses, and the infiltration of the pericapsular fat by large numbers of the cells that destroyed the architecture of the lymph nodes. Eventually, this disorder progresses to all of the lymphoid tissues of the gastrointestinal tract.

TABLE 20.2 Relationship of Leukemias and Lymphomas

Leukemia Type	Solid Tumor Counterpart
Stem cell leukemia	Lymphoma, undifferentiated
Acute lymphoblastic leukemia (ALL)	Lymphoma, poorly differentiated; lymphocytic
Chronic lymphocytic leukemia (CLL)	Lymphoma, well differentiated; lymphocytic
Monocytic leukemia	Reticulum cell sarcoma
Acute myelogenous granulocytic leukemia	Chloroma
Plasma cell leukemia	Myeloma

Categories

Lymphomas have been described in all races and ethnic groups. The gender distribution of these disorders is approximately equal. The major forms of malignant lymphomas are divided into Hodgkin's and non-Hodgkin's types. The non-Hodgkin's lymphomas account for over two thirds of all lymphomas and over 75% of the fatalities due to lymphoma. Rare forms of lymphoma include Burkitt's lymphoma and mycosis fungoides, a variant of Sézary syndrome, which demonstrates skin involvement.

In 1982, the Working Formulation was introduced as a simplified histologic system for classifying non-Hodgkin's lymphomas. This system has proved to be accurate in the majority of cases. The system generalizes that low-grade neoplasms are systemic at the time of earliest detection and hold little potential for cure. In contrast, intermediate- to high-grade neoplasms are more often localized at presentation. These neoplasms are sensitive to intensive cytotoxic therapy, which frequently results in an effective cure.

The application of immunologic techniques has allowed for characterization of variant types of lymphoma. Five categories of non-Hodgkin's lymphomas have been newly recognized. These categories are:

1. Low-grade B cell lymphomas of mucosa-associated lymphoid tissue (MALT), also known as monocytoid B cell lymphoma and extranodal "pseudolymphoma"
2. Centrocytic lymphomas
3. Peripheral T cell lymphomas, also called malignant histiocytosis
4. Sclerosing large cell lymphoma of the mediastinum
5. Large cell anaplastic lymphomas

Etiology

Although the etiology of most lymphomas is unknown, immunological, infectious, environmental, and genetic factors have been implicated. An enhanced understanding of the association of Burkitt's lymphoma and the Epstein-Barr virus, nonhuman leukemias, and the retrovirus associated with adult T cell lymphomas encourages further speculation about the potential role of a virus in the pathogenesis of other lymphomas, including Hodgkin's disease.

Hodgkin's Disease

Although the etiology of Hodgkin's disease remains questionable, it has long been suspected that the cause is an infectious agent with a long latent period. Hodgkin's disease has an age-related incidence, with one peak occurring in the period from 25 to 35 years of age and a second peak after 50 years of age. Sixty percent of adults afflicted with the disease are male, as are 80% of children suffering from the disease.

In the early stages of the disease, both the total leukocyte count and the result of differential examination of leukocytes from peripheral blood are normal. However, as the disease advances, a neutrophilia with total leukocyte counts of 15 to 25 × 10^9/L develops. Neutrophilia, varying degrees of eosinophilia, and monocytosis become apparent on peripheral smears as the disease progresses. In the later stages of the disorder, most patients develop lymphocytopenia and thrombocytopenia.

Hodgkin's disease is characterized by the presence of **Reed-Sternberg cells** (Plate 69) in the lymph nodes. The nodes and other lymphoid tissue are often infiltrated with lymphocytes, reticulum cells, fibrocytes, plasma cells, monocytes, and eosinophils. Fibrosis and necrosis are frequent findings.

Hodgkin's disease is considered a distinct clinical entity. It displays a wide range of features, however, with four histologic subtypes and numerous variant subtypes. The diagnosis is made primarily by examination of sections of lymph nodes. There are no unique phenotypic characteristics and there are no specific genotypic findings or chromosomal abnormalities that can substitute for the diagnostically important histopathological features.

Hodgkin's disease is characterized by a persistent defect in cellular immunity with abnormalities in T lymphocytes, IL-2 production, and increased sensitivity to suppressor monocytes and normal T suppressor cells.

The cellular origin of the Reed-Sternberg (RS) cell is unknown, but RS cells have been shown to function as stimulatory cells in many lymphocyte reactions, as accessory cells in mitogen-induced T cell proliferation, and as antigen-presenting cells in HLA-DR-restricted, antigen-specific T cell activation.

Although little is known about the karyotypic pattern of Hodgkin's disease, it is clear that the involvement of specific chromosomes in numerical and structural abnormalities is nonrandom. **Aneuploidy,** or a deviation from the diploid number of chromosomes, resulting from the gain or loss of chromosomes or from polyploids, is a characteristic feature of Hodgkin's disease. Hyperdiploidy is observed in the majority of Hodgkin's disease tumors that have an abnormal karyotype. A gain of chromosomes 1, 2, 5, 12, and 21 is a recurring numerical abnormality; structural rearrangements involving chromosome 1 are frequently observed.

Characteristics of Other Forms

In non-Hodgkin's lymphoma, Reed-Sternberg cells are absent. The infiltrating cells may be of one type or may have a mixed cell population of lymphocytes, histiocytes, eosinophils, and some plasma cells.

Cytogenetic Analysis

The chromosomal anomalies that have been observed in hematologic malignant disease include structural rearrangement as translocations and deletions and numerical abnormalities with respect to structural rearrangements. Analysis of DNA sequences, located at the chromosomal breakpoint of several of the recurring translocations in leukemias or lymphomas, have revealed that the genes located at these sites are protooncogenes. As a result of the genetic mutation induced by the chromosomal rearrangement, the function of the gene is altered, thereby converting the gene to an oncogene.

The best examples are the translocations observed in Burkitt's lymphoma and CML. In Burkitt's lymphoma, one of three translocations is usually observed. These translocations involve the Myc oncogene normally located on chromosome 8, and either chromosome 14, 2, or 22. These are the sites of the immunoglobulin heavy chain [t(8;14)], kappa light chain [t(2;8)], and lambda light chain [t(8;22)] genes, respectively. In these translocations, Myc oncogene is juxtaposed with the DNA sequence of the immunoglobulin genes, resulting in the unregulated transcriptional activity of the Myc gene.

Sézary Syndrome

The leukemic phase of cutaneous T cell lymphoma, **mycosis fungoides,** is called Sézary syndrome. Diagnosis of Sézary syndrome is dependent on the primary diagnosis of mycosis fungoides in a skin biopsy. Adults between 40 and 60 years old are most frequently afflicted with skin lesions that progress to the tumor stage. In peripheral blood the disease is characterized by the presence of abnormal circulating lymphocytes, **Sézary cells.**

A Sézary cell is typically the size of a small lymphocyte and has a dark-staining, clumped, nuclear chromatin pattern. The distinctive folded, groovelike chromatin pattern is described as **cerebriform.** Mature T lymphocytes in Sézary display a phenotype with reactivity for CD2, CD3, CD4, and CD5.

PLASMA CELL DYSCRASIAS
Multiple Myeloma
Etiology and Symptoms

Multiple myeloma (also referred to as plasma cell myeloma, myelomatosis, or Kahler's disease) is a malignant plasma cell disease. **Plasma cell leukemia** is an increased number of plasma cells in the peripheral blood, and should be considered a form of multiple myeloma and not a separate entity. Multiple myeloma accounts for about 1% of all types of malignant disease and slightly more than 10% of hematological malignancies.

In multiple myeloma, typically, the bone marrow is involved, but the disorder may involve other tissues as well. The etiology is unknown; however, radiation may be a factor, and the possibility of a viral cause has been suggested. The likelihood of a genetic factor in some cases is supported by well-documented reports of 23 familial clusters with multiple myeloma.

The onset of this disorder is between the ages of 40 and 70 years, with a peak incidence in the seventh decade. It is uncommon in patients under 40 years old. Males are affected in about 61% of cases, and blacks are afflicted twice as often as Caucasians.

Symptoms of multiple myeloma include bone pain, typically in the back or chest and present at the time of diagnosis in more than two thirds of patients; weakness; and fatigue. Weight loss and night sweats are not prominent until the disease is advanced. Abnormal bleeding may be a prominent feature. In some patients, the major symptoms result from acute infection, renal insufficiency, hypercalcemia, or amy-

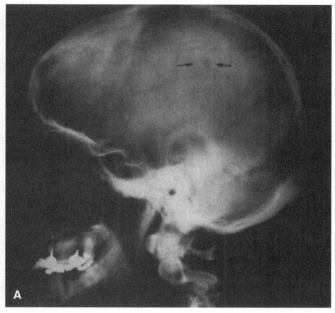

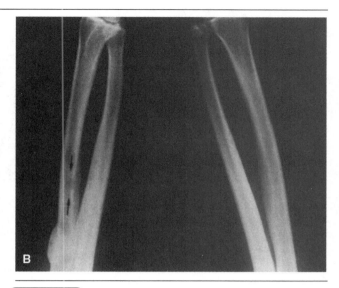

FIGURE 20.2 Lesions in multiple myeloma. **A.** A single osteolytic lesion is detectable in this skull radiograph and exhibits a "punched-out" appearance. **B.** Another osteolytic lesion is detectable in the tibia.

loidosis. In addition to the conclusive laboratory findings, including bone marrow examination results, about 90% of patients suffer from broadly disseminated destruction of the skeleton (Fig. 20.2). This disorder runs a progressive course, and most patients die in 1 to 3 years. The major causes of death are infection and renal insufficiency.

Laboratory Data

Anemia is present at the time of diagnosis in about two thirds of patients. Increased plasma volume due to monoclonal protein commonly produces hypervolemia. The leukocyte count can be normal, although about one third of patients suffer from leukopenia. Relative lymphocytosis is usually present. Sometimes eosinophilia is noted. In rare cases in the terminal stages, plasmablasts and plasma cells (Plate 70) may amount to 50% of the leukocytes in the peripheral blood. Rouleaux formation (discussed in Chapter 6) on peripheral blood smears is common. Other laboratory findings include an increased erythrocyte sedimentation rate (ESR) and the presence of **Bence Jones** protein in the urine.

Bleeding is common. Platelet abnormalities, impaired aggregation of platelets, and interference with platelet function by the abnormal monoclonal protein contribute to bleeding. Inhibitors of coagulation factors and thrombocytopenia from marrow infiltration of plasma cells or chemotherapy may also contribute to bleeding. Some patients have a tendency toward thrombosis, which may be manifested by a shortened coagulation time, increased fibrinogen, and increased factor VIII.

Electrophoresis (Fig. 20.3) of the serum or urine reveals tall sharp peaks on the densitometer tracing; a dense localized band is seen in 75% of myeloma cases. A monoclonal serum protein is detected in 91% of patients. The type of antibody is IgG in the majority of patients. Less frequently IgA is seen, and rarely IgD is demonstrated.

Chromosomal abnormalities are found in at least half of patients with multiple myeloma. Numerous changes and structural abnormalities, including giant chromosomes, translocations, and deletions, have been noted; however, the abnormalities are limited to the plasma cells.

Waldenstrom's Primary Macroglobulinemia

Etiology and Symptoms

Waldenstrom's macroglobulinemia is a malignant lymphocyte–plasma cell proliferative disorder with abnormally large amounts of gamma globulin of the 19S or IgM type. The basic abnormality in this macroglobulinemia is uncontrolled proliferation of lymphocyte–plasma cells. The condition has an age-specific incidence. It is most commonly found in older men; the mean age of onset is about 60 years. The onset is usually insidious.

The symptoms include weakness, fatigue, and bleeding. Bone pain is virtually nonexistent. About one fourth of patients with Waldenstrom's macroglobulinemia have neurological abnormalities. The incidence of infection is twice the normal rate. Patients usually suffer from chronic anemia and bleeding episodes. Thrombocytopenia and hyperviscosity may also contribute to the bleeding disorder. The median survival time is approximately 3 years after diagnosis.

Laboratory Data

The lymphocyte–plasma cells vary morphologically, ranging from small lymphocytes to obvious plasma cells. Their cytoplasm is frequently ragged and may contain periodic acid–Schiff (PAS)–positive material that is probably identical to the circulating macroglobulin.

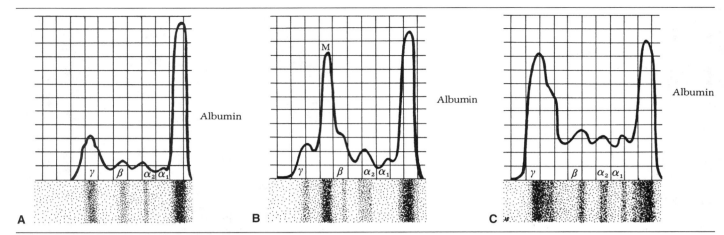

FIGURE 20.3 Serum electrophoresis. Protein electrophoretic patterns are depicted graphically with the corresponding paper electrophoretic mobility pattern stained with blue dye. **A.** Normal. The relationship between the globulin fractions (alpha, beta, gamma). The largest fraction is the gamma fraction. **B.** Multiple myeloma. The pattern in this patient demonstrates a characteristically abnormal M spike. **C.** Waldenstrom's macroglobulinemia. The overall quantity of globulins is increased in the serum of this patient. In addition, the pattern demonstrates globulin with mobility between the beta and gamma fractions.

The total leukocyte count is usually normal, with an absolute lymphocytosis. Moderate to severe degrees of anemia are frequently observed on peripheral blood smears, as well as rouleaux formation. The patient's plasma volume may be greatly increased, and the ESR is increased. Platelet counts are usually normal. Bleeding due to abnormalities in platelet adhesiveness and prothrombin time may be seen, and the values of factor VIII may be low.

Characteristically, blood samples are described as having **hyperviscosity.** Electrophoresis of serum (see Fig. 20.3) usually demonstrates the overproduction of IgM (19S) antibodies. Additionally, **cryoglobulins** can be detected in the patient's serum. Cryoglobulins are proteins that precipitate or gel when cooled to 0°C and dissolve when heated. In most cases, monoclonal cryoglobulins are IgM or IgG.

SUMMARY

Chronic Leukemias

A characteristic feature of chronic leukemias is the presence of increased numbers of mature leukocytes on peripheral blood smears. Supplementary testing for the chronic leukemias can also include electron microscopy and chromosome analysis.

Lymphomas

The lymphomas are closely related to the leukemias. Frequently, the neoplastic cells of leukemia and lymphoma are identical. Initially, lymphomas are confined to the lymph nodes, but they may spill over into the blood in the leukemic phase. Lymphomas are commonly divided into the Hodgkin's and non-Hodgkin's types. The presence or absence of Reed-Sternberg cells is critical in establishing a diagnosis. Cytogenetic analysis is valuable in identifying Burkitt's lymphoma and some other malignant lymphomas.

Plasma Cell Dyscrasias

Multiple myeloma is a malignant plasma cell disease, typically of the bone marrow. Plasma cell leukemia is considered to be a form of multiple myeloma, not a separate entity; however, increased numbers of plasma cells are found in the peripheral blood rather than in the bone marrow. The etiology of multiple myeloma is unknown. The outstanding laboratory characteristics include the presence of Bence Jones protein in the urine and an abnormal serum and/or urinary electrophoretic pattern.

Waldenstrom's macroglobulinemia is a malignant lymphocyte-plasma cell proliferative disorder with abnormally large amounts of the gamma globulin type (19S or IgM). Abnormal serum electrophoresis patterns, and the presence of cryoglobulin, are characteristic.

CASE STUDIES

CASE 1 A 58-year-old female medical records librarian was admitted to the hospital for minor elective surgery. Although the patient had been complaining of general malaise and fatigue, she suspected that it was a work-related problem rather than a physical problem. Physical examination revealed that she had both cervical and supraclavicular lymphadenopathy.

Laboratory Data
Her preoperative blood count revealed that her erythrocytes and hemoglobin were within normal range; however, her total leukocyte count was 26.5 × 10⁹/L. The distribution of leukocytes was as follows:

Bands 6%
Segmented neutrophils 18%

(continued)

Lymphocytes 75%
Monocytes 1%

Some variant lymphocytes and smudge-type cells were present. The distribution of platelets was normal.

Follow-up laboratory tests included an infectious mononucleosis screen, with negative results. Bone marrow examination revealed lymphocytic infiltration of approximately 50% of the cells in the marrow.

Questions

1. What could be the possible explanation for the leukocytosis and concurrent lymphocytosis?
2. What further testing could be done to establish a diagnosis?
3. What is the patient's prognosis?

Discussion

1. Persons over 50 years old with leukocytosis and lymphocytosis may be suffering from the early stages of CLL. The lymphadenopathy further suggests a lymphoproliferative disorder.
2. A lymph node biopsy could be performed in order to study the architecture of the node. This examination would be helpful in differentiating a lymphocytic lymphoma from CLL. Electron microscope studies may be of additional value in demonstrating the ultrastructure of the lymphocytes. Patients with CLL frequently have lymphocytes that vary from normal. Cytogenetic analysis might also be useful. The existence of a trisomy 12 would be helpful in establishing the patient's prognosis.
3. The majority of these patients usually survive for at least 10 years after diagnosis if the karyotype is normal. However, a patient with an abnormal karyotype would have a graver prognosis. The general prognosis in CLL is much more favorable than in other forms of leukemia. Some patients survive for over 30 years, although the median survival time is from 4 to 6 years.

☞ Diagnosis: Chronic lymphocytic leukemia

CASE 2 A 58-year-old male college professor saw his family physician because of increasing fatigue and weakness. He also reported pain in his lower back and arms when he walked. Physical examination revealed that the man had pale mucous membranes and hepatosplenomegaly. The physician ordered a complete blood count (CBC) and urinalysis. A follow-up appointment was scheduled for the following week.

Laboratory Data

The CBC revealed that the patient had anemia. His leukocyte count and differential count were normal, except for a rouleaux (rolled coin) appearance of the red blood cells. The result of urinalysis was normal. The patient was called and requested to return to the laboratory for additional tests. The physician ordered the following tests: ESR, kidney screening profile, liver blood profile, and radiographic skeletal survey, with the following results: ESR, 50 mm/hr; normal kidney profile; and normal liver profile except for increased globular protein. The skeletal survey indicated bone lesions in various sites.

Questions

1. What follow-up laboratory tests might be ordered to assist in establishing a definitive diagnosis?

2. What type of leukocyte disorder could be present?
3. What is the nature of the protein found in the urine?
4. What is the most significant laboratory finding in this disorder?

Discussion

1. In this case, further investigation of the increased ESR and increased serum globular protein was ordered. A serum electrophoresis and immunoelectrophoresis revealed the presence of an abnormal protein, a 7S immunoglobulin. Bence Jones protein was identified in the urine. Subsequent bone marrow examination revealed a remarkable increase in plasma cells.
2. Although an increase in proteins, specifically immunoglobulins, is responsible for the elevated ESR, an absence of cells related to antibody production is frequently noted in this disorder. However, a bone marrow examination would reveal an overproliferation of plasma cells. In rare cases, a leukemic form of myeloma, called **plasma cell leukemia**, develops. In these cases, some plasma cells may be seen in the peripheral blood.
3. Bence Jones protein precipitates when heated to 56°C and dissolves when heated to boiling, and reprecipitates with cooling. On electrophoresis, this protein will reflect its monoclonal nature and appear in the beta or gamma region.
4. Although metastatic carcinoma involving the liver can produce bone marrow plasmacytosis, the presence of increased plasma cells is significant in establishing the diagnosis. Laboratory tests, particularly serum and urine electrophoresis, are important adjuncts.

☞ Diagnosis: Multiple myeloma

BIBLIOGRAPHY

Bell, A., T. Hippel, and H. Goodman. "Use of Cytochemistry and FAB Classification in Leukemia and Other Pathological States." *Am. J. Med. Technol.,* Vol. 47, No. 6, June, 1981, pp. 437–470.

Billing, R. et al. "Cytotoxic Monoclonal Antibodies Against Cell Surface Antigens Useful for the Characterization of Normal Leukocyte Subpopulations and Leukemia Cells." *Complements,* October, 1981.

Bunn, P. A. et al. "Systemic Therapy of Cutaneous T-Cell Lymphomas (Mycosis Fungoides and the Sézary Syndrome)." *Ann. Intern. Med.,* Vol. 121, No. 8, October 15, 1994, pp. 592–602.

Cabanillas, F. et al. "Lymphomatoid Papulois: A T-Cell Dyscrasia With a Propensity to Transform Into Malignant Lymphoma." *Ann. Intern. Med.,* Vol. 122, No.3, February 1, 1995, pp. 210–217.

Carovsky, D., J. V. Melo, and E. Matutes. "Biological Markers in Lymphoproliferative Disorders," in *Chronic and Acute Leukemias in Adults.* C. D. Bloomfield (ed.). Boston: Martinus Nijhoff, 1985, pp. 69–101.

Davis, T. H. et al. "Hodgkin's Disease, Lymphomatoid Papulosis, and Cutaneous T-Cell Lymphoma Derived From a Common T-Cell Clone." *N. Engl. J. Med.,* Vol. 326, No. 17, April 23, 1992, pp. 1115–1122.

DeVita, V. T. and S. M. Hubbard. "Hodgkin's Disease." *N. Engl. J. Med.,* Vol. 328, No. 8, February 25, 1993, pp. 560–565.

Engellenner, W. and M. Golightly. "Large Granular Lymphocyte Leukemia." *Lab. Med.,* Vol. 22, No. 7, July, 1991, pp. 454–456.

French, M. et al. "Plasma Cell Proliferation in Monoclonal Gammopathy: Relations With Other Biologic Variables—Diagnostic and

Prognostic Significance." *Am. J. Med.*, Vol. 98, No. 1, January, 1995, pp. 60–66.

Gill, P. S. et al. "Treatment of Adult T-cell Leukemia-Lymphoma With a Combination of Interferon Alfa and Zidovudine." *N. Engl. J. Med.*, Vol. 332, No. 26, June 29, 1995, pp. 1744–1748.

Hermine, O. et al. "Treatment of Adult T-Cell Leukemia-Lymphoma With Zidovudine and Interferon Alfa." *N. Engl. J. Med.*, Vol. 332, No. 26, June 29, 1995, pp. 1749–1751.

Hoffman, R. A. "Clinical Utility of Cell Surface Antigen Detection." *Am. Clin. Products Rev.*, Vol. 20, April, 1985, pp. 16–31.

Kaminski, M. S. et al. "Radioimmunotherapy of B-Cell Lymphoma with [131I]Anti-B1(Anti-CD20) Antibody." *N. Engl. J. Med.*, Vol. 329, No. 7, August 12, 1993, pp. 459–465.

Kleiler, K. R. "Lymphocytic Leukemia: A Review of the Literature." *Am. J. Med. Technol.*, Vol. 45, No. 6, 1979, pp. 590–599.

Kluin, P. M. "Bcl-6 in Lymphoma—Sorting Out a Wastebasket." *N. Engl. J. Med.*, Vol. 331, No. 2, July 14, 1994, pp. 116–118.

Koepke, J. A. *Laboratory Hematology*, Vol. 1. Edinburgh: Churchill-Livingstone, 1984, pp. 251–357.

Link, M. P. et al. "Treatment of Children and Young Adults With Early-Stage Non-Hodgkin's Lymphoma." *N. Engl. J. Med.*, Vol. 337, No. 18, October 30, 1997, pp. 1259–1266.

Minowada, J. "Marker Utility in the Diagnosis and Management of Leukemias." *Lab. Med.*, Vol. 16, No. 5, May, 1985, pp. 305–309.

Neri, G. "Some Questions on the Significance of Chromosome Alterations in Leukemias and Lymphomas: A Review." *Am. J. Med. Genet.*, Vol. 18, 1984, pp. 471–481.

Pearson, M. and J. D. Rowley. "The Relation of Oncogenetics in Leukemia and Lymphoma." *Annu. Rev. Med.*, Vol. 36, 1985, pp. 471–483.

Press, O. W. et al. "Radiolabeled-Antibody Therapy of B-Cell Lymphoma With Autologous Bone Marrow Support." *N. Engl. J. Med.*, Vol. 229, No. 17, Oct. 21, 1993, pp. 1219–1224.

Reich, P. R. *Hematology* (2nd ed.). Boston: Little, Brown & Co., 1984, pp. 311, 314, 316, 322, 324, 328, 330, 375, 377.

Rowley, J. D. "Consistent Chromosome Abnormalities in Human Leukemia and Lymphoma." *Can. Invest.*, Vol. 1, No. 3, 1983, pp. 267–280.

Rozman, C. and E. Montserrat. "Chronic Lymphocytic Leukemia." *N. Engl. J. Med.*, Vol. 333, No. 16, October 19, 1995, pp. 1052–1057.

Stevenson, F. K. "Hodgkin's Disease—New Insights From Immunoglobulin Genetics." *N. Engl. J. Med.*, Vol. 333, No. 14, October 5, 1995, pp. 934–936.

The International Non-Hodgkin's Lymphoma Prognostic Factors Project. "A Predictive Model for Aggressive Non-Hodgkin's Lymphoma." *N. Engl. J. Med.*, Vol. 329, No. 14, September 30, 1993, pp. 987–994.

Urba, W. J. and D. L. Longo. "Hodgkin's Disease." *N. Engl. J. Med.*, Vol. 326, No. 10, March 5, 1992, pp. 678–687.

Verdonck, L. F. et al. "Comparison of CHOP Chemotherapy with Autologous Bone Marrow Transplantation for Slowly Responding Patients With Aggressive Non-Hodgkin's Lymphoma." *N. Engl. J. Med.*, Vol. 332, No. 16, April 20, 1995, pp. 1045–1051.

REVIEW QUESTIONS

1. The most common form of chronic leukemia is:

   A. Myelogenous.
   B. Lymphocytic.
   C. Monocytic.
   D. Eosinophilic.

2. The median survival time of patients with CLL, compared with patients with chronic monocytic leukemia, is:

   A. Not significantly different.
   B. Shorter.
   C. Longer.
   D. Shorter, if the patient is female.

3. CLL is classically a:

   A. T cell disorder.
   B. B cell disorder.
   C. Null cell disorder.
   D. Disorder of the young.

4. CLL symptoms frequently include:

   A. Weight loss, anemia, and extreme leukocytosis.
   B. Absolute lymphocytosis, edema, and splenic infarction.
   C. Absolute lymphocytosis, malaise, and low-grade fever.
   D. Neutrophilia, splenomegaly, and anemia.

5. Electron microscopy examination of lymphocytes from a patient with CLL can demonstrate:

   A. An increase in specific and azurophilic granules.
   B. A smooth, homogeneous surface with abundant amounts of cytoplasm.
   C. Unusual crystalline inclusions.
   D. Both B and C.

6. Characteristics of malignant lymphoma typically include:

   A. Overproliferation of neutrophils.
   B. Overproliferation of lymphocytes.
   C. Lymph node involvement.
   D. All, except A.

7. Hodgkin's disease:

   A. Is characterized by neutrophilia in the early stages of the disease.
   B. Occurs more frequently in females than males.
   C. Is a lymphoma, characterized by Reed-Sternberg cells, and occurs more frequently in females than males.
   D. Is a lymphoma, characterized by Reed-Sternberg cells, and occurs more frequently in males than females.

8. Rare forms of lymphoma include:

   A. Hodgkin's and non-Hodgkin's lymphoma.
   B. Burkitt's lymphoma and mycosis fungoides.
   C. Hodgkin's and non-Hodgkin's lymphoma and Burkitt's lymphoma.
   D. Non-Hodgkin's lymphoma and mycosis fungoides.

9. Multiple myeloma is a disorder of:

   A. T lymphocytes.
   B. Megakaryocytes.
   C. Plasma cells.
   D. The lymph nodes.

10. The abnormal protein frequently found in the urine of persons with multiple myeloma is:

    A. Albumin.
    B. Globulin.
    C. IgG.
    D. Bence Jones.

11. Waldenstrom's macroglobulinemia is characterized by increased levels of:

    A. IgG.
    B. IgM.
    C. IgD.
    D. IgA.

Chronic Myeloproliferative Disorders

OBJECTIVES

General characteristics and classification
- Name the diseases classified as chronic myeloproliferative disorders.
- Differentiate and compare the peripheral blood characteristics of these disorders.
- Briefly describe the common abnormalities of hemostasis and coagulation in chronic myeloproliferative disorders.
- Report the general prognostic features of chronic myeloproliferative disorders.
- Briefly explain general treatment approaches to chronic myeloproliferative disorders.

Chronic myelogenous leukemia
- Name the subtypes of chronic myelogenous leukemia.
- Describe the epidemiology of chronic myelogenous leukemia.
- Explain the pathophysiology of this leukemia.
- Delineate the usefulness of karyotyping and detection of genetic alterations in chronic myelogenous leukemia.

- Compare the clinical signs and symptoms of this leukemia in the three phases of disease.
- Describe the cellular aspects of chronic myelogenous leukemia.
- Explain the usefulness of electron microscopy and cytochemistry in the diagnosis and prognosis of chronic myelogenous leukemia.
- Characterize the prognostic features and modes of treatment in chronic myelogenous leukemia.

Polycythemia vera
- State the other names that might be used to refer to polycythemia vera.
- Describe the epidemiology of polycythemia vera.
- Name the most striking feature of polycythemia vera.
- Identify the most frequent structural chromosomal abnormality in polycythemia vera.
- Describe the clinical signs and symptoms of polycythemia vera.
- Correlate at least four symptoms related to hyperviscosity.

- List the major and minor criteria as designated by the National Polycythemia Vera Study Group for establishing a diagnosis.
- State the required diagnostic measures in polycythemia vera.
- Describe the cellular alterations seen in polycythemia vera.
- Compare the characteristics of polycythemia vera and other types of polycythemia.
- Explain the factors that influence the prognosis.
- Name the primary control method in the treatment of polycythemia vera.

Idiopathic myelofibrosis

- State the other name for idiopathic myelofibrosis.
- Briefly describe the epidemiology of idiopathic myelofibrosis.
- Name the predominant clinical manifestation in idiopathic myelofibrosis.
- Describe the pathophysiology of idiopathic myelofibrosis.
- Define and describe the consequences of dysmegakaryocytopoiesis.
- Briefly characterize the karyotype profile of idiopathic myelofibrosis.
- Delineate the clinical signs and symptoms of idiopathic myelofibrosis.
- Name the cellular components of a "leukoblastic" peripheral blood picture.
- Describe the life span prognosis in idiopathic myelofibrosis.

- Explain the treatment approach to idiopathic myelofibrosis.

Essential thrombocythemia

- List and describe the major criteria and other findings for the diagnosis of essential thrombocythemia.
- Describe the epidemiology of essential thrombocythemia.
- Outline the major features of essential thrombocythemia.
- Explain the most common disorders in patients with essential thrombocythemia.
- State the classic laboratory findings in essential thrombocythemia.
- Discuss platelet function findings in essential thrombocythemia.
- Compare the bone marrow architecture of essential thrombocythemia with other chronic myeloproliferative disorders.
- Review the relationship between essential thrombocythemia and polycythemia vera.
- Report the treatment approach to essential thrombocythemia.

Case studies

- Apply the laboratory data to the stated case studies and discuss the implications of these cases to the study of hematology.

GENERAL CHARACTERISTICS AND CLASSIFICATION

Chronic myeloproliferative disorders (MPDs) are interrelated clonal abnormalities resulting in the excessive proliferation of various phenotypically normal mature cells.

One type of chronic MPD may evolve into another type during the course of the disease. All of the types of chronic MPDs may evolve into acute leukemia.

Classification

Chronic MPDs are divided into chronic myelogenous leukemia (CML), polycythemia vera, idiopathic myelofibrosis (also known as agnogenic myeloid metaplasia or myelofibrosis with myeloid metaplasia), and essential thrombocythemia. Histopathologists have developed the Hannover classification (Table 21.1) of chronic MPDs. This system of classification subdivides CML into a common type and a type showing an increase of megakaryocytes.

Relationship of the Chronic Myeloproliferative Disorders

Studies with molecular probes and glucose-6-phosphate dehydrogenase (G6PD) indicate that the myeloid leukemias and the various types of chronic MPDs are clonal diseases. No environmental agent has been identified; however, it has been suggested that a genetic susceptibility to MPDs may exist. The findings of G6PD studies indicate that CML, polycythemia vera, and essential thrombocythemia involve progenitor cells for granulocytes, erythrocytes, megakaryocytes, and lymphocytes. Agnogenic myeloid metaplasia is also a clonal disease that involves multipotential hematopoietic cells. However, in myelofibrosis, the predominant clinical manifestation occurs secondarily and is not a component of the abnormal clonal proliferation.

Distinguishing Features

The MPDs are acquired disorders of hematopoiesis that are characterized by an excessive production of phenotypically normal mature cells. The dysfunction in chronic MPDs appears to be a loss of regulatory signals that control the production of mature cells.

Variation in the pattern of cellular proliferation and differentiation can be explained by the clonal mutation of pluripotent stem cells with different lineage potentials. Features that distinguish one category from another are presented in Table 21.2.

Bone marrow examination is useful as an aid in determining the cause of extreme thrombocytosis. The differences between the marrow findings in MPDs and extreme reactive thrombocytosis are the numbers of megakaryocytes, the presence or absence of megakaryocyte clusters, stainable iron, cellularity, and reticulin content.

Common Disorders of Hemostasis and Coagulation

Patients with an MPD suffer from various mild disorders of hemostasis or coagulation. An abnormal coagulation mechanism is believed to be related to a low-grade, possible secondary form of disseminated intravascular coagulation (DIC), a chronic state of abnormal blood coagulation that occurs even after treatment to reduce the platelet count. Other abnormalities include a prolonged activated partial thromboplastin time (APTT) and a significantly decreased level of factor V. In many patients, the levels of D-dimer, thrombin-antithrombin III complex, and plasmin-alpha-2 plasmin inhibitor complex are higher than normal.

TABLE 21.1 Hannover Classification of Primary Categories of Chronic Myeloproliferative Disorders

1. Chronic myelogenous leukemia (CML)—common type
2. Chronic myelogenous leukemia (CML)—megakaryocytic increase
3. Polycythemia vera
4. Primary or idiopathic thrombocythemia
5. Chronic megakaryocytic-granulocytic myelosis

TABLE 21.2 Comparative Peripheral Blood Characteristics of Chronic Myeloproliferative Disorders

	CML	IM	PV	ET
Erythrocytes $\times 10^{12}$/L	Decreased	Decreased	Extremely increased	Normal
Leukocytes $\times 10^9$/L	Extremely increased	Variable	Increased	Normal
Platelets $\times 10^9$/L	Moderately increased	Variable	Moderately increased	Extremely increased
Teardrop-shaped erythrocytes	None	Extremely increased	None	None
Leukocyte alkaline phosphate score	Decreased	Variable	Extremely increased	Normal/increased
Marrow fibrosis	Variable	Very increased	None	None
Ph[1] chromosome	Positive	Negative	Negative	Negative

CML = chronic myelogenous leukemia; IM = idiopathic myelofibrosis; PV = polycythemia vera; ET = essential thrombocythemia.
Source: From J. H. Stein. *Internal Medicine* (3rd ed.). Boston: Little, Brown & Co., 1990.

Patients with an MPD commonly exhibit thrombotic phenomena. This is thought to be associated with an increase in circulating platelets affecting the arterial and venous circulation. In rare cases, the initial manifestation of MPD can be gangrene of the extremities. Numerical and morphological characteristics of the megakaryopoiesis differ in each category of MPD. A triad of qualitative platelet defects (abolished second-wave epinephrine aggregation, increased ADP aggregation threshold, and markedly reduced ATP secretion during collagen-induced aggregation) seems to be a good diagnostic marker of chronic MPD with thrombocytosis.

In addition, arachidonate metabolism is frequently deranged in patients with MPD. The change in thromboxane formation in essential thrombocythemia and polycythemia vera could be one of the factors responsible for the different incidences of thrombotic and hemorrhagic complications in these diseases. When arachidonic acid metabolism in patients with an MPD was evaluated, the generation of thromboxane B_2 was found to be significantly reduced and inversely correlated with the platelet count in patients with essential thrombocythemia. Polycythemia vera patients showed an increased formation of this metabolite of arachidonic acid. The generation of prostaglandin E_2 and 6-keto-prostaglandin $F_{1\alpha}$ was markedly reduced in patients with CML.

Prognosis

Acute leukemic transformation in idiopathic myelofibrosis generally has an insidious presentation, contrasting with its abrupt onset in most patients with polycythemia vera or essential thrombocythemia. Most acute leukemias exhibit a myeloid phenotype. About two thirds of the patients whose illness transforms into acute leukemia develop myelogenous leukemia; the remaining one third develop lymphoblastic leukemia. The patients' median survival time from diagnosis of the acute transformation averages only 3 months. Within the realm of therapeutic possibilities, current therapy may be considered quite satisfactory in terms of survival for patients with polycythemia vera and those with essential thrombocythemia. On the other hand, owing to the poor survival rate of the patients with idiopathic myelofibrosis, new therapeutic approaches for this condition are clearly needed.

Treatment

Interferon alfa has been used in the treatment of MPDs, particularly CML, polycythemia vera, and idiopathic thrombocythemia. Interferons have been shown to suppress the proliferation of human pluripotent and single-lineage hematopoietic progenitor cells. The effectiveness of interferon alfa in idiopathic myelofibrosis (agnogenic myeloid metaplasia), however, needs additional evaluation, although preliminary evidence suggests that it may be more efficacious when it is used in the cellular (i.e., proliferative) phase of disease than when the marrow is fibrotic or osteosclerotic.

Treatment with interferon alfa-2a produces decreased platelet counts within 2 to 12 weeks, from a median value of above $1000 \times 10^9/L$ to $350 \times 10^9/L$. Responses have been reported to be dose-dependent. In addition, a simultaneous reduction in leukocyte count can occur. No primary or secondary resistance has been observed. Side effects can occur in about one fourth of patients and may require a dose reduction or the discontinuation of treatment. Thrombocytosis can recur rapidly when treatment is stopped, but a second remission can be achieved by the resumption of interferon therapy.

Cytogenetic and molecular changes after interferon therapy are apparent in patients with CML, as manifested by a change in the Philadelphia (Ph[1]) chromosome and BCR-*abl* gene, respectively. The exact role of interferon in prolonging the life of CML patients, however, remains to be determined. Interferon treatment seems to be well tolerated, and the frequency of treatment-limiting toxicity is low.

Data to date suggest that interferon alfa may be a new and effective drug for the treatment of MPDs. The mechanism of action of interferon is not completely understood. This biological agent, either alone or in combination with other antineoplastic treatment, may represent a new therapeutic approach for these disorders. However, the long-term benefit of interferon in these disorders remains to be established.

In clinical phase studies, ranimustine showed excellent responses in patients with CML, polycythemia vera, and thrombocythemia. When compared with busulfan, no difference was observed in the remission rate, crisis rate, and survival time. Ranimustine exhibits an efficacy almost equal to that of busulfan, but is superior to busulfan in patients who need rapid responses. Side effects are usually mild. Hydroxyurea is currently the favored therapy because it has less acute leukemogenic potential.

CHRONIC MYELOGENOUS LEUKEMIA

CML, a nonlymphocytic leukemia, is also referred to as chronic myeloid leukemia and chronic granulocytic leukemia. It is one of four primary types of MPDs.

CML is one of the most common forms of chronic leukemia. Chronic lymphocytic leukemia (see Chapter 20) is the other principal type of chronic leukemia.

Classification

CML includes five subtypes. The subtypes of CML are:

1. CML—common type
2. Juvenile CML
3. Chronic neutrophilic leukemia
4. Chronic myelomonocytic leukemia
5. Atypical CML

Chronic myelomonocytic leukemia is classified with the myelodysplastic syndromes (see Chapter 22). Chronic myelomonocytic leukemia with high leukocyte counts, however, is both myelodysplastic and myeloproliferative in character. Atypical CML is intermediate between the common type of CML and chronic myelomonocytic leukemia, but it is an entity that is molecularly distinct from common CML. The clinical characteristics and the high frequency of genetic (*ras*) mutations suggest that atypical CML may constitute a subset of the myelodysplastic syndrome and may be best classified as a variant of chronic myelomonocytic leukemia.

Epidemiology

Ninety-five percent of patients with CML have the common type. The other four subtypes constitute 5% of the cases of CML. Juvenile CML and chronic neutrophilic leukemia are extremely rare.

This is predominantly a leukemia of young and middle-aged adults ranging in age from 30 to 50 years old. CML accounts for 20% to 25% of all leukemia cases, with an estimated incidence of 5000 new cases each year. The incidence of CML in western countries is estimated to be approximately 2 per 100,000 persons annually (all age groups included). The age-specific incidence, however, increases markedly after the age of 50 years.

Males are afflicted more frequently than females. Five to 10% of patients have a history of excessive radiation exposure.

Pathophysiology

CML is a clonal proliferative disorder of the pluripotent hematopoietic progenitor cell that results in a disordered proliferation of the erythroid, myeloid, monocytic, and megakaryocytic cell lines. An excessive increase in mostly mature myeloid cells in the peripheral blood is the hallmark of the initial phase of CML.

CML is characterized by a chronic, indolent disease course that frequently transforms into a terminal, acute "blast crisis" phase. An accelerated phase, when patients become refractive to traditional therapy, may precede the acute phase. Some patients may enter the phase of blast transformation abruptly.

Karyotype

The Ph¹ chromosome (Fig. 21.1), the first aberrant chromosome described in a malignant disorder, was discussed by Nowell and Hungerford in 1960. In 1973 it was shown to result from the reciprocal translocation of DNA between chromosomes 9 and 22. Ninety-two percent of Ph¹-positive patients have the typical t(9;22); the remainder have variant translocations. In about half of the variant translocations, chromosome 9 is not affected; the translocation involves chromosome 22 and some other chromosome.

The Ph¹ chromosome is the first demonstrable hematological change in more than 90% of CML patients and is present in myelogenous and erythroid precursors as well as megakaryocytes. It is usually not found in normal lymphocytes. The t(9;22) alteration, however, is not a specific marker for CML. It can also be found in 3% to 5% of children and adults with acute myelogenous (FAB M1) leukemia, and about 5% of children and 10% to 25% of adults with acute lymphoblastic (FAB L1 and L2 types) leukemia.

The balanced reciprocal translocation t(9;22) is probably not the primary event in the pathogenesis of this disease, at least at a cytogenetic level. The cause of Ph¹ variants in about 5% of patients is still unknown. Ph¹-negative CML represents a heterogeneous group of myeloproliferative or myelodysplastic disorders and perhaps should not be called CML.

Seventy-five to 80% of patients in a blast crisis of CML develop other chromosome aberrations in addition to the Ph¹ chromosome. The most common abnormalities are a duplication of the Ph¹ chromosome and trisomy 8. Nonrandom clonal changes found in 80% of patients, in addition to trisomy 8, include +19 and loss of the Y chromosome.

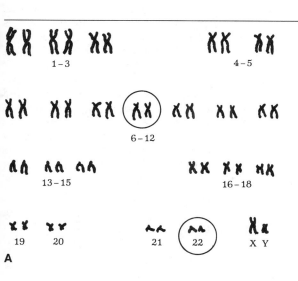

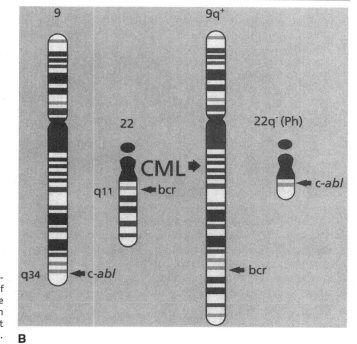

FIGURE 21.1 **A.** Philadelphia chromosome. This chromosomal aberration represents a translocation of the long arm of chromosome 22 to the long arm of chromosome 9. **B.** The Philadelphia translocation in CML. Arrows indicate the chromosome breakpoints at 9q34 and 22q11 and the genes directly involved in the translocation. (From D. Crisan and E. R. Carr, "BCR/*abl* Gene Rearrangement in Chronic Myelogenous Leukemia and Acute Leukemias." *Lab. Med.* Vol. 23, No. 11, November, 1992, p. 731.)

TABLE 21.3 Subtypes of Chronic Myelogenous Leukemia (CML)

Type	Philadelphia (Ph¹) Chromosome	BCR Gene
CML—common	Positive[a]	Positive
Juvenile CML	Negative	Negative
Chronic neutrophilic leukemia	Negative	Negative
Chronic myelomonocytic leukemia	Negative	Negative
Atypical CML	Negative	Negative[b]

[a]5% are Ph¹ chromosome–negative, BCR-positive.
[b]A few patients are BCR-positive.

Genetic Alterations

Patients with CML and acute lymphoblastic leukemia express the BCR gene rearrangement (Table 21.3), which is the molecular counterpart of the Ph¹ chromosome. These reciprocal translocations (see Fig. 21.1) involve the relocation and fusion of the proto-oncogene *c-abl* on the distal arm of chromosome 9 to a break in the newly identified genetic locus of chromosome 22, known as *BCR* (breakpoint cluster region). The significance of the presence of the Ph¹ chromosome is possibly related to amplification of the BCR/*abl* fusion gene product. The BCR/*abl* fusion gene is transcribed into a chimeric BCR/*abl* mRNA, which is in turn translated into a fusion protein with abnormal structure and function. The BCR/*abl* fusion gene, mRNA, and protein are diagnostic markers of CML at the molecular level.

Detecting gene rearrangements involving the BCR and c-*abl* genes is clinically useful for:

1. Confirmation of Ph¹-positive cases of CML
2. Diagnosis of Ph¹-negative cases of CML
3. Diagnosis of CML presenting in blast crisis
4. Monitoring of patients with CML during and after therapy for detection of minimal residual disease
5. Confirmation of remission
6. Early detection of relapse

Clinical Signs and Symptoms

The clinical course of CML can be characterized by three separate progressive phases (Table 21.4). The onset of the early, initial phase (chronic phase) of CML is insidious and may last from 2 to 3 years. Signs and symptoms can include progressive fatigue and malaise, low-grade fever, anorexia, weight loss, and bone pain. Night sweats and fever, associated with an increased metabolism due to granulocytic cell turnover, may occur. Physical examination usually reveals splenic enlargement. Splenic infarction is common because of the abnormal overproduction and accumulation of granulocyte precursors in the bone marrow, spleen, and blood. These infarcts in the spleen may produce left-upper-quadrant pain. Any organ may eventually be infiltrated with myeloid elements. Extramyeloid masses in areas other than the spleen and liver, however, are uncommon findings in the chronic phase. On fresh incision, extramyeloid masses appear green, presumably because of the presence of the myeloid enzyme myeloperoxidase. These greenish tumors have been called **chloromas.**

A transitional, accelerated period may precede blast transformation. This transition is heralded by an increase in splenomegaly, a rising peripheral blood leukocyte count, an increased percentage of basophils, worsening anemia, and thrombocytopenia.

About three fourths of patients eventually enter a gradual transformation to a blast crisis. The "blast crisis" phase is characterized by the appearance of primitive blast cells similar to those seen in acute leukemia. Acute-phase CML is hematologically and clinically indistinguishable from acute leukemia. Excessive bleeding or bruising, and fevers may be manifested in the later stage of CML. Complications are frequent in conjunction with the blast crisis. Bleeding complications are related to thrombocytopenia, impaired platelet function, and low intraplatelet concentrations of beta thromboglobulin and platelet factor 4 (PF4).

Laboratory Data

Cellular Components

The chronic leukemias are usually characterized by the presence of leukocytosis. In the case of CML, the degree of leukocytosis is extreme. In addition, CML can also be identified by the presence of the entire spectrum of immature and mature myelogenous cells in the blood and marrow.

Anemia is a common finding. The total leukocyte count is usually greater than $50 \times 10^9/L$ and may exceed $300 \times 10^9/L$. Peripheral blood smears (Fig. 21.2 and Plate 71) demonstrate increased numbers of mature granulocytic forms, such as segmented neutrophils and band forms, and smaller numbers of immature forms. Myeloblasts rarely exceed 5% of the nucleated cells. Eosinophils and basophils may also be increased. Thrombocytosis may be observed in 40% of patients, although thrombocytopenia often ensues. Nucleated erythrocytes and red blood cells exhibiting anisocytosis and basophilic stippling can be seen.

Patients experiencing the terminal phase of CML may enter a blast crisis, which is indistinguishable from acute myelogenous leukemia, particularly the FAB M2 type. About 30% of patients have cytologic features of CLL.

TABLE 21.4 Typical Phases of Chronic Myelogenous Leukemia

Phase	Approximate Length of Phase	Treatment Status*
Initial (chronic)	2–5 yr	Highly treatable
Accelerated	6–18 mo	Resistance develops
Blast crisis (acute)	3–4 mo	Generally unresponsive

*Conventional chemotherapy.

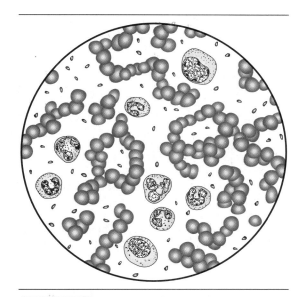

FIGURE 21.2 Chronic myelogenous leukemia (CML). Most of the cells in this field are mature granulocytes (band forms and segmented neutrophils). An increased number of platelets (thrombocytes) is also seen in this field of the smear. (Simulates magnification ×1000.)

Examination of a bone marrow biopsy specimen reveals hypercellularity with prominent granulocytic hyperplasia. An increased number of myeloid cells in the intermediate stage is seen. The myeloid-erythroid (M:E) ratio can be as high as 25:1. The bone marrow may become fibrotic late in the disease and may be mistaken for myelofibrosis (agnogenic myeloid metaplasia).

Electron Microscopy

The study of cellular ultrastructure is less commonly performed for chronic leukemias than for acute leukemias. Electron microscope examination of the blood of a person in the chronic phase of CML usually demonstrates that the majority of the segmented neutrophils appear morphologically normal. The number of specific and azurophilic granules may be slightly decreased but is within the normal range. Occasional cells may exhibit abnormalities such as aggregates of smooth endoplasmic reticulum, several stacked rows of endoplasmic reticulum, and abnormal granules.

Immature myelogenous (granulocytic) precursors, myeloblasts and promyelocytes, frequently manifest abnormalities. These abnormalities include bundles of microfilaments and deep folds in the nucleus.

Cytochemistry

Cytochemical studies are used less frequently for chronic leukemias than for acute leukemias. In special cases, however, these stains may be of diagnostic value. The leukocyte alkaline phosphatase (LAP) procedure is used to differentiate between CML and a **leukemoid reaction.** A leukemoid reaction is produced by a severe infection or inflammation and frequently resembles leukemia on bone marrow or blood smears. In CML, the LAP score is decreased, as compared with a leukemoid reaction, in which a high score is usual.

However, an increased LAP score may be encountered in CML because of subsequent secondary infections or inflammation. Additionally, during remission phases of CML, the LAP score may return to normal limits.

In the LAP (see Chapter 24) or neutrophilic alkaline phosphatase (NAP) reaction, a solution of naphthol AS-MX phosphate alkaline and either fast blue RR or fast red violet LB salt is incubated with a microscopic smear of peripheral blood or bone marrow. Positive reactions are indicated by the deposition of blue or violet pigment at the cellular sites of alkaline phosphate activity within either band-form or segmented neutrophils.

Following staining, 100 bands or segmented neutrophils are counted. Each cell is rated according to the distribution and intensity of staining. The possible range is 0 to 400, although the normal range is from 20 to 100. Increased scores are associated with leukemoid reactions, severe bacterial infections, and polycythemia vera. Decreased scores can be found in viral infections and CML.

Prognosis

Because chronic-phase CML is highly responsive to treatment, many patients experience at least one remission. These remissions can last from several weeks to months, with 60% of patients becoming asymptomatic. Ninety percent of patients experience a decreased total leukocyte count, although the chromosomal abnormality, the Ph^1 chromosome, persists.

The median survival time from the time of diagnosis is about 1 year in patients lacking Ph^1. Those patients with Ph^1 have a better prognosis, with a median survival time of 3 to 4 years. After progression to the blast crisis phase, the prognosis is poor, with patient survival time usually being less than 6 months. Patients with atypical CML, however, have a markedly worse survival rate than patients with common CML and probably worse than patients with chronic myelomonocytic leukemia.

Treatment

Traditionally, treatment for chronic-phase CML has consisted of either hydroxyurea or busulfan therapy. Although these agents may extend the chronic phase, they have not averted the ultimate transformation to the acute phase. Intensive chemotherapy in conjunction with total body irradiation and allogeneic bone marrow transplantation in patients under 50 years old have produced some cures, but the toxicity of cytotoxic therapy and the unavailability of matched donors have limited this approach.

After years of stagnation in the treatment of chronic hematological malignancies, some agents that might improve the prognosis of these diseases have emerged. Interferon alfa seems to be active in CML and to result in occasional cytogenetic remissions in bone marrow. Interferons are a group of glycoproteins produced by a variety of cells in response to viral infections, immune stimulation, and chemical inducers. Currently, two types of interferon alfa are commercially available: interferon alfa-2a and interferon alfa-2b. The mechanisms of action of interferon are multiple, overlapping, and potentially mediated through antiproliferative activity, direct cytotoxic effects, and immunomodulatory effects. The specific anticancer mechanism is presently unknown.

Interferon therapy leads to a reduction in the number of Ph[1] chromosome–positive cells, but additional chromosomal anomalies may be induced by interferon directly or may arise at random and gain a proliferative advantage during interferon therapy. The role and importance of most of these anomalies are not known. In terms of both safety and effectiveness, it has been established that treatment with interferon alfa is an appropriate method of inducing complete hematological remission in early, chronic-phase, Ph[1] chromosome–positive CML.

POLYCYTHEMIA VERA

Polycythemia vera can also be referred to as polycythemia rubra vera, Osler's disease, Vaquez's disease, and erythremia. Erythremia is a benign or incipient form of polycythemia vera that may gradually develop other characteristics of classic polycythemia vera over many years. Polycythemia vera is distinguished from the other kinds of chronic MPDs by the remarkable increases in red cell mass and total blood volume. However, generalized hyperplasia of the bone marrow with subsequent increases in the erythroid, leukocytic, and megakaryocytic series also exists. This is typically reflected in the circulating blood by an absolute increase in erythrocytes, leukocytes, and thrombocytes (platelets).

Epidemiology

The occurrence of polycythemia vera is almost equal in men and women (1.2 : 1.0 ratio). The natural history of polycythemia vera is that it occurs gradually over many decades. The mean age at diagnosis ranges from 60 to 65 years. The most serious complications are arterial and venous complications (vascular accidents) and the transition to acute leukemia. Because the evolution of polycythemia vera occurs gradually and over a period of many years, it is difficult to document the annual incidence accurately. However, the annual incidence is believed to be between 0.6 and 1.6 cases per 100,000 persons.

Etiology

Polycythemia vera is a clonal MPD of the pluripotent hematopoietic stem cell with an unknown etiology. Patterns of increased risk have been observed among chemical plant workers. In addition, kindreds with familial polycythemia vera have been identified. The mode of inheritance is unclear, but genetic factors may be involved in the pathogenesis of this MPD.

Pathophysiology

Although polycythemia vera is a clonal hematopoietic progenitor cell disorder with trilineage hyperplasia, the most constant and striking feature is erythroid hyperplasia of the bone marrow. This very slow evolution of the malignant erythroid clone leads to overexpansion of the red cell mass, hypervolemia, and splenomegalic red cell pooling. These consequences eventually cause generalized marrow hyperplasia with subsequent increases in the quantity of all three cell lines.

Abnormalities in polycythemia vera erythroid progenitors are expressed at the level of both the colony-forming unit-erythroid (CFU-E) and burst-forming unit-erythroid (BFU-E), which suggests multiple changes in the erythroid progenitors. A shift in the cell compartment may occur in polycythemia vera. Interleukin-3 (IL-3) stimulates trilineage hematopoiesis, but a striking hypersensitivity of polycythemia vera BFU-E to recombinant IL-3 has been noted. This may be a major factor in the pathogenesis of increased erythropoiesis without increased erythropoietin concentrations.

In addition, the manganese and zinc contents of the physiologically active erythrocytic microelements demonstrate disturbances in erythrocytes of the peripheral venous blood in patients with polycythemia vera. These changes indicate the neoplastic character of proliferation of bone marrow cells in polycythemia vera.

Karyotype

Chromosomal abnormalities in polycythemia vera can include alterations and partial duplications involving the long arm of chromosome 1, monosomy or partial deletion of chromosome 5, and trisomy 8 and 9. Trisomy 1q is the most frequent structural chromosomal abnormality. Surplus 1q material is commonly translocated to other chromosomes (e.g., particularly to chromosome 9). Other abnormalities overrepresented in polycythemia vera involve chromosomes 12 and 20. Partial deletion of chromosome 20 (20q−) is among the most prevalent cytogenetic findings in polycythemia vera.

Trisomy 8, +9, and a partial deletion of chromosome 20 (20q−) can be found in a small proportion of patients early in the course of diagnosis and treatment, and also among untreated patients. These chromosomal abnormalities seem to be related to the natural course of polycythemia vera rather than resulting from therapy. During the first 10 years of disease, approximately one fourth of patients demonstrate an abnormal clone, but after more than 10 years more than three fourths of patients exhibit an abnormal clone. Patients with a chromosomally abnormal clone at the time of diagnosis have a poorer chance of survival than those exhibiting a normal karyotype in metaphase cells. Cytogenetic results do not predict evolution of the disease, but do provide clues to the hematological phenotype, duration of the disease, and consequences of myelosuppressive therapy.

Clinical Signs and Symptoms

Plethora is the hallmark of polycythemia vera. Splenomegaly is a commonly found sign of disease; it occurs in more than three fourths of patients. Reversible, moderate hypertension frequently occurs as the result of the expanded blood volume. An increased total blood volume (hypervolemia) occurs in polycythemia vera and in disorders such as congestive heart failure, primary aldosteronism, and Cushing's syndrome, and as a result of overtransfusion of donor blood.

Neurological symptoms are reported by 50% to 80% of patients. Symptoms such as headaches, dizziness, paresthesias, and sight alterations are frequently related to hyperviscosity, and respond immediately to a reduction of cell counts, except in ictus patients. Other neurological symptoms seem to result from an associated coagulopathy. Patients with polycythemia tend to develop both arterial and venous thrombosis and are prone to hemorrhages. Polycythemia vera, sickle cell anemia, sickle cell–hemoglobin C disease, and essential thrombocythemia are the major disorders of formed blood elements causing stroke. Hemorrhagic phenomena are frequent among patients with digestive manifestations, including gastrointestinal hemorrhage, abdominal pain, or portal vein thrombosis, or thrombosis of the suprahepatic vein. In addition, thrombophlebitis with pulmonary embolism is a common complication of polycythemia vera and often is unrecognized.

Severe psychotic depression is rare in patients with polycythemia vera. In venography-documented Budd-Chiari syndrome, the underlying diseases include polycythemia vera.

The criteria for the diagnosis of polycythemia vera outlined by the National Polycythemia Vera Study Group are presented in Table 21.5.

Laboratory Data

Cellular Alterations

An increased erythrocyte cell count, packed cell volume, and hemoglobin with normal erythrocytic indices (discussed later in this chapter) are characteristic of polycythemia vera. Peak polycythemic values are a hemoglobin of approximately 20.6 gm/dL, a microhematocrit of about 80%, a total

leukocyte (white blood cell, WBC) count of $28,000 \times 10^9/L$, and a platelet count of $1400 \times 10^9/L$.

In patients with polycythemia vera, as in those with the other diseases, the red blood cell distribution width (RDW) tends to be higher than normal. The RDW transiently increases following administration of a myelosuppressive agent, corresponding to the transition period from microcytes to normal blood cells. The RDW is even higher during polycythemic periods than during the myelofibrotic period. This may be associated with hematopoietic abnormality due to extramedullary hematopoiesis. RDW seems to reflect accurately the pathological status of polycythemia vera.

Lymphocyte populations in patients with polycythemia vera demonstrate an altered CD4/CD8 ratio, mainly due to a decreased CD8 subpopulation. Increased lymphocyte activity has also been observed. Interleukin-2 (IL-2) production is significantly higher; the lymphoproliferative response both to phytohemagglutinin and IL-2 is also greater in lymphocytes from polycythemia vera patients. These observations suggest that patients may also suffer from an altered lymphoid lineage.

Blood Volume, Red Blood Cell Mass, and Viscosity

A diagnosis of polycythemia requires an accurate assessment of plasma volume and red blood cell mass. Total blood volume and erythrocyte volume need to be determined (usually by radioisotope methods) in order to distinguish polycythemia vera from other forms of polycythemia. An increase in both measurements is an important distinction between polycythemia vera and polycythemias resulting from a decrease in plasma volume.

Patients with polycythemia vera frequently demonstrate a complex of hemorrheological disorders (high blood viscosity at different rates of deviation, intensified red blood cell aggregation, and decreased deformability of these cells) and hemocoagulation disorders. These characteristics are considered to be implicated in the disease pathogenesis.

Increased whole blood viscosity contributes to vascular occlusions and reversible lesions including cerebral and myocardial infarction, as well as shortness of breath and hot flushes, probably due to circulatory disturbance. Patients with a blood viscosity higher than twice the normal mean value may be in danger of vascular occlusion. A correlation has been revealed among the parameters of red blood cell rheological properties, hemostasis, and the disease severity.

Abnormalities of Hemostasis and Coagulation

In some cases, disorders in the rheological phenomena of red blood cells are a triggering mechanism in the development of the DIC syndrome.

In the chronic phase of polycythemia vera, patients with thrombohemorrhagic complications have higher platelet counts, more severe platelet aggregation defects, and increased plasma levels of beta thromboglobulin and fibrinopeptide A compared to patients without complications. However, thrombohemorrhagic complications are not predictable by changes in these parameters in individual patients during the chronic disease phase.

TABLE 21.5 National Polycythemia Vera Study Group Criteria for Diagnosis

Major Criteria

Red cell mass	Males > 36 mL/kg
	Females > 32 mL/kg
Normal arterial O_2 saturation	>92%
Splenomegaly	

Minor Criteria

Leukocyte alkaline phosphatase (LAP) activity	>100 units (with no evidence of fever or infection)
Leukocytosis	>1200 × 10⁹/L with no evidence of fever or infection
Serum vitamin B_{12} or	>900 pg/mL
Unbounded vitamin B_{12}–binding capacity	>2200 pg/mL
Thrombocytosis platelet count	> 400,000 × 10⁹/L

Diagnostic Measures
Patient has polycythemia vera if
- All three major criteria are present, or
- The first two major criteria and any two minor criteria are present

---

Source: L. R. Wasserman. "The Management of Polycythemia Vera." *Br. J. Haematol.,* 21:371, 1971.

The plasma level of tissue plasminogen activator antigen (t-PA-Ag) is significantly decreased in patients with polycythemia vera compared to normal individuals. In contrast, patients with spurious polycythemia and secondary polycythemia exhibit significantly increased concentrations of t-PA-Ag. There is no significant difference in t-PA-Ag levels in polycythemic patients with or without thromboembolic disease.

Other Laboratory Assays

Erythropoietin excretion in the urine is decreased in polycythemia vera, in contrast to the other kinds of polycythemias. Radioimmunoassay of erythropoietin has been used to distinguish between polycythemia vera and other forms of erythrocytosis.

Laboratory findings that would support a diagnosis of polycythemia vera as compared to other forms of polycythemia are an absence of hemosiderin from the bone marrow and an increased LAP score. In addition, hyperuricemia and hyperuricosuria are present in over half of polycythemia vera patients at diagnosis due to excess nucleic acid degradation. The level of uric acid parallels increases in severity of polycythemia vera as the disease progresses.

A comparison of the laboratory findings in polycythemia vera and other forms of polycythemia is presented in Table 21.6.

TABLE 21.6 **A Summary of Significant Differences Between Polycythemia Vera and Other Types of Polycythemia**

	Polycythemia Vera	Other Types
Total blood volume	Increased	Normal or decreased
Total leukocytes	Increased	Normal
Immature red blood cells	Occasional	None
Platelets	Increased	Normal
Leukocyte alkaline phosphatase stain	Increased	Normal
Erythrocyte sedimentation rate	Decreased	Normal
Serum iron	Decreased	Normal or increased
Erythropoietin	Decreased or absent	Normal or increased
Blood histamine	Increased	Normal
Unsaturated vitamin B_{12}–binding capacity	Increased	Normal
Basophil count	Increased	Normal
Hyperuricemia	Present or absent	Normal
Hyperuricosuria	Present or absent	Normal

Prognosis and Complications

Polycythemia vera is considered to be a chronic disease, with a 10- to 20-year life expectancy after diagnosis. Certain prognostic factors and treatment strategies have an effect on survival. The clinical course of most patients is characterized by a low rate of acute leukemia and a high rate (approximately 40%) of thromboembolic complications. Some patients develop myelofibrosis.

A high initial hemoglobin concentration in peripheral blood and the use of any myelosuppressive therapy are associated with an increased risk of leukemic transformation. However, the use of hydroxyurea has much less potential for inducing leukemic transformation. Transformation from polycythemia vera to CML is very unusual. However, it does occur in patients who have received either phosphorus 32 (^{32}P) or chemotherapy treatment. This suggests that irradiation and alkylating agents play a role in the transformation to CML. This risk becomes substantial with the use of two or more myelosuppressive agents. Myelosuppressive therapy does prolong survival, especially in patients with elevated platelet counts.

Myelodysplastic syndrome (see Chapter 22) is an increasingly recognized complication of polycythemia vera that often precedes leukemic transformation. Unique characteristics of patients who experience this complication are as follows:

1. History of polycythemia vera
2. Rapidly increasing splenomegaly resistant to standard therapy
3. Absence of overt marrow fibrosis
4. Hypercellularity (greater than or equal to 90% cellular) of the bone marrow with dysplasia in the myeloid, erythroid, and megakaryocytic cell lines
5. Peripheral monocytosis greater than 1×10^9/L
6. Extensive infiltration of the spleen and liver by dysplastic myeloid cells

Treatment

Primary control of polycythemia vera is achieved by phlebotomy. The aim of phlebotomy is to produce an iron deficiency that then limits red blood cell production. This may be performed by the removal of units of whole blood or by large-volume erythrocytopheresis using a cell separator. Cytopheresis produces a long-lasting reduction of red blood cell volume (microhematocrit), hemoglobin, and erythrocyte counts, as well as the immediate disappearance or reduction of clinical symptoms.

The evolution of the process of polycythemia vera is favorably altered by bleedings and chemotherapeutic cytoreduction, which are often performed simultaneously. This may take the form of treatment with chlorambucil supplemented with phlebotomy, or ^{32}P plus phlebotomy. Hydroxyurea is now the preferred agent, and alkylating agents are avoided when possible. Marrow suppression by radioactive phosphorus or low-dose busulfan is usually used only as a second-line therapy or to lower high platelet counts. Whatever treatment is chosen, the aim of therapy should be to reduce the microhematocrit to approximately 40% to 45%.

Recombinant interferon alfa, a natural product with growth-inhibiting capabilities, was recently demonstrated for the first time to have significant therapeutic efficacy in controlling the red blood cell mass in patients with polycythemia vera. The striking advantage in the use of this drug is its presumed absence of leukemogenic effect. Small doses of interferon alfa-2a have been observed to produce a durable normal hematocrit level (microhematocrit less than 48%), a reduction of platelet count, and a reduction in spleen size within 4 to 8 weeks of treatment in some patients. The range of patient responses is from very good to substantially unchanged. In some patients, neurological side effects have been observed and forced the cessation of treatment. The problems with this form of treatment are the necessity of injections and cost.

IDIOPATHIC MYELOFIBROSIS

Idiopathic myelofibrosis is also referred to as agnogenic myeloid metaplasia. It is a chronic MPD of unknown cause, characterized by systemic bone marrow fibrosis and extramedullary hematopoiesis. Secondary myelofibrosis is caused by infiltrative disorders, including malignancies and infections, or exposure to chemical toxins or irradiation.

Epidemiology

Patients with myelofibrosis may undergo temporary or permanent transition to polycythemia vera or may convert to CML. About one fifth of patients with polycythemia vera develop myelofibrosis.

Idiopathic myelofibrosis is uncommon, with the number of new cases estimated at 1000 to 2000 per year in the United States, or an overall rate of 2 per 100,000 worldwide. The incidence of myelofibrosis, however, is known to be increased after exposure to irradiation and chemicals such as benzene.

Although there have been a few reports of patients in the pediatric population, the majority of patients with idiopathic myelofibrosis are in their late 50s, 60s, and 70s. It is also more common in the white population, and men and women are equally affected.

Pathophysiology

Idiopathic myelofibrosis is a clonal disorder of the multipotential progenitor cell compartment. The blood–marrow barrier is disrupted early in the course of myelofibrosis, so that blast cells and committed stem cells such as colony-forming unit-granulocyte-macrophage (CFU-GM), BFU-E, and colony-forming unit-megakaryocyte (CFU-Meg) cells escape into the circulating blood in large numbers.

Sclerosis of the bone develops in about half of patients. However, myelofibrosis, the predominant clinical manifestation, occurs secondarily and is not a component of the abnormal clonal proliferation. The process of fibrosis ensues from proliferation of fibroblasts and increased collagen production in reaction to the abnormal clone of hematopoietic cells. Fibrosis is probably the result of a product secreted by megakaryocytes.

If the constituents of the hematopoietic microenvironment (myeloid stroma) are examined microscopically, an overall increase, particularly in so-called undifferentiated (primitive-pluripotent) and also in transitional (fibroblastic) reticular cells and myofibroblasts, can be observed. Undifferentiated and transitional reticular cells as well as myofibroblasts seem to form an integral part of the hematopoietic microenvironment and are assumed to play an important role in the evolution of disease-specific myelofibrosis. In addition, the evolution of medullary fibrosis is thought to be associated with the striking predominance of large, atypical, possibly overaged and hyperpolyploid megakaryocytes, but not with an increase in precursor cells.

Dysmegakaryocytopoiesis leading to an overproduction of defective platelets is the most constant feature of myelofibrosis. Research findings imply that the marked increase in circulating progenitor cells of the megakaryocyte lineage may be generated by extramedullary, probably splenic hematopoiesis. One abnormality of the megakaryopoiesis in bone marrow tissue, however, is pronounced pleomorphism of the megakaryocytic cell line consisting of giant forms, micromegakaryocytes, and naked (pyknotic) neuclei. Another maturational abnormality is the dissociation of nuclear-cytoplasmic maturation, including the amount of dense granules, and the development of the demarcation membrane system as well as the occurrence of emperipolesis (i.e., internalization of hematopoietic cells) already in immature or megakaryoblastic elements. A striking variety in the appearance of dense granules of the alpha type also frequently exists. Thrombocytes show giant forms with either hypertrophy of the open canalicular system or an abundance of dense granules and beta glycogen accumulation. Other remarkable features include a focal sponge-like proliferation of the open canalicular system in many of the large platelets and giant and fused granules of the alpha and osmiophilic type. These abnormalities in megakaryocytes and thrombocytes may have certain functional implications (e.g., hemorrhage and thrombosis) that are often encountered out of proportion to the platelet counts in this disorder. In addition, those anomalies indicate a disorganization of megakaryopoiesis, which may contribute to the abnormal release of factors (platelet-derived growth factor and PF4) predominantly involved in the process of myelofibrosis. It has been postulated that platelet-derived growth factor and PF4 are involved in the imbalance of the mechanism of medullary stroma maintenance, which triggers off the bone marrow myelofibrotic process. A relationship between the presence of myelofibrosis and abnormal levels of beta thromboglobulin, PF4, and mitogenic activity in platelet-poor plasma and platelet extracts has been observed in patients with idiopathic myelofibrosis.

Karyotype

Idiopathic myelofibrosis is not associated with a specific or unique chromosomal anomaly. However, about 40% of patients acquire recurrent cytogenetic abnormalities and nearly 80% acquire nonspecific aberrations. Several chromosomal abnormalities are overrepresented in patients with myelofibrosis. These alterations involve the long arm of chromosome 1; monosomy and partial deletion of chromosomes 5, 7, 9, 11, and 13; loss of Y chromosome; and trisomy of 8, 9, and 21. Partial trisomy 1q is a karyotypic change detectable in unstimulated peripheral blood cell cultures or bone marrow cultures, which suggests that partial trisomy 1q is a primary chromosome aberration in myelofibrosis and is relevant to the pathogenesis of this disorder.

Karyotypic changes occur as secondary events during the multistep process of leukemogenesis. Therefore, changes such as t(5;17) may represent a therapy-induced abnormality nonrandomly related to the terminal phase of myeloid disorders.

Clinical Signs and Symptoms

Patients with myelofibrosis usually exhibit progressive anemia, splenomegaly, and marrow fibrosis. Splenomegaly and some hepatomegaly are due to extramedullary hematopoiesis. Patients may notice easy bruising or bleeding resulting from thrombocytopenia, abnormal platelet function, or both. About one third of patients manifest purpura. More than 40% of patients have osteosclerosis with accompanying bone pain, malaise, and leukocytosis. A mild degree of jaundice, abdominal fullness, dyspepsia, or weight loss may be manifested in some patients. Portal hypertension may be evident.

In a rare case, one patient presented with a breast mass. Excision biopsy of the mass revealed extramedullary hematopoiesis, as did histopathological examination of the liver and the spleen. This type of presentation demonstrates the complementary character of both diagnostic modalities and the resemblance to lymphoma of the breast, although the findings are too nonspecific to rule out breast carcinoma. Knowledge of the clinical history and histopathology is necessary to make the proper diagnosis. Another rare presentation occurred in a patient with cutaneous extramedullary hematopoiesis. The skin lesions appeared as multiple papules and nodules on the trunk. Histological examination of a lesion showed all three components of the hematopoietic tissue, that is, myeloid, erythroid, and megakaryocytic series.

Cellular Alterations

Hematological findings are variable and nonuniform, but blood morphology provides the best clues to diagnosis. The leukoerythroblastic picture of teardrop-shaped erythrocytes, nucleated erythrocytes, and immature myeloid cells is classic for myelofibrosis. Leukocytosis, mild anemia, thrombocytosis, and panhyperplasia in the marrow are characteristic in the early stages. Extramedullary hematopoiesis, peripheral cytopenias (i.e., anemia, leukopenia, or thrombocytopenia), and myelofibrosis, with or without osteosclerosis, reflect the changes seen in the later stages. Transitions among the different types of chronic MPDs and termination in acute leukemia or marrow failure are common.

Erythrocytes

Mild anemia due to ineffective erythropoiesis, decreased red blood cell survival, and overt hemolysis may occur. Polychromatophilia and an elevated reticulocyte count in the absence of erythropoietic stress provide an important clue to diagnosis because they signify a breakdown in marrow ultrastructure.

Leukocytes

In about 50% of patients, the total leukocyte (WBC) count is increased. Most patients have total WBC counts of less than 30×10^9/L, but the total WBC count can be as high as 100×10^9/L. A high WBC count (neutrophilia) and immature granulocytes on peripheral blood smears including blasts can create a picture that can be confused with leukemia.

Platelets

The concentration of platelets is variable, but giant dysplastic platelets and fragments of megakaryocytes can be seen. Thrombocytosis gradually progresses to thrombocytopenia. As myelofibrosis progresses, the entire morphological picture of myelophthisis (infiltrative myelopathy) unfolds: teardrop-shaped erythrocytes, nucleated erythrocytes, early granulocytic forms, bizarre platelets, and megakaryocyte fragments.

Bone Marrow

The bone marrow is hypocellular and becomes fibrotic with an associated decrease in hematopoiesis. Bone marrow aspiration is unsuccessful in nearly 90% of patients because reticulin and collagen fibrosis lock in the marrow content, causing a "dry tap." A bone marrow biopsy shows fibrosis, generally with increased numbers of megakaryocytes.

Prognosis

The median survival time ranges from 4.3 to 5.0 years. In patients with idiopathic myelofibrosis, hemoglobin concentration, platelet count, and the presence of osteomyelosclerosis have been identified as factors with prognostic significance. Patients with a hemoglobin concentration of less than 10 gm/dL have been identified as having a significantly shorter survival time than those with a hemoglobin concentration greater or equal to 10 gm/dL. A platelet count of less than 100×10^9/L also implies a significantly shorter survival time and is of prognostic significance within the first 6 months from diagnosis. Patients with osteomyelosclerosis, as demonstrated on x-ray film of the skeleton, have a significantly better prognosis compared to those without osteomyelosclerosis. The presence of osteomyelosclerosis emerged as a favorable parameter at 3 and 5 years. Using these three parameters and spleen size, a prognostic scoring system has been designed; it categorizes patients into three prognostic groups with highly different survival times (low-risk group = 69 months; intermediate-risk group = 33 months; high-risk group = 4 months).

In addition, major thromboembolic complications that contribute to shortened survival times are seen in about one fifth of patients.

Treatment

There is no therapy that will affect the basic disease process. Asymptomatic patients require no treatment.

Treatment for myelofibrosis can consist of periodic transfusions of packed red blood cells, androgens, cytotoxic agents, and platelet reduction by plateletpheresis. Administration of prophylactic antibiotics may also be considered. Recombinant interferon alfa may be efficacious when used in the cellular (i.e., proliferative) phase, and less so when the marrow is fibrotic or osteosclerotic. Moderate doses of radiotherapy to the spleen have been effective in controlling symptoms. However, clinical improvement after irradiation is a slow, gradual process.

Splenectomy may be appropriate in some circumstances (e.g., massively enlarged spleen). Splenectomy in patients with myelofibrosis is associated with an operative mortality of 13.4%, an early morbidity of 45.3%, and a late morbidity of 16.3%. Almost all patients with portal hypertension and painful splenomegaly, but only about half of those with thrombopenia and anemia, have been reported to experience a relief in symptoms or signs after splenectomy. There is no evidence that splenectomy affects survival in myelofibrosis. Splenectomy in patients with advanced myelofibrosis is a palliative procedure that carries a substantial risk.

ESSENTIAL THROMBOCYTHEMIA

Essential or primary thrombocythemia (essential thrombocytosis) is characterized by a marked increase in circulating platelets, usually in excess of 1000×10^9/L. However, elevated platelet counts may be encountered as a reactive phenomenon, secondary to a variety of systemic conditions, or they may represent essential thrombocythemia, a primary disorder of the bone marrow.

Diagnostic Characteristics

The diagnosis of essential thrombocythemia is difficult and relies on the exclusion of other myeloproliferative states and nonhematological illnesses associated with an increased concentration of platelets. Major criteria and ancillary findings manifested in essential thrombocythemia are presented in Table 21.7.

TABLE 21.7 Criteria for Diagnosis of Essential Thrombocythemia

Major Criteria
Persistent elevation of platelets in peripheral blood

Marked increase (hyperplasia) of megakaryocytes in the bone marrow.

Absence of other chronic myeloproliferative disorders

Absence of any systemic condition responsible for reactive thrombocytosis (e.g., infection, malignancy, postsplenectomy)

Other Findings
Absence of the Ph[1] chromosome

Expanded red blood cell mass

Mild neutrophilia

Elevation of vitamin B_{12} and vitamin B_{12}–binding proteins

Epidemiology

Essential or primary thrombocythemia (essential thrombocytosis) is the least common MPD. Essential thrombocythemia occurs most frequently among persons in the fifth and sixth decades of life. Men and women are equally affected.

Pathophysiology

Essential thrombocythemia is a clonal disorder of multipotential cell origin and belongs to the chronic MPDs that include polycythemia vera, CML, and idiopathic myelofibrosis. This rare disorder includes a mucocutaneous hemorrhagic diathesis and thromboembolic events. Both thrombocytosis and platelet dysfunction can be responsible for the thrombohemorrhagic phenomena exhibited by patients with this disease. However, qualitative platelet abnormalities rather than thrombocytosis are believed to be the main cause of thromboembolic events.

Karyotype

At least three fourths of patients have a normal karyotype. The balance of patients demonstrate variable chromosomal abnormalities, with aneuploidy being the most common.

Clinical Signs and Symptoms

Thrombotic or bleeding problems are the most commonly seen disorders in patients with thrombocythemia. Patients typically manifest easy bruising, nosebleeds, or gastrointestinal bleeding.

Splenomegaly is found in less than half of patients. Neurological manifestations, however, are frequent and are due to obstruction of the cerebral microvasculature. Cerebral ischemia and digital ischemia or even gangrene relent or respond completely to a reduction of platelet levels. In addition, unexplained hematomas are common.

A benign form free of hemorrhagic or thrombotic presentation can be observed in a subset of patients aged from 15 to 25 years old.

Laboratory Findings

Cellular Abnormalities

The classic laboratory finding in essential thrombocythemia is a markedly elevated peripheral blood platelet count. The number of platelets in the circulating blood is usually in excess of 1000×10^9/L, with a minimum of 600×10^9/L. Platelet morphology reveals a normal discoid-shaped cell; bleeding time is normal. In addition, pseudohyperkalemia may result during the preparation of serum. Potassium from platelets is not released during the aggregation phase but during the degranulation phase of the coagulation process.

Peripheral blood erythrocytes are frequently hypochromic and microcytic. If splenic atrophy is present, abnormal erythrocyte morphology includes target cells, Howell-Jolly bodies, nucleated erythrocytes, and acanthocytes. The total concentration of leukocytes is elevated in about 50% of patients but it seldom exceeds $40 \times 10^9/L$. The LAP value is normal or increased. Concentrations of vitamin B_{12} and uric acid are usually increased.

Platelet Function

In patients with thrombocythemia, the mean extent of aggregation induced by epinephrine, collagen, or ADP is significantly lower than in normal controls. In more than half of patients with thrombocythemia, the platelet-rich plasma does not respond to epinephrine. The total calcium content of platelets is also significantly lower.

Bone Marrow

Bone marrow morphology in primary thrombocythemia is similar to the architecture seen in polycythemia vera and CML with associated extreme thrombocytosis. However, significant differences are observable between the marrow findings in MPD and those in extreme reactive thrombocytosis. These differences include the numbers of megakaryocytes, the presence or absence of megakaryocyte clusters, stainable iron, cellularity, and reticulin content.

In addition to increased marrow cellularity (hyperplasia), megakaryocytic hyperplasia is striking. This conspicuous megakaryocytic proliferation also manifests polyploidy of the nuclei, giant forms, and clusters.

Relationship of Thrombocythemia and Polycythemia Vera

The seminal events responsible for initiating thrombocythemia and polycythemia vera clones are unknown. Both clonal disorders are marked by a low-grade hyperproliferation of two committed stem cell lines plus a marked stimulation of a third cell line. These two disorders are differentiated by a single characteristic—the absence of an expanded red blood cell mass in thrombocythemia.

The mutant stem cell in both disorders has a predisposition to undergo transformation to either myelofibrosis or acute leukemia. The similarities in the natural history of these MPDs suggest that they both begin as very similar, pluripotent stem cell disorders expressed differently only at the colony-forming cell level.

Treatment

The course of the disease is rather benign and resembles that of polycythemia vera. It may evolve into another form of MPD and in some cases into acute leukemia.

Hemapheresis has been used in a variety of clinical states, primarily for its ability to remove an offending component, likely to be either plasma or cellular elements. Therapeutic hemapheresis is useful in certain clinical conditions, but judicious application should be considered.

Alkylating agents and radioactive phosphorus (^{32}P) are effective treatment; however, these agents are associated with an increased risk of leukemia and other neoplasms. Hydroxyurea can be effective, but it can rarely induce severe neutropenia and anemia. If hydroxyurea is ineffective, busulfan can be used with caution.

Although treatment of the symptomatic patient with platelet-lowering agents or antiplatelet drugs may be indicated and effective, the role of therapy in the asymptomatic individual remains highly controversial. No remarkable advances have been made in the treatment of MPDs except for the development of an antiplatelet drug, anagrelide. This agent seems to be highly effective in controlling thrombocytosis. The relative merit of this agent as compared with interferon alfa, as well as the impact of this agent on the survival time and on the quality of life of patients with MPDs, has yet to be defined.

SUMMARY

General Characteristics and Classification

Chronic MPDs are interrelated clonal abnormalities resulting in an excessive proliferation of various phenotypically normal mature cells. Classifications of chronic MPDs include CML, polycythemia vera, idiopathic myelofibrosis (or agnogenic myeloid metaplasia), and essential thrombocythemia.

No environmental causes of MPDs have been identified; however, it has been suggested that a genetic susceptibility may exist. The dysfunction appears to be a loss of regulatory signals that control the production of mature cells.

Patients with an MPD suffer from various mild disorders of hemostasis or coagulation such as DIC. Patients with an MPD commonly exhibit thrombotic phenomena. Many patients with a form of MPD progress to acute leukemia. Interferon may be a new and effective drug for the treatment of the MPDs. This biological agent, either alone or in combination with other antineoplastic treatment, may represent a new therapeutic approach for these disorders.

Chronic Myelogenous Leukemia

CML is one of the most common forms of chronic leukemia. Chronic myeloid leukemia includes five subtypes: CML—common type, juvenile CML, chronic neutrophilic leukemia, chronic myelomonocytic leukemia, and atypical CML.

Ninety-five percent of patients with CML suffer from the common type. This is predominantly a leukemia of young and middle-aged adults and accounts for 20% to 25% of all leukemia cases. Males are afflicted more frequently than females. Five to 10% of patients have a history of excessive radiation exposure.

An excessive increase in mostly mature myeloid cells in the peripheral blood is the hallmark of the initial phase of CML. The disease course is characterized by a chronic, indolent stage that frequently transforms into a terminal, acute "blast crisis" phase. An accelerated phase, when patients become refractory to traditional therapy, may precede the acute phase.

The Philadelphia chromosome, Ph[1], was the first aberrant chromosome described in a malignant disorder. It results from the reciprocal translocation of DNA between chromosomes 9 and 22. It is the first demonstrable hematological change in more than 90% of CML patients and is present in myelogenous and erythroid precursors as well as megakaryocytes. Patients with CML or acute lymphoblastic leukemia (ALL) express the BCR gene rearrangement, which is the molecular counterpart of the Ph[1] chromosome.

The clinical course of CML can be characterized by three separate progressive phases. The onset of the early, initial phase (chronic phase) of CML is insidious and may last from 2 to 3 years. A transitional, accelerated period may precede blast transformation. About three fourths of patients eventually enter a gradual transformation to a blast crisis, which is characterized by the appearance of primitive blast cells similar to those seen in acute leukemia.

The chronic leukemias are usually characterized by the presence of leukocytosis. In CML, the degree of leukocytosis is extreme. CML can also be identified by the presence of the entire spectrum of immature and mature myelogenous cells in the blood and marrow. The total leukocyte count is usually greater than $50 \times 10^9/L$ and may exceed $300 \times 10^9/L$. Bone marrow biopsy reveals hypercellularity with prominent granulocytic hyperplasia.

The study of cellular ultrastructure is less commonly performed for chronic leukemias than for acute leukemias. Electron microscope examination of the blood of a person in the chronic phase of CML usually demonstrates that the majority of segmented neutrophils appear morphologically normal. Cytochemical studies are also used less frequently for chronic leukemias than for acute leukemias. The LAP test is used to differentiate between CML and a leukemoid reaction. In CML, the LAP score is decreased, as compared with a leukemoid reaction in which a high score is usual.

Because chronic-phase CML is highly responsive to treatment, many patients experience at least one remission. After progression to the blast crisis phase, the prognosis is poor, with the patient surviving usually less than 6 months.

Traditionally, treatment for chronic-phase CML has consisted of either hydroxyurea or busulfan therapy. Although these agents can extend the chronic phase, they have not averted the ultimate transformation to the acute phase. Intensive chemotherapy in conjunction with total body irradiation and allogeneic bone marrow transplantation in patients under 50 years old have produced some cures, but the toxicity of cytotoxic therapy and the unavailability of matched donors have limited this approach. In terms of both safety and effectiveness, it has been established that interferon alfa is an appropriate method of inducing complete hematological remission in Ph[1] chromosome–positive patients with early chronic-phase CML.

Polycythemia Vera

Polycythemia vera is distinguished from the other kinds of chronic MPD by the remarkable increases in red blood cell mass and total blood volume. Polycythemia vera occurs gradually over many decades. The mean age at diagnosis ranges from 60 to 65 years. The most serious complications are vascular accidents and the transition to acute leukemia.

Polycythemia vera is a clonal MPD of the pluripotent hematopoietic stem cell, with an unknown etiology. Although it is a clonal hematopoietic stem cell disorder with trilineage hyperplasia, the most constant and striking feature is erythroid hyperplasia of the bone marrow. Abnormalities in polycythemia vera erythroid progenitors are expressed at the level of both the CFU-E and BFU-E, which suggests multiple changes in the erythroid progenitors. A shift in the stem cell compartment may occur. IL-3 stimulates trilineage hematopoiesis, but a striking hypersensitivity of polycythemia BFU-E to recombinant IL-3 has been noted. This may be a major factor in the pathogenesis of increased erythropoiesis without increased erythropoietin concentrations.

Chromosomal abnormalities can include alterations and partial duplications involving the long arm of chromosome 1, monosomy or partial deletion of chromosome 5, and trisomy 8 and 9. Trisomy 1q is the most frequent structural chromosomal abnormality.

An increased total blood volume (hypervolemia) occurs in polycythemia vera. Neurological symptoms are reported by 50% to 80% of patients. The criteria for diagnosis has been outlined by the National Polycythemia Vera Study Group.

An increased erythrocyte cell count, packed cell volume, and hemoglobin with normal erythrocytic indices are characteristic of polycythemia vera. Peak polycythemic values are a hemoglobin of approximately 20.6 gm/dL, a microhematocrit of about 80%, a total leukocyte (WBC) count of $28,000 \times 10^9/L$, and a platelet count of $1400 \times 10^9/L$. A diagnosis of polycythemia, however, requires an accurate assessment of plasma volume and red blood cell mass. In some cases, disorders in the rheological phenomena of red blood cells are a triggering mechanism in the development of DIC syndrome. In the chronic phase of polycythemia vera, patients with thrombohemorrhagic complications have higher platelet counts, more severe platelet aggregation defects, and increased plasma levels of beta thromboglobulin and fibrinopeptide A compared to patients without complications.

Polycythemia vera is considered to be a chronic disease with a 10- to 20-year life expectancy after diagnosis. Certain prognostic factors and treatment strategies have an effect on survival. Primary control is achieved by phlebotomy. Recombinant interferon alfa, a natural product with growth-inhibiting capabilities, was recently demonstrated for the first time to have significant therapeutic efficacy in controlling the red blood cell mass in patients with polycythemia vera. The striking advantage in the use of this drug is its presumed absence of antileukemic effect.

Idiopathic Myelofibrosis

Idiopathic myelofibrosis is also referred to as agnogenic myeloid metaplasia. It is a chronic MPD of unknown cause, characterized by systemic bone marrow fibrosis and extramedullary hematopoiesis. Secondary myelofibrosis is caused by infiltrative disorders, including malignancies and infections, or exposure to chemical toxins or irradiation. Idiopathic myelofibrosis is uncommon.

Idiopathic myelofibrosis is a clonal disorder of the multipotential progenitor cell compartment. The blood–marrow barrier is disrupted early in the course of myelofibrosis so that blast cells and committed stem cells such as CFU-GM, BFU-E, and CFU-Meg escape into the circulating blood in large numbers. Sclerosis of the bone develops in about half of patients. However, myelofibrosis, the predominant clinical manifestation, occurs secondarily and is not a component of the abnormal clonal proliferation. The process of fibrosis ensues from the proliferation of fibroblasts and increased collagen production in reaction to the abnormal clone of hematopoietic cells. Dysmegakaryocytopoiesis leading to an overproduction of defective platelets is the most constant feature of myelofibrosis.

Idiopathic myelofibrosis is not associated with a specific or unique chromosomal anomaly. Karyotypic changes occur as secondary events during the multistep process of leukemogenesis.

Patients with myelofibrosis usually exhibit progressive anemia, splenomegaly, and marrow fibrosis. Splenomegaly and some hepatomegaly are due to extramedullary hematopoiesis. Patients may notice easy bruising or bleeding, resulting from thrombocytopenia, abnormal platelet function, or both. More than 40% of patients suffer from osteosclerosis with accompanying bone pain, malaise, and leukocytosis.

Hematological findings are variable and nonuniform, but blood morphology provides the best clues to diagnosis. The leukoerythroblastic picture of teardrop-shaped erythrocytes, nucleated erythrocytes, and immature myeloid cells is classic for myelofibrosis. The bone marrow is hypocellular and becomes fibrotic with an associated decrease in hematopoiesis.

The median survival time ranges from 4.3 to 5.0 years. Major thromboembolic complications that contribute to shortened survival are seen in about one fifth of patients.

There is no therapy that will affect the basic disease process. Asymptomatic patients require no treatment. Treatment for myelofibrosis can consist of periodic transfusions of packed red blood cells, androgens, cytotoxic agents, and platelet reduction by plateletpheresis. Administration of prophylactic antibiotics may also be considered. Recombinant interferon alfa may be more efficacious when used in the cellular (i.e., proliferative) phase than when the marrow is fibrotic or osteosclerotic. Moderate doses of radiotherapy to the spleen have been effective in controlling symptoms. However, clinical improvement after irradiation is a slow, gradual process.

Essential Thrombocythemia

Essential or primary thrombocythemia (essential thrombocytosis) is characterized by a marked increased in circulating platelets, usually in excess of 1000×10^9/L. The diagnosis of essential thrombocythemia is difficult and relies on the exclusion of other myeloproliferative states and nonhematological illnesses associated with an increased concentration of platelets.

Essential thrombocythemia occurs most frequently among persons in the fifth and sixth decades of life. Men and women are equally affected.

Essential thrombocythemia is a clonal disorder of multipotential stem cell origin and belongs to the chronic MPDs that include polycythemia vera, CML, and idiopathic myelofibrosis. It is a rare disorder.

Thrombotic or bleeding problems are the most commonly seen disorders in patients with thrombocythemia. Patients typically manifest easy bruising, nosebleeds, or gastrointestinal bleeding.

The classic laboratory finding in essential thrombocythemia is a markedly elevated peripheral blood platelet count. The number of platelets in the circulating blood is usually in excess of 1000×10^9/L, with a minimum of 600×10^9/L. In patients with thrombocythemia, the mean extent of aggregation induced by epinephrine, collagen, or ADP is significantly lower than in normal controls. Bone marrow morphology is similar to the architecture seen in polycythemia vera and CML with associated extreme thrombocytosis.

The course of the disease is rather benign and resembles that of polycythemia vera. It may evolve into another form of MPD and in some cases into acute leukemia. Hemapheresis has been used in a variety of clinical states, primarily for its ability to remove an offending component, likely to be either plasma or cellular elements. Therapeutic hemapheresis is useful in certain clinical conditions, but judicious application should be considered. Alkylating agents and radioactive phosphorus (^{32}P) are effective treatment, but these agents are associated with an increased risk of leukemia and other neoplasms. Hydroxyurea can be effective, but it can induce severe neutropenia and anemia. Although treatment of the symptomatic patient with platelet-lowering agents or antiplatelet drugs may be indicated and effective, the role of therapy in the asymptomatic individual remains highly controversial. No remarkable advances have been made in the treatment of MPDs except for the development of an antiplatelet drug, anagrelide. This agent seems to be highly effective in controlling thrombocytosis. The relative merit of this agent as compared with interferon alfa, as well as the impact of this agent on the survival time and quality of life of patients with MPDs, has yet to be defined.

CASE STUDIES

CASE 1 This 51-year-old, white male construction worker was taken to the emergency room by a fellow worker after injuring his wrist at work. On physical examination, an elevated blood pressure was noted. No other abnormalities were found. The patient reported that he had been diagnosed as suffering from hypertension about 5 years ago. The emergency room physician ordered a routine blood count (CBC), urinalysis, and an x-ray film of his wrist.

Laboratory Data
Hemoglobin 21.5 gm/dL
Hematocrit 64% (0.64 L/L)
Erythrocyte count 9.2×10^{12}/L
Total leukocyte count 14.0×10^9/L

An increase in neutrophilic bands and segmented neutrophils was observed, as well as an increase in the number of thrombocytes. The erythrocytic indices were all within the normal range.

Follow-up testing revealed a total blood volume of 79 mL/kg (normal: adult males 61.5 ± 8.5 mL/kg, adult females 59.0 ± 5 mL/kg of body weight) and a total red cell volume of 48 mL/kg (normal: 20 to 36 mL/kg of body weight). A urinary erythropoietin assay revealed the absence of measurable erythropoietin in the urine.

(continued)

Questions
1. What quantitative cellular abnormalities were revealed by laboratory testing?
2. What do the laboratory data suggest in this case?
3. Name other tests that would support a differential diagnosis of polycythemia vera.

Discussion
1. The erythrocyte count, hematocrit, and hemoglobin were all extremely elevated. The total leukocyte count was slightly elevated and the platelet count was also increased.
2. An increased total blood volume (hypervolemia) occurs in disorders such as congestive heart failure, primary aldosteronism, Cushing's syndrome, and polycythemia vera and after an overtransfusion of donor blood. This patient's increased total blood volume is undoubtedly producing his hypertension.

   Additionally, an increased erythrocyte count, hematocrit, and hemoglobin with normal erythrocytic indices are suggestive of polycythemia. A red cell volume greater than 36 mL/kg in males and 32 mL/kg in females is considered to be in the polycythemic range. The absence of erythropoietin in this patient's urine further suggests that the patient is suffering from polycythemia vera.
3. Further testing that would differentiate polycythemia vera from other forms of polycythemia would be:

   LAP score
   Erythrocyte sedimentation rate
   Serum iron determination
   Blood histamine assay
   Vitamin B$_{12}$ binding capacity
   Basophil count
   Examination of the bone marrow for hemosiderin

✏ **Diagnosis: Polycythemia vera, hypertension**

CASE 2 A 64-year-old white man saw his physician because he was experiencing pain in the shoulders and wrists since returning from his winter home in Florida 6 weeks before. Physical examination revealed that the patient was pale but in otherwise good health. The physician sent the patient to the outpatient laboratory for a CBC, and prescribed an analgesic for the joint discomfort.

Laboratory Data
The patient's erythrocytes and hemoglobin were moderately decreased. His total leukocyte count was 68 × 10^9/L. The leukocyte distribution was as follows:

Promyelocytes 1%
Myelocytes 8%
Metamyelocytes 15%
Bands 35%
Segmented neutrophils 25%
Lymphocytes 14%
Monocytes 2%

Some immature erythrocytes were noted, and the number of platelets was increased.

A subsequent bone marrow examination revealed both granulocytic and megakaryocytic overproliferation. Cytochemistry staining resulted in the following LAP scores:

Patient 6
Control 43

Questions
1. What is the most probable diagnosis in this case?
2. Would any additional tests be of value?
3. Why did this patient exhibit a thrombocytosis on the peripheral blood smear?

Discussion
1. Based on the findings of a leukocytosis, many immature and mature granulocytic forms, and a severely diminished LAP score, a diagnosis of CML can be established.
2. Yes, cytogenetic analysis would be of value in confirming the other test results. In 1960, Nowell and Hungerford demonstrated the presence of the Philadelphia chromosome in the karyotype of patients with CML. This chromosome represents a partly deleted G portion of chromosome 22. Approximately 85% of patients with CML carry Ph^1. CML patients can be subdivided into Ph^1-positive and Ph^1-negative types. Ph^1-negative patients with CML are correlated with a shorter survival time, lower leukocyte and platelet counts, and a younger age of incidence.
3. Thrombocytosis is common in patients with CML. Frequently, the platelet count reaches into the millions. Thrombotic and hemorrhagic tendencies may complicate the clinical course of this type of leukemia.

✏ **Diagnosis: Chronic myelogenous (granulocytic) leukemia**

CASE 3 A 55-year-old white man was taken by the local volunteer ambulance service to the hospital emergency room. His chief complaint was severe pain in the abdomen and diarrhea for the last 3 days. Physical examination revealed extensive abdominal distention, fresh blood in the stool, an elevated oral temperature, decreased blood pressure, and a rapid pulse. The physician admitted the patient and ordered a stat CBC and serum electrolyte determinations. An intravenous physiological saline solution was started after the blood had been drawn for examination. A full-body computed tomography (CT) scan was scheduled for the next morning because a conventional lower gastrointestinal radiographic series was contraindicated owing to the fresh bleeding.

Laboratory Data
The patient's erythrocyte and hemoglobin parameters were within normal range; however, the total leukocyte count was 63 × 10^9/L. The leukocyte differential results were as follows:

Blast forms 2%
Promyelocytes 5%
Myelocytes 13%
Metamyelocytes 20%
Bands 20%
Segmented neutrophils 35%

(continued)

CASE STUDIES (*continued*)

Lymphocytes 4%
Monocytes 1%

The platelet estimate from the differential smear indicated a slightly increased number. The serum electrolyte values indicated a state of dehydration.

Additional Clinical Data
The patient's temperature continued to remain elevated during the night of admission. A broad-spectrum antibiotic was added to the intravenous infusion. The patient's blood pressure became unstable during the night. A repeat CBC was ordered the next morning. At that time, the leukocyte count had risen to 118×10^9/L with essentially the same differential distribution of leukocytes. At 10 A.M. the laboratory was notified that the patient had expired and an autopsy had been requested.

The autopsy revealed that the patient had a mesenteric thrombosis and had subsequently developed acute peritonitis.

Questions
1. What disorder is suggested by the peripheral blood film?
2. What other hematological test could differentiate between various types of leukocytosis?

Discussion
1. CMLs and leukemoid reactions are indistinguishable on a peripheral blood smear. The sudden elevation of the total leukocyte count and marked increase (to the left) of granulocytic precursors could have suggested a serious infection with or without an underlying leukemic state.
2. The LAP test is of diagnostic importance in distinguishing between CML and a leukemoid reaction. The LAP score is high in leukemoid reactions and usually low in the CMLs.

✏️ **Diagnosis: Leukemoid reaction**

BIBLIOGRAPHY

Anger, B. et al. "Polycythemia Vera. A Clinical Study of 141 Patients." *Blut,* Vol. 59, No. 6, December, 1989, pp. 493–500.

Anger, B. et al. "Idiopathic Myelofibrosis: A Retrospective Study of 103 Patients." *Haematologica,* Vol. 75, No. 3, May–June, 1990, pp. 228–234.

Appelbaum, F. R. "Introduction and Overview of Interferon Alfa in Myeloproliferative and Hemangiomatous Diseases." *Semin. Hematol.,* Vol. 27, No. 3, Suppl. 4, July, 1990, pp. 1–5.

Arnaud, J. et al. "Consequences of Moderate Hypoxia on Red Cell Glycolytic Metabolism in Polycythemia Rubra Vera." *Ann. Biol. Clin. Paris,* Vol. 91, No. 1, 1991, pp. 9–13.

Aulbert, E. and H. Fromm. "Ferritin in Myeloproliferative Diseases." *Med. Klin.,* Vol. 85, No. 3, March 15, 1990, pp. 125–131.

Averbuch, M. et al. "Budd-Chiari Syndrome in Israel: Predisposing Factors, Prognosis, and Early Identification on High-Risk Patients. *J. Clin. Gastroenterol.,* Vol. 13, No. 3, June, 1991, pp. 321–324.

Baglin, T. P., S. M. Price, and B. J. Boughton. "Circulating High Molecular Weight IgG Fibronectin Complexes in Myeloproliferative Disorders." *J. Clin. Pathol.,* Vol. 43, No. 2, February, 1990, pp. 102–105.

Benbassat, J., D. Gilon, and S. Penchas. "The Choice Between Sple-

nectomy and Medical Treatment in Patients With Advanced Agnogenic Myeloid Metaplasia." *Am. J. Hematol.,* Vol. 33, No. 2, February, 1990, pp. 128–135.

Bernstein, R. "Cytogenetics of Chronic Myelogenous Leukemia." *Semin. Hematol.,* Vol. 25, No. 1, January, 1988, pp. 20–34.

Bertino, J. R., et al. "Chronic Myelogenous Leukemia." Public education and information department booklet. New York: Leukemia Society of America, 1988.

Bessmel'tsev, S. S., Z. D. Fedorova, and K. M. Abdulkadyrov. "Rheologic Properties of the Erythrocytes and Hemostatic System in Patients With Polycythemia Vera." *Gematol. Transfuziol.,* Vol. 34, No. 11, November, 1989, pp. 29–33.

Bettelheim, P. and P. Valent. "Radioimmunometric Determination of Histamine in Myeloproliferative Syndromes." *Wein. Klin. Wochenschr.,* Vol. 101, No. 20, October 27, 1989, pp. 706–710.

Bick, R. L. and W. R. Laughlin. "Myeloproliferative Syndromes." *Lab. Med.,* Vol. 24, No. 12, December, 1993, pp. 770–776.

Biljanovic-Paunovic, L., R. Ruvidic, and V. Pavlovic-Kentera. "Endogenous BFU-E in Peripheral Blood in Diagnosis of Polycythemia Vera." *Eur. J. Haematol.,* Vol. 45, No. 5, November, 1990, pp. 262–266.

Botelho-de-Sousa, A. and J. Gouveia. "Coexistent Chronic Lymphocytic Leukemia and Polycythemia Vera Requiring No Treatment." *Med. Oncol. Tumor Pharmacother.,* Vol. 6, No. 3, 1989, pp. 239–240.

Buss, D. H. et al. "Bone Marrow and Peripheral Blood Findings in Patients With Extreme Thrombocytosis. A Report of 63 Cases." *Arch. Pathol. Lab. Med.,* Vol. 115, No. 5, May, 1991, pp. 475–480.

Cervantes, F. et al. "Acute Transformation in Nonleukemic Chronic Myeloproliferative Disorders: Actuarial Probability and Main Characteristics in a Series of 218 Patients." *Acta Haematol.,* Vol. 85, No. 3, 1991, pp. 124–127.

Chott, A. et al. "Interferon-Alpha-Induced Morphological Changes of Megakaryocytes: A Histomorphometrical Study on Bone Marrow Biopsies in Chronic Myeloproliferative Disorders With Excessive Thrombocytosis." *Br. J. Haematol.,* Vol. 74, No. 1, January, 1990, pp. 10–16.

Chow, M. P. et al. "Clinical Application of Therapeutic Hemapheresis." *Chung Hua I Hsueh Tsa Chih,* Vol. 45, No. 2, February, 1990, pp. 87–92.

Cogswell, P. C. et al. "Mutations of the ras Protooncogenes in Chronic Myelogenous Leukemia: A High Frequency of ras Mutations in bcr/*abl* Rearrangement-Negative Chronic Myelogenous Leukemia." *Blood,* Vol. 74, No. 8, December, 1989, pp. 2629–2633.

Cohen, A. M. et al. "Tissue Plasminogen Activator Levels in Different Types of Polycythemia." *Eur. J. Haematol.,* Vol. 45, No. 1, July, 1990, pp. 48–51.

Cohen, J. R., H. R. Sterman, and L. Wise. "Arterial Reconstruction in Patients With Polycythemia Vera." *Surg. Gynecol. Obstet.,* Vol. 170, No. 4, April, 1990, pp. 314–316.

Conley, C. L. "Polycythemia Vera." *JAMA,* Vol. 263, No. 18, May 9, 1990, pp. 2481–2483.

Corredoira, J. C. et al. "A Clinical and Biological Study of 33 Cases of Polycythemia Vera." *Rev. Clin. Esp.,* Vol. 186, No. 8, May, 1990, pp. 378–382.

Corredoira-Sanchez, J. C. et al. "Neurologic Manifestations of Polycythemia Vera. Analysis of 24 Cases and Review of the Literature." *Ann. Med. Interne* (Paris), Vol. 7, No. 2, February, 1990, pp. 67–70.

Crisan, D. and E. R. Carr. "BCR/*abl* Gene Rearrangement in Chronic Myelogenous Leukemia and Acute Leukemias." *Lab. Med.,* Vol. 23, No. 11, November, 1992, pp. 730–735.

Dai, C. H. et al. "Polycythemia Vera Blood Burst-Forming Units–Erythroid Are Hypersensitive to Interleukin-3." *J. Clin. Invest.,* Vol. 87, No. 2, February, 1991, pp. 391–396.

Del-Forno, C. et al. "Cutaneous Extramedullary Hematopoiesis in Idiopathic Myelofibrosis: Description of a Case." *G. Ital. Dermatol. Venereol.*, Vol. 125, No. 5, May, 1990, pp. 205–209.

Derderian, P. M. et al. "Chronic Myelogenous Leukemia in the Lymphoid Blastic Phase: Characteristics, Treatment Response, and Prognosis." *Am. J. Med.*, Vol. 94, January, 1993, pp. 69–74.

de-Wolf, J. T. et al. "Erythroid Progenitors in Polycythemia Vera Demonstrate a Different Response Pattern to IL-4 Compared to the Normal BFU-E From Peripheral Blood." *Exp. Hematol.*, Vol. 19, No. 9, October, 1991, pp. 888–892.

"Diagnostic and Therapeutic Technology Assessment. Alpha-Interferon and Chronic Myelogenous Leukemia." *JAMA*, Vol. 264, No. 16, 1990, pp. 2137–2139.

Diez-Martin, J. L. et al. "Chromosome Studies in 104 Patients with Polycythemia Vera." *Mayo Clin. Proc.*, Vol. 66, No. 3, March, 1991, pp. 287–299.

Dini, D., T. Artusi, and U. Di-Prisco. "Idiopathic Myelofibrosis Associated With an IgM-Secreting Immunocytoma." *Recenti Prog. Med.*, Vol. 82, No. 2, February, 1991, pp. 77–79.

Donti, E. et al. "Partial Trisomy 1q in Idiopathic Myelofibrosis." *Leuk. Res.*, Vol. 14, No. 11–12, 1990, pp. 1035–1040.

Fialkow, P. J. "Stem Cell Origin of Human Myeloid Blood Cell Neoplasms." *Verh. Dtsch. Ges. Pathol.*, Vol. 74, 1990, pp. 43–47.

Finelli, C. et al. "Ticlopidine Lowers Plasma Fibrinogen in Patients With Polycythaemia Rubra Vera and Additional Thrombotic Risk Factors. A Double-Blind Controlled Study." *Acta Haematol.*, Vol. 85, No. 3, 1991, pp. 113–118.

Froom, P. et al. "Decreased Natural Killer (NK) Activity in Patients With Myeloproliferative Disorders." *Cancer*, Vol. 64, No. 5, September 1, 1989, pp. 1038–1040.

Fujioka, S. "Rheological Study on Vascular Occlusion and Cellular Hyperviscosity Syndrome in Polycythemia Vera." *Nippon Ketsueki Gakkai Zasshi*, Vol. 52, No. 4, July, 1989, pp. 688–695.

Garcia, S., et al. "Heparin-Associated Thrombocytopenia in a Patient With Polycythemia Vera: The Importance of a Marked Drop in Platelet Count." *Acta Haematol.*, Vol. 85, No. 3, 1991, pp. 169–170.

Gilliland, D. G., et al. "Clonality in Myeloproliferative Disorders: Analysis by Means of the Polymerase Chain Reaction." *Proc. Natl. Acad. Sci. USA*, Vol. 88, No. 15, August 1, 1991, pp. 6848–6852.

Gisslinger, H. et al. "Long-Term Interferon Therapy for Thrombocytosis in Myeloproliferative Diseases." *Lancet*, Vol. 1, March 25, 1989, pp. 634–637.

Griffin, C. G. and B. W. Grant. "Effects of Recombinant Interferons on Human Megakaryocyte Growth." *Exp. Hematol.*, Vol. 18, No. 9, October, 1990, pp. 1013–1018.

Guilhot, F. et al. "Interferon Alfa-2b Combined With Cytarabine Versus Interferon Alone in Chronic Myelogenous Leukemia." *N. Engl. J. Med.*, Vol. 337, No. 4, July 24, 1997, pp. 223–228.

Haq, A. U. "Transformation of Polycythemia Vera to ph-Positive Chronic Myelogenous Leukemia." *Am. J. Hematol.*, Vol. 35, No. 2, October, 1990, pp. 110–113.

Hart, R. G. and M. C. Kanter. "Hematologic Disorders and Ischemic Stroke. A Selective Review." *Stroke*, Vol. 21, No. 8, August 1990, pp. 1111–1121.

Hasselbalch, H. and B. A. Jensen. "Prognostic Factors in Idiopathic Myelofibrosis: A Simple Scoring System With Prognostic Significance." *Eur. J. Haematol.*, Vol. 44, No. 3, 1990, pp. 172–178.

Hild, F., M. Freund, and C. Fonatsch. "Chromosomal Aberrations During Interferon Therapy for Chronic Myelogenous Leukemia." *N. Engl. J. Med.*, Vol. 325, No. 2, July, 1991, p. 324.

Ho, A. D. "Chemotherapy of Chronic Haematological Malignancies." *Baillieres Clin. Haematol.*, Vol. 19, No. 2, 1991, pp. 99–130.

Hochhaus, A. et al. "Megakaryocytic Myelosis—Clinical Aspects, Morphology and Platelet Function." *Klin. Wochenschr.*, Vol. 67, No. 2, January 20, 1989, pp. 51–59.

Hochhaus, A., et al. "Aggregative Behavior and Calcium Content of Platelets in Thrombocythemia and Thrombocytosis." *Folia Haematol. (Leipz)*, Vol. 117, No. 6, 1990, pp. 765–770.

Holcombe, R. F., P. A. Treseler, and D. S. Rosenthal. "Chronic Myelomonocytic Leukemia Transformation in Polycythemia Vera." *Leukemia*, Vol. 5, No. 7, July, 1991, pp. 606–610.

Hyun, B. H., G. L. Gulati, and J. K. Ashton. "Myeloproliferative Disorders. Classification and Diagnostic Features With Special Emphasis on Chronic Myelogenous Leukemia and Agnogenic Myeloid Metaplasia." *Clin. Lab. Med.*, Vol. 10, No. 4, December, 1990, pp. 825–838.

Im, T., et al. "Evaluation of Serum Sialyl Acid-i in Hematologic Disorders." *Osaka City Med. J.*, Vol. 36, No. 2, November, 1990, pp. 141–147.

Islam, M. S., et al. "Captopril Induces Correction of Postrenal Transplant Erythemia." *Transplant. Int.*, Vol. 3, No. 4, December, 1990, pp. 222–225.

Kaboth, U. et al. "Treatment of Polycythemia Vera by Isovolemic Large-Volume Erythrocytapheresis." *Klin. Wochenschr.*, Vol. 68, No. 1, January 4, 1990, pp. 18–25.

Kaloutsi, V., et al. "Megakaryocytes in Chronic Myeloproliferative Disorders: Numerical Density Correlated Between Different Entities." *Virchows Arch. A. Pathol. Anat. Histopathol.*, Vol. 418, No. 6, 1991, pp. 493–497.

Kantarjian, H. M. et al. "Prolonged Survival in Chronic Myelogenous Leukemia After Cytogenetic Response to Interferon-alpha Therapy." *Ann. Internal Med.*, Vol. 122, No. 4, February 15, 1995, pp. 254, 261.

Kanz, L. et al. "Analysis of Megakaryocyte Ploidy in Patients With Thrombocytosis." *Int. J. Cell Cloning*, Vol. 8, No. 4, July, 1990, pp. 299–306.

Kerim, S. et al. "Trisomy 8 and an Unbalanced t(5;17) (q11;p11) Characterize Two Karyotypically Independent Clones in a Case of Idiopathic Myelofibrosis Evolving to Acute Nonlymphoid Leukemia." *Cancer Genet. Cytogenet.*, Vol. 52, No. 1, March, 1991, pp. 63–69.

Kimura, S. et al. "Polycythemia Vera Terminating in Myelodysplastic Syndrome." *Rinsho Ketsueki*, Vol. 31, No. 1, January, 1990, pp. 100–104.

Kobayashi, M. et al. "Polycythemia Vera With an Inhibitor Against Factor XII." *Rinsho Ketsueki*, Vol. 30, No. 8, August, 1989, pp. 1271–1274.

Kyritsis, A. P., E. C. Williams, and H. S. Schutta. "Cerebral Venous Thrombosis Due to Heparin-Induced Thrombocytopenia." *Stroke*, Vol. 21, No. 10, October, 1990, pp. 1503–1505.

Lambertenghi-Deliliers, G. et al. "Myelodysplastic Syndrome With Increased Marrow Fibrosis: A Distinct Clinico-pathological Entity." *Br. J. Haematol.*, Vol. 78, No. 2, June, 1991, pp. 161–166.

Landaw, S. A. "Polycythemia Vera and Other Polycythemic States." *Clin. Lab. Med.*, Vol. 10, No. 4, December, 1990, pp. 857–871.

Lara, J. F. and P. P. Rosen. "Extramedullary Hematopoiesis in a Bronchial Carcinoid Tumor. An Unusual Complication of Agnogenic Myeloid Metaplasia." *Arch. Pathol. Lab. Med.*, Vol. 114, No. 12, December, 1990, pp. 1283–1285.

Lazzarino, M. et al. "Interferon Alpha-2b as Treatment for Philadelphia-Negative Chronic Myeloproliferative Disorders With Excessive Thrombocytosis." *Br. J. Haematol.*, Vol. 72, No. 2, June, 1989, pp. 173–177.

Leinweber, C., S. E. Order, and A. R. Calkins. "Whole-Abdominal Irradiation for the Management of Gastrointestinal and Abdominal Manifestations of Agnogenic Myeloid Metaplasia." *Cancer*, Vol. 68, No. 6, September 15, 1991, pp. 1251–1254.

Likhovetskaia, Z. M., et al. "Blood Rheologic Disorders in Patients With Polycythemia Vera and Their Correction by Therapeutic Erythrocytapheresis." *Gematol. Transfuziol.*, Vol. 34, No. 11, November, 1989, pp. 33–36.

Lofvenberg, E. and T. K. Nilsson. "Qualitative Platelet Defects in Chronic Myeloproliferative Disorders: Evidence for Reduced ATP Secretion." *Eur. J. Haematol.*, Vol. 43, No. 5, November, 1989, pp. 435–440.

Lofvenberg, E. et al. "Reversal of Myelofibrosis by Hydroxyurea." *Eur. J. Haematol.*, Vol. 44, No. 1, January, 1990, pp. 33–38.

Lopez-Guillermo, A. et al. "Idiopathic Myelofibrosis: Clinical Course, Survival, and Causes of Death in a Series of 60 Patients." *Sangre (Barc)*, Vol. 35, No. 2, April, 1990, pp. 114–118.

Macavei, I. and N. Galatar. "Bone Marrow Biopsy (BMB). II. Bone Marrow Biopsy in Myeloproliferative Disorders." *Morphol. Embryol. Bucur.*, Vol. 35, No. 2, April–June, 1989, pp. 117–127.

Maeda, S. et al. "Therapeutic Effect of Ranimustine (MCNU) on Myeloproliferative Disorder and Chronic Myelomonocytic Leukemia." *Gan To Kagaku Ryoho*, Vol. 18, No. 2, February, 1991, pp. 251–258.

Majer, R. V. et al. "Which Tests Are Most Useful in Distinguishing Between Reactive Thrombocytosis and the Thrombocytosis of Myeloproliferative Disease?" *Clin. Lab. Haematol.*, Vol. 13, No. 1, 1991, pp. 9–15.

Mamiya, S. et al. "Abnormal Blood Coagulation and Fibrinolysis in Chronic Myeloproliferative Disorders." *Rinsho Ketsueki*, Vol. 32, No. 5, May, 1991, pp. 527–536.

Marsh, G. M., P. E. Enterline, and D. McCraw. "Mortality Patterns Among Petroleum Refinery and Chemical Plant Workers." *Am. J. Ind. Med.*, Vol. 19, No. 1, January, 1991, pp. 29–42.

Masaoka, T. "Ranimustine." *Gan To Kagaku Ryoho*, Vol. 17, No. 2, February, 1990, pp. 301–307.

McDonald, E. et al. "Gangrene of the Fingers Secondary to Myeloproliferative Disease." *Postgrad. Med.*, Vol. 90, No. 1, July, 1991, pp. 115–118.

Mertens, F. et al. "Karyotypic Patterns in Chronic Myeloproliferative Disorders: Report on 74 Cases and Review of the Literature." *Leukemia*, Vol. 5, No. 3, March, 1991, pp. 214–220.

Miller, R. L., J. D. Purvis, III, and J. K. Weick. "Familial Polycythemia Vera." *Cleve. Clin. J. Med.*, Vol. 56, No. 8, November–December, 1989, pp. 813–818.

Mitus, A. J. and A. I. Schafer. "Thrombocytosis and Thrombocythemia." *Hematol. Oncol. Clin. North Am.*, Vol. 4, No. 1, February, 1990, pp. 157–178.

Murray, D. and R. Hodgson. "Polycythaemia Rubra Vera, Cerebral Ischaemia and Depression." *Br. J. Psychiatry*, Vol. 158, June, 1991, pp. 842–844.

Nafe, R. et al. "Quantitative Cytomorphology of Megakaryocytes in Chronic Myeloproliferative Disorders—Analysis of Planimetric and Numeric Characteristics by Means of a Knowledge Based System." *Exp. Pathol.*, Vol. 40, No. 4, 1990, pp. 213–219.

Najean, Y. et al. "Clinical Significance of Serum Pro-collagen III in Chronic Myeloproliferative Disorders." *Eur. J. Haematol.*, Vol. 45, No. 5, November, 1990, pp. 239–243.

Najean, Y. et al. "Radioimmunoassay of Immunoreactive Erythropoietin as a Clinical Tool for the Classification of Polycythaemias." *Nouv. Rev. Fr. Hematol.*, Vol. 32, No. 4, 1990, pp. 237–240.

Nand, S. et al. "Leukemic Transformation in Polycythemia Vera: Analysis of Risk Factors." *Am. J. Hematol.*, Vol. 34, No. 1, May, 1990, pp. 32–36.

Newton, L. K. "Neurologic Complications of Polycythemia and Their Impact on Therapy." *Oncology (Williston Park)*, Vol. 4, No. 3, March, 1990, pp. 59–66.

Nielsen, H. and H. Nordin. "Polycythemia Vera in a Danish Family." *Ugeskr. Laeger*, Vol. 153, No. 29, July 15, 1991, pp. 2072–2073.

Parise, P., et al. "Generation of Arachidonic Acid Metabolites from Stimulated Whole Blood in Patients With Chronic Myeloproliferative Disorders." *Acta Haematol.*, Vol. 85, No. 2, 1991, pp. 88–92.

Radin, A. I., P. Buckley, and T. P. Duffy. "Interferon Therapy For Agnogenic Myeloid Metaplasia Complicated by Immune Hemolytic Anemia." *Haematol. Pathol.*, Vol. 5, No. 2, 1991, pp. 83–88.

Randi, M. L. et al. "Haematological Complications in Polycythaemia Vera and Thrombocythaemia Patients Treated With Radiophosphorus (^{32}P)." *Folia Haematol. (Leipz)*, Vol. 117, No. 3, 1990, pp. 461–467.

Remaley, A. T., J. M. Kennedy, and M. Laposata. "Evaluation of the Clinical Utility of Platelet Aggregation Studies." *Am. J. Hematol.*, Vol. 31, No. 3, July, 1989, pp. 188–193.

Rozman, C. et al. "Life Expectancy of Patients With Chronic Nonleukemic Myeloproliferative Disorders." *Cancer*, Vol. 67, No. 10, May 15, 1991, pp. 2658–2663.

Rueda, F. et al. "Abnormal Levels of Platelet-Specific Proteins and Mitogenic Activity in Myeloproliferative Disease." *Acta Haematol.*, Vol. 85, No. 1, 1991, pp. 12–15.

Rueda, F. et al. "Different Lymphocyte Activity in Patients With Polycythaemia Vera Versus Secondary Polycythaemia and Healthy Blood Donors." *Acta Haematol. (Basel)*, Vol. 83, No. 1, 1990, pp. 31–34.

Saad, G. M. and T. V. de-Almeida. "Idiopathic Myelofibrosis." *Rev. Paul. Med.*, Vol. 109, No. 2, March–April, 1991, pp. 47–50.

Scheithauer, W. et al. "Effect of Recombinant Interferon-Alpha-2C on Reticuloendothelial Function in Patients With Thrombocytosis." *J. Interferon Res.*, Vol. 10, No. 2, April, 1990, pp. 237–242.

Shamdas, G. J., C. M. Spier, and A. F. List. "Myelodysplastic Transformation of Polycythemia Vera: Case Report and Review of the Literature." *Am. J. Hematol.*, Vol. 37, No. 1, May, 1991, pp. 45–48.

Shepherd, P. C., T. S. Ganesan, and D. A. Galton. "Haematological Classification of the Chronic Myeloid Leukaemias." *Baillieres Clin. Haematol.*, Vol. 1, No. 4, December, 1987, pp. 887–906.

Shimizu, K. and T. Hotta. "Spontaneous Remission of Agnogenic Myeloid Metaplasia in a Splenectomized Patient: A Case Report With Erythrokinetic Studies." *Acta Haematol. (Basel)*, Vol. 83, No. 1, 1990, pp. 45–48.

Silver, R. T. "A New Treatment for Polycythemia Vera: Recombinant Interferon Alfa." *Blood*, Vol. 76, No. 4, August 15, 1990, pp. 664–665.

Silver, R. T. "Interferon in the Treatment of Myeloproliferative Diseases." *Semin. Hematol.*, Vol. 27, No. 3, Suppl. 4, July, 1990, pp. 6–14.

Sinzinger, H., et al. "Defects in the Prostaglandin System. IX. Lipoxygenase Defect of Thrombocytes in a Patient With Polycythemia Vera." *Wien. Klin. Wochenschr.*, Vol. 102, No. 3, February 2, 1990, pp. 74–76.

Steelman, R. et al. "Idiopathic Myelofibrosis: Dental Treatment Considerations." *Spec. Care Dentist.*, Vol. 11, No. 2, March–April, 1991, pp. 68–70.

Stewart, K. et al. "Neutrophilic Myelofibrosis Presenting as Philadelphia Chromosome Negative BCR Non-rearranged Chronic Myeloid Leukemia." *Am. J. Hematol.*, Vol. 34, No. 1, May, 1990, pp. 59–63.

Sugiyama, H. et al. "Cytogenetic Evidence for a Clonal Disorder Involving CFU-GEMM, BFU-E and CFU-C in Patients With Myeloproliferative Disorders." *Nippon Ketsueki Gakkai Zasshi*, Vol. 52, No. 6, September, 1989, pp. 1022–1032.

Tassies, D. et al. "Tuberculosis in Chronic Myeloproliferative Syndromes: Its Incidence and Principle Characteristics in a Series of 562 Patients." *Med. Clin. (Barc)*, Vol. 96, No. 9, March 9, 1991, pp. 321–323.

Thiele, J. et al. "Ultrastructure of Bone Marrow Tissue in So-called Primary (Idiopathic) Myelofibrosis-Osteomyelosclerosis (Agnogenic Myeloid Metaplasia). I. Abnormalities of Megakaryopoiesis and Thrombocytes." *J. Submicrosc. Cytol. Pathol.*, Vol. 23, No. 1, January, 1991, pp. 93–107.

Thiele, J. et al. "Ultrastructure of Bone Marrow Tissue in So-called Primary (Idiopathic) Myelofibrosis-Osteomyelosclerosis (Agnogenic Myeloid Metaplasia). II. The Myeloid Stroma (Hematopoietic Microenvironment)." *J. Submicrosc. Cytol. Pathol.*, Vol. 23, No. 1, January, 1991, pp. 109–121.

Thiele, J. et al. "Pro-megakaryoblasts in Bone Marrow Tissue From Patients With Primary (Idiopathic) Osteo-myelofibrosis (Agnogenic Myeloid Metaplasia). An Immunomorphometric Study on Trephine Biopsies." *Pathol. Res. Pract.*, Vol. 186, No. 5, October, 1990, pp. 589–596.

Tichelli, A. et al. "Treatment of Thrombocytosis in Myeloproliferative Disorders With Interferon Alpha-2a." *Blut*, Vol. 58, No. 1, January, 1989, pp. 15–19.

Tichelli, A. et al. "Therapy of Thrombocytosis in Myeloproliferative Syndromes Using Recombinant Interferon-alpha-2a." *Schweiz Med. Wochenschr.*, Vol. 119, No. 39, September, 1989, pp. 1347–1352.

Turri, D. et al. "Alpha-interferon in Polycythemia Vera and Essential Thrombocythemia." *Haematologica*, Vol. 76, No. 1, January–February, 1991, pp. 75–77.

Turtureanu-Hanganu, E. and E. Ungureanu. "Polycythaemia Rubra Vera. Analysis of 20 Cases." *Rev. Med. Chir. Soc. Med. Nat. Iasi*, Vol. 93, No. 3, July–September, 1989, pp. 481–483.

Van-Camp, G. "Essential Thrombocytosis." *Acta Clin. Belg.*, Vol. 44, No. 1, 1989, pp. 31–36.

Vydyborets, S. V. and L. M. Tishchenko. "The Chemical Element Content of the Erythrocytes in Polycythemia Vera." *Vrach. Delo*, No. 10, October, 1989, pp. 80–81.

Wanless, I. R. et al. "Hepatic Vascular Disease and Portal Hypertension in Polycythemia Vera and Agnogenic Myeloid Metaplasia: A Clinicopathological Study of 145 Patients Examined at Autopsy." *Hepatology*, Vol. 12, No. 5, November, 1990, pp. 1166–1174.

Wehmeier, A. et al. "A Prospective Study of Haemostatic Parameters in Relation to the Clinical Course of Myeloproliferative Disorders." *Eur. J. Haematol.*, Vol. 45, No. 4, October, 1990, pp. 191–197.

Wulkan, R. W. and J. J. Michiels. "Pseudohyperkalaemia in Thrombocythaemia." *J. Clin. Chem. Clin. Biochem.* Vol. 28, No. 7, July, 1990, pp. 489–491.

Yonemitsu, H. et al. "Clinical Significance of Red Cell Distribution Width in Polycythemia Vera." *Rinsho Byori*, Vol. 37, No. 7, July, 1989, pp. 813–818.

Yoshida, N. et al. "An Erythremia With Acquired HbH Disease and Chromosomal Abnormality." *Rinsho Ketsueki*, Vol. 31, No. 7, July, 1990, pp. 963–968.

Zonderland, H. M., J. J. Michiels, and F. J. ten-Kate. "Case Report: Mammographic and Sonographic Demonstration of Extramedullary Haematopoiesis of the Breast." *Clin. Radiol.*, Vol. 44, No. 1, July, 1991, pp. 64–65.

REVIEW QUESTIONS

1. Myeloproliferative disorders (MPDs) are characterized by all of the following *except:*

    A. Clonal disorders.
    B. May evolve into acute leukemia.
    C. Initial increase of immature cells.
    D. Increased production of mature cells.

2. In chronic myelogenous leukemia (CML), the total leukocyte (WBC) count is:

    A. Extremely increased.   C. Extremely variable.
    B. Slightly increased.   D. Usually normal.

3. Idiopathic myelofibrosis differs from other types of chronic MPD in which of the following ways:

    A. Ph¹ chromosome is present.
    B. Marrow fibrosis is greatly increased.
    C. LAP score is increased.
    D. Platelet count is increased.

4. Which of the following is a remarkable characteristic of polycythemia vera compared to other types of chronic MPD?

    A. Extremely increased erythrocyte mass.
    B. Extremely increased leukocyte count.
    C. Extremely increased platelet count.
    D. Teardrop-shaped erythrocytes.

5. Which of the following is a predominant feature of essential thrombocythemia compared to other types of chronic MPD?

    A. Variable number of platelets.
    B. Moderately increased number of platelets.
    C. Extremely increased number of platelets.
    D. Increased marrow fibrosis.

6. In MPD, the test results of disorders of hemostatis and coagulation that are most likely to be abnormal are:

    A. Decreased platelet count, increased activated partial thromboplastin time, and increased factor V level.
    B. Increased activated partial thromboplastin time, decreased factor V level, and increased concentration of antithrombin III in many.
    C. Decreased activated partial thromboplastin time, decreased factor V level, and increased concentration of D-dimers.
    D. Decreased concentration of D-dimers, decreased concentration of antithrombin III, increased concentration of plasmin-alpha-2 plasmin inhibitor complex.

7. Interferon alfa has been shown to:

    A. Stimulate trilineage cell proliferation.
    B. Suppress proliferation of progenitor cells.
    C. Subdue erythropoiesis only.
    D. Suppress megakaryocytopoiesis only.

8. A leukemia of long duration that affects the neutrophilic granulocytes is referred to as:

    A. Acute lymphoblastic leukemia.
    B. Acute myelogenous leukemia.
    C. Acute monocytic leukemia.
    D. Chronic myelogenous leukemia.

9. The alkaline phosphatase cytochemical staining reaction is used to differentiate between:

    A. Chronic lymphoblastic leukemia and acute myelogenous leukemia.
    B. Acute lymphoblastic leukemia and acute myelogenous leukemia.
    C. Chronic myelogenous leukemia and severe bacterial infections.
    D. Leukemoid reactions and severe bacterial infections.

10. Patients with CML are prone to:
    A. Weight gain, edema, and fatigue.
    B. Edema, anemia, and splenic infarction.
    C. Low-grade fevers, night sweats, and splenic infarction.
    D. Prominent lymphadenopathy and night sweats.

11. The total leukocyte count in CML is ___ $\times$ 10^9/L.
    A. Normal.
    C. Less than 50.
    B. Less than 25.
    D. Greater than 50.

12. The Philadelphia chromosome is typically associated with:
    A. Acute myelogenous leukemia.
    B. Leukemoid reactions.
    C. Acute lymphoblastic leukemia.
    D. Chronic myelogenous leukemia.

13. Patients with polycythemia vera suffer from:
    A. Leukemic infiltration.
    C. Hypervolemia.
    B. Bone marrow fibrosis.
    D. Anemia.

14. The most frequent structural chromosomal abnormality in polycythemia vera is:
    A. Trisomy 1q.
    B. Partial deletion of chromosome 5.
    C. Trisomy 8.
    D. Trisomy 9.

15. In polycythemia vera, cytogenetic results do *not* predict/provide:
    A. Duration of the disease.
    B. Consequences of myelosuppressive therapy.
    C. Clues to hematological phenotype.
    D. Evolution of the disease.

16. Hyperviscosity can produce:
    A. Anemia.
    C. Hemorrhages.
    B. Dizziness.
    D. Psychotic depression.

17. The *major* criteria established by the National Polycythemia Vera Study Group for diagnosis includes all of the following *except:*
    A. Increased red blood cell mass.
    B. Arterial O_2 saturation (greater than 92%).
    C. Leukocytosis.
    D. Splenomegaly.

18. Increased blood viscosity in patients with polycythemia vera can cause a dangerous condition of:
    A. Hot flushes.
    C. High RDW.
    B. Shortness of breath.
    D. Vascular occlusion.

19. The level of erythropoietin in the urine is ___ in patients with polycythemia vera compared to other kinds of polycythemia.
    A. Increased.
    C. Variable.
    B. The same.
    D. Decreased.

20. Patients with polycythemia vera demonstrate a(n) ___ of hemosiderin in the bone marrow.
    A. Absence.
    B. Normal amount.
    C. Slightly increased amount.
    D. Extremely increased amount.

21. Patients with polycythemia vera have a ___ life expectancy after diagnosis.
    A. 1- to 6-month.
    C. 1- to 5-year.
    B. 6- to 12-month.
    D. 10- to 20-year.

22. The primary treatment for polycythemia vera is:
    A. Phlebotomy.
    B. Myelosuppressive agents.
    C. Radioactive phosphorus.
    D. Low-dose busulfan.

23. Idiopathic myelofibrosis is also called:
    A. Essential thrombocythemia.
    B. Chronic myelogenous leukemia.
    C. Polycythemia vera.
    D. Agnogenic myeloid metaplasia.

24. The incidence of idiopathic myelofibrosis is known to increase after exposure to:
    A. Sunshine.
    C. Antibiotics.
    B. Benzene.
    D. Interferon.

25. The predominant clinical manifestation of idiopathic myelofibrosis is:
    A. Anemia.
    C. Medullary fibrosis.
    B. Splenomegaly.
    D. All of the above.

26. The most constant feature of idiopathic myelofibrosis is:
    A. Dyserythropoiesis.
    B. Dysleukopoiesis.
    C. Dysmegakaryocytopoiesis.
    D. Trilineage maturational disruption.

27. Which of the following is a specific chromosomal anomaly associated with idiopathic myelofibrosis?
    A. Alteration of chromosome 1.
    B. Loss of the X chromosome.
    C. Trisomy 8.
    D. There is no unique chromosomal anomaly.

28. In idiopathic myelofibrosis, splenomegaly is due to:
    A. Extramedullary hematopoiesis.
    B. Increased red blood cell production.
    C. Increased platelet production.
    D. Leukemic infiltration of organs.

29. A leukoerythroblastic picture includes all of the following *except:*
    A. Teardrop-shaped erythrocytes.
    B. Nucleated erythrocytes.
    C. Immature lymphocytes.
    D. Immature myeloid cells.

30. The median survival time for patients with idiopathic myelofibrosis is about ___ years.
    A. 1.
    C. 5.
    B. 3.
    D. 10.

31. The least common form of chronic MPD is:
    A. Polycythemia vera.
    B. CML.
    C. Idiopathic myelofibrosis.
    D. Essential thrombocythemia.

32. A *major* criterion for the diagnosis of essential thrombocythemia is:

    A. Absence of Ph¹ chromosome.
    B. Increased red blood cell mass.
    C. Mild neutrophilia in peripheral blood.
    D. Persistent increase of platelets in peripheral blood.

33. The most common disorder in patients with essential thrombocythemia is:

    A. Splenomegaly.
    B. Thrombotic or bleeding problems.
    C. Abnormal karyotype.
    D. Anemia.

34. The bone marrow architecture in essential thrombocythemia exhibits:

    A. Erythroid hyperplasia.
    B. Leukocyte hyperplasia.
    C. Megakaryocytic hyperplasia.
    D. Hypoplastic marrow.

22

Myelodysplastic Syndromes

OBJECTIVES

Terminology
- Name several terms that were previously used to recognize the myelodysplastic syndromes.
- Describe the need for a new nomenclature for myelodysplastic syndromes.

Pathophysiology
- Explain the pathophysiology of myelodysplastic syndromes.

Classification
- Name and describe the comparative characteristics of the FAB classification of myelodysplastic syndromes.

Etiology
- Explain the causes or predisposing factors of primary and secondary myelodysplastic syndromes.

Epidemiology
- Describe the age and gender distribution of myelodysplastic syndromes.

Chromosomal abnormalities
- Briefly describe the causes, types, and consequences of chromosomal abnormalities in myelodysplastic syndromes.
- List the incidence of chromosomal abnormalities.
- Describe the relationship of karyotype to prognosis in myelodysplastic syndromes.

Clinical signs and symptoms
- Explain the clinical signs and symptoms of myelodysplastic syndromes.

Laboratory manifestations
- Itemize the cellular alterations, with an emphasis on the prominent features and additional hematological features in myelodysplastic syndromes.
- Compare the laboratory features of specific types of myelodysplastic syndromes.
- Calculate the percentage of myeloblasts in the bone marrow.

Treatment
- Compare and contrast the forms of treatment and supportive care for the myelodysplastic syndromes.

Prognosis
- Discuss factors that can affect prognosis in the myelodysplastic syndromes, including FAB classification and karyotype.
- Compare the parameters used in the Bournemouth and Sanz prognostic scores.

Case Study
- Apply the laboratory data to the stated case study and discuss the implications of this case to the study of hematology.

TERMINOLOGY

Prior to the meeting of international researchers and subsequent formation of the French-American-British (FAB) group in 1982, the myelodysplastic syndromes (MDSs), which encompass a variety of hematological disorders, were described by a variety of terms. Historically, the terms preleukemia and preleukemia syndrome were used to categorize some of these disorders. Other terms of MDSs included hematopoietic dysplasia, dysmyelopoietic syndrome, myelodysplasia, smoldering leukemia, subacute leukemia, atypical chronic myelocytic leukemia, sideroblastic anemia, and refractory anemia. Because the use of so many terms created confusion among clinicians and researchers, the need for a uniform nomenclature was recognized.

The use of many of the older terms also contributed to the erroneous impression that all of the disorders classified under the MDS umbrella progressed to acute leukemia (acute nonlymphocytic leukemia, ANLL) as the major cause of death. Although patients with some varieties of MDS are at an increased risk of transformation to ANLL, the degree of risk varies within and between each type of MDS.

PATHOPHYSIOLOGY

The MDSs are a heterogeneous group of clonal disorders of the bone marrow. The clonal nature of MDS is supported by research studies, even in the absence of detectable cytogenetic abnormalities.

Isoenzyme and cytogenetic analyses suggest that the pathogenesis of MDS is a multistep process beginning with the destabilization of the multipotential progenitor cell, causing proliferation of a divergent clone of genetically unstable pluripotential stem cells that produce morphologically variable but clonally related progeny. This type of aberration becomes permanent when the acquisition of a clonal chromosome abnormality exists.

If the cell abnormality persists, additional subclones with recurrent chromosome abnormalities emerge. This precedes either failure of effective hematopoiesis or acute transformation (clonal escape) to ANNL or both. Hematopoiesis is "dysplastic" because of inefficient maturation of a slowly expanding or sometimes of a stable population of blood cell precursors.

CLASSIFICATION

The development of the FAB classification for MDS has provided classification continuity and may be helpful as a guideline for prognosis. This classification is, however, of limited value as a guide for therapy. The major value of the system is in providing a common language to hematologists when discussing the syndrome. A disadvantage of the current terminology is that it is confused and inconsistent in childhood MDS.

The MDSs are classified into five subcategories: four types of refractory anemias and chronic myelomonocytic leukemia (CMML). The five specific subtypes are refractory anemia (RA), refractory anemia with ringed sideroblasts (RARS), refractory anemia with excess of blasts (RAEB), CMML, and refractory anemia with excess of blasts in transition (RAEB-T). The FAB classification for MDS is based on the number of blasts in the bone marrow in conjunction with other features such as dysplastic maturation in one or more cell lines, ringed sideroblasts in the marrow, blasts in the peripheral blood, Auer rods in granulocyte precursors, and absolute monocytosis (Table 22.1).

ETIOLOGY

The etiology of primary MDS is unknown. Most cases of primary MDS occur without a known exposure to a leukemogenic agent. Secondary MDS can sometimes be directly related to a known agent. Examples of diseases that precede MDS include ovarian carcinoma treated with alkylating agents (10% to 15% of MDS cases), Hodgkin's disease treated with combined therapy (8% to 10% of MDS cases), and multi-

TABLE 22.1 French-American-British Cooperative Group Classification of Myelodysplastic Syndromes

Subtype	Peripheral Blood Monocytes ($\times 10^9$/L)	Ringed Sideroblasts (%)	Blast Cells (%) peripheral blood	bone marrow	Auer Bodies in Marrow
RA	No	<15	<1	<5	No
RARS	No	>15	<1	<5	No
RAEB	No	No	<5	5–20	No
CMML	>1000	No	<5	<20	No
RAEB-T	No	No	>5	20–30	Yes or no

RA = refractory anemia; RARS = refractory anemia with ringed sideroblasts; RAEB = refractory anemia with excess of blasts; CMML = chronic myelomonocytic leukemia; RAEB-T = refractory anemia with excess of blasts in transition.

Source: Reproduced with permission from Pierre Noël, "Management of Patients With Myelodysplastic Syndromes." *Mayo Clin. Proc.,* Vol. 66, 1991, pp. 485–497.

ple myeloma (approximately 15% of MDS cases). The greatest incidence of MDS follows combined chemotherapy and radiation therapy. It should also be noted that secondary MDS precedes ANLL, as a late consequence of chemotherapy or radiotherapy or both in many treated patients.

Chemical agents that have been implicated in MDS include alkylating agents and phenylbutazone. Environmental mutagens might also be involved in primary MDS. Exposures to genotoxic agents such as insecticides, pesticides, and solvents have been correlated with abnormal karyotypes and the development of ANLL, but to a lesser degree when compared to exposures to irradiation and alkylating drugs. However, a previously believed strong association between exposures to organic solvents and the development of MDS has not been supported by recent studies. Because of the progression of MDS to ANLL in many patients, it is difficult to implicate a relationship between exposure to pesticides and solvents in ANLL and MDS.

Some predisposing factors for MDS may be genetic. In some patients there is chromosomal fragility or an inability of DNA to repair itself effectively after exposure to ionizing radiation. One theory to explain the induction of MDS and perhaps eventual ANLL is that alkylating agents induce DNA cross-linkages, which because of unequal crossing over may place DNA in juxtaposition to certain oncogenes. The oncogenes may then become activated and lead to the development of a malignant clone of bone marrow cells, which develops into MDS.

EPIDEMIOLOGY

MDS is rare in childhood. The adult form usually occurs in persons over 50 years old (most patients are 60 to 75 years old). MDS is more common in males.

The incidence of MDS is still unknown but is probably similar to that of acute leukemia. There are estimated to be at least 1500 to 2000 cases annually in the United States. The prevalence of MDS, however, may be as high as 1:500 in individuals over the age of 55 years.

CMML develops at a median age of 66 years and the male-female ratio is 2.4:1. CMML is preceded by an MDS of a different subtype in about one fourth of patients and is transformed into acute leukemia in one fourth.

The most common time interval from treatment for a preexisting condition to the development of MDS is 2 to 5 years. Transformation to leukemia has a variable frequency. In about one third of patients, the condition evolves into ANLL, as the result of either a progressive expansion of the original clone or a new mutation producing a more malignant subclone. The majority of patients suffer from the results of bone marrow insufficiency, with pancytopenia and possibly immune deficiency.

CHROMOSOMAL ABNORMALITIES

Chromosomal abnormalities have been observed in a significant proportion of patients with MDS. Karyotype differences exist between primary (de novo) and secondary MDS, and may be observed on initial bone marrow observation or during evolution of the disease.

Causes

The cause of de novo MDS resulting from genetically unstable pluripotential stem cells is unclear. Secondary MDS frequently results from exposure to alkylating agents or radiation. A history of previous exposure to toxic products, such as alkylating agents, or environmental factors of occupational origin is common. Alkylating agents are used in the treatment of patients with disorders such as multiple myeloma. A period of MDS often precedes ANLL in patients who have been treated with ionizing irradiation or with alkylating agents.

Abuse of prescription or over-the-counter drugs may also be causative of MDS. Although no firm relationship has been established to date, drugs such as analgesics, tranquilizers, and nonsteroidal antiinflammatory drugs may eventually be linked to the pathogenesis of MDS (sideroblastic anemia).

Types

Clonal chromosomal anomalies may be observed during initial bone marrow analysis or seen as the result of karyotypic evolution during disease progression. Chromosome abnormalities may be monosomic or trisomic in nature and may involve partial or total chromosomal alterations. Most chromosomes display a recurrent loss of chromosomal material rather than the translocations or inversions commonly found in ANLL. In many instances, the cytogenetic abnormalities become complex and involve more than one chromosome. Some of these chromosomal alterations seem to be consistently involved in the pathogenetic mechanisms of secondary leukemia and MDS.

Characteristic karyotype anomalies involve mainly chromosomes 5, 7, and 8. These same chromosomes are known to carry different oncogenes. The most frequent alterations are in the marker chromosomes: 5 (monosomy or 5q−), 7 (either monosomy, partial loss of the long arm, 7q−, or rearrangement), and 8 (trisomy or rearrangement). Other implicated chromosomes are 1, 3 (monosomy), 4 (monosomy), 9, 12, 17, 20 (20 q−), and 21, as well as the Y chromosome (loss).

The most frequent abnormalities in children are trisomy 8, monosomy 7, and deletions involving the long arms of chromosomes 20 and X. In children with MDS, an abnormality like monosomy 7 is typical and probably indicates an unfavorable prognosis.

Consequences

Chromosomal alterations, mostly of the deleted type, are assumed to play a specific role in the genesis of MDS. These abnormalities are perhaps reflections of an alteration of oncogene function and alterations of production of growth factors and their receptors that may lead to proliferation of the abnormal clone. Some theories suggest that abnormalities in the production of growth factors or receptors relate to the development of MDS.

In primary MDS, abnormal (colony-forming unit–granulocyte-macrophage) growth of the granulocyte-macrophage precursor, CFU-GM, occurs in approximately 79% of patients and clonal chromosome abnormalities occur in an average of 34%.

Incidence

One or more clones of chromosomally abnormal cells may exist in the bone marrow. These abnormalities occur most commonly in younger age groups.

Forty to 90% of patients with MDS have chromosomal abnormalities. Different rates of occurrence exist between de novo and secondary MDS. The majority of patients with de novo MDS have recurrent chromosomal defects, with alterations of chromosomes 5, 7, and 8 being seen in one third to one half of patients. In secondary MDS and ANLL, chromosomal abnormalities are more frequent in patients with a history of multiple myeloma or macroglobulinemia, and myeloproliferative disorders.

Relationship of Karyotype to Prognosis

Survival of patients with MDS is better for those with normal chromosomal patterns.

Both single-chromosome anomalies and multiple cytogenetic changes are significant. Sequential cytogenetic studies demonstrate that most patients whose condition transforms to acute leukemia exhibit a karyotypic evolution. The existence of monosomy 5 or monosomy 7 can be useful in identifying patients who will develop acute leukemia.

The occurrence of trisomy 11 in MDS and in ANLL suggests that this abnormality can be specifically associated with the subsequent development of ANLL. Patients with a long-arm deletion of chromosome 20 (20q−) usually have intractable dysplastic syndromes, and many progress to leukemia.

Although de novo and secondary MDSs share certain clinical and cytogenetic features, over 20% of patients with de novo MDS have a normal karyotype and nearly all of these patients survive beyond 5 years. In contrast, secondary MDS is frequently associated with clonal chromosome abnormalities and overt leukemia generally occurs within 1 year.

CLINICAL SIGNS AND SYMPTOMS

A history of infections, bleeding, weight loss, or cardiovascular symptoms may be reported by a patient. Infections are due to dysfunctional granulocytic neutrophils or absolute granulocytopenia. Hemorrhages can occur due to decreased or dysfunctional platelets. Anemia is a common initial presenting symptom. A paucity of other physical symptoms is usually present.

Neutrophilic dermatosis has occurred occasionally in MDS patients. In these patients, biopsy specimens of skin lesions showed marked infiltration by neutrophils with nuclear anomalies, that is, hyposegmentation (pseudo–Pelger-Huët anomaly) or hypersegmentation.

LABORATORY MANIFESTATIONS

Cellular Abnormalities

Anemia, low platelet count, and low total leukocyte count, usually with an absolute neutropenia, are commonly pres-

---

TABLE 22.2 Prominent Hematological Findings in Myelodysplastic Syndromes

Dyserythropoiesis
  Sideroblasts*
  Multinuclearity
  Howell-Jolly bodies and nuclear fragments
  Basophilic stippling
  Uneven cytoplasmic staining
  Anisocytosis and poikilocytosis
Dysgranulocytopoiesis
  Hypogranulation
  Pseudo–Pelger Huët anomaly
  Hypersegmentation
Dysmegakaryopoiesis
  Micromegakaryocytes
  Abnormal segmentation (hyposegmentation or hypersegmentation)
  Giant platelets

*Type I (1–5 granules), type II (5–10 granules), and type III (numerous granules forming a ring around the nucleus).

---

ent. Peripheral blood smears frequently exhibit red blood cell abnormalities and large dysfunctional platelets. MDS is characteristically manifested by pancytopenia in the peripheral blood, dysplasia of two or three cell lines (Table 22.2) that may initially be in just one cell line, and a low leukemic blast count in the bone marrow and peripheral blood. Pancytopenia occurs in more than 50% of patients.

Some categorical characteristics of MDS types are overlapping. The hematopoietic disorders comprising MDS (Table 22.3) also share some common features with the early phases of myeloproliferative diseases, especially ANLL. However, the bone marrow of many pancytopenic patients may reveal acute leukemia, de novo or from other causes, including MDS. In addition, pancytopenia may represent an aplastic anemia. Distinguishing between MDS and aplastic anemia can be difficult, because both of these disorders can have similar clinical and morphological features (see Chapter 9 for a discussion of aplastic anemia). MDS must also be differentiated from secondary anemias (e.g., vitamin B_{12} deficiency).

Patients with "aggressive" subtypes of MDS (i.e., RAEB, RAEB-T, and CMML) frequently have thrombocytopenia and neutropenia, and their marrow demonstrates dysmegakaryocytopoiesis and dysgranulocytopoiesis as compared to the more "benign" subtypes (i.e., RA and RARS). In addition, leukemic transformation most frequently comes from the "aggressive" subtypes.

Children with a primary MDS can have clinical and laboratory features of "juvenile chronic myeloid leukemia." Some pediatric patients could be considered to have either the monosomy 7 syndrome or "juvenile chronic myeloid leukemia," indicating that these two entities are not mutually exclusive. In these patients, abnormal frequencies of hematopoietic progenitors or differentiation patterns in culture or both can occur. Abnormalities often affect the erythroid as well as the granulopoietic lineages, predominantly abnormal-appearing macrophage colonies. Clinical outcomes are poor, with rapid transformation to ANLL in most patients.

TABLE 22.3 Characteristics of Myelodysplastic Syndromes

Blood and Bone Marrow	RA	RARS	RAEB	CMML	RAEB-T
Blood morphology					
Dyserythropoiesis	+/−	+	+	+/−	+
Dysgranulocytopoiesis	+/−	+/−	+	+/−	+
Dysmegakaryocytopoiesis	+/−	+/−	+	+/−	+
Bone marrow morphology					
Cellularity	N/↑	N/↑	N/↑	N/↑	N/↑ *
Dyserythropoiesis	+	+	+	+	+
Dysgranulocytopoiesis	+/−	+/−	+	+	+
Dysmegakaryocytopoiesis	+/−	+/−	+	+	+
Ringed sideroblasts in bone marrow (% of total erythroblasts)	<15%	>15%	+/−	+/−	+/−

*Some are hypocellular.

RA = refractory anemia; RARS = refractory anemia with ringed sideroblasts; RAEB = refractory anemia with excess of blasts; CMML = chronic myelomonocytic leukemia; RAEB-T = refractory anemia with excess of blasts in transition; N = normal.

A Summary of Cell Line Abnormalities

Erythrocyte Abnormalities

Erythroid abnormalities of blood and bone marrow are common because MDS is dominated by ineffective hematopoiesis. Islands of erythroid hyperplasia with erythroblastic deformities can be seen in the bone marrow. The megaloblastic changes (e.g., nuclear-cytoplasmic dyssynchrony) often are similar to those of nutritional megaloblastic anemias. Erythroblasts (rubriblasts) may be multinucleated, fragmented, or misshaped. Abnormal nuclear shapes include indentations, lobes, or an irregular outline. Cytoplasmic staining is often uneven, and the cell margins may be ragged or indistinct and may display punctate basophilic stippling.

About one fourth of patients with RA demonstrate ringed sideroblasts similar to those of sideroblastic anemias in the bone marrow. Ringed sideroblasts are scarce in megaloblastic anemias. Patients with RARS usually present with a dual population of red cells: a minor one that is hypochromic and microcytic, often displaying basophilic stippling, and a major one that is macrocytic with a high mean corpuscular volume and megaloblastoid changes. An occasional nucleated red blood cell may be seen in the peripheral blood.

Leukocyte Abnormalities

Abnormalities of the myeloid series are generally more subtle than those of dyserythropoiesis. Neutrophils are often agranular or hypogranular. Precursor marrow myelocytes may also lack secondary granules. A dense rim of basophilia may occur at the cell periphery. Primary granules may be absent from promyelocytes.

Myelocytes and promyelocytes can have central, round nuclei. Nuclear anomalies include the pseudo–Pelger-Huët anomaly and the twinning deformity. The twinning deformity involves two discrete segmented strands in a tetraploid cell, which also produces an abnormally large cell. Hypersegmentation may also be seen. Peripheral blood and bone marrow neutrophils have similar anomalies.

Low lymphocyte counts in bone marrow can be observed. A significant decrease of CD3-defined pan-T lymphocytes in peripheral blood can be exhibited. This reduction is primarily confined to the CD4-defined helper subset, but there can be a relative increase in the CD8-defined suppressor subpopulation. As a result, the ratio of CD4-CD8 lymphocytes is reversed. Consequently, abnormalities of cell-mediated immunity function can occur in patients.

Platelet Abnormalities

The megakaryocyte population may be decreased, normal, or increased. Micromegakaryocytes, mononuclear megakaryocytes, multiple small separated nuclei, and giant granules can be seen in the peripheral blood. Large bizarre platelets are a frequent finding in the peripheral blood. A distinct subpopulation of platelets in MDS, which by phase contrast microscopic examination seem to have a balloon-shaped bulge of the cell membrane, has been observed. Increased numbers of these atypical platelets can be observed in the majority of patients with MDS. Normal platelet morphology may be observed in patients with RARS. The number of atypical platelets is negatively correlated with the peripheral platelet counts in MDS. The atypical platelets most likely reflect maturation disturbances of megakaryocytopoiesis. Unless associated with recent cytotoxic therapy, an increased value (greater than 1%) in a cytopenic patient would suggest a diagnosis of MDS.

Additional Hematological Features

Numerous morphological features have been observed in the bone marrow and peripheral blood of patients with MDS. In addition, a subtle morphological feature, **internuclear bridging** (INB), was recently recognized in MDS. The occurrence of INB in MDS suggests an underlying abnormality of mitotic division that could explain the impaired production of hematopoietic cells, the cytogenetic changes of addition and deletion, and the stepwise disease progression and cytogenetic progression characteristic of MDS. Lack of awareness that INB occurs in MDS may cause a confusion of MDS with congenital dyserythropoietic anemia type I, a congenital process also characterized by INB.

Intracellular alkaline phosphatase activities in peripheral neutrophils are decreased in MDS compared to normal controls. The measurement of intracellular alkaline phosphatase activity is useful for supporting a diagnosis of MDS.

Lymphoid agglutination or cell clusters of blast cells are also seen in biopsy specimens from patients with MDS.

Features of Specific Types of Myelodysplastic Syndromes

Refractory anemia (RA) is the mildest form of all types of MDS. About 20% of patients have this type of MDS. Most patients exhibit pancytopenia. The percentage of reticulocytes and the total peripheral red blood count are typically decreased. Peripheral erythrocytes have a tendency to be macrocytic. Decreased hemoglobin levels are caused by an impaired release of erythrocytes from the bone marrow. The total peripheral blood leukocyte and platelet counts are either normal or decreased. Some neutrophils are agranular or tetraploid. Giant platelets are common. The level of bone marrow storage iron is increased.

Refractory anemia with ringed sideroblasts (RARS) is similar to RA but differs because of the presence of ringed sideroblasts (Plate 72). Ringed sideroblasts, which exceed 15% of the nucleated erythroid cells of the bone marrow, are formed when iron deposits encircle the nuclei of erythroid precursors. Over time, the number of dysplastic sideroblasts and the medullary iron levels increase in parallel, and serum ferritin levels steadily rise. A small number of patients eventually develop hemochromatosis. In these patients, the incidence of HLA-A3 is significantly higher (71%) than in the general population, which suggests that patients in this subgroup inherited a gene for hemochromatosis and later acquired a mutant one for RARS.

The percentage of reticulocytes and the total peripheral red blood cell count are typically decreased, although few patients manifest leukocytopenia or thrombocytopenia. Erythroid dimorphism is present, with macrocytosis predominating.

It is important to note that RARS is not related etiologically to congenital forms of sideroblastic anemia or to acquired, secondary sideroblastic anemias.

Refractory anemia with excess blasts (RAEB) (Plate 73) is the first MDS type to demonstrate an overt classic relationship to ANLL, that is, an elevated percentage of type I and type II* myeloblasts in the bone marrow and the presence of myeloblasts in the circulating blood. RAEB is the most frequent of the MDS types, representing 40% to 50% of all new cases.

Dyserythropoiesis, dysgranulocytopoiesis, and dysmegakaryocytopoiesis are common. Anemia is usually macrocytic

and often dimorphic, and oval macrocytes may be present. A variable number of ringed sideroblasts are also present. Granulocytic abnormalities can include pseudo–Pelger-Huët anomaly, ring-shaped nuclei, and agranular or hypergranular forms. About half of RAEB patients exhibit giant platelets and micromegakaryocytes.

The percentage of reticulocytes and the total peripheral red blood cell count, white blood cell count, and platelet count are typically decreased. The presence of cytopenias and dyspoiesis distinguishes RAEB from chronic myelogenous leukemia.

Chronic myelomonocytic leukemia (CMML) is a leukemic disorder. This form of myelomonocytic leukemia is much less frequent than the acute variety. Diagnosis of CMML according to the FAB classification criteria distinguishes the two forms. One shows only an increase of mature monocytes, and it has no relationship to the type that transforms into ANLL. It is considered as a reactive monocytosis. The other form, in addition to an increase of mature monocytes, shows an increase of a few monoblasts and promonocytes. This is considered to be a true CMML and usually quickly develops into the M4 or M5 forms of leukemia (ANLL).

The clinical symptoms closely resemble those of subacute myelogenous leukemia. However, the presence of monocytosis distinguishes it from RAEB. Peripheral blood smears usually demonstrate a persistent monocyte count greater than 1×10^9/L. Neutrophilia is commonly observed, with morphological abnormalities being present. Fewer than 5% blast cells are usually seen in the peripheral blood. The bone marrow often has increased promonocytes, which may be distinguished from abnormal myelocytes by **nonspecific esterase staining.**

Dyshematopoiesis of all three cell lines is present. The percentage of reticulocytes, the total peripheral red blood cell count, and the platelet count are typically decreased, although the total peripheral white blood cell count may be decreased or increased.

Refractory anemia with excess blasts in transformation (RAEB-T) is similar to RAEB, but includes patients in whom leukemic transformation appears to be in progress. However, the percentage of myeloblastic cells in the bone marrow must exceed 20% but be less than 30% (see calculation section that follows), or 5% or more of myeloid cells in the blood must be myeloblasts. The presence of Auer rods in the blasts may also distinguish this category. All of the cellular elements of the peripheral blood are decreased. Patients with this type of MDS have the highest rate of progression to ANLL (usually 100%); therefore, they have the poorest prognosis of all of the categories.

Calculation of Myeloblast Percentage in Bone Marrow

The FAB classification of ANLL (M1 to M7) and MDS necessitates the determination of the percentage of myeloblasts in the bone marrow. This is particularly important in distinguishing FAB M2, FAB M6, RAEB, and RAEB-T.

With the formula given below, the current proposal is:

More than 30% myeloblasts and an actual percentage of erythroblasts over 50% = M6

---

*The FAB group introduced the distinction between type I and type II blasts. The historically well-defined myeloblast (see Plate 27 and Chapter 14) became a type I blast. A type II blast is slightly larger with a lower nucleus-cytoplasm ratio and always contains one to six nonspecific azurophilic granules. More mature cells with a greater number of granules are classified as promyelocytes.

More than 30% myeloblasts and an actual percentage of erythroblasts under 50% = M2

Twenty to 30% myeloblasts and a real percentage of erythroblasts under 50% = RAEB − T

Five to 20% myeloblasts and a real percentage of erythroblasts under 50% = RAEB

The accepted FAB standard for the calculation of the percentage of myeloblasts is accomplished by subtracting all nucleated erythroid precursors in the bone marrow from the differential count. The calculation is performed as follows:

Example 1

1. Count all nucleated cells in the bone marrow:

$$Total = 100\ cells$$

2. If the erythroid precursors are over 50%,[†] subtract the erythroid precursors (E) from the total (100) count:

$$100\ total\ cells - 55\ (E) = 45\ cells$$

3. List the number of myeloblasts in the 100 cell count:

$$Number\ of\ myeloblasts = 25\ cells$$

4. Calculate the percentage of myeloblasts in the nonerythroid cell count. Twenty-five myeloblasts were included in the nonerythroid count of 45 cells. Therefore the percentage of myeloblasts in this count is:

$$(25/45) \times 100 = 55\%$$

Note: This patient has acute myelogenous leukemia, FAB M6.

Example 2

100 total cells − 55 (E) = 45 cells
Number of myeloblasts = 10 cells
Calculation:

$$(10/45) \times 100 = 22\%$$

Note: This patient has MDS (RAEB).

TREATMENT

Treatment consideration in MDS must weigh the risk of therapy versus the risk of problems associated with the existing cytopenias, and the likelihood and imminence of leukemic transformation. The risk of progression to acute leukemia ranges from 10% to 100%. Progression is least likely in RA and RARS, and inevitable in RAEB-T.

In patients with ANLL transforming from MDS, the clinical responses to the standard therapy are poor. The greatly decreased hematopoiesis in these patients is considered responsible for their clinical picture. Leukemia-associated inhibitory activity, which inhibits human granulocyte-macrophage progenitors, may be responsible for the suppression of normal granulocytopoiesis in some patients. In addition, the profound derangement of normal hematopoietic capabil-

[†]If the percentage of erythroblasts is greater than 50, the diagnosis of M6 is based on the nonerythroid cell (NEC) blast count, which must be 30% or greater.

ity in these cases may be due to multiple complex factors. Although MDS is rare in children, these represent some of the most difficult dyscrasias to treat. Children treated for MDS respond poorly to conventional chemotherapy. Infrequently children may achieve remission with intensive therapy and allogeneic bone marrow transplantation.

Forms of Therapy

At present, no generally accepted form of therapy has been established for MDS. A variety of treatment strategies used either alone or in combination are commonly employed (Table 22.4).

Vitamin Supplementation

Patients should receive a trial course of folate and vitamin B_{12} in large doses, regardless of serum assay results. Patients with MDS generally manifest megaloblastoid features, and in rare instances, blood counts may improve. Transfusion-dependent requirements may lessen after long-term (3-month) treatment with pyridoxine. Long-term benefits as the result of pyridoxine are uncommon.

Androgens

Androgens are ineffective in patients with MDS and may actually hasten the progression to acute leukemia. Elevated values on liver function assay may necessitate the discontinuation of androgen therapy.

Corticosteroids

Corticosteroids are generally ineffective and often risky. In a small proportion of the population, remission is induced; however, protracted administration of corticosteroids increases the risk of infection. Therapy should be pursued with caution. Other complications associated with high doses of steroids include hyperglycemia, hypertension, fluid retention, gastrointestinal hemorrhage, and aseptic necrosis at the hip. Other conditions possibly associated with steroid administration include seizures, arrhythmias, and headache with papilledema.

Cytotoxic Drugs

Combination chemotherapeutic regimens are conventionally used for treating ANLL. This approach is often successful in inducing remission in young (less than 50 years old) MDS

TABLE 22.4 Forms of Therapy for Myelodysplastic Syndromes

- Vitamin supplementation (folate, vitamin B_{12}, and pyridoxine in high doses, 150 mg/day)
- Androgens (including danazol for a subset of patients with cell-bound platelet antibodies present)
- Steroids
- Cytotoxic drugs: 13-*cis* retinoic acid, low-dose cytosine arabinoside, other low-dose chemotherapy, aggressive chemotherapy
- Recombinant growth factors
- Bone marrow transplantation

patients, but in older patients the results have been dismal. However, 13-*cis* retinoic acid has not been found to exert a beneficial therapeutic effect in patients with MDS.

The cytoreductive effect of aclacinomycin A has been demonstrated to be minor compared to therapy with small doses of cytosine arabinoside. Therefore, aclacinomycin A warrants further consideration for the treatment of patients with MDS.

Cytosine arabinoside and other compounds have been used in the aggressive ANLL induction regimen. However, remission has been of a short duration and has culminated in death with progressive marrow failure or evolution to ANLL. This indicates the limitations of the current treatment strategies for MDS and highlights the need for exploring new therapeutic approaches.

Recombinant Colony-Stimulating Growth Factors

The applications of recombinant colony-stimulating growth factors are an extremely active area of clinical research. The family of colony-stimulating factors and interleukins influence all aspects of hematopoietic cell proliferation and differentiation. In most instances, these hematopoietic growth factors have overlapping, pleiotropic effects and frequently regulate early progenitor cell proliferation and mature cell function.

Colony-stimulating factors are a family of regulatory glycoprotein hormones that promote the proliferation and differentiation of hematopoietic progenitor cells and also augment the functions of mature effector cells in vitro. The recent cloning of human genes and the availability of sufficient quantities of recombinant purified growth factors have made it possible to evaluate their therapeutic potential in cytopenic states.

These growth factors include erythropoietin, granulocyte colony–stimulating factors (G-CSF), and granulocyte-macrophage colony-stimulating factors (GM-CSF). The use of growth factors can lead to a normalization of blood counts and bone marrow, with a concurrent decrease or eradication of the need for blood transfusions. Initial studies with GM-CSF have demonstrated its ability to increase neutrophil, monocyte, and eosinophil counts in patients with MDS, acquired immunodeficiency syndrome (AIDS), and aplastic anemia. Both GM-CSF and G-CSF reduce the duration of neutropenia following chemotherapy and accelerate hematopoietic recovery in patients undergoing intensive chemotherapy and autologous bone marrow transplantation. In addition, the increase in absolute numbers of functionally active neutrophils may have a profound effect on the rate and severity of neutropenia-related sepsis. Studies are ongoing to determine the optimal dose, route, schedule of administration, and long-term effects of G-CSF and GM-CSF.

Observations of the responsiveness of bone marrow erythropoietic stem cells (colony-forming units–erythroid [CFU-E], and burst-forming units–erythroid [BFU-E]) to recombinant human erythropoietin in patients with MDS have demonstrated that the responses of CFU-E to erythropoietin were relatively good in RA and primary acquired sideroblastic anemia. On the other hand, the responses of CFU-E to erythropoietin were poor for patients with RAEB or RAEB

in transformation who were younger than 55 years and who never experienced cytopenia.

The status of underlying disease at the time of transplantation is prognostic for 2-year disease-free survival. Results are significantly less favorable for those patients with more advanced disease who only partially responded to prior intensive chemotherapy (2-year disease-free survival rate 18%). No patients who either relapse or are resistant to chemotherapy survive bone marrow transplantation for 2 years. The disease-free survival rate at 2 years after bone marrow transplantation has been demonstrated in one study to be related to the FAB classification. The survival rates are approximately 38% to 78% for patients with RA, 60% to 88% for patients with RAEB, 34% to 66% for patients with RAEB-T, and 7% to 39% for patients with secondary ANLL. Allogeneic bone marrow transplantation can therefore be considered as curative treatment for patients with MDS. Patients with AML who have a histocompatible donor should be given chemotherapy intensive enough to induce complete remission. If this is achieved, these individuals have a prognosis comparable to those with de novo ANLL in first remission after bone marrow transplantation.

Since 1985, the results of transplantation from human leukocyte antigen (HLA)–matched siblings have improved and the 3-year survival rate is now more than 90% for patients under 20 years old. The chance of survival is influenced by the conditioning regimen and the recipient's age. For MDS, the actuarial survival rate at 3 years was 42%. When HLA status bone marrow transplantation is considered, the probabilities of survival at 5 years are 70% for patients with grafts from HLA-matched siblings and 100% for the patients with grafts from monozygous twins. The survival rate at 3 years for the patients with grafts from family members other than HLA-matched siblings was 46%. Recipients with sustained engraftment had a significantly higher survival rate than those with graft failure (83% versus 11%).

Supportive Care

Supportive care includes transfusions and antibiotics.

Transfusion Therapy

The most common problem in MDS is anemia. Therefore, red cell transfusion is the main form of supportive therapy. Platelet transfusions during active bleeding episodes and granulocyte transfusions may also be necessary.

Antibiotics

Findings suggest that GM-CSF may be useful in regulating the host response to infection when it is used in combination with antimicrobial therapy in neutropenic patients.

PROGNOSIS

Survival is generally good for patients with RA and RARS, and intermediate for those with RAEB and CMML. Unfortunately, the prognosis is extremely poor for patients with RAEB-T.

In most FAB groups, deaths due to the complications of bone marrow failure are more common than those caused by transformation to ANLL. Complications of bone marrow failure, including infections and hemorrhage, are major causes of death. The overall rate of 0.96 infection per patient-year is slightly lower than rates for multiple myeloma and hairy cell leukemia. Patients with RAEB and RAEB-T are at particularly high risk, as are patients who are neutropenic or receiving immunosuppressive therapy.

The median survival time for all patients with MDS is about 2 years. In the types of MDS with 5% to 30% or more bone marrow blasts, the risk of progression to ANLL is high, especially in childhood, and usually leads to death.

FAB Classification and Prognosis

Refractory Anemia

The average survival time after diagnosis is about 32 months, with infection causing nearly one fourth of deaths. Patients in this category have a good prognosis, with about 11% terminating in ANLL.

Refractory Anemia With Ringed Sideroblasts

This FAB form progresses slowly at first, intensifying after a period of years to a stage of intractable, transfusion-dependent anemia in almost 40% of patients. About 5% of patients with RARS terminate in ANLL. The median survival time after diagnosis is about 76 months, but many patients appear to have a prolonged subclinical phase for many years.

Refractory Anemia With Excess Blasts

The average survival time after diagnosis is less than 12 months, with death from infection or hemorrhage occurring in about half of the patients. About 30% of patients in this category terminate in ANLL. The median length of survival is 10.5 months.

Chronic Myelomonocytic Leukemia

Although patients with CMML have a more chronic and capricious course than patients with some of the other forms, about 13% of patients terminate in ANLL. The median length of survival is 22 months.

Refractory Anemia With Excess Blasts in Transformation

Patients with this form of MDS have a very short median survival time of 5 months. More than half of patients succumb to ANLL. Infections and bleeding or anemia or both claim the lives of the other patients.

Relationship of Karyotype to Prognosis

MDS patients with multiple karyotypic anomalies have a shorter survival time (average 8 months) than do patients with single anomalies (average 18 months) or those with a normal karyotype (average 36 months). Transformation to ANLL can be observed in about 25% of patients with a normal karyotype, an average of 40% of patients with single anomalies, and 50% of patients with multiple changes. Therefore, an unstable karyotype can be associated with a poor prognosis.

Patients with MDS and patients with ANLL share certain specific karyotypes. Patients with "unfavorable" karyotypes have similarly short survival times regardless of whether they are classified as having RAEB, RAEBT, or ANLL. Patients with diploid karyotypes survive significantly longer, again with relatively minor differences between patients with RAEB, RAEBT, and ANLL. Therefore, classification of patients with excess myeloblasts in the marrow might more appropriately be based on cytogenetics than on the distinction between MDS and ANLL.

The absence of cytogenetically normal cells indicates a poor prognosis with frequent progression to ANLL, which is resistant to chemotherapy. Progression to ANLL depends not only on chromosomal abnormalities but also on FAB subtype. Patients with monosomy 7, del(7q), trisomy 8, or i(17q), have shorter survival times, more frequent progression to leukemia, and less response to treatment with 13-*cis* retinoic acid than patients with del(20q) or t(2;11).

Prognostic Scales

Prognostic scores determined by Bournemouth or Sanz (Table 22.5) scoring systems may be of some value in predicting longevity as well as modes of treatment such as low-dose cytarabine or 13-*cis* retinoic acid. The survival time according

TABLE 22.5 Examples of Scoring Systems

	Score
Bournemouth	
Hemoglobin	
>10 gm/dL	0
≤10 gm/dL	1
Platelet count	
>100 × 10⁹/L	0
≤100 × 10⁹/L	1
Absolute neutrophil count	
>2.5 × 10⁹/L	0
≤2.5 × 10⁹/L	1
Bone marrow blast count	
<5%	0
≥5%	1
Sum of scores: 0 or 1—group A; 2 or 3—group B; 4—group C	
Sanz	
Bone marrow blast count	
<5%	0
≥5–≤10%	1
>10%	2
Platelet count	
≥100 × 10⁹/L	0
>50–<100 × 10⁹/L	1
≤50 × 10⁹/L	2
Age	
≤60 yr	0
>60 yr	1
Sum of scores: 0 or 1—group A; 2 or 3—group B; 4—group C	

Source: M. A. Shifman. "FAB Help: A Rule-Based Consultation Program." *Lab. Med.*, Vol. 22, 1991, p. 642.

to the Bournemouth score ranges from 8.5 months to 62 months. Another study suggests that the Bournemouth score gives excessive prognostic importance to peripheral cytopenias, gives insufficient weight to the percentage of blasts in the bone marrow, and does not take into account a host-related factor such as age. In addition, changes in therapeutic strategies over time may modify the natural history of the disease and also affect the relative importance of different prognostic factors.

To calculate either the Bournemouth or the Sanz score, several parameters need to be weighted. These parameters are hemoglobin concentration, total platelet count, absolute neutrophil count, bone marrow blast count, and the patient's age. The Bournemouth system scores a patient based on hemoglobin, absolute neutrophil count, bone marrow blast count, and platelet count. The Sanz system uses the bone marrow blast count, the platelet count, and the patient's age. Based on the result of each scoring system, patients can be placed into prognostic groups.

SUMMARY
Terminology

The FAB group established a classification for MDSs in 1982. There have been many terms for MDS, which resulted in an inconsistent terminology used among clinicians and the erroneous impression that all of the disorders classified under the MDS umbrella progressed to acute leukemia as the major cause of death.

Pathophysiology

The MDSs are a heterogeneous group of clonal disorders of the bone marrow. Analyses suggest that the pathogenesis of MDS is a multistep process beginning with the destabilization of the multipotential stem cell, causing proliferation of a divergent clone of genetically unstable pluripotential stem cells that produce morphologically variable but clonally related progeny. Hematopoiesis is "dysplastic" because of inefficient maturation of a slowly expanding or sometimes of a stable population of blood cell precursors.

Classification

The major value of the FAB classification is in providing a common language for hematologists when discussing the syndrome. A disadvantage of the current terminology is that it is confused and inconsistent in childhood MDS.

The MDSs are classified into five specific subtypes: RA, RARS, RAEB, CMML, and RAEB-T.

Etiology

The etiology of primary MDS is unknown. Secondary MDS can sometimes be directly related to a known agent. The greatest incidence of MDS follows combined chemotherapy and radiation therapy. Chemical agents that have been implicated in MDSs include alkylating agents and phenylbutazone. Environmental mutagens might also be involved in primary MDS. In addition, some predisposing factors for MDS may be genetic.

Epidemiology

MDS is rare in childhood. It occurs mainly in older individuals and is more common in males. It is estimated that at least 1500 to 2000 cases of MDS are diagnosed annually in the United States. The prevalence of MDS, however, may be as high as 1:500 in individuals over 55 years of age.

Chromosomal Abnormalities

Chromosomal abnormalities have been observed in a significant proportion of patients with MDS. Karyotype differences exist between primary (de novo) and secondary MDS, and may be observed on initial bone marrow observation or during evolution of the disease. The cause of de novo MDS resulting from genetically unstable pluripotential stem cells is unclear. Secondary MDS frequently results from exposures to alkylating agents or radiation. Abuse of prescription or over-the-counter drugs may also be causative in MDS. Chromosome abnormalities may be monosomic or trisomic in nature and involve partial or total chromosomal alterations. Most chromosomes display a recurrent loss of chromosomal material rather than the translocations or inversions commonly found in ANLL. In many instances, the cytogenetic abnormalities become complex and involve more than one chromosome. Characteristic karyotype anomalies involve mainly chromosomes 5, 7, and 8. The most frequent abnormalities in children with MDS are trisomy 8, monosomy 7, and deletions involving the long arms of chromosomes 20 and X.

Forty to 90% of patients with MDS have chromosomal abnormalities. Different rates of occurrence exist between de novo and secondary MDS. The majority of patients with de novo MDS have recurrent chromosomal defects, with alterations of chromosomes 5, 7, and 8 being seen in one third to one half of patients. In secondary MDS and ANLL, chromosomal abnormalities are more frequent in patients with a history of multiple myeloma or macroglobulinemia, and myeloproliferative disorders. Survival of patients with MDS is better for those with normal chromosomal patterns.

Clinical Signs and Symptoms

A history of infections, bleeding, weight loss, or cardiovascular symptoms may be reported by a patient. Anemia is a common initial presenting symptom.

Laboratory Manifestations

MDS is characteristically manifested by pancytopenia in the peripheral blood, dysplasia of two or three cell lines that may initially be in just one cell line, and a low leukemic blast count in the bone marrow and peripheral blood. Pancytopenia occurs in more than 50% of patients.

RA is the mildest form of all types of MDS. About 20% of patients with MDS have this type. Most patients exhibit pancytopenia. Some neutrophils are agranular or tetraploid.

Giant platelets are common. The level of bone marrow storage iron is increased.

RARS is similar to RA but differs because of the presence of ringed sideroblasts. Erythroid dimorphism is present, with macrocytosis predominating.

RAEB is the most frequent of the MDS types, representing 40% to 50% of all new cases. Dyserythropoiesis, dysgranulocytopoiesis, and dysmegakaryocytopoiesis are common. Anemia is usually macrocytic and often dimorphic, and oval macrocytes may be present. Granulocytic abnormalities can include pseudo–Pelger-Huët anomaly, ring-shaped nuclei, and agranular or hypergranular forms. About half of RAEB patients exhibit giant platelets and micromegakaryocytes. The presence of cytopenias and dyspoiesis distinguishes RAEB from chronic myelogenous leukemia.

CMML is a leukemic disorder. This form of myelomonocytic leukemia is much less frequent than the acute variety. The presence of monocytosis distinguishes it from RAEB. Fewer than 5% blast cells are usually seen in the peripheral blood, and the bone marrow often has increased promonocytes, which may be distinguished from abnormal myelocytes by nonspecific esterase staining.

RAEB-T is similar to RAEB, but includes patients in whom leukemic transformation appears to be in progress. The percentage of myeloblastic cells in the bone marrow must exceed 20% but be less than 30%, or 5% or more of myeloid cells in the blood must be myeloblasts. The presence of Auer rods in the blasts may also distinguish this category.

Treatment

Treatment considerations in MDS must weigh the risk of therapy against the risk of problems associated with the existing cytopenias, and the likelihood and imminence of leukemic transformation. In patients with acute leukemia transforming from MDS, the clinical responses to the standard therapy are poor. Although MDS is rare in children, these represent some of the most difficult dyscrasias to treat. Children treated for MDS respond poorly to conventional chemotherapy.

At present, no generally accepted form of therapy has been established for MDS. A variety of treatment strategies used either alone or in combination are commonly employed. These include vitamin supplementation, androgens, corticosteroids, cytotoxic drugs, recombinant colony-stimulating growth factors, and allogeneic bone marrow transplantation. Bone marrow transplantation is a viable option for patients younger than 55 years who have never experienced cytopenia. Supportive care includes transfusions and antibiotics.

Prognosis

Survival is generally good for patients with RA and RARS and intermediate for those with RAEB and CMML. Unfortunately, the prognosis is extremely poor for patients with RAEB-T. In most FAB groups, deaths due to the complications of bone marrow failure are more common than those caused by transformation to ANLL. The median survival time for all patients with MDS is about 2 years. MDS patients with multiple karyotypic anomalies have a shorter survival

time (average of 8 months) than patients with single anomalies (average of 18 months) or those with a normal karyotype (average of 36 months). Prognostic scores determined by the Bournemouth or Sanz scoring system may be of some value in predicting longevity as well as modes of treatment.

CASE STUDY

This 65-year-old white male retired painter consulted his primary care physician because of increasing fatigue. His medical history was unremarkable. Physical examination revealed no gross abnormalities. A complete blood count (CBC) was ordered.

Laboratory Data
Hemoglobin 8.0 g/dL
Hematocrit 20%
RBC count 1.9×10^{12}/L
WBC count 2.5×10^9/L
Platelet count 90×10^9/L
RDW 23.5%
MCV 96 fL

Examination of the peripheral blood film showed 3% blasts, few Pelger-Huët neutrophils, occasional giant platelets, marked anisocytosis, marked macrocytosis, and occasional basophilic stippling.

A subsequent bone marrow aspiration revealed a hypercellular marrow with 25% leukocytic blasts; a few of these blasts had Auer rods. Myeloid dysplasia was present with asynchronous maturation of the nucleus and cytoplasm. Erythroblasts comprised 38% of the cells; some exhibited megaloblastic characteristics. Micromegakaryocytes were also present.

Additional testing: A Prussian blue stain of the marrow revealed 12% ringed sideroblasts. Cytogenetic studies disclosed a monosomy 7 abnormality.

Questions
1. What would the presumed diagnosis be in this case?
2. What is the significance of the presence of Auer rods?
3. What is the probable prognosis for this patient?

Discussion
1. A diagnosis of RAEB-t was confirmed based on the percentage of bone marrow blasts being less than 30% and the presence of trilineage dysplasia.
2. Although the presence of Auer rods was not critical to this patient's diagnosis, the presence of Auer rods would have been diagnostic for RAEB-t even if bone marrow blasts had been less than 20%.
3. The presence of the chromosomal abnormality, monosomy 7, is suggestive of a short survival because of expected leukemic transformation.

➮ **Diagnosis: RAEB-t**

BIBLIOGRAPHY

Abrams, C. "Demographic Trends Reshape Frequency of Diseases." *Adv. Med. Lab. Professionals*, Vol. 3, January 7, 1991, pp. 19, 30.
Advani, S. H. et al. "Limitations of the Therapeutic Regimens for Myelodysplastic Syndrome." *Indian J. Med. Res.*, Vol. 90, August, 1989, pp. 248–253.

Antin, J. H., D. S. Weinberg, and D. S. Rosenthal. "Variable Effect of Recombinant Human Granulocyte-Macrophage Colony-Stimulating Factor on Bone Marrow Fibrosis in Patients With Myelodysplasia." *Exp. Hematol.*, Vol. 18, No. 4, May, 1990, pp. 266–270.

Aoki, I. et al. "Responsiveness of Bone Marrow Erythropoietic Stem Cells (CFU-E and BFU-E) to Recombinant Human Erythropoietin (rh-Ep) In Vitro in Aplastic Anemia and Myelodysplastic Syndrome." *Am J. Hematol.*, Vol. 35, No. 1, September, 1990, pp. 6–12.

Balinski, C. "Researchers Sub-Divide Myelodysplastic Syndrome to Five Sub-Categories." *Adv. Med. Technol.*, Vol. 1, No. 36, November 6, 1989, pp. 1–2.

Bennett, J. M. et al. "Proposals for the Classification of Myelodysplastic Syndromes." *Br. J. Haematol.*, Vol. 51, 1982, pp. 189–199.

Bennett, J. M. et al. "Acute Myeloid Leukemia and Other Myelopathic Disorders Following Treatment With Alkylating Agents." *Hematol. Pathol.*, Vol. 1, No. 2, 1987, pp. 99–104.

Beverstock, G. C. et al. "Trisomy 13 and Myelodysplastic Syndrome." *Cancer Genet. Cytogenet.*, Vol. 48, No. 2, September, 1990, pp. 179–182.

Borbenyi, Z. et al. "Factors Influencing Leukemic Transformation in Myelodysplastic Syndrome." *Orv. Hetil.*, Vol. 131, No. 23, June 10, 1990, pp. 1231–1236, 1239–1240.

Brandwein, J. M. et al. "Childhood Myelodysplasia: Suggested Classification as Myelodysplastic Syndromes Based on Laboratory and Clinical Findings." *Am. J. Pediatr. Hematol. Oncol.*, Vol. 12, No. 1, Spring, 1990, pp. 63–70.

Broun, E. R., N. A. Heerema, and G. Tricot. "Spontaneous Remission in Myelodysplastic Syndrome. A Case Report." *Cancer Genet. Cytogenet.*, Vol. 46, No. 1, May, 1990, pp. 125–128.

Bursztyn, M., D. Douer, and B. Ramot. "Myelodysplastic Syndrome: A Review of 35 Patients." *Isr. J. Med. Sci.*, Vol. 23, No. 11, November, 1987, pp. 1140–1144.

Carter, G. et al. "RAS Mutations in Patients Following Cytotoxic Therapy for Lymphoma." *Oncogene*, Vol. 5, No. 3, March, 1990, pp. 411–416.

Cournoyer, D. et al. "Trisomy 9 in Hematologic Disorders: Possible Association With Primary Thrombocytosis." *Cancer Genet. Cytogenet.*, Vol. 27, No, 1, July, 1987, pp. 73–78.

Creutzig, U. and D. T. I. Hoelzer. "Myelodysplastic Syndrome: A Review." *Klin. Pediatr.*, Vol. 199, No. 35, May–June, 1987, pp. 169–172.

D'Angelo, G. et al. "Acquired Idiopathic Sideroblastic Anemia With Cyclic Hypereosinophilia of Unclear Significance. A Case Report." *Minerva Med.*, Vol. 81, No. 5, May, 1990, pp. 433–437.

De-Witte, T. et al. "Allogeneic Bone Marrow Transplantation for Secondary Leukaemia and Myelodysplastic Syndrome: A Survey by the Leukaemia Working Party of the European Bone Marrow Transplantation Group (EBMTG)." *Br. J. Haematol.*, Vol. 74, No. 2, February, 1990, pp. 151–155.

De-Witte, T. et al. "Intensive Antileukemic Treatment of Patients Younger Than 65 Years With Myelodysplastic Syndromes and Secondary Acute Myelogenous Leukemia." *Cancer*, Vol. 66, No. 5, September 1, 1990, pp. 831–837.

Doney, K. et al. "Treatment of Aplastic Anemia With Antithymocyte Globulin, High-Dose Corticosteroids, and Androgens." *Exp. Hematol.*, Vol. 15, No. 3, March, 1987, pp. 239–242.

Donti, E. et al. "Evolution of Multiple Cytogenetic Clones and Leukemic Transformation in a Case of Myelodysplastic Syndrome." *Med. Oncol. Tumor Pharmacother.*, Vol. 6, No. 3, 1989, pp. 233–238.

Egli, F. et al. "Combined GM-CSF and Erythropoietin Therapy in Myelodysplastic Syndrome." *Schweiz Med. Wochenschr.*, Vol. 119, No. 49, December 9, 1989, pp. 1777–1780.

Estey, E. H. et al. "Karyotype Is Prognostically More Important Than the FAB System's Distinction Between Myelodysplastic Syndrome and Acute Myelogenous Leukemia." *Hematol. Pathol.*, Vol. 1, No. 4, 1987, pp. 203–208.

Fukuoka, T. and S. Fujita. "Leukemia-Associated Inhibitory Activity in Acute Leukemia Developed From Myelodysplastic Syndrome." *Jpn. J. Med.*, Vol. 26, No. 3, August, 1987, pp. 314–318.

Gisslinger, H. et al. "Long-Term Alpha-Interferon Therapy in Myelodysplastic Syndromes." *Leukemia*, Vol. 4, No. 2, February, 1990, pp. 91–94.

Gold, E. J. et al. "Marrow Cytogenetic and Cell-Culture Analyses of the Myelodysplastic Syndromes: Insights to Pathophysiology and Prognosis." *J. Clin. Oncol.*, Vol. 1, 1983, pp. 627–634.

Goldberg, H. et al. "Survey of Exposure to Genotoxic Agents in Primary Myelodysplastic Syndrome: Correlation With Chromosome Patterns and Data on Patients Without Hematological Disease." *Cancer Res.*, Vol. 50, No. 21, November 1, 1990, pp. 6876–6881.

Gutterman, J. et al. "Effects of Granulocyte-Macrophage Colony-Stimulating Factor in Iatrogenic Myelosuppression, Bone Marrow Failure, and Regulation of Host Defense." *Semin. Hematol.*, Vol. 27, No. 3, Suppl. 3, July, 1990, pp. 15–24.

Head, D. R. et al. "Pathogenetic Implications of Internuclear Bridging in Myelodysplastic Syndrome. An Eastern Cooperative Oncology Group/Southwest Oncology Group Cooperative Study." *Cancer*, Vol. 64, No. 11, December 1, 1989, pp. 2199–2202.

Holmes, J. et al. "Glutathione-s-Transferase Pi Expression in Leukaemia: A Comparative Analysis With mdr-1 Data." *Br. J. Cancer*, Vol. 62, No. 2, August, 1990, pp. 209–212.

Horiike, S. et al. "The Unbalanced 1;7 Translocation in De Novo Myelodysplastic Syndrome and Its Clinical Implication." *Cancer*, Vol. 65, No. 6, March 15, 1990, pp. 1350–1354.

Humphries, J. E., M. S. Wheby, and J. Jandl. "Trisomy 19 in a Patient With Myelodysplastic Syndrome and Thrombocytosis." *Cancer Genet. Cytogenet.*, Vol. 44, No. 2, February, 1990, pp. 187–191.

Iurlo, A. et al. "Cytogenetic and Clinical Investigations in 76 Cases With Therapy-Related Leukemia and Myelodysplastic Syndrome." *Cancer Genet. Cytogenet.*, Vol. 43, No. 2, December, 1989, pp. 227–241.

Jacob, A. K. et al. "Translocation (1;6) (p12;p23) in ANLL." *Cancer Genet. Cytogenet.*, Vol. 45, No. 1, March, 1990, pp. 67–71.

Jiang, Y. L., Y. H. Hou, and X. R. Li. "A Clinical Study on Myelodysplastic Syndrome. Report of 64 Cases." *Chung Hua Nei Ko Tsa Chih*, Vol. 28, No. 7, July, 1989, pp. 413–417, 444.

Jotterand-Bellomo, M. et al. "A New Case of Myelodysplastic Syndrome with 6p Rearrangement." *Cancer Genet. Cytogenet.*, Vol. 44, No. 2, February, 1990, pp. 271–274.

Jotterand-Bellomo, M. et al. "Cytogenetic Analysis of 54 Cases of Myelodysplastic Syndrome." *Cancer Genet. Cytogenet.*, Vol. 46, No. 2, June, 1990, pp. 157–172.

Kabutomori, O. et al. "Intracellular Alkaline Phosphatase Activities in Myelodysplastic Syndrome." *Rinsho Byori*, Vol. 38, No. 3, March, 1990, pp. 328–329.

Kai, S. and Y. Shinohara. "Bone Marrow Transplantation for Patients With Severe Aplastic Anemia and Myelodysplastic Syndrome." *Nippon Ketsueki Gakkai Zasshi*, Vol. 52, No. 8, December, 1989, pp. 1402–1411.

Kere, J. et al. "Molecular Characterization of Chromosome 7 Long Arm Deletions in Myeloid Disorders." *Blood*, Vol. 70, No. 5, November, 1987, pp. 1349–1353.

Kerim, S. et al. "Molecular Cytogenetic Analysis Discloses Complex Genetic Imbalance in a t(11;21) Myelodysplastic Syndrome." *Cancer Genet. Cytogenet.*, Vol. 46, No. 2, June, 1990, pp. 243–250.

Kerkhofs, H. et al. "Utility of the FAB Classification for Myelodysplastic Syndromes: Investigation of Prognostic Factors in 237 Cases." *Br. J. Haematol.*, Vol. 65, No. 1, January, 1987, pp. 73–81.

Kerndrup, G., K. Bendix-Hansen, and B. Pedersen. "The Prognostic Significance of Cytological, Histological and Cytogenetic Findings in Refractory Anaemia (RA) and RA with Sideroblasts. A Follow Up Study." *Blut*, Vol. 54, No. 4, April, 1987, pp. 231–238.

Kimura, S. et al. "Polycythemia Vera Terminating in Myelodysplastic Syndrome." *Rinsho Ketsueki,* Vol. 31, No. 1, January, 1990, pp. 100–104.

Koeffler, H. P. et al. "Randomized Study of 13-*cis* Retinoic Acid v. Placebo in the Myelodysplastic Disorders." *Blood,* Vol. 71, No. 3, March, 1988, pp. 703–708.

Kuwazuru, Y. et al. "Expression of the Multidrug Transporter, P-Glycoprotein, in Acute Leukemia Cells and Correlation to Clinical Drug Resistance." *Cancer,* Vol. 66, No. 5, September 1, 1990, pp. 868–873.

Lai, J. L. et al. "Translocations (5;17) and (7;17) in Patients with De Novo or Therapy-Related Myelodysplastic Syndromes or Acute Nonlymphocytic Leukemia. A Possible Association With Acquired Pseudo–Pelger-Huët Anomaly and Small Vacuolated Granulocytes." *Cancer Genet. Cytogenet.,* Vol. 46, No. 2, June, 1990, pp. 173–183.

Mecucci, C. et al. "11q-Chromosome Is Associated With Abnormal Iron Stores in Myelodysplastic Syndromes." *Cancer Genet. Cytogenet.,* Vol. 27, No. 1, July, 1987, pp. 39–44.

Mertens, F. et al. "A Case of Myelodysplastic Syndrome With High Platelet Counts and a t(3;8) (q26;q24)." *Cancer Genet. Cytogenet.,* Vol. 27, No. 1, July, 1987, pp. 1–4.

Michiels, J. J., A. Hagemeyer, and M. E. Prins. "Thrombocythaemic Erythromelalgia in Chronic Myeloproliferative and Myelodysplastic Disorders." *Neth. J. Med.,* Vol. 35, No. 1–2, August, 1989, pp. 4–10.

Miller, J. A. "Myelodysplastic Syndromes: New Classifications, New Concerns." *Testrends,* New Jersey: Roche Diagnostics, Vol. 7, No. 2, November, 1993, pp. 1, 3, 11.

Moore, M. A. "Hematopoietic Growth Factors in Cancer." *Cancer,* Vol. 65, No. 3, Suppl., February 1, 1990, pp. 836–844.

Morgan, R., M. H. Greene, and A. A. Sandberg. "Trisomy 11 in Myelodysplasia." *Cancer Genet. Cytogenet.,* Vol. 3, No. 1, January, 1988, pp. 159–162.

Morioka, N. et al. "Neutrophilic Dermatosis With Myelodysplastic Syndrome: Nuclear Segmentation Anomalies of Neutrophils in the Skin Lesion and in Peripheral Blood." *J. Am. Acad. Dermatol.,* Vol. 23, No. 2, Pt. 1, August, 1990, pp. 247–249.

Mufti, G. J. et al. "Myelodysplastic Syndromes: A Scoring System With Prognostic Significance." *Br. J. Haematol.,* Vol. 15, 1985, pp. 425–433.

Nagler, A. et al. "Effects of Recombinant Human Granulocyte Colony Stimulating Factor and Granulocyte-Monocyte Colony Stimulating Factor on In Vitro Hemopoiesis in the Myelodysplastic Syndromes." *Leukemia,* Vol. 4, No. 3, March, 1990, pp. 193–202.

Najean, Y. and T. Lecompte. "Chronic Pure Thrombocytopenia in Elderly Patients. An Aspect of the Myelodysplastic Syndrome." *Cancer,* Vol. 64, No. 12, December 15, 1989, pp. 2506–2510.

Ng, S. C. et al. "Myelodysplastic Syndrome: A Review From University Hospital, Kuala Lumpur." *Singapore Med. J.,* Vol. 31, No. 2, April, 1990, pp. 153–158.

Niikura, H. et al. "Acquisition of Philadelphia Chromosome With bcr Rearrangement Concomitant With Transformation of Refractory Anemia With Excess of Blasts With 8 Trisomy Into Acute Myelogenous Leukemia." *Rinsho Ketsueki,* Vol. 31, No. 3, March, 1990, pp. 335–340.

Noel, P. "Management of Patients With Myelodysplastic Syndromes." *Mayo Clin. Proc.,* Vol. 66, 1991, pp. 485–497.

Nowell, P. C. and E. C. Besa. "Prognostic Significance of Single Chromosome Abnormalities in Preleukemic States." *Cancer Genet. Cytogenet.,* Vol. 42, No. 1, October 1, 1989, pp. 1–7.

Ohata, M. et al. "Combination Assay of IAP and ADA in Hematologic Malignancies." *Rinsho Byori,* Vol. 38, No. 6, June, 1990, pp. 703–710.

Ohyashiki, K. et al. "In Vitro Cytogenetic Effects of Recombinant Human Hematopoietic Growth Factors on Cells Derived From Myelodysplastic Syndromes." *Cancer Genet. Cytogenet.,* Vol. 48, No. 2, September, 1990, pp. 169–178.

Ohyashiki, K. et al. "Phenylbutazone-Induced Myelodysplastic Syndrome With Philadelphia Translocation." *Cancer Genet. Cytogenet.,* Vol. 26, No. 2, June, 1987, pp. 213–216.

Ohyashiki, K. et al. "Translocation Between Chromosomes 7 and 11 in Nonlymphocytic Neoplasia." *Cancer Genet. Cytogenet.,* Vol. 26, No. 2, June, 1987, pp. 191–197.

Ohyashiki, K. et al. "Hematologic and Cytogenetic Findings in Myelodysplastic Syndromes Treated With Recombinant Human Granulocyte Colony-Stimulating Factor." *Jpn. J. Cancer Res.,* Vol. 80, No. 9, September, 1989, pp. 848–854.

Pomeroy, C. et al. "Infection in the Myelodysplastic Syndrome." *Am. J. Med.,* Vol. 90, March, 1991, pp. 338–344.

Powers, L. W. "Myelodysplastic Syndromes: State of Confusion." *Clin. Lab. Sci.,* Vol. 1, No. 3, May/June, 1988, pp. 150–151.

Rappaport, E. S. et al. "Myelodysplastic Syndrome: Identification in the Routine Hematology Laboratory." *South. Med. J.,* Vol. 80, No. 8, August, 1987, pp. 969–974.

Rosenthal, D. S. and W. C. Moloney. "Refractory Dysmyelopoietic Anemia and Acute Leukemia." *Blood,* Vol. 63, 1984, pp. 314–318.

Ross, F. M. et al. "A Myelodysplastic Syndrome With Eosinophilia Associated With a Break in the Short Arm of Chromosome 16." *Leukemia,* Vol. 1, No. 9, September, 1987, pp. 680–681.

Rosti, V. et al. "In Vitro and In Vivo Effects of Recombinant Interferon Gamma on the Growth of Hematopoietic Progenitor Cells From Patients With Myelodysplastic Syndrome." *Haematologica (Pavia),* Vol. 74, No. 5, September–October, 1989, pp. 435–440.

Sanz, G. F. et al. "Two Regression Models and a Scoring System for Predicting Survival and Planning Treatment in Myelodysplastic Syndromes: A Multi-Variant Analysis of Prognostic Factors in 370 Patients." *Blood,* Vol. 74, No. 1, July, 1989, pp. 395–408.

Sardeo, G. et al. "Aplastic Anemia and Myelodysplasia: A Not-Always-Easy Distinction." *Minerva Med.,* Vol. 78, No. 20, October 31, 1987, pp. 1519–1522.

Sato, K. et al. "Atypical Infiltration of Megakaryocytes Into the Liver and Spleen in a Case of Refractory Anemia." *Rinsho Ketsueki,* Vol. 31, No. 7, July, 1990, pp. 1004–1007.

Seo, I. S. and C. Y. Li. "Myelodysplastic Syndrome: Diagnostic Implications of Cytochemical and Immunocytochemical Studies." *Mayo Clin. Proc.,* Vol. 68, No. 1, January, 1993, pp. 47–53.

Shibuya, T. et al. "Treatment of Four Patients With Myelodysplastic Syndrome With a Small Dose of Aclacinomycin-A." *Leuk. Res.,* Vol. 11, No. 10, 1987, pp. 851–854.

Smadja, N. et al. "Refractory Anemia With Excess of Blasts in Transformation. Clinical, Hematologic, and Cytogenetic Findings in Nine Patients." *Cancer Genet. Cytogenet.,* Vol. 42, No. 1, October 1, 1989, pp. 55–65.

Suciu, S. et al. "Results of Chromosome Studies and Their Relation to Morphology, Course, and Prognosis in 120 Patients With De Novo Myelodysplastic Syndrome." *Cancer Genet. Cytogenet.,* Vol. 44, No. 1, January, 1990, pp. 15–26.

Swolin, B., S. Rodjer, and J. Westin. "Bone Marrow In Vitro Growth and Cytogenetic Studies in Patients With FAB-Classified Primary Myelodysplastic Syndromes." *Am. J. Hematol.,* Vol. 34, No. 3, July, 1990, pp. 175–180.

Takaku, F. "Colony Stimulating Factor." *Gan To Kagaku Ryoho,* Vol. 16, No. 11, November, 1989, pp. 3550–3553.

Takaku, F., H. Hirai, and J. Nishida. "Transforming Gene in the Preleukemic State." *Gao To Kagaku Ryoho,* Vol. 14, No. 6, Pt. 2, June, 1987, pp. 2170–2175.

Tanzer, J. et al. "Rearrangement of the Short Arm of Chromosome 12 in Chronic Myelomonocytic Leukemias." *Nouv. Rev. Fr. Hematol.,* Vol. 29, No. 1, 1987, pp. 65–68.

Tefferi, A. et al. "Chronic Myelomonocytic Leukemia: Natural History and Prognostic Determinants." *Mayo Clin. Proc.,* Vol. 64, No. 10, October, 1989, pp. 1246–1254.

Testoni, N. et al. "Sequential Observation of Clinical and Karyotypic Evolution in a Patient With Myelodysplastic Syndrome." *Haematologica*, Vol. 74, No. 6, November–December, 1989, pp. 595–599.

Tian, D., W. Sun, and Z. Z. Long. "Study of Mechanisms in the Pathogenesis of Myelodysplastic Syndrome: Changes in Lymphocyte Subpopulations." *Chung Hua Nei Ko Tsa Chih*, Vol. 28, No. 3, March, 1989, pp. 153–155, 186.

Turgeon, M. L. "Myelodysplastic Syndromes." *Guthrie J.*, Vol. 61, No. 4, Fall, 1992, pp. 149–159.

Vadhan-Raj, S. "Clinical Applications of Colony-Stimulating Factors." *Oncol. Nurs. Forum*, Vol. 16, No. 6, Suppl., November–December, 1989, pp. 21–26.

Vadhan-Raj, S. et al. "Effects of Recombinant Human Granulocyte-Macrophage Colony-Stimulating Factor in Patients With Myelodysplastic Syndromes." *N. Engl. J. Med.*, Vol. 317, No. 25, December 17, 1987, pp. 1545–1552.

Verwilghen, R. L. and M. A. Boogaerts. "The Myelodysplastic Syndromes." *Blood Rev.*, Vol. 1, No. 1, March, 1987, pp. 34–43.

Vineis, P. et al., "Cytogenetics and Occupational Exposure to Solvents: A Pilot Study on Leukemias and Myelodysplastic Disorders. Dipartimento di Scienze Biomediche e Oncologia Umana, Universita di Torino." *Tumori*, Vol. 76, No. 4, August 31, 1990, pp. 350–352.

Vozobulova, V. et al. "Treatment of Myelodysplastic Syndrome Using Continual Subcutaneous Infusion of Low Doses of Cytosine Arabinoside." *Vnitr. Lek.*, Vol. 36, No. 5, May, 1990, pp. 483–488.

Welte, K. et al. "Recombinant Human Granulocyte-Colony Stimulating Factor: In Vitro and In Vivo Effects on Myelopoiesis." *Blood Cells*, Vol. 13, No. 1–2, 1987, pp. 17–30.

Widell, S. and R. Hast. "Balloon-Like Platelets in Myelodysplastic Syndromes—A Feature of Dysmegakaryopoiesis?" *Leuk. Res.*, Vol. 11, No. 8, 1987, pp. 747–752.

REVIEW QUESTIONS

1. Which of the following terms was *not* used to refer to myelodysplastic syndromes?

    A. Myeloproliferative syndrome.
    B. Refractory anemia.
    C. Smoldering leukemia.
    D. Myelodysplasia.

2. Patients with some variety of myelodysplastic syndrome are at increased risk of developing:

    A. Acute lymphoblastic leukemia.
    B. Acute nonlymphocytic leukemia.
    C. Chronic lymphocytic leukemia.
    D. Chronic myelogenous leukemia.

Questions 3 through 7: match the following myelodysplastic syndrome with the appropriate description (use an answer *only* once).

3. ___ RA
4. ___ RARS
5. ___ RAEB
6. ___ CMML
7. ___ RAEB-T

    A. May exhibit Auer rods.
    B. More than 15% ringed sideroblasts.
    C. More than 100×10^9/L monocytes in peripheral blood.
    D. Less than 15% ringed sideroblasts.
    E. Less than 5% peripheral blood blasts and 5 to 20% bone marrow blasts.

8. Which of the following agents has not been supported by scientific research as being associated with the development of secondary myelodysplastic syndrome?

    A. Alkylating agents.
    B. Organic solvents.
    C. Radiation.
    D. Insecticides.

9. An increased incidence of myelodysplastic syndromes is seen in:

    A. Males less than 55 years old.
    B. Females less than 55 years old.
    C. Males more than 55 years old.
    D. Females more than 55 years old.

10. The *most* frequently involved chromosomes in adults with myelodysplastic syndrome are:

    A. 1, 5, and 7.
    B. 3, 5, and 8.
    C. 5, 7, and 8.
    D. 8, 12, and 13.

11. The most frequent chromosomal abnormalities in children with myelodysplastic syndrome include all of the following except:

    A. Trisomy 8.
    B. Monosomy 7.
    C. Deletion of long arm of chromosome 20.
    D. Deletion of the entire X chromosome.

12. The incidence of chromosomal abnormality in adults with myelodysplastic syndrome is:

    A. 5 to 15%.
    B. 15 to 25%.
    C. 25 to 60%.
    D. 40 to 90%.

13. The karyotype associated with a high probability of transforming to ANLL is:

    A. Monosomy 5.
    B. Monosomy 7.
    C. Trisomy 11.
    D. All of the above.

14. Patients with myelodysplastic syndromes commonly suffer from ___ initially.

    A. A rash.
    B. Anemia.
    C. Visual disturbances.
    D. Vertigo.

15. Myelodysplastic syndromes and ___ can have similar clinical and morphological features.

    A. Aplastic anemia.
    B. Iron deficiency anemia.
    C. Chronic lymphocytic leukemia.
    D. Acute lymphoblastic leukemia.

Questions 16 through 20: match the following cellular abnormalities with the respective cell line (an answer can be used more than once).

16. ___ Can resemble the nuclear-cytoplasmic dyssynchrony of a nutritional deficiency.

17. ___ Pseudo–Pelger-Huët anomaly.

18. ___ Balloon-shaped bulge of cell membrane.

19. ___ Howell-Jolly bodies and nuclear fragments.

20. ___ Hypogranulation.

A. Erythrocytes.

B. Leukocytes.

C. Megakaryocytes (platelets).

Questions 21 through 25: match the type of myelodysplastic syndrome and the appropriate description.

21. ___ Iron deposits encircle the nuclei of red blood cell precursors; serum ferritin increases over time, with a small number of patients developing hemochromatosis; not related to sideroblastic anemia.

22. ___ Demonstrates overt classic relationship to ANLL; increased type I and II myeloblasts in bone marrow; 50% of patients demonstrate giant platelets and micromegakaryocytes; presence of cytopenias and dyspoiesis from CMML.

23. ___ Mildest form of all types of myelodysplastic syndromes; decreased reticulocytes; pancytopenias.

A. RA.

B. RARS.

C. RAE B.

D. CMML.

E. RAEB-T.

24. ___ Includes patients who suffer from a leukemic transformation in progress; highest rate of progression to ANLL.

25. ___ A leukemic disorder; dyshematopoiesis of all three cell lines.

26. Calculate the percentage of myeloblasts in the bone marrow, given that 55 erythroid precursors and 17 myeloblasts are counted in a total cell count of 100.

A. 15.

B. 25.

C. 35.

D. 38.

27. In young patients, the therapy of choice for myelodysplastic syndromes involves:

A. Vitamins.

B. Allogeneic bone marrow transplantation.

C. Cytotoxic drugs.

D. Colony-stimulating growth factors.

28. Patients with ___ have the best prognosis.

A. RA or RARS.

B. RARS or CMML.

C. RA or CMML.

D. CMML or RAER.

29. The Bournemouth and Sans prognosis scales use some of the variables listed below as indicators.

A. Hemoglobin concentration, total platelet count, and absolute neutrophil count.

B. Hemoglobin concentration, total platelet count, and bone marrow blast count.

C. Total platelet count, bone marrow blast count, and patient's age.

D. All of the above.

PART 5

Fundamentals of Hematologic Analysis

CHAPTER 23

Body Fluid Analysis

Cerebrospinal fluid
Anatomy and physiology
Laboratory analysis
Pleural, peritoneal, and pericardial fluids
Effusions: transudates and exudates
Pleural fluid
Peritoneal fluid

Pericardial fluid
Seminal fluid
Anatomy and physiology
Analysis of seminal fluid
Synovial fluid
Anatomy and physiology of joints
Purpose of arthrocentesis

Aspiration
Laboratory assays
Body fluid slide preparation
Staining of body fluid sediment
Summary
Bibliography
Review questions

OBJECTIVES

Associate the various terms for body fluids with their respective synonyms.

Cerebrospinal fluid
- Describe the anatomical structures involved in the circulation of cerebrospinal fluid.
- Explain how cerebrospinal fluid is produced.
- Describe the collection procedure for cerebrospinal fluid.
- Name the appropriate type or types of testing for each of the aliquots of a specimen.
- Compare the descriptive characteristics of cerebrospinal fluid on gross examination and the respective associated abnormalities.
- Describe the characteristics seen on microscopic examination and the associated disorders.
- Name and describe cells unique to the cerebrospinal fluid.

Pleural, peritoneal, and pericardial fluids
- Define the term **effusion.**
- Compare the major characteristics of transudates and exudates.
- Identify the location of the pleura.
- Name at least three disorders associated with the existence of pleural exudate.
- Associate the various colors of exudate with the typical disorders.
- Name at least two reasons for turbidity in pleural fluid.
- Name the disorder that produces an extremely elevated total leukocyte count in pleural fluid.

- Name the types of cells that can be encountered in pleural fluid.
- Name the characteristics of malignant cells that can be found in a pleural effusion.
- Discuss the cellular abnormalities encountered in pleural and peritoneal fluid.
- Identify the location of the peritoneum.
- Name at least three disorders or diseases that can cause a peritoneal effusion.
- List at least two reasons for a turbid peritoneal effusion.
- Associate a variety of conditions with various colors or appearances of peritoneal effusion.
- Name several conditions that can produce a high total leukocyte count in peritoneal fluid.
- List the types of cells that can be seen in peritoneal effusion and associate these cell types with a representative disorder.
- Describe the anatomy of the pericardium.
- Associate the various types and causes of pericardial effusion.
- Name a cause of an increased total leukocyte count with mostly segmented neutrophils (PMNs).

Seminal fluid
- Describe the anatomical structures and their respective cellular and/or chemical components.
- Discuss the proper collection and handling of seminal fluid.
- Name the normal number of sperm cells per milliliter or per liter.

- Name the types of microscopic assays and the respective normal values.

Synovial fluid

- Define the term **arthrocentesis.**
- List at least three disorders that can be diagnosed definitively by synovial fluid analysis.
- List several sites that may be aspirated.
- Name the tests that should be included in the routine analysis of synovial fluid.
- Name the procedures included in the gross examination of synovial fluid.

- List and describe the types of crystals that may be observed in synovial fluid.
- Describe the normal total cell count and differential in synovial fluid.
- Compare the laboratory findings in noninflammatory and inflammatory arthritis.

Body fluid slide preparation

- Compare the features of various methods of body fluid sediment preparation.
- Differentiate the characteristics of Wright-Giemsa and Papanicolaou stains.

Except in large, dedicated laboratory facilities, the analysis of body fluids is assigned to the hematology laboratory. Gross physical examination, total cell count, microscopic examination, and other special testing are generally within the job responsibility of hematology technicians and technologists. Because clinical correlations of body fluid analyses are diagnostically important, clinical information is presented in each section of this chapter.

Chemical analyses and microbial and cytological examinations are generally performed in the chemistry, microbiology, and cytology departments, respectively. For this reason, specific procedures in these disciplines are not included in this chapter.

Sterile body fluid can be found in various body cavities under normal conditions. In diverse disorders and disease processes, the quantity of these fluids can increase significantly. Fluid specimens aspirated from different anatomical sites (Table 23.1) can be analyzed for the total number of cells, differentiation of cell types, chemical composition, and microbial contents. All body fluids should be handled with caution. Universal precautions must be practiced.

The type of examination performed on the body fluid depends on the source of the specimen. However, a portion of the examination of cerebrospinal fluid (CSF); serous fluids from the pleural, pericardial, and peritoneal cavities; synovial fluid; and seminal fluid is frequently performed in the hematology laboratory.

CEREBROSPINAL FLUID

Anatomy and Physiology

CSF acts as a shock absorber for the brain and spinal cord, circulates nutrients, lubricates the central nervous system (CNS), and may also contribute to the nourishment of brain tissue. The CSF circulates through the ventricles and subarachnoid space that surrounds both the brain and the spinal cord. The ventricles (Fig. 23.1) consist of four hollow, fluid-filled spaces inside the brain. A lateral ventricle lies inside each hemisphere of the cerebrum. The two lateral ventricles communicate with the third ventricle through the foramen of Monro. The third ventricle, a narrow channel between the hemispheres through the area of the thalamus, communicates with the fourth ventricle, located in the pons and medulla, by means of the aqueduct of Sylvius in the midbrain portion of the brainstem. This ventricle is continuous with the central canal of the spinal cord.

Three openings in the roof of the fourth ventricle, a pair of lateral apertures (foramina of Luschka) and a median aperture (foramen of Magendie), allow CSF to flow into the basal cisterns and subarachnoid space of the spinal cord. From these basal cisterns, CSF migrates over the convexities toward the cerebral sinuses.

Production

CSF production is primarily a function of the choroid plexus, with a smaller proportion being derived from the ependymal lining and perivascular spaces. The plexus is composed of two layers: the ependyma (the lining epithelium of the ventricle) and the pia mater. The folded projections of the highly vascularized pia lined with epithelium are referred to as the choroidal epithelium. Choroidal epithelium, blood vessels, and interstitial connective tissue form the choroid plexus. The plexuses in the lateral ventricles are the largest and produce most of the CSF. The choroid plexus epithelium and the endothelium of capillaries in contact with CSF constitute the anatomical structure of the **blood–brain barrier.** The **ependyma** is a single layer of cells with villous projections and cilia on its surface. **Tanycytes** are specialized ependymal cells without cilia, located on the floor of the third ventricle. The main portion of this cell is directed toward the ventricle, and the neck and tail portions contact the capillary wall. These cells are not thought to be involved in the production of CSF.

Specimen Collection: Lumbar Puncture

CSF is found inside all the ventricles, in the central canal of the spinal cord, and in the subarachnoid space around both the brain and the spinal cord. The subarachnoid space is the area between the arachnoid mater, the middle meningeal membrane covering the brain and spinal cord, and the innermost meningeal membrane, the pia mater. The total maximum volume of CSF in adults is about 150 mL. The maximum volume in neonates is approximately 60 mL. The rate of formation in adults is approximately 500 mL/day or 20 mL/hour and is reabsorbed at the same rate, so the volume remains constant.

Introducing a needle into the subarachnoid space makes

TABLE 23.1 Body Fluids

Fluids	Synonyms
Bronchoalveolar lavage	Bronchial washings
Cerebrospinal fluid (CSF)	Spinal fluid Lumbar puncture fluid Ventricular fluid Meningeal fluid
Synovial fluid	Joint fluid
Peritoneal fluid	Dialysate fluid Paracentesis fluid Ascitic fluid
Pericardial fluid	Fluid from around the heart Pericardiocentesis fluid
Pleural fluid	Chest fluid Thoracic fluid Thoracentesis fluid
Seminal fluid	Semen

TABLE 23.2 Reasons for Performance of a Lumbar Puncture and Removal of an Aliquot of Cerebrospinal Fluid

Therapeutic	Relief of increased intracranial pressure
Diagnostic	Identification of conditions such as subarachnoid hemorrhage, meningeal infection (meningitis), multiple sclerosis, and neoplasms

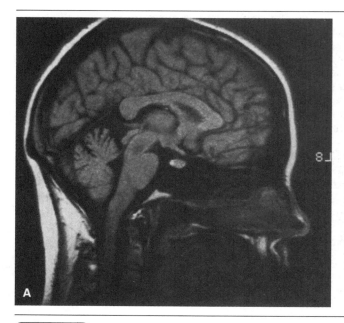
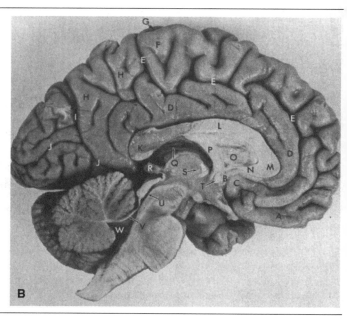

FIGURE 23.1 **A.** Normal T1-weighted MRI scan. **B.** Medial view of the brain, arachnoid and pia mater removed. Median section (×1.5). A = Straight gyrus (gyrus rectus); B = paraterminal gyrus; C = subcallosal area; D = cingulate gyrus; E = cingulate sulcus (and its marginal ramus); F = paracentral lobule; G = central sulcus; H = precuneus; I = parieto-occipital sulcus; J = calcarine sulcus; K = splenium of corpus callosum; L = trunk of corpus callosum; M = genu of corpus callosum; N = rostrum of corpus callosum; O = septum pellucidum; P = body of fornix; Q = choroid plexus of lateral ventricle; R = pineal body; S = interthalamic adhesion; T = anterior commissure; U = cerebral aqueduct; V = superior medullary velum; W = fourth ventricle. (From C. Watson, *Basic Human Neuroanatomy* [4th ed.] Boston: Little, Brown & Co., 1991.)

it possible to measure CSF pressure and to obtain fluid for analysis (Table 23.2). This procedure is contraindicated when there is a skin infection at the puncture site or when the patient has septicemia or a general systemic infection, because of the risk of spreading the infection into the meninges.

The patient is placed in a horizontal position, and the site is thoroughly cleansed to reduce the possibility of contamination with normal skin microbial flora. A stylet needle is introduced by a physician into the intervertebral space between the L4 and L5 (lumbar) vertebrae. Up to 20 mL of fluid can be removed if the patient has a normal opening pressure. The specimen should be placed into sterile tubes. After CSF collection, the closing pressure is measured, the stylet replaced, and the needle removed. Specimens must be *promptly* delivered to the laboratory for analysis. The patient should be given appropriate aftercare because the procedure is not without risk.

Indications for spinal fluid examination are changing as other diagnostic methods are improved. Only in a few conditions, such as meningitis, is the lumbar puncture essential and often diagnostic. It may be of differential value in other cases.

Laboratory Analysis

General Principle

A specimen of CSF is examined visually and microscopically. The total number of cells can be enumerated and the types of cells can be morphologically distinguished.

Specimen

From three to five samples of 2 to 4 mL each are collected in sterile tubes by a physician. The number of tubes depends on institutional protocol. Typically, tube 1 is for chemical and serological examination; tube 2 is for microbiological examination; and tube 3 is for gross examination, cell count, and morphology. Because cells disintegrate rapidly, they *must be counted within 1 hour* of specimen collection. *Caution:* All CSF specimens should be handled with extreme care. These specimens could potentially harbor viruses or other infectious organisms.

Gross Physical Examination

The spinal fluid is examined visually for turbidity (cloudiness), color, and viscosity. Normal CSF is clear and colorless. Its appearance and viscosity are comparable to those of water.

Turbidity

If any turbidity exists, it should be graded using a scale of 0 to 4+. In the absence of a set of known standards for comparison, the rating scale is subjective. This scale ranges from 1+, slight cloudiness, to 4+, where newsprint cannot be seen through the tube. Cloudiness or turbidity may be due to pleocytosis (increased concentrations of leukocytes, erythrocytes, or microorganisms), or less commonly, radiographic contrast media or the presence of fat globules.

Grossly bloody specimens can result from a traumatic tap or from conditions such as a bleeding subarachnoid

TABLE 23.3 Changes in Cerebrospinal Fluid Following Hemorrhage

Gross Examination

2–12 hr	Xanthochromia (pink to orange)
12–24 hr	Xanthochromia (yellow color, disappears in 2–4 wk)

Microscopic Examination

2–24 hr	Neutrophilic granulocytes (PMNs), mononuclear phagocytes, lymphocytes, erythrocytes
12–48 hr	Mononuclear phagocytes, lymphocytes, erythrophagocytosis
≥ 48 hr	Mononuclear phagocytes, erythrophagocytosis, siderophages (may persist for 2–8 wk)

Source: M. Oehmichen, D. Domasch, and H. Wietholter. "Origin, Proliferation and Fate of Cerebrospinal Fluid Cells." *J. Neurol.* Vol. 227, 1982, pp. 145–150.

hemorrhage or intracerebral hemorrhage. Traumatic taps more commonly occur in children because of movement during the procedure.

It is important to differentiate between specimens from a traumatic tap and those that are related to the patient's clinical condition. A freshly collected specimen should be examined *immediately*. If the reddish color diminishes between the first and the last tube, the blood in the specimen is due to a traumatic tap. In addition, clots may be observed in traumatically collected specimens due to the presence of an increased concentration of protein or blood, or in a specimen from a patient with a subarachnoid block or meningitis.

Color

Any presence of color should be noted. A yellow coloring of a specimen or the supernatant of a centrifuged specimen is referred to as **xanthochromia.** The release of hemoglobin from hemolyzed erythrocytes (red blood cells [RBCs]) in the CSF is a potential cause of xanthochromia. The lysis of RBCs in CSF begins about 2 hours after the occurrence of a subarachnoid hemorrhage (Table 23.3). Other conditions (Table 23.4) as well as a delay in the examination of a specimen (which can cause a false-positive result) can produce xanthochromia.

Viscosity

Normal CSF has the viscosity of water. Clotting in CSF can be due to a variety of conditions, including increased protein or gel formation on standing due to an increased fibrinogen content.

Microscopic Examination: Cellular Enumeration

Cell counts should be performed by manual methods (see procedure in Chapter 24). Electronic cell counters should be used with care. RBC counts are of limited value, and observations as to whether the RBCs are crenated are not useful in developing a differential diagnosis. Total white blood cell (WBC) counts, however, are useful in developing a differential diagnosis. Very few leukocytes should be seen in normal CSF. The generally accepted total number of WBCs in the CSF ranges from 0 to 5 cells/μL or 0 to 5×10^6/L. A value of up to 20×10^6/L can be considered within the range of normal for children and adults. Neonates have a higher normal range, 0 to 30 cells $\times 10^6$/L.

Occasionally, the WBC count may be very low (0 to 20×10^6/L) but the CSF is turbid because of a high concentration of bacteria. In acute, untreated bacterial meningitis, the CSF leukocyte count usually ranges from 100 to 10,000 cells $\times 10^6$/L. Very high WBC counts (greater than $50,000 \times 10^6$/L) are unusual and suggest intraventricular rupture of a brain abscess.

Microscopic Examination: Cellular Differentiation

Normal CSF contains a few mononuclear cells (lymphocytes and monocytes) and rare ependymal cells. There is no gen-

TABLE 23.4 Potential Causes of Xanthochromic Cerebrospinal Fluid (CSF)

Clinical Conditions (In Vivo)

Oxyhemoglobin from RBCs lysed "in vivo" (e.g., recent subarachnoid hemorrhage)

Bilirubin from RBCs lysed "in vivo" (e.g., older subarachnoid hemorrhage)

Increased direct bilirubin with normal blood–brain barrier (e.g., marked jaundice)

Premature infants with an underdeveloped blood–CSF barrier and hyperbilirubinemia (e.g., hemolytic disease of the newborn)

Increased CSF protein levels (> 150 mg/dL) (e.g., severe meningeal inflammation or infection)

Carotenoids in CSF (uncommon) (e.g., systemic hypercarotemia)

Melanin pigment in CSF (uncommon) (e.g., meningeal melanosarcoma)

Technical Conditions (In Vitro)

Traumatic tap with "in vitro" lysis (e.g., detergent in needle, delay in examination)

Traumatic tap with blood plasma contamination that produces an elevated (>150 mg/dL) protein concentration

Antiseptic contamination of CSF (e.g., Merthiolate or Mercurochrome)

Delayed examination of CSF specimen (e.g., lysis of intact RBCs)

CELL COUNTING PROCEDURE

Total Leukocyte Count

Principle
To enumerate the number of WBCs in order to assist in the development of a differential diagnosis (e.g., bacterial meningitis, viral meningitis, ruptured brain abscess).

Reagents, Supplies, and Equipment
1. 10% acetic acid: Prepare by filling a 100-mL volumetric flask about half-full with distilled water. Using a safety bulb, pipette 10 mL of glacial acetic acid into the flask. Add distilled water to the calibration mark and mix.
2. Wright-Giemsa or Wright stain or 1% methylene blue in methyl alcohol: Prepare by weighing 1 gm of methylene blue and transferring it to a 100-mL volumetric flask. Dilute to the calibration mark with methyl alcohol. Mix.
3. Small (12 × 75-mm) test tubes, Pasteur pipettes, rubber bulb, and microscope slides
4. Neubauer hemocytometer
5. Centrifuge, microscope, and immersion oil
6. Disinfectant solution

Procedure
1. Mix the spinal fluid by inversion. With a Pasteur pipette, transfer 9 drops of spinal fluid to a small test tube. Add 1 drop of 10% acetic acid. Mix by gently tapping the tube.
2. Allow this mixture to stand for 5 minutes. Mix again.
3. To each side of the chamber of a clean hemocytometer with a coverslip, load a small amount of the diluted spinal fluid. Allow the counting chamber to sit covered, with a moistened filter paper in half of a Petri plate, for a few minutes to allow the cells to settle and the erythrocytes to completely lyse.
4. Place the hemocytometer under the 10× microscopic objective (low power). Erythrocytes should either be absent or appear as ghost cells. The nucleus of segmented neutrophils will be bright, while the lymphocyte nucleus will be round.
5. The leukocytes in all nine squares of each side of the chamber should be counted (refer to the leukocyte procedure for whole blood in Chapter 24 for an illustration of the chamber rulings). Average the count from both sides.

Calculations

Total leukocyte count = average number of cells counted $\times \dfrac{10}{9}$

Example: If an average of 9 cells were counted, the total count =

$$9 \times \frac{10}{9} = 11 \text{ leukocytes}/\mu L$$

(These calculations may need to be adjusted if the quantity of specimen varies.)

Reporting Results
Normal values: 0 to 5 cells/μL or 0 to 5 × 10^6/L (lymphocytes and monocytes).

Some use a reference value of 0 to 10/μL or 0 to 10 × 10^6/L.

Neonates have a higher normal range, 0 to 30 mononuclear cells × 10^6/L.

Values in children are comparable to those in adults.

If many RBCs are present, the WBC count can be corrected by subtracting 1 WBC for each 700 RBCs/mm^3 counted in the CSF if the complete cell count (CBC) is normal. If there is significant anemia or leukocytosis, the following formula can be used:

$$\text{Corrected WBC count} = \text{WBC in bloody CSF} - \frac{\text{WBC (blood)} \times \text{RBC (CFS)}}{\text{RBC (blood)}}$$

Total Erythrocyte Count

Principle
The number of RBCs can be determined by placing a sample of undiluted specimen on the counting chamber and counting *all* cells within the nine-square ruled area on one side of the chamber. The WBC count (as described previously) is subtracted from the total cell count of the undiluted specimen.

Reporting Results
Normal CSF is crystal clear and colorless. No clots or red blood cells should be observed. In addition, normal CSF has the viscosity of water.

Cellular Enumeration Procedure Notes

Sources of Error
If the specimen is not examined promptly after collection, WBC lysis will give a false impression of the number of WBCs present. If a delay is anticipated, the specimen should be refrigerated.

Clotted specimens result in a falsely low cell count because RBCs and WBCs will be trapped in the clot.

eral agreement as to the significance of a few neutrophilic leukocytes in a CSF specimen.

Cells observed in the CSF resemble comparable cells seen in the peripheral blood or bone marrow in terms of size and nuclear and cytoplasmic features. However, the appearance of cells in the CSF that are also seen in peripheral blood may vary in some details. A Wright-Giemsa stain is recommended for the microscopic differentiation of cells.

Cells that may be encountered in CSF include granulocytes (mature and immature neutrophils, eosinophils, and basophils), mature lymphocytes or reactive lymphocytes, mononuclear phagocytes (monocytes, histiocytes, and macrophages), plasma cells, ependymal cells and choroidal cells, leukemic blasts, and malignant cells (e.g., lymphoma cells or tumor cells). Other types of cells can include immature, nucleated erythrocytes and intracellular bacteria. Lupus erythematosus (LE) cells are rarely observed in CSF.

Lymphocytes

The features of CSF lymphocytes are similar to those of small lymphocytes in peripheral blood. Normal CSF has a few observable lymphocytes. Large lymphocytes and lymphocytes with a darker blue cytoplasm are occasionally seen in normal CSF.

Degenerative changes such as vacuolization, pyknotic nuclear changes, and variations in the staining pattern may be present. Artifactual changes can include overall cell shrinkage, a shrunken nucleus or dense clumps of very dark coloration in the nucleus, and an irregular cytoplasmic border due to slow drying of the specimen on the slide.

An increased number of lymphocytes in the CSF is typically associated with viral infections but may be seen in a variety of disorders. These disorders include viral meningoencephalitis, aseptic meningitis syndrome (the majority of cases), fungal meningitis, syphilitic meningoencephalitis, and partially treated bacterial meningitis. Noninfectious causes of increased numbers of lymphocytes include conditions such as multiple sclerosis.

CSF specimens from patients with acute viral meningitis may contain reactive lymphocytes, which must be differentiated from lymphoblasts associated with leukemia, as well as a large number of lymphocytes. In addition, patients who have undergone chemotherapy and irradiation for conditions such as leukemia may have reactive lymphocytes in their CSF subsequent to treatment. Reactive lymphocytes are variable in shape and maturation, compared to blasts, which are uniform in shape and degree of maturation. Reactive lymphocytes are also larger, have more cytoplasm, and usually lack the large nucleoli of lymphoblasts.

Patients with disorders other than acute viral meningitis or who have received chemotherapy or radiation therapy can manifest reactive lymphocytes in their CSF. These conditions include subacute and chronic meningoencephalitis, tuberculous meningitis, listeriosis, cerebral phlegmona, purulent encephalitis, subacute sclerosing panencephalitis, multiple sclerosis, and bacterial meningitis (recuperative phase).

In addition, viral inclusions may be seen in patients with viral meningoencephalitis, but they are rare.

Mononuclear Phagocytes

Monocytes. The morphological appearance of CSF monocytes is similar to that of blood monocytes. These cells do, however, degenerate more rapidly than lymphocytes in vitro. Young monocytic cells have less cytoplasm than do mature cells and the cytoplasm is more basophilic. The nucleus may be rounder or more convoluted in younger cells. Activated monocytic cells are larger in overall size and nucleoli may be observed in the nucleus. The cytoplasm may be vacuolated and cytoplasmic pseudopods may be seen.

Less than 2% of the cells seen in normal CSF should be monocytes. They are more numerous, especially degener-

ated and stimulated forms, in infants and small children than in adults. Disease states that can produce an increase in monocytes in CSF include tuberculous meningitis, syphilis, and viral encephalitis. In addition, meningeal irritation and subarachnoid hemorrhage can induce increased numbers of monocytes. Monocytes also may be seen in leukemic infiltration of the meninges and infectious states.

Macrophages. The morphological characteristics of macrophages (histiocytes) are described in detail in the section describing pleural fluids. Macrophages can be seen in the CSF from patients with meningitis or meningeal inflammation, infectious diseases, CNS leukemia, lymphoma, malignant melanoma, or other metastatic tumors that have spread to the meninges of the brain or spinal cord. In addition, macrophages can be seen in patients who have had hemorrhage in the CSF space or who have undergone pneumoencephalography, intrathecal chemotherapy, or irradiation therapy of the brain. Macrophages with ingested leukocytes can be observed following a surgical procedure that involves the CNS.

Polymorphonuclear Segmented Neutrophils (PMNs). Very few, if any, PMNs should be observed in the CSF. PMNs may demonstrate rapid disintegration if the specimen is not examined promptly. The cells may appear as shadows or totally disappear in an aged specimen. In addition, the cytoplasm is usually pale-staining and azurophilic granulation may not be evident in a specimen that is a few hours old. Vacuolization of PMNs may be noticed in abnormal or old specimens.

The overall size of PMNs may be enlarged if the cell is in the process of phagocytosis. The nucleus may be hyperlobulated with long and narrow filaments. Older neutrophils can exhibit pyknosis or karyorrhexis (one or more spherical, densely staining nuclear fragments) and be mistaken for nucleated RBCs.

The observation of more than an occasional PMN in the CSF classically suggests bacterial infection. However, an increase in the number of segmented neutrophils can be due to infectious and noninfectious agents. Infectious disorders with a predominance of PMNs include acute, untreated bacterial meningitis; viral meningoencephalitis during the first few days; early tuberculosis; and mycotic meningitis. Aseptic meningitis can exist in cases where the septic focus is adjacent to the meninges. Noninfectious causes of increased PMN numbers include a reaction to CNS hemorrhage (3 to 4 days afterward), injection of foreign substances such as lidocaine into the subarachnoid space, and leukemic infiltration.

Other Granulocytic Cells

Eosinophils and basophils are not normally seen in the CSF. Their appearance in CSF is similar to that in peripheral blood.

Eosinophils may be increased due to causes similar to those of an increase in PMNs (e.g., bacterial infection). However, unique causes of an increase in eosinophils include systemic parasitic or fungal infections, systemic drug reaction, and idiopathic eosinophilic meningitis.

Increased basophil numbers can be observed in chronic basophilic leukemia, which involves the meninges; chronic granulocytic leukemia; purulent meningitis; inflammatory processes; and parasitic infections.

Plasma Cells

Plasma cells are normally absent in the CSF. They may be found in association with viral disorders such as herpes simplex virus infection, meningoencephalitis, syphilitic involvement of the CNS, and Hodgkin's disease, and after a subarachnoid hemorrhage.

Erythrocytes

A few erythrocytes (RBCs) may be seen. An increased concentration of RBCs may be seen in traumatic tap specimens or in CSF from patients who have conditions such as a bleeding subarachnoid hemorrhage or intracerebral hemorrhage (see the discussion of gross examination). The number of RBCs may also be increased in chronic myelogenous leukemia or leukoerythroblastic conditions.

Mesothelial Cells

Mesothelial cells are not found in normal CSF. If seen, they can resemble pia arachnoidal or ependymal cells. Both monocytes and mesothelial cells may be transformed into macrophages and the morphological distinction is not always obvious.

Immature Cells

Immature cells can be seen in patients with leukemias or malignant lymphomas. Although a single blast is insignificant unless accompanied by clinical symptoms, the demonstration of a number of leukemic cells is strongly suggestive of involvement of the subarachnoid space in patients with leukemia or lymphoma.

Malignant Cells

The presence of even a few cells with malignant features is diagnostic of metastatic involvement of the subarachnoid space. These cells may also originate from primary tumors of the brain or spinal cord. About 25% of primary tumors of the CNS shed identifiable malignant cells into the CSF.

Malignant cells are recognizable by the dyssynchrony in maturation between cells. In addition, malignant cells occur singly or in clusters. Malignant cells are usually accompanied by many histiocytes.

Medulloblastoma, a highly malignant tumor, often invades the subarachnoid space and sheds cells into the CSF. The cells of medulloblastoma are small and hyperchromatic. They can occur singly, in rosette formations, or in clumps. These malignant cells are very similar in appearance to neuroblastoma, retinoblastoma, and oat cell carcinoma cells.

Cells Unique to the Cerebrospinal Fluid

Ependymal Cells. A few ependymal cells, the cuboidal epithelial cells that cover the surface of the cerebral ventricles and the choroid plexus, may be seen in normal CSF. These cells become rounded in appearance after separating from the lining and resemble lymphocytes or monocytoid cells.

Ependymal cells are medium in size and may appear in clusters or as individual cells (Plate 80). The nucleus is round and generally in the center of the cell. The chromatin is dense and may be slightly grainy or pyknotic. In addition, nucleoli may be seen. The nuclear-cytoplasmic ratio is 1:2 to 1:3. Cellular cytoplasm is usually abundant in amount and stains a cloudy gray-blue or pinkish color with Wright-Giemsa stain. The cytoplasm displays indefinite borders, and fragmented projections of cytoplasm or pseudopods may be seen.

Although ependymal cells appear similar to choroidal cells on light microscopy, they differ from choroidal epithelial cells because of the absence of intracytoplasm inclusions, and the border of cilia extending into the ventricular cavity.

An increased number of ependymal cells in the CSF is rare. However, they may be observed in specimens from small children and in patients with hydrocephalus, or following pneumoencephalography. Finding these cells in the CSF is of limited diagnostic value.

Choroidal Cells. Choroidal cells are medium in size (about the size of a mature lymphocyte) and usually occur in a clump of similar cells (Plate 81). The nucleus is round or cuboidal and eccentrically located. It has a loose chromatin structure and nucleoli are not visible. A generous amount of cytoplasm is evident and is gray or slightly basophilic.

The nucleus changes from a blue to pink-tinted color in older samples. In addition, peripheral vacuolization in the cytoplasm can be observed in an aging specimen.

PLEURAL, PERITONEAL, AND PERICARDIAL FLUIDS

Effusions: Transudates and Exudates

An **effusion** is an abnormal accumulation of fluid in a particular space of the body. Effusions in the pleural, pericardial, and peritoneal cavities are divided into **transudates** and **exudates**. Transudates generally indicate that fluid has accumulated because of the presence of a systemic disease. In contrast, exudates are usually associated with disorders such as inflammation, infection, and malignant conditions involving the cells that line the surfaces of organs (e.g., lung or abdominal organs).

Transudates and exudates frequently differ in characteristics such as color and clarity and in total leukocyte cell count. Classically, transudates have been considered to differ from exudates based on the properties of specific gravity and total protein. These characteristics, however, are unreliable in consistently differentiating the two categories of effusions. For example, the mean values of total protein display considerable overlap between transudates and exudates.

A variety of physical and chemical properties need to be considered when fluids are categorized as transudates or exudates (Table 23.5).

Pleural Fluid

Anatomy of the Pleura

The lungs lie in the thoracic (chest) cavity, where they are separated by the heart in the mediastinum. Each lung

PROCEDURE FOR DIFFERENTIATION OF CELLS IN SPINAL FLUID

Principle
Slide preparations are routinely performed on all CSF specimens. If the total leukocyte count exceeds the normal value, a differential count is usually performed.

Reagents, Supplies, and Equipment
1. Conical centrifuge tubes
2. Microscope slides and Pasteur pipettes
3. Centrifuge
4. Methylene blue or Wright stain

Procedure
The sediment to be examined should be prepared using a cytocentrifuge, filtration, or sedimentation technique. The cytocentrifuge is the preferred method for concentrating CSF specimens. If these methods are not available, an older alternative can be used.

Alternative Method for Sediment Preparation
1. Pour 1 to 2 mL of fresh undiluted spinal fluid into a conical centrifuge. Balance the centrifuge and centrifuge at 2500 rpm for 10 minutes.
2. Following centrifugation, remove the supernatant fluid with a Pasteur pipette and either save at 4° to 6°C or freeze for other analyses, if needed. Resuspend the precipitate by gently tapping the tip of the centrifuge tube against the palm of the hand.
3. Transfer a small drop of the resuspended sediment onto a glass slide and smear out as a blood smear. Air-dry thoroughly.
4. Stain with either methylene blue or Wright stain. The methylene blue stain is preferred and should be applied to the smear for approximately 12 minutes. Gently wash off the stain with distilled water.
5. Allow the smear to air-dry. Examine using the 100× (oil immersion) objective. Count the number of different cells observed on a total count of 100 leukocytes.

Reporting Results
Few mononuclear cells (lymphocytes and monocytes) and a rare ependymal cell are considered normal findings.

Procedure Notes
Sources of Error
Artifactual distortion of cells prepared with a cytocentrifuge can lead to misidentification. Specimens should be prepared with a cytocentrifuge, but these preparations may demonstrate artifacts. Portions of fragmented nuclei or cytoplasm can be seen. In addition, cells may assume distorted shapes, granules may become localized in the cytoplasm, and vacuoles may appear in the cytoplasm. Abnormal cells are more prone to exhibit artifactual disruptions, perhaps because of increased cellular fragility. In addition, cellular size can be distorted by cytocentrifuge preparation. Cells in the interior of a specimen may be smaller and have a denser nucleus than cells at the periphery.

Clinical Applications
Normal CSF is crystal clear and colorless. Gross blood may be observed in traumatic tap specimens or in cases of pathological bleeding due to spontaneous subarachnoid hemorrhage or intracerebral hemorrhage.

Xanthochromia may be indicative of the pathological condition subarachnoid hemorrhage, if the erythrocytes have been present long enough to hemolyze.

Clotting can be due to the presence of peripheral blood, increased protein, or gel formation on standing due to an increased fibrinogen content.

Turbidity is seen if at least 200 leukocytes × 10^6/L, or 400 erythrocytes × 10^6/L, or microorganisms are present. Increased segmented neutrophil counts classically suggest bacterial infection; however, increased segmented neutrophils can be from infectious and noninfectious agents. Infectious disorders include bacterial meningitis, viral meningoencephalitis (the first few days), early tuberculosis, and mycotic meningitis. Aseptic meningitis can exist in cases where the septic focus is adjacent to the meninges. Noninfectious causes of increases in segmented neutrophils include reaction to CNS hemorrhage (3 to 4 days afterward), injection of foreign substances such as lidocaine into the subarachnoid space, and leukemic infiltration.

Increased numbers of lymphocytes are typically associated with viral infections but may be seen in a variety of disorders. These disorders include viral meningoencephalitis, fungal meningitis, syphilitic meningoencephalitis, and partially treated bacterial meningitis. Noninfectious causes of increased lymphocyte numbers include conditions such as multiple sclerosis.

Other types of cells are rarely encountered. Plasma cells are normally absent. Eosinophils may be increased due to causes similar to those of an increase in segmented neutrophils; increased basophils can be seen in chronic basophilic leukemia, which involves the meninges; and monocytes may be seen in leukemic infiltration of the meninges and infectious states.

Associated Findings
Glucose and protein values are important to correlate with gross and microscopic findings in the CSF. In general, a decreased glucose level in the CSF in the presence of a normal blood glucose level indicates bacterial utilization of glucose. In addition, an elevated total protein concentration is also suggestive of an inflammatory reaction or a bacterial infection. A viral infection will not have a dramatic effect on CSF glucose levels and may not affect the total protein level significantly.

---

is covered by a serous membrane, the visceral pleura (Fig. 23.2). The interior of the chest wall, the superior surface of the diaphragm, and the lateral portion of the mediastinum are also lined by a thin membrane, the parietal pleura. The layers of the visceral and parietal pleurae are contiguous and the potential space between them on each side of the thorax forms the pleural cavity. However, the pleural cavity is not a true cavity. It becomes a cavity if an abnormal condition creates an excess accumulation of fluid or air in it.

The pleural cavity is lined by a single-cell layer of mesothelial cells that form the mesothelium. Mesothelial cells are supported by layers of connective tissue that contain an extensive network of lymphatic vessels and blood capillaries. Although the function of the pleural space is obscure, the stretchable mesothelial cells that line this potential space

TABLE 23.5 Comparison of Transudates and Exudates[a]

Characteristics	Transudate	Exudate
Physical Characteristics		
pH	7.4–7.5	7.35–7.45
Specific gravity	<1.016	>1.016
Cellular Characteristics		
Erythrocytes	Few	Variable
Leukocytes	<1000	>1000
Chemical Analyses		
Glucose level	Equal to serum	Possibly decreased
Protein level	<3.0 gm/dL	>3.0 gm/dL
Pleural fluid–serum ratio of protein	<0.5	>0.5
LDH level	<200	>200 IU/L
Pleural fluid–serum ratio of LDH[b]	<2:3 (<0.6)	>2:3 (>0.6)

[a]Variations can be observed in examples of various conditions.

[b]If nonhemolyzed, nonbloody effusion.

LDH = lactic dehydrogenase.

provide the lungs and other intrathoracic organs with the flexibility to expand and retract.

Pleural fluid is normally produced by the parietal pleura and absorbed by the visceral pleura, as a continuous process. Although healthy individuals form 600 to 800 mL of fluid daily, the normal volume of fluid in each pleural space is estimated at less than 10 mL. This fluid is formed by the filtration of blood plasma through the capillary endothelium. The fluid is reabsorbed by lymphatic vessels and venules in the pleura. Transport in and out of the pleural space is dependent on the balance of hydrostatic pressure in the capillary network of the parietal and visceral pleurae, and capillary permeability, plasma oncotic pressure, and lymphatic reabsorption.

Pleural Effusion

The accumulation of fluid in the pleural space is referred to as a **pleural effusion.** Excess fluid accumulates if the balance of fluid formation and absorption is in disequilibrium. This may be due to an increased production or a decreased absorption of fluid. Large quantities may need to be drained. Aspiration of pleural fluid is referred to as **thoracentesis** (Fig. 23.3). Failure to remove an increased accumulation of leukocytes or blood from the pleural space may lead to the

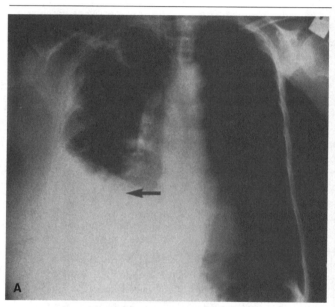

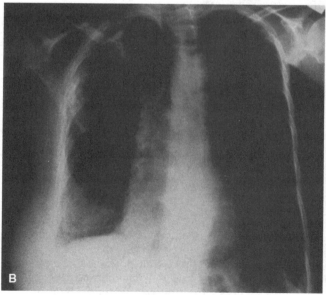

FIGURE 23.2 Pleurae from above and in front. Note position of mediastinum and root of each lung. (From R. S. Snell, *Clinical Anatomy for Medical Students* [4th ed.]. Boston: Little, Brown & Co., 1992.)

FIGURE 23.3 **A.** A substantial amount of pleural fluid has accumulated in this patient's right chest cavity (*arrow*). **B.** After draining off more than 100 mL, the patient's chest radiograph reveals a decreased amount of fluid in the right chest cavity.

TABLE 23.6 Clinical Correlations (Pleural Fluid)

Transudates
    Congestive heart failure
    Cirrhosis with ascites
Exudates
    Infectious diseases
    Empyema
    Tuberculosis
    Malignant neoplasms
    Lymphoma
    Mesothelioma
    Pancreatitis
    Rheumatoid arthritis

formation of fibrothorax and a subsequent impairment of pulmonary function.

The location of a pleural effusion may be suggestive of the type of disorder involved in causing the effusion (Table 23.6). Typically, left-sided effusions are associated with conditions such as a ruptured esophagus or acute pancreatitis.

If a fluid has the general characteristics of an exudate, at a minimum a Gram stain and culture and cytological studies need to be performed. An open lung biopsy of tissue for examination with histochemical stains and electron microscopy may be required for a diagnosis in suspected malignant conditions.

Laboratory Analysis

Physical Characteristics

Transudates are usually clear, are pale yellow, and do not clot. In comparison, exudates can display a range of colors depending on the associated disorder (Table 23.7). Only 2 mL of circulating blood in 1 L of pleural fluid will produce a blood-tinged appearance. Very viscous fluids, clear or bloody, are characteristic of mesothelioma. In addition, exudates may be cloudy or purulent, and frequently clot on standing because of the presence of fibrinogen.

TABLE 23.7 Representative Exudate Appearance

Appearance	Typical Associated Disorder
Dark red-brown	Amebiasis
Greenish to greenish-yellow and turbid	Classic rheumatoid effusion
Yellow and turbid	Infectious process
Milky	Chylothorax (chylous or pseudochylous)
Bloody (hemorrhagic)	Traumatic tap, malignancy, pulmonary infarction, trauma, pancreatitis, tuberculosis
Clearly visible pus (WBCs)	Empyema
Foul odor	Anaerobic bacterial infection

Specimen turbidity may be due to lipids or result from an increased number of leukocytes. A clear supernatant after centrifugation indicates the presence of an abundant number of leukocytes, but a white supernatant is due to chylomicrons. In contrast, chyliform or pseudochylous pleural effusions resemble a chylous effect. These effusions have a milky or greenish appearance and might have a pearly opalescent sheen. This appearance results from cellular debris and cholesterol crystals.

Cell Count

Erythrocyte and leukocyte counts are of limited value in the differential diagnosis of pleural effusions. A massively bloody (hemorrhagic) effusion in the absence of trauma almost always suggests malignancy, or occasionally pulmonary infarct. Pure blood in the pleural cavity, true hemothorax, results from severe chest injuries. In these cases, a microhematocrit determination will confirm that the microhematocrit value is similar to the patient's peripheral blood packed RBC volume.

Extremely elevated total leukocyte (WBC) counts of $50.0 \times 10^9/L$ or higher are consistent with a diagnosis of empyema. In general, WBC counts less than $1.0 \times 10^9/L$ are associated with transudates and WBC counts above 1000 are associated with exudates.

Use undiluted fluid to perform the cell count (refer to the spinal fluid cell count procedure). Electronic counting instruments should be used with caution, because debris may cause falsely increased counts.

Cell Differential Examination

Smears should be prepared for microscopic examination by cytocentrifugation, filter preparation (Millipore), or sedimentation methods. Following preparation of the sediment, the smears should be properly stained with Wright or Wright-Giemsa stain for differential leukocyte evaluation, or stained with Papanicolaou stain for cytological evaluation.

Cell types that can be encountered in the examination of a Wright-Giemsa–stained specimen include PMNs, eosinophils, basophils, lymphocytes, plasma cells, mononuclear phagocytes (monocytes, histiocytes, and macrophages), mesothelial cells (normal, reactive, atypical, and malignant), and metastatic tumor (malignant) cells. In addition, in vivo LE cells have also been observed in pleural fluids.

If a cytocentrifuge is used for sediment preparation, artifacts may be encountered. Cells in the interior of a specimen may be smaller in overall size with a denser nucleus than cells at the periphery. Abnormal cells in particular are more likely to be affected because of their propensity to be more fragile. In addition, nuclear-induced changes can include distorted shape and segmentation, fragmentation, or holes. Cytoplasmic artifacts can include irregular fragmentation, localization of granules, and peripheral vacuolization.

PMNs should be distinguished from mononuclear cells. It can be difficult to differentiate lymphocytes from monocytes.

Polymorphonuclear Neutrophils. PMNs in pleural fluid may appear morphologically identical to those in the circulating blood or may be difficult to recognize. Immature neutrophils are rarely seen except in chronic granulocytic leukemia or a leukoerythroblastic condition.

In long-standing effusions, signs of cellular degeneration such as vacuolization and a decreased number of granules can occur in the cytoplasm. The nuclei may appear as densely stained spherical fragments and resemble nucleated erythrocytes (RBCs). Occasionally, the cytoplasm may have a bluish color and resemble the cytoplasm of a lymphocyte.

An increase in PMNs (Table 23.8) is associated with exudates from patients with infectious diseases of a bacterial etiology.

Lymphocytes. Lymphocytes resembling small peripheral blood lymphocytes are seen in variable numbers in most body fluids. However, lymphocytes may be variable in size and have an immature appearance. The cellular nucleus can be cleaved and exhibit nucleoli that are often more prominent than those in peripheral blood lymphocytes.

Degenerative changes in aged specimens can include vacuolization, pyknotic nuclear changes, and variations in the staining pattern. Artifactual changes can include a shrunken nucleus or dense clumps of very dark coloration, overall cell shrinkage, and an irregular cytoplasmic border due to slow drying of the specimen on the slide.

Effusions from patients with tuberculosis or malignancies frequently show a predominance of lymphocytes. Effusions from patients with non-Hodgkin's lymphoma can manifest malignant lymphocytes that are generally uniform in comparison to benign conditions in which there is usually a mixture of different types of lymphocytes (small, medium, and large).

Detection of lymphocyte subsets (T and B lymphocytes) in pleural effusion may aid in the differential diagnosis. The T subset is considerably higher in fluids from patients with pulmonary tuberculosis than in their blood. The B subset is usually significantly lower in pleural fluid than in the circulating blood in patients with pulmonary tuberculosis, pulmonary malignant disorders, or nonspecific pleuritis. The presence of a monoclonal B cell population is usually associated with malignant lymphoma.

Mononuclear Cells. Mononuclear phagocytes (monocytes, histiocytes, and macrophages) are seen in variable numbers in both benign and malignant effusions. The terms macrophage and histiocyte are used synonymously. Both monocytes and mesothelial cells may be transformed into macro-

---

TABLE 23.8 **Examples of Cellular Abnormalities Encountered in Pleural and Peritoneal Fluids**

Condition	Cellular Characteristics
Bacterial inflammation	
Acute	Many neutrophils, histiocytes, and mesothelial cells
	May display bacteria
Chronic	Some neutrophils and eosinophils
	Many lymphocytes, plasma cells, and histiocytes
	Reactive mesothelial cells
	May display bacteria
Chronic granulomatous inflammation (e.g., tuberculosis, sarcoidosis, fungal infections, rheumatoid arthritis)	Elongated or round multinuclear giant cells
	Histiocytes, lymphocytes, and plasma cells
	Some neutrophils
	Many reactive mesothelial cells
	Amorphous background material from the center of granulomas
	May display fungi (special stain), if fungal inflammations
	May display tuberculous bacilli (special stains), if tuberculosis
Malignant mesothelioma	Abundant number of cells (single or cluster)
	Gland-like peculiar multinucleated cells present
	Clusters of cells are made of more than 4–5 cells
	Calcified bodies
	Occasional psammoma bodies
Metastatic tumors	Malignant cells (single or clusters)
	Cytoplasm may display intracellular vacuole, associated with mucin in adenocarcinoma, or squamous cell carcinoma
	Intracellular mucin appears as large paranuclear vacuole containing granular blue material
	Nucleus may be marginated
	Sarcomas have very large elongated cells with oval to rod-shaped nuclei, small nucleoli and coarse chromatin, abundant cytoplasm—elongated and finely reticular to granular
	Poorly differentiated sarcomas have very large tumor cells with large pleomorphic nuclei
After chemotherapy or radiation therapy	Atypical mesothelial cells
	Increased number of histiocytes
Viral infections	Many lymphocytes, plasma cells, histiocytes, and mesothelial cells

phages; the morphological distinction is not always obvious.

Macrophages (see Plate 36) vary in size, with a diameter ranging from 15 to 25 μm. The cytoplasm is pale gray and frequently vacuolated. Macrophages may contain phagocytized material such as RBC particles. The nucleus is eccentrically located, with one or more observable nucleoli. **Signet ring cells** are a type of macrophage that forms when the small vacuoles of the cell fuse and form one or two large vacuoles that push the nucleus against the side of the cell membrane. The nucleus forms the "stone" component of the ring. Signet ring macrophages with a normal-size nucleus are commonly seen in sterile inflammatory effusions.

The degeneration and death of a macrophage are characterized by an irregular nuclear shape and pyknosis, and cytoplasmic vacuolization and inclusions, with peripheral fraying.

The number of mononuclear cells usually increases as an inflammatory process becomes chronic. Mononuclear cells predominate in early inflammatory effusions (e.g., pneumonia, pulmonary infarct, pancreatitis, and subphrenic abscess). After several days, macrophages, lymphocytes, and mesothelial cells may predominate.

Eosinophils. An increased number of eosinophils (eosinophilia) in pleural fluid is nonspecific. Eosinophilia in pleural fluid (greater than 10% of total WBCs) may signify that air or blood has been introduced into the pleural space (e.g., repeated thoracenteses, pneumothorax, and traumatic hemothorax). However, it is not diagnostically significant. Eosinophilia may also be manifested in parasitic or fungal diseases, pulmonary infarction, and polyarteritis nodosa.

Plasma Cells. The plasma cells resemble those encountered in the bone marrow. An increase in plasma cells accompanies an increase in lymphocytes in patients with multiple myeloma. Plasma cells may also be seen in effusions from patients with tuberculosis, rheumatoid arthritis, malignancy, Hodgkin's disease, or other conditions associated with lymphocytosis.

Mesothelial Cells. Mesothelial cells (middle lining of cells) form the lining of the pleural, pericardial, and peritoneal cavities. In vivo the cells form a single-cell layer or sheet of uniform cells. Normally, a small number of cells is sloughed into the serous cavities.

These cells vary in appearance, frequently manifesting atypical or reactive changes, and usually cause the most difficulty during the evaluation of cell types. It is extremely difficult to distinguish between mononuclear phagocytes and intermediate forms of mesothelial cells. Therefore, they may be mistaken for malignant cells.

Mesothelial cells may appear as single cells, in clusters, or as sheets. Clustering of cells may be caused by centrifugation and may closely resemble malignant cells. Clumps of benign mesothelial cells can be differentiated from malignant cells by comparing the appearance of the cells in the clump with other more easily distinguished mesothelial cells in the same smear. In addition, a uniform, regular arrangement of cells that display fenestrations (openings or windows)

between the cytoplasmic membranes of these cells usually indicates that they are benign.

Mesothelial cells have a large overall size and average from 12 to 30 μm in diameter. Benign mesothelial cells can have various appearances; some resemble large plasma cells. The nucleus or nuclei have a round to oval appearance and occupy about one third to one half of the cell's diameter. Although one to three nucleoli may be seen, cells may be multinucleated. Occasionally a cell may contain 20 or more nuclei. The nuclear contour is usually smooth and regular, with stippled and dark-purple nuclear chromatin.

The cytoplasm is abundant and varies from light gray to deep blue. Localized basophilic areas are often seen in the center of the cell. This perinuclear zone of pallor resembles a fried egg in appearance. Cytoplasmic vacuoles of various sizes are often seen. Vacuoles or clear areas at the periphery of the cytoplasm probably represent glycogen.

Degenerative mesothelial cells may show pyknosis and karyorrhexis. They may also exhibit phagocytosis and transform into macrophages. Tiny projections of microvilli may be observed extending from the periphery of the cytoplasm; this is an artifact.

Mesothelial cells are seen in variable numbers in most effusions and are increased in sterile inflammations caused by such conditions as pleurisy associated with pulmonary infarction. Few cells, if any, are seen in effusions from patients with tubercular pleurisy or when an increased number of pyogenic organisms are present in the effusion. If the number of large mesothelial cells, differing from macrophages, is more than 5%, tuberculosis is ruled out.

Cytological Examination

Most malignant effusions are caused by metastatic adenocarcinoma because of its peripheral location and high incidence. Analysis of body fluids, secretions, and tissue biopsy specimens can be of value in the diagnosis of carcinoma. Another source for the diagnosis of pleural malignancy is sputum.

The presence of a massive bloody (hemorrhagic) effusion in the absence of trauma is highly suggestive of malignancy. The number of malignant cells varies. On microscopic examination, tumor cells frequently aggregate in clumps and sometimes show gland-like formation. Characteristics of malignant cells include the following:

1. Variation in cell sizes and shapes (pleomorphic) or similar in appearance (monomorphic)
2. Multiple, round aggregates of cells
3. High nuclear-cytoplasmic (N:C) ratio
4. Irregularity in nuclear size and shape
5. Coarseness and clumping of chromatin
6. Large, prominent, irregular nucleoli
7. Possible giant vacuoles
8. Basophilic or vacuolated (mucin-containing) cytoplasm
9. Irregular and abnormal mitosis
10. Engulfment of malignant cells by other malignant cells

Peritoneal Fluid

Anatomy of the Peritoneum

The peritoneum is a smooth membrane that covers the abdominal walls and viscera of the abdomen and pelvis (Fig.

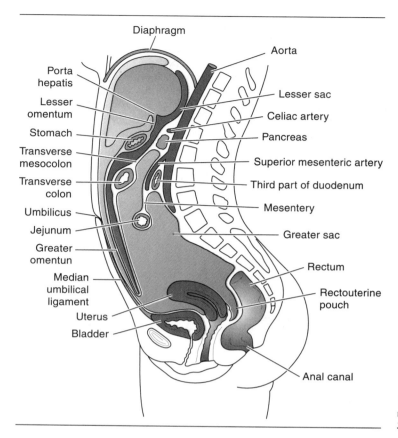

FIGURE 23.4 Sagittal section of female abdomen, showing arrangement of peritoneum. (From R. S. Snell, *Clinical Anatomy for Medical Students* [4th ed.]. Boston: Little, Brown & Co., 1992.)

23.4). The continuous sheet of single-cell layers of mesothelial cells supported by connective tissue forms the visceral and parietal peritoneum. The potential space between the parietal and visceral layers of the peritoneum is the peritoneal cavity. The parietal peritoneum lines the entire abdominal cavity. At the posterior midline, the left and right sheets of the membrane come together to form a double membrane, the mesentery. Each of the abdominal organs is suspended by this mesentery. As the sheets separate to surround an organ, they become the visceral peritoneum of the organ. In two places within the abdominal cavity, mesenteries extend beyond the organs and form a four-layered thickness, the omenta. Omenta contain phagocytic cells that protect the abdominal cavity from infection. However, peritonitis, an inflammation of these membranes, can result from infection or chemical irritation.

A small amount of fluid, formed by the ultrafiltration of plasma, lubricates the peritoneum. The presence of this fluid, peritoneal fluid, reduces friction between the visceral and parietal peritonea as they move against each other.

Peritoneal Effusion

An abnormal amount of fluid (an effusion) can accumulate in the peritoneal cavity if the balance between fluid formation and reabsorption is altered by a disease process. The collection of fluid in the peritoneal cavity, **ascites,** results from increased hydrostatic pressure in the systemic circulation, increased peritoneal capillary permeability, decreased plasma oncotic pressure, or decreased fluid reabsorption by

the lymphatic system. The procedure for removing fluid from the peritoneal cavity is **paracentesis.**

Causes of Peritoneal Effusions

The causes of peritoneal effusions range from disorders and diseases that directly represent involvement of the peritoneum, such as bacterial peritonitis, to abdominal conditions that do not directly involve the peritoneum, such as hepatic cirrhosis, cirrhosis, congestive heart failure, Budd-Chiari syndrome, hypoalbuminemia (due to nephrotic syndrome or protein-losing enteropathy malnutrition), and miscellaneous disorders such as myxedema, ovarian diseases, pancreatic disease, and chylous ascites.

Effusions that may conform with the definition of transudates can be associated with congestive heart failure, hepatic cirrhosis, and hypoproteinemia.

Effusions that may conform with the definition of exudates can be associated with primary or secondary peritonitis, malignant disorders, trauma, and pancreatitis.

Laboratory Analysis

The laboratory criteria for distinguishing transudates from exudates are less clearly defined for peritoneal (ascitic) fluid than for pleural fluid. Transudates are usually clear and pale yellow. Exudates are cloudy or turbid due to an increased concentration of leukocytes, elevated protein levels, and occasionally microorganisms. Exudates may be seen in peritonitis, cases of perforated or infarcted intestine, and pancreatitis. An evaluation of ascitic fluid includes gross inspection,

TABLE 23.9 Variations in Peritoneal Fluid Appearance

	Examples of Conditions
Color	
Pale yellow	Normal
Straw-colored	Normal
	Congestive heart failure
	Cirrhosis
	Neoplasm
Reddish-brown or bloody	Neoplasm
	Pancreatitis
	Pulmonary infarct
	Trauma
	Traumatic thoracentesis
	Tuberculous peritonitis
Appearance	
Clear	Normal
	Tuberculous peritonitis
Turbid (cloudy)	Bacterial peritonitis
	Pancreatitis
	Conditions with increased cellular components
Mucinous	Neoplasm
Chylous* (milky)	Obstruction of lymphatic duct (e.g., lymphoma)
	Tuberculous peritonitis
	Trauma
	Pancreatitis
Purulent	Bacterial peritonitis

*Supernatant is white due to chylomicrons.

total cell count, microscopic examination of sediment for cell differentiation, cytological studies, chemical analysis for constituents such as total protein and lactic dehydrogenase, and microbial culture.

Physical Characteristics

A variety of clinical conditions (Table 23.9) can produce a deviation from the anticipated yellow or straw-colored fluid.

Grossly bloody (hemorrhagic) peritoneal fluid may be seen in trauma patients with a ruptured spleen or liver, intestinal infarction, pancreatitis, or malignancies. Green-colored effusion results from the presence of bile. This type of discoloration may be seen in patients with perforated gallbladders or intestines, or in those with duodenal ulcers. Greenish fluid, however, may also be present in patients with cholecystitis (inflammation of the gallbladder) or acute pancreatitis. The presence of bile can be confirmed with a spot test for bilirubin.

Chylous (milky-appearing) peritoneal fluid is rare. Chylous ascites is caused by a leakage of lymphatic vessels resulting from trauma, lymphoma, tuberculosis, hepatic cirrhosis, or carcinoma. Malignant lymphoma and carcinoma are the two most common causes of chylous peritoneal fluid. In contrast, pseudochylous fluid has a milky or greenish appearance because of the presence of cellular debris and cholesterol crystals. This abnormality may be associated with chronic effusions produced by a wide variety of causes.

Total Cell Count

Total erythrocyte (RBC) and leukocyte (WBC) counts are usually performed on ascitic fluid. Use undiluted fluid to perform the cell count (refer to the spinal fluid cell count procedure). Use electronic counting instruments with care because debris may cause falsely increased counts. Smears should be prepared for microscopic examination by cytocentrifugation, filter preparation (Millipore), or sedimentation methods.

Cell counts improve the accuracy and specificity of diagnosis by peritoneal lavage (flushing of space with Ringer's lactate solution). However, the total cell count is of less accuracy in the diagnosis of penetrating trauma (gunshot and stab wounds) of the abdomen than in other conditions (Table 23.10). A positive result by lavage is indicative of laparotomy. If the test results are equivocal, another lavage may be indicated in 1 to 2 hours.

Total WBC counts are of limited value in differential diagnosis but a total WBC count higher than $0.3 \times 10^9/L$ is considered to be abnormal. More than half of patients with infected ascites have a total WBC count higher than $0.3 \times$

TABLE 23.10 Criteria for Diagnosing Blunt and Penetrating Trauma by Analysis of Peritoneal Lavage Fluid

Diagnosis	Gross	Laboratory Analysis
Positive	Blood in aspirate or lavage	RBC count $>0.1 \times 10^{12}/L$; $>0.05 \times 10^{12}/L$ in cases of penetrating trauma
	Lavage fluid retrieved via Foley catheter or chest tube Evidence of food, foreign particle, or bile	WBC count $>0.5 \times 10^9/L$ Amylase level $>2 \times$ serum amylase level
Indeterminate	Small amount of bloody fluid noted in dialysis catheter on insertion	RBC count $0.05-0.1 \times 10^{12}/L$; $0.01-0.05 \times 10^{12}/L$ in cases of penetrating trauma WBC count $0.001-0.005 \times 10^9/L$ Amylase levels slightly higher than serum amylase levels
Negative		RBC count $<0.025 \times 10^{12}/L$ WBC count $<0.001 \times 10^9/L$ Amylase level lower than serum amylase level

10^9/L, with more than 25% segmented PMNs on the leukocyte differential smear. Leukocyte counts above 0.5×10^9/L are considered to be useful presumptive evidence in distinguishing between bacterial peritonitis and cirrhosis. In bacterial peritonitis, the total WBC count is higher than 0.5×10^9/L, with more than 50% PMNs.

A wide variation in the peritoneal WBC count is seen in patients with chronic liver disease because of extracellular shifts in fluid associated with ascites formation or resolution. During diuresis, the total leukocyte concentration may increase dramatically, but the concentration of PMNs usually remains low. Therefore, the variance of the total WBC count usually does not lead to confusion between cirrhosis and bacterial peritonitis.

Total WBC counts may occasionally be elevated in peritoneal fluid independently of the RBC count. This is particularly true in patients with penetrating abdominal trauma with visceral injury. If lavage is performed immediately after the injury occurs, the WBC count may not yet be elevated (Table 23.11).

Cellular Differential Examination

Following preparation of the sediment, the smears should be properly stained with Wright or Wright-Giemsa stain for differential leukocyte evaluation or with Papanicolaou stain for cytological evaluation.

A differential cell count should be performed on the Wright-Giemsa stained smear. If a cytocentrifuge is used for sediment preparation, artifacts may be encountered (see Pleural Fluid for a discussion of the artifact induced by cytocentrifuge preparation).

Although the quantities of some cells in peritoneal fluid compared to pleural fluid may vary in some disorders, the cell types that can be encountered are the same as those that can be seen in pleural fluids. These cells include PMNs, eosinophils, basophils, lymphocytes, plasma cells, mononuclear phagocytes (monocytes, histiocytes, and macrophages), mesothelial cells (normal, reactive, atypical, or malignant), and metastatic tumor (malignant) cells. In addition, in vivo LE cells have also been observed.

Segmented Polymorphonuclear Neutrophils. A distribution of PMNs higher than 25% is considered abnormal. A high proportion of PMNs is suggestive of bacterial infection, although about one third of patients with alcoholic cirrhosis demonstrate a ratio of PMNs in excess of 30%.

In addition, an absolute neutrophil count may also be helpful. A count above 0.25×10^9/L is a fairly sensitive indicator of spontaneous or secondary bacterial peritonitis.

Eosinophils. Eosinophilia of the peritoneal fluid is less common than that of the pleural fluid. Eosinophilic ascites is rare, but when present, more than 50% of the cells in the peritoneal fluid are eosinophils. Eosinophilic ascites manifests in patients with eosinophilic gastroenteritis, ruptured hydatid cysts, lymphoma, or vasculitis. In addition, patients with chronic peritoneal dialysis may also exhibit eosinophilic ascites.

Lymphocytes. A predominance of lymphocytes is seen in transudates from patients with congestive heart failure, cirrhosis, or nephrotic syndrome. On differential examination, lymphocytes may represent the majority of leukocytes in chylous effusions, and in patients with tuberculous peritonitis or malignancies.

Mesothelial Cells. In contrast to pleural effusions, tuberculous peritoneal effusions may contain many mesothelial cells. Ascitic fluid associated with cirrhosis may contain many highly atypical mesothelial cells.

Malignant Cells. It is possible to observe malignant tumor cells in peritoneal fluids. Cytological examination should be performed if a malignancy is suspected. It is important to distinguish between malignant and mesothelial cells because the cells most difficult to differentiate from malignant cells are mesothelial cells.

Diagnosis of Ascites

Ascites is a condition in which fluid accumulates within the peritoneal space (cavity). This constitutes a peritoneal effusion. More than several hundred milliliters of peritoneal fluid must usually be present before the effusion can be detected by physical examination. Small amounts of effusion may be asymptomatic. Increasing amounts, however, cause abdominal distention and discomfort, anorexia, nausea, early satiety, heartburn, frank pain, and respiratory distress in patients.

Radiographic studies such as ultrasonography and computerized axial tomography (CAT scan) are very sensitive and allow the radiologist to observe the presence of an effusion and to distinguish it from a cystic mass. Rarely is a laparoscopy or exploratory laparotomy required.

Diagnostic abdominal paracentesis with the removal of 50 to 100 mL of fluid is essential for the establishment of a differential diagnosis. Aspiration may be combined with lavage.

Patients with abdominal pain who have chronic ascites or ascites of unknown origin, sudden onset of ascites (intraperitoneal hemorrhage, infarct, or pancreatic ascites), suspected perforation of a peptic ulcer or bowel perforation, or blunt trauma to the abdomen need to have a paracentesis performed. Two of the most common indications for para-

TABLE 23.11 Examples of Cell Count Variations

Erythrocytes (RBCs)	
High	Neoplasm, tuberculous peritonitis
Variable	Pancreatitis
Low	Cirrhosis, bacterial peritonitis, congestive heart failure
Leukocytes (WBCs)	
High	Bacterial peritonitis (PMNs)
	Congestive heart failure (mesothelial)
	Neoplasm (>50% lymphocytes)
	Tuberculous peritonitis (>70% lymphocytes)

centesis are complications of cirrhosis (e.g., spontaneous bacterial peritonitis and suspected intraabdominal malignancy).

The effusion specimen needs to be promptly analyzed. Laboratory assessment includes gross examination for characteristics such as color and clarity; total erythrocyte and leukocyte cell counts; differential leukocyte examination; chemical assays such as total protein, amylase, and lactic dehydrogenase; and microbial studies including Gram stain, routine cultures, anaerobic cultures, tuberculosis cultures, and cytological examination.

Pericardial Fluid

Anatomy of the Pericardium

The pericardium (Fig. 23.5) is a fibroserous sac, composed of external (fibrous) and internal (serous) layers, that encloses the heart and roots of the great blood vessels. The inner serous portion of the pericardium consists of the parietal and visceral layers. The outer parietal layer is in contact with the fibrous pericardium; the inner visceral layer, also referred to as the epicardium, is in contact with the heart and roots of the great blood vessels. The potential space between the parietal and visceral layers, which is filled with a small amount of fluid to reduce friction between the layers, is the pericardial cavity.

Pericardial Effusion

An abnormal accumulation of fluid in the cavity, a **pericardial effusion,** is most frequently caused by damage to the lining of the cavity and increased capillary permeability. In addition, in acute pericarditis, interference with pericardial venous and lymphatic drainage predisposes the patient to the development of an effusion.

The physiological function of the normal pericardium is considered to be pericardial restraint, which tends to oppose dilatation of the heart. In many circumstances, the restraining effect of the pericardium is essentially reflected by the mean central venous pressure. The term **cardiac tamponade** is often used to indicate a critical state of cardiovascular compromise, usually with hypotension, due to pericardial fluid under increased pressure. It is widely accepted that any elevation of central venous pressure that is due to pericardial effusion constitutes cardiac tamponade. Therapeutic removal of pericardial fluid, pericardiocentesis, is usually indicated if the central venous pressure rises to approximately 10 mm Hg.

Pericardial effusion is usually accurately assessed by echocardiography, but there are pitfalls in the interpretation of such studies. For example, tamponade can be produced by localized pockets of pericardial effusion that may not be evident by echocardiography, particularly if the pocket is located adjacent to the right atrium laterally. Computerized axial tomography (CAT scan) and magnetic resonance imaging (MRI) are also accurate means of demonstrating pericardial effusion and are less subject to the limitations of echocardiography in localized effusions. Pericardial disease causes effusions that are left-sided or bilateral; they are rarely exclusively right-sided. Patients with congestive heart failure typically manifest right-sided or bilateral effusions.

Causes of Pericardial Effusion

A wide variety of diseases and disorders can produce pericardial effusion (Table 23.12). Neoplastic disease produces a significant volume of fluid in the pericardium and is one of the most common causes of pericardial effusion. Primary tumors of the pericardium (mesothelioma) are rare. However, metastatic tumors of the pericardium and heart are common in patients with advanced malignant disease from primary sites such as the lung and breast, and in patients with leukemia or lymphoma. These types of metastasis are the most common causes of malignant effusions. Therefore, one of the most important parts of the laboratory examination of pericardial fluid is cytological studies for malignant cells.

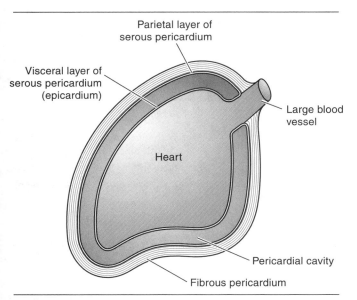

FIGURE 23.5 Different layers of the pericardium. (From R. S. Snell, *Clinical Anatomy for Medical Students* [4th ed.]. Boston: Little, Brown & Co., 1992.)

TABLE 23.12 **Causes of Pericardial Effusion**

Type	Cause
Infectious agents	Viruses, especially Coxsackie group viruses, bacteria (e.g., tubercular, fungal)
Cardiovascular disease	Myocardial infarction, Dressler's (postinfarction) syndrome, cardiac rupture, congestive heart failure, acute aortic dissection
Collagen vascular disease	Rheumatic disease
Hemorrhagic	Trauma, anticoagulant therapy, leakage of aortic aneurysm
Renal disease	Kidney failure and uremia (common), long-term dialysis
Neoplastic disease	Mesothelioma, metastatic carcinoma, leukemia, lymphoma

Laboratory Analysis

Gross Examination

Normal fluid is transparent and pale yellow. Hemorrhagic (bloody) effusions may result from a variety of abnormal conditions or from aspiration of intracardiac blood into the specimen. On visible examination, a hemorrhagic effusion should not form clots in a plain (nonanticoagulant) tube, but aspirated blood usually exhibits clotting. A milky-appearing effusion may be a true or pseudochylous fluid (see Pleural Fluid for a discussion of milky effusions).

The value of the measurement of pH is not well established. However, specimens with a pH less than 7.0 may be associated with infectious or rheumatoid disease. In addition, hemorrhagic specimens typically demonstrate a pH that is lower than the pH in circulating blood.

Cell Counts

Erythrocyte and leukocyte cell counts are of limited value in the differential diagnosis of a pericardial effusion. Erythrocyte counts or a determination of packed cell volume (microhematocrit), however, can be of value in distinguishing a hemorrhagic effusion from aspirated blood in a specimen. The quantity of erythrocytes is usually lower in a hemorrhagic effusion than in a simultaneously assayed circulating blood specimen. In contrast, aspirated blood, if sufficient in quantity, will exhibit an erythrocyte volume that is comparable to that in the circulating blood.

Pericardial fluid is relatively acellular. An increase (more than $1 \times 10^9/L$) is suggestive of microbial infection or malignancy.

Evaluation of Smears

Sediment should be prepared for microscopic examination as previously described in the Pleural Fluid section. The sediment should be stained and examined for leukocytic cells and malignant mesothelial cells.

Leukocyte Differential. The value of a differential leukocyte count in establishing a differential diagnosis is debatable. However, an elevated total leukocyte count in conjunction with mostly polysegmented neutrophils (PMNs) can be observed in bacterial pericarditis. In contrast, pericardial fluid may demonstrate increased lymphocytes in viral pericarditis.

Mononuclear phagocytes (monocytes, histiocytes, and macrophages) can be seen in variable numbers in pericardial effusions. In addition, in vivo LE cell formation has been observed in pericardial fluids.

Cytological Examination. Smears should be closely examined for the presence of malignant mesothelial cells. The appearance of these cells was previously described in the section on pleural fluids.

SEMINAL FLUID

The main function of seminal fluid is to transport sperm to female cervical mucus. After deposition in the female reproductive tract, sperm remain in seminal plasma for a short time while attempting to enter the mucus.

Anatomy and Physiology

Each of the male reproductive structures (Fig. 23.6) contributes specific components to seminal fluid. In addition to spermatozoa, which constitute only a small part of the total volume of seminal fluid, this fluid has a highly varied composition (Table 23.13).

Analysis of Seminal Fluid

Principle

Seminal fluid is examined physically, chemically, and microscopically. These procedures are performed in order to determine the physical and chemical properties, to quantitate the number of sperm cells, and to examine cellular motility and morphology. Seminal fluid can be analyzed for a variety of reasons, including infertility studies, artificial insemination protocols, postvasectomy assessment, and evaluation of probable sexual assault.

Specimen Collection

A fresh specimen is needed. The specimen may be collected in a clean, sterile, glass or plastic container. Ideally, seminal fluid should be analyzed within 30 minutes of collection. It is mandatory that the specimen be kept at 37°C and examined within 1 to 2 hours of collection. However, after 60 minutes of storage in a plastic container, sperm motility is significantly reduced.

Most laboratories examine two specimens collected a few days apart. Collection, proper transport, and prompt examination are critical factors in the analysis of seminal fluid. Universal precautions should be adhered to when handling semen, blood, and other body fluids.

It is recommended that a 3- to 5-day period of sexual abstinence be observed prior to specimen collection. Two days may be sufficient; the period should not exceed 5 days. Condoms treated with spermicide or lubricants with spermicidal properties must be avoided during specimen collection. In addition, patients need to be advised to keep

TABLE 23.13 Composition of Seminal Fluid

Structure	Component
Testicle	Sperm, steroids: testosterone and dihydrotestosterone
Testicle or epididymus	Androgen-binding protein
Testicle (most probable source)	Proteins (enzymes), lipids, electrolytes
Epididymus	Carnitine, acetylcarnitine, glyceryl phosphorylcholine
Seminal vesicles	Flavin, fructose, prostaglandins
Seminal vesicles and prostate	Magnesium
Prostate	Citric acid, enzymes, zinc, p30 glycoprotein
Cowper's glands, glands of Littre	Unknown

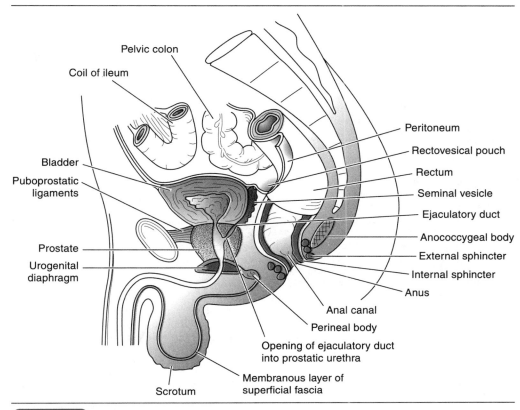

FIGURE 23.6 Sagittal section of male pelvis. (From R. S. Snell, *Clinical Anatomy for Medical Students* [4th ed.]. Boston: Little, Brown & Co., 1992.)

the specimen warm, if it is collected at home. In addition, they must be aware that it must be promptly delivered to the laboratory.

Gross Examination

Fresh specimens should be examined for color, pH, volume, and viscosity. These procedures are described in the following analysis section. The results may be useful not only in the assessment of fertility, but also in the detection of other disorders.

Microscopic Examination

Several microscopic procedures may be of value in the assessment of seminal fluid. Enumeration of the number of sperm and examination of the morphological characteristics of the cells are routinely performed procedures. Other microscopic procedures may include motility, viability, and agglutination studies.

Agglutination may indicate sperm-agglutinating antibodies or prostatitis. A significant increase in abnormal movements of sperm, notably immobilizing-type motion, is highly suggestive of the presence of sperm-immobilizing antibodies in the fluid. Viability and mobility studies should also be correlated.

Morphological characteristics, the commonly encountered variant forms, are presented in Table 23.14. Increases in the number of tapered spermatozoa and immature forms are frequently characteristic of patients with a varicocele and

those who have been under extreme stress. Increases in both of these variants are referred to as a "nonspecific stress pattern." Other variants have no direct correlation with specific disorders.

Additional Laboratory Procedures

Other techniques for the examination of semen may be requested in various situations. In cases of infertility, cervical mucus–sperm compatibility tests may be warranted to determine whether the sperm cells are able to penetrate the cervical mucus.

In medicolegal cases, for example, identification and security are paramount, and the procedural protocol is deter-

TABLE 23.14 Sperm Morphology (Variant Forms)

Type	% Normal Limits
Immature sperm cells (spermatids)	<15
Tapered heads	<15
Poorly formed heads	<15
Double heads	<5
Large heads	<5
Small heads	<5
Double or broken tails	<5

PROCEDURES FOR GROSS EXAMINATION

Measurement of Color

Procedure
Observe the color of a freshly collected specimen. Normal seminal fluid ranges in color from gray-white to translucent.

Clinical Significance
A dense white, cloudy specimen can be associated with increased numbers of leukocytes due to inflammation of structures such as the urethra or ejaculatory ducts.

A brown or red color suggests the presence of blood in the specimen. This can be associated with prostatitis.

A yellow color may be indicative of a variety of conditions including prostatovesiculitis, the use of certain oral antibiotics or medications, and the presence of urine in the semen.

Note: The color of semen can vary, depending on the length of abstinence from sexual activities. More transparent fluid is observed if the length of time is short; the fluid will be more yellow in color if the length of time has been long.

Measurement of pH

Procedure
1. Transfer a drop of seminal fluid to a piece of pH paper.
2. Observe the color of the strip and compare it to the color chart.
3. Record the results.

Reporting Results
Normal seminal fluid has a pH range of 7.5 to 8.0. The average pH is 7.7.

Clinical Significance
Determination of seminal fluid pH is rarely useful in the evaluation for fertility potential. However, low pH values can identify seminal fluid that is mainly composed of prostatic secretions. pH values less than 7.5 can be observed in patients with chronic prostatitis or other semen-related infections, inflammatory blockage of the ejaculatory ducts, or congenital aplasia of the vas deferens and seminal vesicles.

Measurement of Viscosity

Materials
1. A clean test tube marked at intervals of 0.5 mL
2. Pasteur pipette and safety bulb

Procedure
1. Transfer the specimen to the test tube with the Pasteur pipette.

2. Allow a portion of the specimen to be expelled slowly from the pipette.
3. Observe the viscosity (thickness or thinness) of the specimen by seeing if it forms discrete droplets.

Reporting Results
If a specimen is abnormal, a notation should be made of the type and degree of viscosity abnormality (e.g., minor, moderate, severe).

Reference value: Following ejaculation, seminal fluid (semen) is a thin liquid. Within a few minutes, it forms a gel (coagulum). If the specimen is kept at 37°C, the gel will spontaneously liquify to form a translucent, turbid, viscous fluid.

Normal seminal fluid (normal viscosity) should form discrete droplets as it falls from the pipette tip. Increased viscosity varies from progressive stringiness to a jelly-like coagulum that cannot be poured.

Liquefaction should be complete within 30 minutes. Lack of liquefaction is very rare. Incomplete liquefaction can take two forms: liquid viscosity or particulate viscosity. In liquid viscosity, the liquid portion of the fluid remains more viscous than normal for more than 1 hour after collection. Particulate viscosity represents particles in the fluid that prevent it from forming normal discrete droplets.

Clinical Significance
In the rare cases of lack of liquefaction, infertility could result because of the gelatinous character of the semen. Increased viscosity can be of significance if it impedes sperm motility. Increased viscosity is associated with poor invasion of the cervical mucus in postcoital studies and may be the only demonstrable defect in an infertile couple.

Measurement of Volume

Procedure
1. Observe the level of the meniscus of the fluid in the calibrated tube used for observation of viscosity.
2. Record the measurement to the nearest 0.5 mL.

Reporting Results
Reference value: 2 to 5 mL.

Clinical Significance
An absolute correlation between volume and fertility does not exist. If the volume is consistently less than 1.0 mL, problems with fertility should be suspected.

Note: The volume of seminal fluid usually increases as the frequency of intercourse decreases. However, a large ejaculate volume is not believed to have a negative effect on fertility if other measurements (e.g., sperm count) are normal.

MICROSCOPY PROCEDURES

Counting Sperm Cells

Principle
Following liquefaction of the semen, the spermatozoa can be counted in a hemocytometer chamber following an initial dilution in a Thoma leukocyte pipette.

Procedure
1. Mix the semen sample thoroughly and draw an aliquot up to the 0.5 mark on the pipette. Dilute to the 11 mark* with the following solution: 5 gm sodium bicarbonate, 1 mL formalin (neutral), and 100 mL distilled water.
2. Expel the first few drops from the pipette and fill the chamber. Allow the chamber to rest for 2 minutes on a piece of moistened filter paper under an inverted Petri dish cover in order for the immobilized sperm to settle.
3. Count the spermatozoa in 2 mm^2 (two large squares).
4. This number is multiplied by a factor of 100,000 to calculate the number of sperm per milliliter.† The entire counting procedure including the initial dilution should be repeated at least once and the results averaged. If viscosity is increased, dilute 1:1 with a mucolytic agent prior to dilution, with the final count being multiplied by 2.

Reporting Results
Reference values: 60 to 150 million/mL or 60 to 150 × 10^9/L. Sperm counts increase with abstinence for up to 10 days. In addition, the sperm count does not change significantly with age.

Clinical Significance
A decreased sperm count is considered abnormal, but it does not necessarily indicate infertility. Sperm concentration may decline seasonally (i.e., summer). In azoospermic (no observable sperm) specimens, a fructose assay should be conducted to verify the integrity of the vas deferens and seminal vesicles.

Examining Motility

Specimen
To evaluate motility, a small drop of liquefied semen is placed on a microscope slide that has been prewarmed to 37° C. The specimen is coverslipped and the edge sealed with petroleum jelly.

Procedure
Motility can be evaluated by scanning several fields with the high (43 to 44×) objective, until a total of 200 sperm cells have been observed. It is essential to focus through the entire depth of a given field in order to include nonmotile sperm that have settled to the bottom. The percentage of sperm cells showing actual progressive motion is recorded.

Reporting Results
Reference value: The normal motility for a fresh specimen is greater than 60%. If specimens are observed over a period of 24

---

*Alternate dilutions may be prepared but the calculation factor must be altered to reflect any alteration in the dilution.

†The number of sperm per milliliter can be multiplied by the total volume of the ejaculated specimen to determine the total number of spermatozoa in the specimen.

---

hours (e.g., at 3, 6, 12, and 24 hours), the motile forms will decrease by about 5%/hr after the fourth hour following collection.

Alternate Reporting System: Total Motility Score
Motility can be evaluated by observing the spermatozoa fields with the high (43 to 44x) objective, until a total of 100 sperm cells have been observed. It is essential to focus through the entire depth of a given field in order to include nonmotile sperm that have settled to the bottom. The speed of movement is determined (graded) for each of the 100 sperm cells.

Grade	Description of Movement
0	Not moving
1	Moving with no forward progression
2	Moving with slow, forward direction
3	Moving rapidly in almost a straight line
4	Moving with high speed in a straight line

Calculation
1. List the number of sperm at each grade (e.g., 0 = 35, 1 = 20, 2 = 15, 3 = 15, 4 = 15).
2. Multiply the number of cells at each grade by the numerical level of the grade (e.g., 0 × 35 = 0, 1 × 20 = 20, 2 × 15 = 30, 3 × 15 = 45, and 4 × 15 = 60).
3. Add the product of each of the grades to determine the total motility score (e.g., 0 + 20 + 30 + 45 + 60 = 155).

Sample Calculation:

Grade ×	Number of Sperm =	Motility
0	35	0
1	20	20
2	15	30
3	15	45
4	15	60
Total	100	155

Total motility score = 155

Reporting Results
Reference value: The total motility score for spermatozoa should be 150 or higher.

Examination of Sperm Morphology

Principle
Sperm morphology is evaluated by performing a differential count of morphologically normal and abnormal sperm types on a stained smear. The best stain for morphological detail is the Papanicolaou stain or Bryan-Leishman stain. Hematoxylin-eosin gives satisfactory but somewhat poorer differentiation of morphological detail.

Specimen Preparation
1. Smears are prepared on clean slides in a manner identical to blood smears.
2. It is essential that the smear be placed immediately into a fixative, either 95% (vol/vol) ethanol or 50% (vol/vol) ethanol/ether, before drying has occurred.

(continued)

MICROSCOPY PROCEDURES (continued)

Procedure: Hematoxylin-eosin
1. Air-dry the prepared smear (5 to 10 minutes at room temperature).
2. Place in 10% formalin for 1 minute.
3. Rinse gently with distilled water.
4. Place in Meyer's or Harris hematoxylin for 2 minutes.
5. Rinse gently with distilled water and air-dry.
6. Using the oil (100×) objective, at least 200 sperm should be examined and the percentage of forms recorded.

Note: In addition to sperm morphology, the presence of RBCs, leukocytes, and epithelial cells should be noted. Immature cells of the germinal line can appear in the semen and must be differentiated from macrophages or leukocytes. The immature spermatozoan may consist of spermatogonia, primary or secondary spermatocytes, and different spermatids. Numerous granules and globulins are normally present in semen.

Reporting Results
Reference value: Normal seminal fluid has a mean of 73% morphologically mature and normal oval-headed sperm (normal range 40% to 90%). Abnormal forms can include spermatids, small or giant heads, poorly formed heads, double heads, double tails, and broken tails. Table 23-14 enumerates the distribution and variations of morphological types in normal specimens.

Procedure for Sperm Viability Examination

Principle
To determine the number of sperm cells that are alive in a fresh specimen of seminal fluid.

Specimen
A freshly collected seminal specimen that has been kept at 37°C since collection.

Materials
1. Three microscope slides
2. Wooden applicator stick
3. 10% aqueous nigrosin
4. 5% aqueous eosin Y

Procedure
1. Label two slides with the patient's name and identification number.
2. Place a drop of semen on each slide, using a Pasteur pipette.
3. Add 2 drops of freshly filtered 5% eosin Y solution and mix for 30 seconds with a wooden applicator stick.
4. Add 3 drops of freshly filtered 10% nigrosin solution.
5. With a Pasteur pipette, transfer half of the volume on the slide to a second slide.
6. Smear each slide by pushing the blank slide at a 45-degree angle on the specimen-containing slide. The smear should occupy most of the length of the slide.
7. Air-dry. The slides may be dried at 37°C but they must be removed immediately on drying.
8. Examine a total of 200 sperm cells on each slide using the high-power (45×) objective.
9. Record the number of cells that are white and the number that are pink.
10. Determine the percentage of white and pink cells.

Reporting Results
Interpretation: Live sperm cells will not stain and appear white; dead sperm cells stain pink.

Reference value: At least 50% of spermatozoa should be alive in a properly collected and promptly examined specimen.

Procedure Notes
Sources of Error
Collection of a specimen into a container with spermicide (e.g., standard condom) or contaminated with soap or detergent residue will produce falsely decreased results.

Old specimens or specimens that have been improperly stored from the time of collection to the time of examination will also produce falsely decreased results.

Determination of Agglutination

Procedure
A drop of seminal fluid is placed on a microscope slide and coverslipped. The pattern of the sperm can then be observed in several high-power (45×) fields.

Reporting Results
Agglutination is present if the cells display a definite pattern of head-to-head, head-to-tail, or tail-to-tail. The degree of association should be reported as slight, moderate, or severe.

Reference value: no agglutination.

Note: If sperm are clumped, no definite pattern exists.

Clinical Significance
If agglutination is observed in more than one specimen from the same person, further investigation is warranted. Causes of agglutination can include chronic prostatitis and the presence of sperm-agglutinating antibodies.

mined by local jurisdiction. In cases of alleged rape or suspected sexual assault, vaginal smears may be submitted for evaluation of the presence of sperm. Sperm can be detected in the vagina for 24 to 72 hours after intercourse. However, the absence of sperm does not mean that intercourse has not taken place. Procedures for the identification of semen stains on clothing may also be requested. These procedures can include screening for A, B, or H blood group substances, the labile enzyme marker peptidase A, and phosphoglucomutase in combination with ABO typing. Other procedures can include examination for fluorescence under ultraviolet light, acid phosphatase test, and enzyme-linked immunosorbent assay for p30 male-specific semen glycoprotein of prostatic origin or an immunological precipitin test to identify semen of human origin on clothing.

Other Microscopic Features

When sperm are being examined for morphological characteristics, the presence of other cellular elements (e.g., erythrocytes, leukocytes, or bacteria) in the specimen should be observed. Debris (e.g., precipitated stain) should not be mistaken for bacteria. All specimens should be observed for *Trichomonas* parasites, particularly donor semen.

Technical Notes: If bacteria are observed, a sterile portion of the specimen should be cultured. However, the probability of a positive finding is low. Semen for artificial insemination should be tested for infectious diseases (e.g., *Neisseria gonorrhoeae*). If a man is being studied for infertility, the specimen should be cultured for *Mycoplasma*.

SYNOVIAL FLUID

Synovial (joint) fluid is a transparent, viscous fluid secreted by the synovial membrane. This fluid is found in joint cavities, bursae, and tendon sheaths (Fig. 23.7). Its function is to lubricate the joint space and transport nutrients to the articular cartilage. Impaired function of synovial fluid with age or disease may play a role in the development of degenerative joint disease (osteoarthritis). A variety of disorders produce changes in the number and types of cells and the chemical composition of the fluid. Analysis of synovial fluid plays a major role in the diagnosis of joint diseases.

Anatomy and Physiology of Joints

Diarthrodial joints are lined at their margins by a synovial membrane (synovium), with synovial cells lining this space. The lining cells synthesize protein and are phagocytic. Mechanical, chemical, immunological, or bacteriological damage may alter the permeability of the membrane and capillaries to produce varying degrees of inflammatory response. In addition, inflammatory joint fluids contain lytic enzymes that produce depolymerization of hyaluronic acid, which greatly impairs the lubricating ability of the fluid.

Purpose of Arthrocentesis

Arthrocentesis constitutes a liquid biopsy of the joint. It is a fundamental part of the clinical data base, together with the medical history, physical examination, and plain radiographic films. Analysis of aspirated synovial fluid is essential in the evaluation of any patient with joint disease because it provides a better reflection of the events in the articular cavity, compared to blood tests. For example, abnormal test results such as antinuclear antibody (ANA), increased erythrocyte sedimentation rate (ESR), elevated uric acid concentration, and rheumatoid factor can be seen in normal individuals or in unrelated joint diseases.

Disorders such as gout, calcium pyrophosphate dihydrate (CPPD) deposition disease, and septic arthritis can be diagnosed definitively by synovial fluid analysis and may allow for consideration or exclusion of rheumatoid arthritis and systemic lupus erythematosus (SLE). Synovial fluid analysis can also support a diagnosis of diseases as disparate as amyloidosis, hypothyroidism, ochronosis, hemochromatosis, and even simple edema.

In addition, arthrocentesis may alleviate elevated intraarticular pressure. The removal of fluid will relieve symptoms and potentially decrease joint damage. Removal of the products of inflammation is an important component in the treatment of infectious arthritis and may be beneficial in other forms of arthritis.

Aspiration

Arthrocentesis is the process performed by a physician for obtaining synovial fluid. It is readily obtained by aspiration

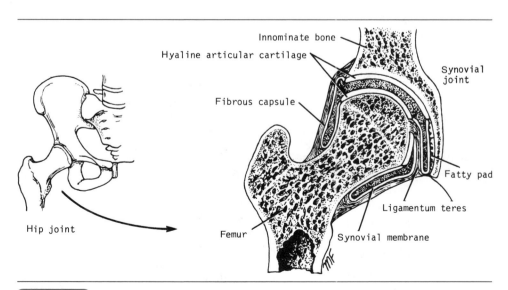

FIGURE 23.7 Example of synovial joint (hip joint). (From R. S. Snell, *Clinical Anatomy for Medical Students* [4th ed.]. Boston: Little, Brown & Co., 1992.)

from most joints. Frequent sites of aspiration include the knee, shoulder, elbow, wrist, interphalangeal joints, hip, and ankle.

Although aspiration was once performed in surgery, it is now considered to be a bedside procedure. As with other procedures involving potentially infectious fluids, gloves should be worn when performing an aspiration or handling the fluid. Infiltration of the site with lidocaine to decrease pain into the deeper, pain-sensitive structures of the capsule or periosteum increases the risk of injecting anesthetic into the joint space and can interfere with the results of some assays.

Laboratory Assays

Routine analysis of synovial fluid should include microscopic examination of a wet preparation, crystals, Gram stain, and microbiological culture. If the fluid is very turbid, or if septic arthritis is considered for other reasons, the specimen should be sent for Gram stain and culture. A Gram stain is needed if a high likelihood of infection exists.

Gross Examination

Other observations or procedures can include volume and appearance, viscosity, mucin test, chemical analysis for protein, and glucose.

Appearance

Synovial fluid is a plasma dialysate; however, certain molecules are preferentially excluded from the joint. Normal, noninflamed joints have small quantities of clear or transparent fluid. This fluid is viscous and slightly alkaline, and if normal, does not clot.

Inflammatory fluid can be translucent or opaque. In general, the more inflammatory the fluid is, the more opaque or purulent its appearance is, but there is no discrete gross appearance that separates infected from noninfected fluid. Cloudiness is not always the result of leukocytes. Fluids can also be opaque because of crystals or other materials (Table 23.15).

The color of synovial fluid ranges from pale yellow to straw-colored depending on the amount of albumin, bilirubin, cells, and other debris present. Edema produces relatively colorless fluid because of its low protein content. The presence of a grossly bloody fluid should raise the suspicion of a number of disorders (Table 23.16).

TABLE 23.15 Particulate Matter Found in Synovial Fluid

Adipose tissue fragments	Immune complexes
Amyloid fibrils	Lipid
Bacteria and fungi	Metal and plastic fragments
Cartilage fragments	Parasites
Cells	Rice bodies
Collagen fibrils	Synovial fragments
Crystals	Unrecognizable junk
Fibrin strands and clumps	

TABLE 23.16 Conditions Associated With Hemarthrosis

Amyloidosis (xanthochromia only)
Anticoagulant therapy
Ehlers-Danlos syndrome
Gaucher's disease
Hemangioma or arteriovenous malformation
Hereditary deficiency of clotting factors (e.g., hemophilia or von Willebrand's disease)
Idiopathic hemarthrosis
Infection
Metallic joint prostheses
Metastatic neoplasm of joints
Munchausen's syndrome
Myeloproliferative disease
Neuropathic joints
Osteoarthritis
Pigmented villonodular synovitis
Popliteal artery aneurysm
Postsurgery or prosthesis
Preexisting arthritis
Primary neoplasm of joints
Pseudogout
Pseudoxanthoma elasticum
Rheumatoid arthritis
Scurvy
Sickle cell disease (crisis)
Synovial hemangioma
Thrombocytopenia
Thrombocytosis
Trauma with or without fracture
Tumor

Source: Adapted from H. R. Schumacher, Jr. (ed.), Arthritis and Synovial Fluid Analysis, in *Primer on the Rheumatic Diseases* (9th ed.). Atlanta: Arthritis Foundation, 1988, p. 55.

Viscosity

The description of viscosity is a time-honored test. In fact, this property gave synovial fluid its name. If synovial fluid is allowed to drip from the aspirating needle, a long string implies high viscosity and an absent or short string implies low viscosity. An implied justification for estimating viscosity is to differentiate between noninflammatory (high-viscosity) and inflammatory (low-viscosity) fluids. Unusually viscous fluids are obtained from ganglia, hypothyroid effusions, and patients with SLE.

Mucin Clot

The best use of the mucin clot test is to distinguish the anatomical origin of bloody or other fluids. The presence of a mucin clot implies that it is synovial fluid.

The mucin clot procedure estimates the density and friability of the precipitate that forms when synovial fluid is placed in dilute acetic acid. The addition of several drops of normal synovial fluid to a dilute (2% to 5%) acetic acid solution results in the formation of a tight, sticky, ropelike mass (polymerization of synovial fluid hyaluronate) that remains intact when shaken. A good or excellent clot implies high–molecular-weight hyaluronic acid and normal hyaluronate-protein interactions. A fair or poor clot implies an inflammatory arthritis. There are, however, no standard criteria for performance of the test, and the end point is subjective.

Microscopic Examination

Wet Preparation Examination

Fresh synovial fluid should be examined under a clean coverslip by routine microscopy for cells and particulate material. Cytoplasmic inclusions within granulocytes sparkle and can appear to be light or dark. These inclusions are believed to represent distended phagosomes or droplets containing lipid. It is important to note whether crystalline material is intracellular or extracellular. In acute attacks of gout and pseudogout, crystals are engulfed by leukocytes. During intercritical periods, crystals may lie free in the fluid. Immunofluorescent studies have demonstrated that some inclusions contain immunoglobulins and complement.

Fracture or trauma to a joint can produce free lipid droplets in the synovial fluid, which can also be seen in aseptic necrosis and fat embolism. These droplets are rarely seen in inflammatory effusions. Irregular strands of fibrin or fibrillar fragments of cartilage may be observed in specimens from patients with degenerative arthritis.

Cells and other particulate matter should not be confused with crystalline materials. One basis for differentiation is that crystals have straight, parallel edges. In addition to routine light microscopy, examination with a polarized light microscope is recommended for the identification of crystals (Table 23.17).

Basic calcium phosphate (BCP) crystals include hydroxyapatite (HA), octacalcium phosphate, and tricalcium phosphate. The size of BCP crystals is below the limits of resolution of optical microscopy. If aggregated, they are visible by light microscopy and appear as shiny, laminated, printed coins. With a polarized microscope, BCP crystals are nonbirefringent.

BCP crystals are associated with subcutaneous calcification and calcific periarthritis and tendinitis. In addition, BCP crystals can be found in both acute and chronic synovitis.

Monosodium urate (MSU) (Plate 74) crystals are 8 to 10 μ in length and are needle- or rod-shaped. The crystals may be pointed and intracellular or extracellular. With a polarization microscope, MSU crystals appear as strongly birefringent rods or needles that are bright against a dark, fully polarized background. With a red compensator, they appear yellow in color when the longitudinal crystal axis is parallel (negative birefringence) to the slow component of the compensator. The crystals appear to be blue when perpendicular to the axis of the compensator.

MSU crystals are pathognomonic for gouty arthritis.

Calcium pyrophosphate dihydrate (CPPD) (Plate 75) crystals are more easily seen with a good light microscope.

CPPD crystals assume multiple, three-dimensional forms: rods, rhomboids, and parallel pipeds occur simultaneously.

With a polarizing microscope, CPPD crystals are less birefringent than MSU crystals and more difficult to identify. With a red compensator, CPPD crystals appear blue when the longitudinal axis is parallel to the slow component of the compensator. They exhibit positive birefringence. CPPD crystals are yellow when perpendicular to the axis of the compensator.

CPPD crystals are associated with CPPD deposition disease. However, they may be identified in effusions from a number of inflammatory joint diseases, particularly rheumatoid arthritis.

Cholesterol crystals are usually easy to distinguish because of their large size and flat, platelike shape. Characteristically, these rectangular plates have notched corners. They may, however, appear as long, birefringent needles or as rhomboids, resembling MSU or CPPD crystals.

The presence of cholesterol crystals is considered to be nonspecific. However, they are usually found in chronic effusions from patients with rheumatoid arthritis.

Artifacts can be mistaken for crystals, although crystals have sharp, clearly defined edges and straight sides. Particulate matter that can be confused with crystals include plastic joint prostheses, nail polish, dust particles, immersion oil droplets, and refractile collagen fibrils.

CPPD and MSU crystals can be confused with other birefringent materials including crystalline anticoagulants, such as calcium oxalate, ethylenediaminetetraacetic acid (EDTA), and lithium heparin; certain corticosteroid preparations; and talcum powder.

BODY FLUID SLIDE PREPARATION

A differential cell count on a body fluid should be performed on stained smears prepared from a concentrated preparation—not in a hemocytometer. Some of the techniques of sediment preparation and staining are different for body fluids than for blood.

Ordinary centrifugation can be used to concentrate cellular elements in the sediment and slides can be prepared with the traditional push method. This method has the advantage of requiring no special equipment, but the recovery of cells is variable and a considerable amount of cellular damage is produced.

More effective methods of concentrating cells include sedimentation, cytocentrifugation, and filtration. Filter techniques using Millipore (Millipore Corp.), Nucleopore (Nucleopore), or Gelman (Gelman Instrument Co.) products produce cell recovery but are more time-consuming than other methods and require more skill.

Staining of Body Fluid Sediment

Morphological descriptions of cells encountered in body fluids reflect their microscopic appearance with Wright or Wright-Giemsa stain. The coloration of cells with Papanicolaou stain (Table 23.20) is somewhat different. However, the Papanicolaou stain is a commonly used cytological stain.

The Wright-Giemsa stain is basically a cytoplasmic stain with moderate nuclear staining ability. In contrast, the Papa-

(*text continues on page 307*)

TABLE 23.17 Characteristics of Synovial Fluid Crystals

Crystal	Microscopic Appearance	With Polarization	Results of Alizarin Red Stain	Associated Disorders
Monosodium urate (MSU)	Acicular	Strongly negatively birefringent	Negative	Acute gouty arthritis Tophaceous gout
Calcium pyrophosphate dihydrate (CPPD)	Polymorphic	Weakly positively birefringent	Some are positive	CPPD deposition disease
Calcium hydroxyapatite	Too small to identify; with electron microscopy, as small needles or rods	Not birefringent	Positive red clumps are "putative" apatite crystals	Calcific tendinitis Apatite-associated destructive arthritis Soft tissue calcifications in the connective tissue diseases
Calcium oxalate	Polymorphic, classically bipyramidal	Variable; positively birefringent or strongly to weakly birefringent	Variable or positive	Chronic renal disease Oxalosis
Lipid liquid	"Maltese cross"	Strongly positively birefringent	Negative	Acute and chronic arthritis
Cholesterol	Large, platelike, with punched-out corners	Strongly variably birefringent	Negative	Chronic rheumatoid effusions
Corticosteroids	Polymorphic clumps, rods, or rhomboids	Strongly variably birefringent	Negative	Iatrogenic
Talc	Varying size	Strongly positively birefringent	Negative	Contaminant

Source: From P. R. Krey and D. M. Lazorra. *Analysis of Synovial Fluid.* Summit, NJ: Ciba-Geigy, 1992.

SYNOVIAL FLUID EXAMINATION PROCEDURE

Principle

Examination of synovial fluid can be diagnostic for several important disorders such as infectious (septic) or crystal-induced arthritis. This information may not be available in any other way. The most frequent use of synovial fluid analysis is to differentiate between inflammatory and noninflammatory arthritis. There is no other sufficiently reliable method for differentiating septic arthritis from acute crystal-induced arthritis or from severe episodes of idiopathic inflammatory arthritis.

The most commonly ordered routine procedures include Gram stain and culture, total leukocyte (WBC) and differential counts, and wet preparation for examination of crystals.

Specimen Collection and Preparation

Universal precautions (see Chapter 2) should be adhered to when performing and examining synovial fluid.

Aspiration of fluid is performed by a physician. The syringe should be moistened with an anticoagulant (25 units of sodium heparin/mL of synovial fluid). If adequate fluid is available, it should be collected into three tubes: 5 to 10 mL in a sterile tube for microbiology; 5 mL in an anticoagulated tube (heparin or liquid EDTA); and the last aliquot, which is allowed to clot, into a plain tube (no anticoagulant). The physician should perform a gross inspection of the fluid at the time of aspiration and note if any blood appeared in the syringe during aspiration or if the fluid was uniformly bloody.

The anticoagulated tube should be centrifuged promptly to remove all cells. The supernatant can be used for assays of rheumatoid factor, ANA, and complement and various biochemical procedures. If the specimen is unusually viscous, it may be difficult to perform several tests. The fluid may be digested with hyaluronidase for several hours prior to analysis.

If a dry tap occurs, a few drops of fluid in the needle can be used for microscopic examination or culture. In this case, leave the needle in the syringe and transport the specimens with the needle inserted into a sterile cork.

Visual and Microscopic Examination

Routine evaluation should consist of visual inspection of the color and clarity of the specimen, microbiological studies, total leukocyte and differential counts, and examination with a simple light and polarizing light microscope for crystals. In addition, other procedures may be helpful.

Volume effusions from all arthritides produce variable volumes of synovial fluid. An aspirated volume of more than 3.5 mL from the knee is considered abnormal. However, a very weak correlation exists between the volume and the origin or severity of the joint disease.

Normal synovial fluid does not clot. In inflammatory conditions, fibrinogen and other coagulation factors are present; clot formation does occur.

Normally, this fluid is clear and pale-yellow to straw-colored. A specimen that is uniformly bloody indicates prior hemarthrosis. A dark red or brown supernatant (in the centrifuged specimen) in the presence of grossly observed blood suggests hemarthrosis rather than a traumatic tap.

Turbidity (cloudiness) should be graded on a scale of 0 to 4+. Turbidity due to increased leukocytes suggests inflammation caused by septic or nonseptic conditions, such as bacterial infection, active gout, and rheumatoid arthritis. Crystal-induced synovitis may be demonstrated by purulent, milky, and occasionally greenish fluid. The presence of "rice bodies," products of de-generating, proliferative, synovial lining cells or of microinfarction of the synovium, may cause the fluid to resemble pus on gross examination. Cloudy, fatty fluid usually indicates the presence of cholesterol crystals, often seen in chronic arthritides. Droplets of free-floating fat frequently occur in trauma with or without fracture.

Microscopic Examination

Wet Preparation for Crystals

Compound light microscopy and phase contrast microscopy are good for distinguishing leukocytes from erythrocytes and for examining crystals. Polarized light microscopic examination usually reveals no crystals. Refer to the preceding discussion of the types, shapes, and clinical significance of the presence of various crystals.

Total Cell Count

Normal specimens have less than 0.2×10^9/L total leukocytes. If turbidity exists, a total leukocyte count should be performed. The total count can be performed with undiluted fluid unless the count is very high (more than 50.0×10^9/L). Physiological saline solution should be used as a diluent. Mix thoroughly. If the specimen is heavily contaminated with blood, the erythrocytes (RBCs) should be lysed using a diluent. Erythrocytes may or may not be counted. Because the concentration of erythrocytes is rarely of clinical significance, there is usually no point in having an RBC count.

A standard hemocytometer or a Fuchs-Rosenthal chamber can be used for counting. If the fluid is highly viscous, it may need to stand in the hemocytometer for more than 30 minutes before the cells settle and can be counted. Electronic counting equipment can be used, but may give spuriously high cell counts because it may count extracellular material such as crystals and fat globules.

Differential Cell Count

If the total leukocyte count is elevated, a differential count should be performed. The leukocyte differential is the most important clue to differential diagnosis in synovial fluid analysis. Although 0.5% methylene blue can be added to the total cell diluent, a differential cell count is most accurately obtained by using a Wright-stained preparation. The smears should be made as soon as possible. Smears should be as thin as possible because mucopolysaccharide and mucoproteins may obscure the cell structure.

Although synovial fluid is relatively acellular, the normal differential count is reported as the percentage of segmented neutrophils per 100 leukocytes. Normal values are less than 25%. The normal distribution of other cellular elements consists of more than 65% mononuclear phagocytes (monocytes and histiocytes) and a variable number of lymphocytes. No cartilaginous or inclusion-bearing cells are normally seen. The number of erythrocytes varies, but an increased number may result from a traumatic tap.

An increased percentage (more than 75 or 80%) of segmented neutrophils (PMNs) is characteristic of septic arthritis. Lymphocytes, including transformed lymphocytes (immunoblasts), are the predominant cell type in the early stages of rheumatoid arthritis, but in later stages a predominance of PMNs develops. The percentage of mononuclear cells (monocytes) in synovial fluid can be increased in arthritis, serum sick-

(continued)

SYNOVIAL FLUID EXAMINATION PROCEDURE (continued)

ness, and certain viral infections such as hepatitis and rubella. An increased representation of eosinophils can be observed in chronic urticaria and angioedema, rheumatic fever, parasitic infestation, metastatic disease, and rheumatoid arthritis, as well as after arthrography and radiation therapy.

Sources of Error
Specimens should be examined promptly. Synovial cells may alter the chemical composition of the fluid, which is an important consideration if a complement assay is requested. Complement levels should be determined within 2 to 3 hours after collection of the specimen, or the specimen should be frozen and stored at $-70°$ C until examination because complement is heat-labile.

Oxalate, powdered EDTA, and lithium heparin can produce artifacts in the microscopic examination for crystals.

Technical Notes: Staining presents some technical difficulties and false-positive reports are common. Precipitated stain, pyknotic extracellular nuclear material, and debris can be mistaken for microbial organisms. In particular, bacteria can be confused with precipitated hyaluronate mucin.

Total Leukocyte Count
Normal fluid is relatively acellular with less than 200×10^9/L leukocytes (WBC). The degree of elevation of the WBC count and the distribution of cell types (percentage of polymorphonuclear cells) in synovial fluid perform well as discriminators between inflammatory and noninflammatory disease (Table 23.18). These measurements indicate the severity of inflammation, suggest the likelihood of bacterial infection, and may help estimate the rate of potential joint destruction. The absolute cell count of PMNs is the major discriminating factor between an inflammatory and noninflammatory fluid. This information is essential to alert the physician as to how quickly a decision to initiate treatment is needed.

Fluids with fewer than 2.0×10^9/L leukocytes (WBC) are considered to be noninflammatory, although normal levels may be seen in some patients with systemic inflammatory diseases such as SLE or scleroderma. Many disorders other than osteoarthritis or mechanical conditions that exhibit noninflammatory fluids, as defined by the WBC count, are important to recognize. These disorders include sickle cell disease, hypertrophic pulmonary disorder, osteoarthropathy, hypothyroidism, and amyloidosis. Patients with active rheumatoid arthritis are unlikely to have synovial fluid with a WBC count less than 2.0×10^9/L.

Assessment of the clinical significance of synovial fluids with total leukocyte counts between 50 and 100×10^9/L is more difficult. Some septic fluids have counts in this range, or even

lower, especially in compromised or partially treated patients. In addition, gonococcal and tuberculosis infections do not elicit very high total WBC counts either. Fluids from patients with crystal-induced or idiopathic inflammatory arthritis, such as rheumatoid arthritis and Reiter's disease, commonly have counts in this intermediate range or even higher. However, a WBC count above 2.0×10^9/L in synovial fluid rules out simple osteoarthritis.

Fluids with severely elevated total WBC counts (higher than 100×10^9/L) should be considered septic until proved otherwise. In addition, the presence of crystals in such a highly inflammatory fluid does not rule out coexisting infection. Synovial fluids with leukocyte counts of more than 100×10^9/L demand a prompt therapeutic decision because of the high possibility of infectious arthritis and the potential for joint destruction.

Differential Leukocyte Count
Many different types of normal and abnormal cells and transient cell types have been identified in synovial fluid. Usually, there is no clinical reason to attempt to differentiate these cells beyond determining the percentages of neutrophils (PMNs) and mononuclear cells.

PMNs should constitute less than 25% of the total leukocyte count. The proportion of PMNs, not infrequently accounting for more than 90% of the total leukocyte count, is increased in inflammatory and septic conditions. In the early stages of rheumatoid arthritis or in certain infections such as tuberculosis, mononuclear cells may predominate, although patients with rheumatoid arthritis usually have less than 90%, even when the absolute cell count is very high. Many crystal-induced effusions also have a high proportion of neutrophils.

Cytology
The cellular characteristics of synovial fluid are independent of those in the peripheral blood. Cells such as neutrophils, lymphocytes, monocytes, eosinophils, plasma cells, macrophages, synovial lining cells, and LE cells can be observed in centrifuged specimens.

Erythrocytes (RBCs) and platelets are normally absent. The presence of sickled RBCs indicates the existence of a hemoglobinopathy in either the homozygous or the heterozygous state.

PMNs may contain inclusions such as fat droplets, crystals, bacteria, and vacuoles. It is common for nuclei to show pyknosis and karyorrhexis. **Ragocytes** or RA cells are neutrophils with small, dark cytoplasmic refractile granules. They are best identified by phase contrast microscopy. Immunofluorescent techniques have demonstrated that these peripheral inclusions consist of immune complexes such as IgG and IgM, complement, and rheumatoid factor. RA cells were originally described in rheumatoid arthritis but are considered to be nonspecific and are not diagnostically significant for rheumatoid arthritis.

Mononuclear phagocytes (monocytes, macrophages, and histiocytes) may be similar to blood monocytes. However, they frequently exhibit variable morphological structure and may be difficult to distinguish from the synovial lining cells that resemble mesothelial cells.

Occasionally, large synoviocytes are seen. These large mononuclear cells are derived from the synovial lining (synoviocytes) and do not appear to have any specific diagnostic significance.

Reiter's cells may be observed. These cells are vacuolated macrophages that contain neutrophilic or basophilic globular

TABLE 23.18   **Synovial Fluid Tests**

	Test Results	
Category	total WBC count	**PMN**
Noninflammatory	$<2 \times 10^9$/L	<75%
Inflammatory	$>2 \times 10^9$/L	>75%

Source: From R. H. Shmerling et al. Synovial fluid tests. *JAMA,* Vol. 264, 1990, pp. 1009–1014. Copyright 1990, American Medical Association.

(continued)

material or both. Reiter's cells may have ingested neutrophils or other cells. Although these cells were originally found in Reiter's disease, they also occur in other conditions. Therefore, they are not a specific indicator of Reiter's disease.

Cartilage cells are giant, multinucleated cells. They are typically seen in patients with osteoarthritis but may also appear in a number of arthritides.

The presence of LE cells (Plate 76) in freshly smeared and Wright-stained synovial fluid strongly suggests SLE. Typically LE cells may be found in centrifuged specimens from SLE effusions and, occasionally, in synovial fluid from patients with Felty's syndrome.

Clinical Applications
The distinction between various types of arthritis is not always easy to make on clinical grounds. In addition, the coexistence of two or more types of arthritis is not uncommon and correctly diagnosing the presence of more than one form of arthritis in a single joint is virtually impossible without synovial fluid analy-

TABLE 23.19	**Classification of Synovial Fluid**	
Group	**Description**
I	Noninflammatory
II	Inflammatory
III	Infectious
IV	Crystal-induced
V	Hemorrhagic

sis. Traditionally, synovial fluids have been classified into several categories (Table 23.19) based on gross appearance, total leukocyte and differential cell counts, and physical and chemical examination.

SLIDE PREPARATION

Push Method
Procedure
Refer to Chapter 2, page 25.

Coverslip Method
Procedure
Refer to Chapter 2, page 26.

Cytocentrifuge Method

Principle and Specimens
The cytospin centrifuge concentrates cells on a microscope slide into a uniform monolayer in an area 6 mm in diameter. The amount of required specimen varies, depending on the type of fluid. If the specimen is clear, 5 to 10 mL is needed; if it is cloudy, only a few drops are needed. Bloody specimens should be diluted 1:5 with saline solution before centrifugation. If a specimen is grossly bloody, a push smear is recommended.

Materials List
See Chapter 2 for materials.

Procedure
1. Place the cytocentrifuge cups into the centrifuge (Shandon cytocentrifuge, Shandon Southern Instrument Inc.) opposite each other. Smears should be prepared in duplicate.
2. Label the microscope slides with identifying information. Slides coated with 22% albumin and allowed to air-dry prior to use reduce the amount of cell distortion and increase the cell yield because the albumin enhances the laying down of filter fibers all over the slide. Slides should be rinsed in alcohol and dried prior to coating.
3. Place special white filter paper (if fluid is pleural, pericardial, peritoneal, or synovial) against a glass slide (hole toward the frosted end of the slide) in back of the cup. Brown filter cards should be used for CSF and fluids of small volume. These cards are thinner than white cards and will not absorb as much of the overall sample fluid.

   To delay fluid absorption and increase the cell yield, a small amount of immersion oil may be spread around the hole of the filter paper (1 cm in diameter) prior to centrifugation.
4. Make sure that the hole in the cup lines up with the hole in the carrier. You should be able to see the slide and filter pad through the outside window when placed in the centrifuge.
5. Set the timer for 10 minutes before placing the fluid in the cuvette.
6. Pour the fluid into the cup and cap the specimen. Pouring enhances the formation of an air block, which prevents seepage of the fluid out to the filter card until spinning begins. If a pipette is used, transfer the fluid gently by using a squeeze bulb. Too much pressure causes cellular damage and may cause fluid to run out to the filter card immediately before the concentration process begins.
7. A bumper rubber cork should be on each cuvette to maintain proper pressure on the cuvette-filter card-slide sandwich. If it is missing, leakage of fluid and loss of nucleated cells may occur. The bumpers can be left in cuvettes at all times.
8. Lock the safety lid into position. Start the centrifugation *immediately* to separate the cells from the fluid and deposit the concentrated specimen on the glass slide as soon as possible. The usual centrifugation speed is 600 to 1000 rpm for approximately 5 minutes. However, the speed and time of centrifugation may be varied to ensure maximum cell yield.

(continued)

SLIDE PREPARATION (continued)

9. Carefully remove the slide and filter paper together. If the specimen is difficult to see, with a wax pencil make a circle on the back of the slide around the concentrate. Discard the filter paper (treat as infectious waste).
10. Air-dry the slide before staining with Wright-Giemsa or Wright stain or fix the slide immediately in 95% alcohol for Papanicolaou staining.
11. Soak the cytocentrifuge cups in a dilute bleach solution for at least 15 minutes for decontamination. Then wash and rinse the cups in tap and distilled water and air-dry.

Sedimentation Method

Procedure

1. Punch a round hole approximately 1 cm in diameter in the center of 9-cm (Whatman No. 2 W&R) filter paper.
2. Wrap the filter paper around a microscope slide so that the hole is in the center of the slide.
3. Transfer 0.2 to 1.0 mL of fresh fluid into a shallow, disposable, 1.8-mL plastic cup (available from Matheson Scientific Co.). The amount of required fluid varies, depending on the cell concentration in the specimen.
4. Center the hole of the wrapped slide over the mouth of the cup. The slide should cover the cup mouth completely.
5. Hold the slide and cup together with one hand. With the other hand, place a No. 18 ball-and-socket-joint pinch clamp onto the slide. Place one side of the clamp above the slide and the other beneath the ledge around the lip of the cup.
6. When the cup and slide are secure, turn the entire setup over so the cup is inverted.
7. Allow the fluid to settle for 20 to 30 minutes. The fluid should be absorbed by the filter paper and the cells should settle on the exposed surface of the slide.
8. When the cup is empty, carefully remove the cup and paper. Discard the cup and paper as infectious waste.
9. Allow the slide to air-dry for a few minutes before staining with Wright-Giemsa or Wright stain. Place the slide in alcohol fixative if a Papanicolaou stain is to be performed.

TABLE 23.20 **Papanicolaou Stained Morphology**

Cell Type	Nucleus	Cytoplasm
Neutrophils (mature)	Multilobulated; hyperchromatic	Green or pink; granules not evident
Neutrophils (immature)		Green or pink; primary granules not visible; secondary granules present
Lymphocytes	Round with finely granular chromatin; no nucleolus visible	Green; absent or scanty
Lymphocytes (reactive)	Oval to cleaved; finely granular with evenly distributed chromatin; small chromocenter	Green; moderate amount
Monocyte (usually macrophages in pleural fluid)	Lacy	Some color; modrate amount; slightly vacuolated
Macrophage	Lacy chromatin pattern; irregular shape	Green; degenerating cell may be pink
Mesothelial cell	Size variable (may occupy up to 50% of cell); round to oval; usually central; well-defined membrane; evenly distributed granular chromatin; small nucleoli may be present; multinucleated	Deep pink or green; homogeneous distribution; may be more densely stained in center of cell and around the nucleus; pale cytoplasmic vacuoles may be seen
Ependymal cells	Round; central dense chromatin; may be grainy or possible nucleoli	Green or pink; may have "brush" borders; generous amount
Choroidal cells	Round; central, smooth, dense chromatin	Pale green; moderate amount
Plasma cells	Round to oval; eccentrically located; clumped chromatin	Dense and green; abundant; paranuclear area present; may contain small vacuoles (e.g., Russell bodies, "grape cells")
Basophils		Granules do not stain

STAINING PROCEDURES

Wright-Giemsa Stain or Wright Stain

Either manual or automated techniques can be used to stain body fluid sediments (see Chapter 2 for a discussion of the staining procedure).

Papanicolaou Stain

Reagents and Equipment
1. Alcohol solutions prepared with reagent-grade ethyl alcohol:
   A. 95% ethyl alcohol: Dilute 950 mL of reagent alcohol to 1 L with distilled water.
   B. 80% ethyl alcohol: Dilute 840 mL of reagent alcohol to 1 L with distilled water.
   C. 70% ethyl alcohol: Dilute 737 mL of reagent alcohol to 1 L with distilled water.
   D. 50% ethyl alcohol: Dilute 526 mL of reagent alcohol to 1 L with distilled water.
2. Xylol, reagent grade (use in a well-ventilated area)
3. 1.0% hydrochloric acid (HCl): Add 1 mL of concentrated HCl to approximately 95 mL of distilled water. Mix and dilute to 100 mL with distilled water.
4. Dilute lithium carbonate ($LiCO_3$)
   Stock solution:
   A. Add approximately 950 mL of distilled water to a volumetric flask.
   B. Weigh out 200 gm of $LiCO_3$, add to the distilled water, and shake vigorously to mix. Some sediment will appear on the bottom of the flask.
   C. Dilute this solution to 1 L with distilled water. Mix and transfer to an appropriately labeled brown bottle with a cap, for storage.
   Working solution (prepare fresh daily or as needed):
   A. Thoroughly mix (by shaking) the stock solution prior to use.
   B. Add 8 drops of stock solution to 400 mL of distilled water and mix.
   C. Add the needed quantity to the staining jar.

5. Papanicolaou stains (hematoxylin, EA 65, and orange G-6) are usually purchased in a ready-to-use form.
6. Staining rack or Coplin staining jars
7. Automatic timer
8. Coverslips and mounting fluid

   Note: Store all flammable reagents in an appropriately designated area.

Procedure
Prestain fixation: Place slides into a slide carrier and insert into a Coplin jar containing 95% ethyl alcohol for a *minimum* of 5 minutes.
   Staining:
1. 80% ethyl alcohol—10 dips
2. 70% ethyl alcohol—10 dips
3. 50% ethyl alcohol—10 dips
4. Distilled water—10 dips
5. Hematoxylin—3-1/2 minutes (blood and body fluids)
6. Tap water—2 changes
7. 1.0% HCl—4 quick dips
8. Tap water—2 changes
9. Dilute lithium carbonate—1 minute
10. Running tap water—5 minutes
11. Distilled water—10 dips
12. 50% ethyl alcohol—10 dips
13. 70% ethyl alcohol—10 dips
14. 80% ethyl alcohol—10 dips
15. 95% ethyl alcohol—10 dips
16. Orange G-6—1-1/2 minutes
17. 95% ethyl alcohol—10 dips
18. 95% ethyl alcohol—10 dips
19. EA 65—3 minutes
20. 95% ethyl alcohol—10 dips
21. 95% ethyl alcohol—10 dips
22. Absolute alcohol—10 dips
23. Absolute alcohol—10 dips
24. Absolute xylol (50-50)—10 dips
25. Xylol—10 dips
26. Xylol—5 minutes
27. Xylol—5 minutes
28. Air-dry and coverslip specimen with mounting fluid

nicolaou stain is predominantly a nuclear stain with a modest ability for cytoplasmic differentiation. The Wright-Giemsa staining method is simpler than the Papanicolaou method because it requires no immediate fixation of the slide and therefore fewer steps in the staining procedure. However, a difference in cell size is evident between the two staining protocols. Cells appear larger when prepared by the air-dried, Wright-Giemsa procedure. It is most helpful, if possible, to prepare and stain specimens by both methods in order to gain as much information as possible. The criteria for diagnosis are exactly the same for normal or abnormal cells by either method.

SUMMARY

Sterile body fluid can be found in various body cavities under normal conditions. In diverse disorders and disease processes, the quantity of these fluids can increase significantly. Specimens can be analyzed for the total number of cells, differentiation of cell types, chemical composition, and microbial contents depending on the source of the aspirate. Universal precautions must be practiced.

Cerebrospinal Fluid

Cerebrospinal fluid (CSF) acts as a shock absorber for the brain and spinal cord, circulates nutrients, lubricates the central nervous system (CNS), and may also contribute to the nourishment of brain tissue. CSF is found inside all the ventricles, in the central canal of the spinal cord, and in the subarachnoid space around both the brain and the spinal cord. The total maximum volume of CSF is about 150 mL in adults and approximately 60 mL in neonates. In the laboratory, a specimen of CSF is examined visually and microscopically. Clinically, the examination of spinal fluid is useful in diagnosing a variety of disorders including subarachnoid hemorrhage, meningeal infection (meningitis), multiple sclerosis, and neoplasms.

Normal CSF is crystal clear and colorless. Any presence of color should be noted. A yellow coloring of a specimen or the supernatant of a centrifuged specimen is referred to as xanthochromia. This discoloration is caused by the release of hemoglobin from hemolyzed erythrocytes (RBCs) in the CSF. Gross blood may also be observed in traumatic tap specimens or in cases of pathological bleeding due to spontaneous subarachnoid hemorrhage or intracerebral hemorrhage. Normal CSF has the viscosity of water. Clotting can be due to increased protein. Gel formation on standing is due to an increased fibrinogen content.

Total WBC counts are useful in developing a differential diagnosis. Very few leukocytes should be seen in normal CSF. Elevated WBC counts can be observed in acute, untreated, bacterial meningitis. Very high WBC counts are unusual and suggest intraventricular rupture of a brain abscess. Normal CSF contains a few mononuclear cells (lymphocytes and monocytes) and rare ependymal cells. Cells that may be encountered in CSF include granulocytic leukocytes (mature and immature neutrophils, eosinophils, and basophils), mature lymphocytes or reactive lymphocytes, mononuclear phagocytes (monocytes, histiocytes, and macrophages), plasma cells, ependymal cells and choroidal cells, leukemic blasts, and malignant cells (e.g., lymphoma cells or tumor cells). Other types of cells can include immature, nucleated erythrocytes or intracellular bacteria. LE cells are rarely observed in the CSF.

Glucose and protein values are important to correlate with gross and microscopic findings. In general, a decreased glucose level in the CSF in the presence of a normal blood glucose level indicates bacterial utilization of glucose. In addition, an elevated total protein concentration is suggestive of an inflammatory reaction or a bacterial infection. A viral infection will not have a dramatic effect on CSF glucose levels and may not affect the total protein level significantly.

Pleural, Peritoneal, and Pericardial Fluids

An **effusion** is an abnormal accumulation of fluid in a particular space of the body. Effusions in the plural, pericardial, and peritoneal cavities are divided into transudates or exudates. **Transudates** generally indicate that fluid has accumu-

lated because of the presence of a systemic disease. In contrast, **exudates** are usually associated with disorders such as inflammation, infection, and malignant conditions involving the cells that line the surfaces of organs (e.g., lung or abdominal organs). Transudates and exudates frequently differ in characteristics such as color and clarity and total leukocyte cell count.

Pleural fluid is normally produced by the parietal pleura and absorbed by the visceral pleura, as a continuous process. Although healthy individuals form 600 to 800 mL of fluid daily, the normal volume of fluid in each pleural space is estimated to be less than 10 mL. The accumulation of fluid in the pleural space is referred to as a pleural effusion. Aspiration of pleural fluid is referred to as **thoracentesis.** The location of a pleural effusion may be suggestive of the type of disorder involved in causing the effusion. Erythrocyte and leukocyte counts are of limited value in the differential diagnosis of pleural effusions. A massively bloody (hemorrhagic) effusion in the absence of trauma almost always suggests malignancy or occasionally pulmonary infarct. Pure blood in pleural cavity, true hemothorax, results from severe chest injuries. Extremely elevated total WBC counts are consistent with a diagnosis of empyema. Cell types that can be encountered in the examination of a Wright-Giemsa–stained specimen include polymorphonuclear neutrophils (PMNs), eosinophils, basophils, lymphocytes, plasma cells, mononuclear phagocytes (monocytes, histiocytes, and macrophages), mesothelial cells (normal, reactive, atypical, or malignant), and metastatic tumor (malignant) cells. In addition, in vivo LE cells have also been observed in pleural fluids.

The presence of peritoneal fluid reduces friction between the visceral and parietal peritonea as they move against each other. An abnormal amount of fluid (an effusion) can accumulate in the peritoneal cavity if the balance between fluid formation and reabsorption is altered by a disease process. The collection of fluid in the peritoneal cavity is called **ascites.** The procedure for removing fluid from the peritoneal cavity is paracentesis. The causes of peritoneal effusions range from disorders and diseases that directly represent involvement of the peritoneum, such as bacterial peritonitis, to abdominal conditions that do not directly involve the peritoneum, such as hepatic cirrhosis, cirrhosis, congestive heart failure, Budd-Chiari syndrome, hypoalbuminemia (due to nephrotic syndrome or protein-losing enteropathy malnutrition), and miscellaneous disorders such as myxedema, ovarian diseases, pancreatic disease, and chylous ascites. A variety of clinical conditions can produce a deviation from the anticipated yellow or straw-colored fluid seen on gross examination. For example, grossly bloody (hemorrhagic) peritoneal fluid may be seen in trauma patients with a ruptured spleen or liver, intestinal infarction, pancreatitis, or malignancies. Total RBC and WBC counts are usually performed on ascitic fluid. Smears should be prepared for microscopic examination and properly stained with Wright or Wright-Giemsa stain for differential leukocyte evaluation or stained with Papanicolaou stain for cytological evaluation.

Although the quantities of some cells in peritoneal fluid compared to pleural fluid may vary in some disorders, the cell types that can be encountered are the same as those that can be seen in pleural fluids. These cells include PMNs, eosinophils, basophils, lymphocytes, plasma cells, mononuclear phagocytes (monocytes, histiocytes, and macrophages), mesothelial cells (normal, reactive, atypical, or malignant), and metastatic tumor (malignant) cells. In addition, in vivo LE cells have also been observed.

The pericardium is filled with a small amount of fluid to reduce friction between the layers of the pericardial cavity. An abnormal accumulation of fluid in the cavity is called a **pericardial effusion.** Pericardial effusion is usually accurately assessed by echocardiography. A wide variety of diseases and disorders can produce pericardial effusion. Neoplastic disease, which produces a significant volume of fluid in the pericardium, is one of the most common causes of pericardial effusion. Normal fluid is transparent and pale yellow. Hemorrhagic (bloody) effusions may result from a variety of abnormal conditions or from aspiration of intracardiac blood into the specimen. Pericardial fluid is relatively acellular.

Seminal Fluid

The main function of seminal fluid is to transport sperm to the female cervical mucus. Seminal fluid is examined physically, chemically, and microscopically. These procedures are performed in order to determine the physical and chemical properties, to quantitate the number of sperm cells, and to examine cellular motility and morphology. Fresh specimens should be examined for color, pH, volume, and viscosity. Increased viscosity can be of significance if it impedes sperm motility. Several microscopic procedures may be of value in the assessment of seminal fluid. Enumeration of the number of sperm and examination of the morphological characteristics of the cells are routinely performed procedures. Other microscopic procedures may include motility, viability, and agglutination studies. Other techniques for the examination of semen may be requested in various situations. In cases of infertility, cervical mucus–sperm compatibility tests may be warranted to determine whether the sperm cells are able to penetrate the cervical mucus.

Seminal fluid can be analyzed for a variety of reasons, including infertility studies, artificial insemination protocols, postvasectomy assessment, and evaluation of probable sexual assault. In cases of alleged rape or suspected sexual assault, vaginal smears may be submitted for evaluation of the presence of sperm.

Synovial Fluid

Synovial fluid is a transparent, viscous fluid secreted by the synovial membrane. This fluid is found in joint cavities, bursae, and tendon sheaths. Its function is to lubricate the joint space and transport nutrients to the articular cartilage. Impaired function of synovial fluid with age or disease may play a role in the development of degenerative joint disease (osteoarthritis). A variety of disorders produce changes in the number and types of cells and the chemical composition of the fluid.

Analysis of synovial fluid plays a major role in the diagnosis of joint diseases. Arthrocentesis constitutes a liquid biopsy of the joint. Analysis of aspirated synovial fluid is essential in the evaluation of any patient with joint disease because it provides a better reflection of the events in the articular cavity than blood tests do. For example, abnormal test results such as antinuclear antibody (ANA), increased erythrocyte sedimentation rate (ESR), elevated uric acid level, and rheumatoid factor can be seen in normal individuals or in unrelated joint diseases. Disorders such as gout, CPPD deposition disease, and septic arthritis can be diagnosed definitively by synovial fluid analysis and may allow for consideration or exclusion of rheumatoid arthritis and SLE. Synovial fluid analysis can also support a diagnosis of diseases as disparate as amyloidosis, hypothyroidism, ochronosis, hemochromatosis, and even simple edema. In addition, arthrocentesis may alleviate elevated intraarticular pressure.

Body Fluid Slide Preparation

A differential cell count on a body fluid should be performed on stained smears prepared from a concentrated preparation—not in a hemocytometer. Ordinary centrifugation can be used to concentrate cellular elements in the sediment and slides can be prepared with the traditional push method. More effective methods of concentrating cells include sedimentation, cytocentrifugation, and filtration.

BIBLIOGRAPHY

Baer, Daniel M. "Semen Analysis." *Med. Lab. Observer,* Vol. 18, No. 5, May, 1991, p. 11.

Barrett, Richard E. "Differences in the Quality of Semen in Outdoor Workers During Summer and Winter Months." *N. Engl. J. Med.,* Vol. 323, No. 22, 1990, pp. 1563–1564.

Bradstock, K. F., E. S. Papgeorgiou, and G. Janossy. "Diagnosis of Meningeal Involvement in Patients With Acute Lymphoblastic Leukemia." *Cancer,* Vol. 47, 1981, pp. 2478–2481.

Braunwald, Eugene et al. "Ascites," in *Harrison's Principles of Internal Medicine* (12th edition). Jean D. Wilson (ed.). New York: McGraw-Hill, 1988, pp. 70–74.

Cannon, Donald C. and John B. Henry. "Seminal Fluid," in *Clinical Diagnosis and Management by Laboratory Methods* (18th edition). John B. Henry (ed.). Philadelphia: Saunders, 1991, pp. 497–503.

Chopra, Sanjiv. "Diseases of the Peritoneum, Mesentery, and Omentum," in *Internal Medicine.* Jay H. Stein (ed.). Boston: Little, Brown & Co., 1990, pp. 556–559.

Creager, Joan G. *Human Anatomy and Physiology.* Belmont, CA: Wadsworth Publishing, 1983, pp. 543–544.

Cush, John J. and Peter E. Lipsky. "Approach to Articular and Musculoskeletal Disorders," in *Harrison's Principles of Internal Medicine* (12th edition). Jean D. Wilson (ed.). New York: McGraw-Hill, 1990, pp. 1472–1473.

Cutler, R. W. P. and R. B. Spertell. "Cerebrospinal Fluid: A Selective Review." *Ann. Neurol.,* Vol. 11, 1982, pp. 1–10.

Dacey, Ralph G., Jr. and H. Richard Winn. "Brain Abscess and Perimeningeal Infections," in *Internal Medicine.* Jay H. Stein (ed.). Boston: Little, Brown & Co., 1990, pp. 1291–1292.

Dever, Bill. "Visualizing Brain Hemorrhage Is Tricky, Even With MR and CT." *Radiol. Today,* December, 1990, p. 13.

Dowdeswell, R. G. "Pleural Diseases," in *Internal Medicine.* Boston: Little, Brown & Co., 1990, pp. 737–744.

Dyken, P. R. "Cerebrospinal Fluid Cytology: Practical Clinical Usefulness." *Neurology,* Vol. 25, 1975, pp. 210–217.

Eastern, J. Donald. "Spinal Fluid Examination," in Jay H. Stein (ed.). *Internal Medicine.* Boston: Little, Brown & Co., 1990, pp. 1870–1871.

Finegold, Sydney M. and Ellen J. Barron (eds.). "Microorganisms Encountered in Solid Tissue, Bone, Bone Marrow, and Body Fluids," in *Diagnostic Microbiology* (7th edition). St. Louis: Mosby-Year Book, 1986, pp. 315–321.

Hoffman, Gary S. "Arthritis Due to Deposition of Calcium Crystals," in *Harrison's Principles of Internal Medicine* (12th edition). Jean D. Wilson (ed.). New York: McGraw-Hill, 1990, pp. 1479–1482.

Izzat, N. N. et al. "Validity of the VDRL Test on Cerebrospinal Fluid Contaminated by Blood." *Br. J. Vener. Dis.*, Vol. 47, 1971, pp. 162–164.

Jones, C. D. and P. J. Cornbleet. "Wright-Giemsa Cytology of Body Fluids." *Lab. Med.*, Vol. 28, No. 11, November, 1997, pp. 713–716.

Judkins, S. W. and P. J. Cornbleet. "Synovial Fluid Crystal Analysis." *Lab. Med.*, Vol. 28, No. 12, December, 1997, pp. 774–779.

Krieg, Arthur F. and C. R. Kjeldsberg. "Cerebrospinal Fluid and Other Body Fluids," in *Clinical Management and Diagnosis by Laboratory Methods*. J. B. Henry (ed.). Philadelphia: Saunders, 1991, pp. 445–457, 463–469.

Lipsky, Peter E. "Rheumatoid Arthritis," in *Harrison's Principles of Internal Medicine* (12th edition). Jean D. Wilson (ed.). New York: McGraw-Hill, 1990, pp. 1437–1471.

Lyons, Mark K. and Fredric B. Meyer. "Cerebrospinal Fluid Physiology and the Management of Increased Intracranial Pressure." *Mayo Clin. Proc.*, Vol. 65, May, 1990, pp. 684–707.

McCarty, Daniel J. "Arthritis Associated With Calcium-Containing Crystals," in *Internal Medicine*. Jay H. Stein (ed.). Boston: Little, Brown & Co., 1990, pp. 1809–1813.

Miller, S. M. "Saliva: New Interest in a Non-Traditional Specimen." *MLO*, April, 1993, pp. 31–35.

Nakamura, Robert M. "Spermatid." *Med. Lab. Observer*, Vol. 18, No. 9, September, 1991, p. 13.

Nosanchuck, J. S. and C. W. Kim. "Lupus Erythematosus Cells in CSF." *JAMA*, Vol. 25, 1976, pp. 2883–2884.

Oehmichen, M., D. Domasch, and H. Wietholter. "Origin, Proliferation and Fate of Cerebrospinal Fluid Cells." *J. Neurol.*, Vol. 227, 1982, pp. 145–150.

"Pericardial Diseases," in *Medical Knowledge Self-Assessment Program VIII, Cardiovascular Medicine*, Part C, Book 3. Philadelphia: American College of Physicians, 1988, pp. 836–837.

"Pleural Effusions," in *Medical Knowledge Self-Assessment Program VIII, Pulmonary Medicine*, Part A, Book 6. Philadelphia: American College of Physicians, 1988, p. 231.

"Rheumatology," in *Medical Knowledge Self-Assessment Program VIII*, Part B, Book 6. Philadelphia: American College of Physicians, 1988.

Rotrosen, Daniel. "Infectious Arthritis," in *Harrison's Principles of Internal Medicine* (12th edition). Jean D. Wilson (ed.). New York: McGraw-Hill, 1990, pp. 544–549.

Sampson, J. H. and N. J. Alexander. "Semen Analysis: A Laboratory Approach." *Lab. Med.*, Vol. 13, 1982, pp. 218–223.

Schumacher, H. Ralph, Jr. (ed.). "Arthrocentesis and Synovial Fluid Analysis," in *Primer on the Rheumatic Diseases* (9th edition). Atlanta: Arthritis Foundation, 1988, pp. 55–60, 79–80.

Schumacher, H. Ralph, Jr. "Synovial Fluid Analysis," in *Textbook of Rheumatology*. William N. Kelley et al. (eds.). Philadelphia: Saunders, 1985, pp. 561–568.

Schumann, G. B. and G. Linker. "Cytopreparatory Techniques for Bronchoalveolar Lavage Specimens." *Lab. Med.*, Vol. 23, No. 2, February, 1992, pp. 115–119.

Shabetai, Ralph and Martin M. Le Winter. "Pericardial Disease and Pericardial Heart Disease," in *Internal Medicine*. Jay H. Stein (ed.). Boston: Little, Brown & Co., 1990, pp. 189–193.

Shmerling, Robert H. et al. "Synovial Fluid Tests—What Should Be Ordered?" *JAMA*, Vol. 264, No. 8, August 22/29, 1990, pp. 1201–1203.

Strickland, Daniel M. and Paul R. Ziaya. "Reduced Sperm Motility in Plastic Containers." *Lab. Med.*, Vol. 18, No. 5, May, 1987, pp. 310–312.

Tunkel, Allan R. and W. Michael Scheld. "Acute Meningitis," in *Internal Medicine*. Jay H. Stein (ed.). Boston: Little, Brown & Co., 1990, pp. 1281–1290.

Tur-Kaspa, Ilan and Alan B. Dudkiewicz. "Differences in the Quality of Semen in Outdoor Workers During Summer and Winter Months." *N. Engl. J. Med.*, Vol. 323, No. 22, 1990, p. 1564.

Vaitkus, P. T., H. C. Herrmann, and M. M. LeWinter. "Treatment of Malignant Pericardial Effusion." *JAMA*, Vol. 272, No. 1, July 6, 1994, pp. 59–64.

Wallach, Jacques. *Interpretation of Diagnostic Tests* (5th edition). Boston: Little, Brown & Co., 1991.

Walters, J. "Hematology and the Analysis of Body Fluids." *Advance for Medical Laboratory Professionals*, Vol. 8, No. 9, April 29, 1996, pp. 10–11, 18–19.

Weisman, Michael H. and Adolf W. Karchmer. "Infections of the Joints," in *Internal Medicine*. Jay H. Stein (ed.). Boston: Little, Brown & Co., 1990, pp. 1780–1786.

WHO Laboratory Manual for Examination of Human Semen and Semen–Cervical Mucus Interaction. New York: Cambridge University Press, 1987.

Zvaifler, Nathan J. "Synovial Fluid Analysis," in *Internal Medicine*. Jay H. Stein (ed.). Boston: Little, Brown & Co., 1990, pp. 1681–1684.

REVIEW QUESTIONS

Questions 1 to 5: match each of the respective terms with their appropriate synonyms.

1. ___ Cerebrospinal fluid.
2. ___ Synovial fluid.
3. ___ Peritoneal fluid.
4. ___ Pericardial fluid.
5. ___ Pleural fluid.

A. Lumbar puncture fluid.

B. Joint fluid.

C. Chest fluid.

D. Ascitic fluid.

E. Fluid from around the heart.

Questions 6 to 8: match the fluids with the appropriate normal characteristics.

6. ___ Cerebrospinal fluid.
7. ___ Synovial fluid.
8. ___ Seminal fluid.

A. Clear and yellow.

B. Turbid and viscous.

C. Clear and colorless.

Questions 9 to 11: match the fluids and normal total leukocyte or total sperm count.

9. ___ Cerebrospinal fluid.
10. ___ Synovial fluid.
11. ___ Seminal fluid.

A. 0 to 10×10^6/L.

B. 60 to 150×10^9/L.

C. Less than 200/μL.

12. The anatomical structures associated with the circulation of cerebrospinal fluid (CSF) are:
    A. Ventricles and subarachnoid spaces.
    B. Subarachnoid space and pia mater.
    C. Ependyma and pia mater.
    D. Arachnoid mater and pia mater.

13. CSF production is associated with the:
    A. Arachnoid mater and pia mater.
    B. Choroid plexus and ependymal lining.
    C. Arachnoid mater and subarachnoid space.
    D. Subarachnoid space and pia mater.

14. CSF is collected from an intervertebral space between the ___ and ___ vertebrae.
    A. T4, T5.   C. L3, L4.
    B. L2, L3.   D. L4, L5.

Questions 15 to 17: match the following test tube aliquots of CSF with the typical type of testing that should be performed.

15. ___ Tube 1.
16. ___ Tube 2.
17. ___ Tube 3.

    A. Gross examination, cell count, and morphology.
    B. Microbial examination.
    C. Chemical and serological examination.

Questions 18 to 21: match the following gross examination findings of CSF with the appropriate diagnosis.

18. ___ Cloudy and turbid.
19. ___ Grossly bloody specimen.
20. ___ Xanthochromia (yellow color).
21. ___ Gel formation.

    A. Increased fibrinogen.
    B. Subarachnoid hemorrhage.
    C. Subarachnoid hemorrhage (more than 12 hours after the bleed).
    D. Pleocytosis.

Questions 22 to 26: match the following microscopic findings of CSF with the associated condition.

22. ___ Intraventricular rupture of brain abscess.
23. ___ Viral infection.
24. ___ 0 to 5 × 10⁶/L.
25. ___ Bacterial infection.
26. ___ CNS leukemia or lymphoma.

    A. Lymphocytosis.
    B. Increased segmented neutrophils (PMNs).
    C. Macrophages.
    D. Extremely elevated leukocyte count in CSF.
    E. Normal leukocyte reference range for CSF.

27. Normal CSF contains:
    A. Lymphocytes and ependymal cells.
    B. Ependymal and choroidal cells.
    C. Mesothelial and ependymal cells.
    D. Erythrocytes and leukocytes.

28. The cell count on a CSF specimen should be performed within ___ of collection.
    A. 30 minutes.   D. 12 hours.
    B. 1 hour.   E. 24 hours.
    C. 2 hours.

29. Clotting in CSF may be due to:
    A. Increased protein concentration.
    B. Increased electrolyte concentration.
    C. Increased glucose concentration.
    D. The presence of bacteria.

30. An increased total leukocyte count in a CSF specimen can be due to:
    A. Bacterial meningitis.
    B. Viral meningoencephalitis.
    C. Intravascular rupture of a brain abscess.
    D. Both A and C.

31. An increase in the number of lymphocytes in a CSF specimen can be caused by:
    A. Multiple sclerosis.
    B. Viral meningoencephalitis.
    C. Fungal meningitis.
    D. All of the above.

32. Which of the following is (are) characteristic of an effusion?
    A. Abnormal accumulation of fluid.
    B. Can be a transudate.
    C. Can be an exudate.
    D. All of the above.

33. A transudate can be described as:
    A. Specific gravity >1.016, low to moderate number of leukocytes, and lactic dehydrogenase <200 IU/L.
    B. Specific gravity <1.016, pH 7.4 to 7.5, and lactic dehydrogenase <200 IU/L.
    C. pH 7.35 to 7.45 and protein concentration >3.0 gm/dL.
    D. Lactic dehydrogenase <200 IU/L and protein concentration >3.0 gm/dL.

Questions 34 to 36: match the term with the appropriate physical description.

34. ___ Pleura.
35. ___ Peritoneum.
36. ___ Pericardium.

    A. Covers abdominal walls and viscera of the abdomen.
    B. Covers the lungs.
    C. A fibrous sac around the heart.

37. Conditions not associated with pleural effusion include:
    A. Tuberculosis.
    B. Infectious diseases.
    C. Mesothelioma.
    D. Viral pneumonia.

Questions 38 to 42: match the representative exudate appearance with a typical associated disorder.

38. ___ Yellow and turbid.
39. ___ Milky.
40. ___ Bloody.
41. ___ Clearly visible pus.
42. ___ Foul odor.

    A. Empyema.
    B. Infectious process.
    C. Anaerobic bacterial infection.
    D. Chylothorax.
    E. Malignancy in the absence of trauma.

43. Pleural fluid can have a white supernatant fluid after centrifugation due to:
    A. Increased concentration of leukocytes.
    B. Presence of lipids.
    C. Presence of chylomicrons.
    D. Both A and B.

44. An extremely elevated leukocyte concentration in pleural fluid is typically associated with:
    A. Hemothorax.
    B. Malignancy.
    C. Empyema.
    D. Classic rheumatoid effusion.

45. Which of the following cells can be seen in pleural fluid?
    A. LE cells.
    B. Mononuclear phagocytes.
    C. Mesothelial cells.
    D. All of the above can be seen.

46. All of the following describe the characteristics of malignant cells except:
    A. Multiple round aggregates of cells.
    B. High N:C ratio.
    C. Large, irregular nucleoli.
    D. Smooth chromatin.

Questions 47 to 50: match the cellular abnormality encountered in pleural and peritoneal fluids with a representative disorder. (Use an answer only once.)

47. ___ Many neutrophils, histiocytes, and mesothelial cells.
48. ___ Abundant, multinuclear cells, and clusters of cells.
49. ___ Many malignant cells (in clusters).
50. ___ Many lymphocytes, mesothelial cells, histiocytes, and plasma cells.

A. Viral infection.
B. Acute bacterial inflammation.
C. Metastatic adenocarcinoma.
D. Malignant mesothelioma.
E. Chronic granulomatous inflammation.

Questions 51 and 52: in a pleural effusion, the percentage of (51) ___ is extremely high in pneumonia and the percentage of (52) ___ is extremely high in viral peritonitis.

51.
    A. Segmented neutrophils.   C. Basophils.
    B. Eosinophils.   D. Monocytes.

52.
    A. Segmented neutrophils.   C. Basophils.
    B. Eosinophils.   D. Lymphocytes.

53. The causes of peritoneal effusion include all of the following except:
    A. Bacterial peritonitis.
    B. Hepatic cirrhosis.
    C. Congestive heart failure.
    D. Tuberculosis.

54. An abnormal-appearing peritoneal effusion can be caused by all of the following except:
    A. Bacterial peritonitis.
    B. Pancreatitis.
    C. Neoplasm.
    D. Tuberculous peritonitis.

Questions 55 to 57: match the following peritoneal effusion colors with the respective condition. Use each answer once.

55. ___ Pale yellow.   A. Normal.
56. ___ Straw-colored.   B. Pulmonary infarct.
57. ___ Bloody.   C. Congestive heart failure.

58. An extremely increased leukocyte concentration in peritoneal fluid can be caused by:
    A. Bacterial peritonitis.   C. Cirrhosis.
    B. Pancreatitis.   D. None of the above.

Questions 59 to 61: match an increase in the following cells in peritoneal fluid with the representative abnormality.

59. ___ Eosinophils.
60. ___ Lymphocytes.
61. ___ Mesothelial cells.

A. Chronic peritoneal dialysis.
B. Congestive heart failure, cirrhosis, and nephrotic syndrome.
C. Tuberculous peritonitis.

Questions 62 to 64: match the various types and respective causes of pericardial effusion.

62. ___ Infectious agents.
63. ___ Collagen vascular disease.
64. ___ Neoplastic disease.

A. Rheumatic disease.
B. Mesothelioma.
C. Dressler's postinfarction syndrome.
D. Coxsackie group viruses.

65. A cause of an increased concentration of cells in pericardial fluid is:
    A. Microbial infection.
    B. Malignancy.
    C. Congestive heart failure.
    D. Both A and B.

Questions 66 to 69: match the following male reproductive structures with their respective constituents.

66. ___ Testicle.
67. ___ Seminal vesicles.
68. ___ Prostate.
69. ___ Cowper's glands.

A. Fructose and prostaglandins.
B. Unknown.
C. Sperm.
D. p30 glycoprotein.

70. Sperm motility can become decreased if the specimen is:
    A. Stored at room temperature.
    B. Stored in a plastic container for more than 1 hour.
    C. Examined after 2 hours of storage.
    D. All of the above.

71. The normal value of sperm cells is ___ $\times 10^9$/L.
    A. 15 to 30.   C. 30 to 60.
    B. 30 to 45.   D. 60 to 150.

Questions 72 to 76: match the normal values or appropriate term.

72. ___ Motility (fresh specimen).

73. ___ Sperm morphology.

74. ___ Viability (fresh specimen).

75. ___ Agglutination.

76. ___ Artificial insemination.

A. At least 50%.

B. 40% to 90% (mature and oval headed).

C. Test for infectious disease.

D. Prostatitis or sperm-agglutinating antibodies.

E. Greater than 60%.

77. Arthrocentesis is:

A. A bone biopsy.
B. A liquid biopsy.
C. Not as accurate as blood testing.
D. A good test to monitor the effects of chemotherapy.

78. Disorders that can be diagnosed definitively by synovial fluid analysis are:

A. Gout, CPPD deposit disease, and rheumatoid arthritis.
B. CPPD deposit disease, rheumatoid arthritis, and SLE.
C. Rheumatoid arthritis, SLE, and septic arthritis.
D. Gout, CPPD deposit disease, and septic arthritis.

79. Which of the following would *not* be an aspiration site for synovial fluid?

A. Knee.
B. Elbow.
C. Posterior iliac crest.
D. Ankle.

80. If a synovial fluid aspirate is very turbid and septic arthritis is suspected, a ___ should definitely be performed.

A. Total cell count and differential count.
B. Crystal examination.
C. Gram stain and culture.
D. All of the above.

81. Crystals that are multiple three-dimensional forms are:

A. CPPD crystals.
B. Basic calcium phosphate crystals.
C. Monosodium urate crystals.
D. Cholesterol.

82. An increased percentage of segmented neutrophils (PMNs) is characteristic of:

A. Chronic urticaria.
B. Septic arthritis.
C. Rheumatoid arthritis.
D. Rheumatic fever.

Questions 83 to 86: match the following crystals with an associated disorder. Use each answer once.

83. ___ Monosodium urate.

84. ___ Calcium oxalate.

85. ___ Cholesterol.

86. ___ Lipid liquid "Maltese cross."

A. Chronic renal disease.

B. Chronic rheumatoid effusions.

C. Acute and chronic arthritis.

D. Acute gouty arthritis.

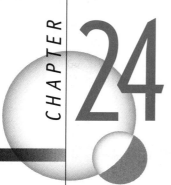

24 Manual Procedures in Hematology and Coagulation

Basic procedures
Erythrocyte count
Hemoglobin determination
Leukocyte differential count
Leukocyte count
Packed cell volume of whole blood
Platelet count
Red blood cell indices
Reticulocyte count
Sedimentation rate of erythrocytes
Special hematology procedures
Acidified serum lysis test
Bone marrow examination
Donath-Landsteiner screening test
Glucose-6-phosphate dehydrogenase
   activity in erythrocytes
Hemoglobin electrophoresis
Hemoglobin F determination by
   alkaline denaturation
Hemoglobin S screening test
Malarial smears
Monospot test
Osmotic fragility of erythrocytes
Sucrose hemolysis test
Special stains
Acid phosphatase in leukocytes

Alkaline phosphatase in
   leukocytes
Esterase (alpha-naphthyl acetate
   esterase) in leukocytes
Double staining esterase
Alpha-naphthyl acetate esterase
   with fluoride inhibition
Esterase (naphthol AS-D
   chloroacetate esterase) in
   leukocytes
Heinz bodies
Hemoglobin F determination by acid
   elution
Lymphocyte enzyme stains: alpha-
   naphthyl butyrate esterase and
   beta-glucuronidase
Periodic acid–Schiff (PAS) in
   leukocytes
Peroxidase (myeloperoxidase) in
   leukocytes
Siderocyte stain
Sudan black B stain
Terminal deoxynucleotidyl
   transferase test
Coagulation procedures
Specimen quality

Special collection techniques
Anticoagulants
Specimen handling
Specimen preparation
General sources of error
Quality control
Coagulation procedures
Activated partial thromboplastin
   time
Antithrombin III
Bleeding time
Circulating anticoagulants
Clot retraction
Clot lysis
Ethanol gelation test
Euglobulin lysis time
Substitution studies and factor
   assays
Fibrin split products
Fibrin-stabilizing factor
Fibrinogen assay
Platelet aggregation
Protamine sulfate assay
Prothrombin time
Thrombin time
Review questions

OBJECTIVES

- Describe the general principles of basic and specialized procedures in hematology, analysis of body fluids, and coagulation procedures.
- Describe the proper type of specimen collection and handling for the stated procedure.
- Prepare the necessary reagents for the stated procedure.
- Describe the quality control steps needed for the procedure.

- Perform the stated procedure.
- Perform any calculations needed for reporting the results in the procedure.
- State the normal values for the parameters measured by the procedure.
- Describe the sources of error and clinical applications of the procedure.

*T*he procedures in this chapter are presented in a format that is consistent with the guidelines set forth by the National Committee for Clinical Laboratory Standards (NCCLS). This format is as follows:

1. Procedure title and specific method
2. Test principle including type of reaction and the clinical reasons for the test
3. Specimen collection and preparation
4. Reagents, supplies, and equipment
5. Calibration of a standard curve
6. Quality control
7. Procedure
8. Calculations
9. Reporting results (normal values)

10. Procedure notes including sources of error, clinical applications, and limitations of the procedure
11. References

All specimens should be treated with caution (see Chapter 2, p. 17). All blood, tissues, and blood derivatives should be considered potentially infectious. Specimen handling notes that are particularly important to coagulation studies are presented on page 353 immediately preceding the Coagulation Procedures section. Many of the procedures in this chapter are classic methods that are infrequently performed in the working clinical laboratory. These procedures are included for use in special circumstances such as in the student laboratory or small clinical laboratories.

BASIC PROCEDURES

Erythrocyte Count

Principle
A specimen containing formed cellular elements, such as erythrocytes and leukocytes, is diluted in specific volumes. The isotonic diluting fluid will not lyse erythrocytes, which facilitates enumeration. Manual determinations of erythrocytes may be performed if an automated cell counter is not available or in cases of extremely low erythrocyte counts.

Specimen
Anticoagulated whole blood or capillary blood can be used. EDTA is the preferred anticoagulant. A *hemolyzed* specimen is inappropriate for an accurate erythrocyte count.

Reagents, Supplies, and Equipment
1. Gower's red cell diluting fluid
   A. Weigh out 6.25 gm of crystalline sodium sulfate. Transfer to 100-mL volumetric flask. Add approximately 50 mL of distilled water to the flask.
   B. Move to a *safety hood* and put on *protective safety glasses* for the next step.
   C. Using a rubber *safety bulb*, slowly pipette 16.7 mL of glacial acetic acid into the flask.
   D. Add distilled water up to the 100-mL calibration mark. Mix. Transfer to a stoppered bottle. Label with the solution name, date, and name of the person who prepared the solution. *Keeps best under refrigeration.*
2. Two Thoma erythrocyte (RBC) pipettes (Fig. 24.1) and manual aspirating device
   Note: A Unopette system may be used to replace the reagent and equipment mentioned in steps 1 and 2.
3. Neubauer hemocytometer and coverslip, and lens paper
4. Hand-held cell counter (optional)
5. Conventional microscope

Quality Control
A normal control specimen should be counted.

Procedure
1. Mix the specimen gently by rotation on a mixer.
2. Place a few milliliters of diluting fluid into a small test tube or container.

3. Using an RBC pipette, the specimen is drawn up to the 0.5 mark. This must be an exact measurement. Wipe the pipette with a disposable wipe. (Do not touch the tip of the pipette.)
4. Carefully transfer the tip of the pipette to the diluent container. Slowly draw the diluent up into the RBC pipette, until it reaches the 101 calibration mark on the pipette. This produces a 1:200 dilution of the patient's specimen in the bulb. By slightly turning the pipette as the fluid is being drawn into it, the small red bead in the bulb of the pipette will be kept from blocking the entrance to the bulb. Avoid introducing air bubbles into the pipette. Using a second RBC pipette, prepare a duplicate sample.
5. Remove the aspirating device, label, and place the pipettes on a pipette shaker for a minimum of 5 to 10 minutes.
6. Clean the Neubauer hemocytometer and coverslip.
7. Remove the pipette from the shaker and discard the first 4 to 5 drops of diluting fluid. Load one side of the counting chamber with the first pipette. Repeat this procedure with the second pipette and load the opposite side of the hemocytometer. Do not allow the dilution to run over into the grooved area of the chamber and exercise care to avoid introducing air bubbles. Label the sample.
8. Allow the hemocytometer to sit for several minutes (it may be covered with a Petri dish cover). During this time, the erythrocytes will settle in the chamber.

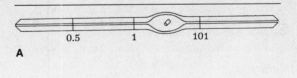

0.5   1   101

A

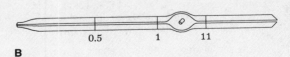

0.5   1   11

B

FIGURE 24.1 **A.** Erythrocyte (RBC) pipette. **B.** Leukocyte (WBC) pipette. (Note: These pipettes should be used with a safety aspiration.)

(continued)

BASIC PROCEDURES (continued)

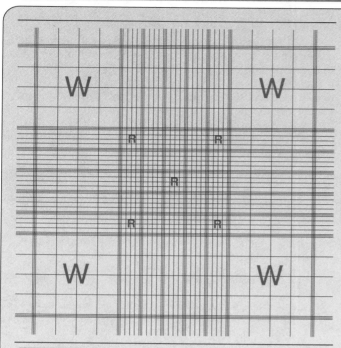

FIGURE 24.2 Neubauer counting chamber. R = red cell area; w = white cell area.

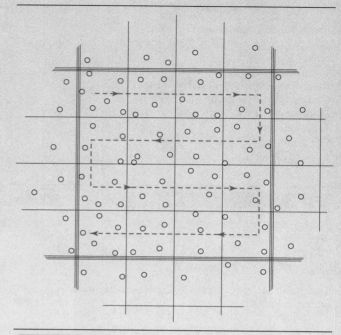

FIGURE 24.3 RBC counting square.

9. Place the hemocytometer on the microscope stage and focus with the 10× objective (low power) on the large central red cell counting area (Fig. 24.2). This central area is ruled off into 25 small squares, each of which is further subdivided into 16 smaller squares. Of the 25 squares, the 4 corner squares and 1 middle square are used for the erythrocyte count (Fig. 24.3).
10. Switch to the 43 to 44× objective (high power) and begin counting the appropriate cells in the five squares designated with Rs (see Fig. 24.2). The number of cells counted in each of the five small squares should not vary by more than 10 cells. It is important to note that the distribution of cells should be roughly equivalent and no clumps of cells should be seen. If clumping is seen, another dilution must be made. Count the erythrocytes on the other side of the hemocytometer. This total should be within 20 to 30 cells of the other side. The total erythrocytes counted on each side are added together and divided by 2 to obtain the average.
11. Soak the hemocytometer in a bleach solution to disinfect.

Calculation

No. of erythrocytes = average total of RBCs counted in 5 squares
× dilution correction factor
× volume correction factor

1. Five of the 25 squares in the large 1-mm square are counted.
2. The specimen dilution factor is 200.
3. The volume correction factor is 50. This number represents the total volume of five squares reported in terms of 1.00 μL. This is calculated by dividing the volume desired (1.00 μL) by the volume used (0.02 μL).

Example: If the average number of erythrocytes counted is 400, the total erythrocyte count would be:

$$400 \times 200 \times 50 = 4.0 \times 10^6/\mu L \text{ or } 4.0 \times 10^{12}/L$$

A simplification of this formula is to use a factor of 10,000, which represents 200 × 50. The total average of 400 erythrocytes × the factor of 10,000 = 4,000,000 or 4 × 10^{12}/L.

Reporting Results
Reference values: Males—4.6 to 6.2 × 10^{12}/L; females—4.2 to 5.4 × 10^{12}/L.

Procedure Notes
In a low count, the specimen may be drawn up to the 1 mark on the RBC pipette to produce a 1:100 dilution, or a white blood cell (WBC) pipette can be used to produce either a 1:20 or 1:10 dilution (see Leukocyte Count section for dilutional details using a WBC pipette). If the dilution is altered from the traditional 1:200 dilution used in the erythrocyte count, the new dilutional factor must be *substituted* in the calculation formula.

Sources of Error
Increased or erratic results may be seen if contaminated diluting fluid, wet or dirty pipettes, a dirty hemocytometer, or drying of the dilution in the hemocytometer occurs.

Clinical Applications
A manual count may be appropriate in specimens with low erythrocyte counts.

References
Henry, John B. (ed.). *Clinical Diagnosis and Management by Laboratory Methods* (17th edition). Philadelphia: Saunders, 1984, p. 1444.

(continued)

Seivard, Charles E. *Hematology for Medical Technologists* (4th edition). Philadelphia: Lea & Febiger, 1972, pp. 170–171.

Turgeon, Mary L. and J. L. Bender. *Hematology and Coagulation Laboratory Manual.* Corning, NY: Corning Community College Press, 1985, pp. 16–17.

· ·

Hemoglobin Determination: Cyanmethemoglobin Quantitative Method

Principle

In a reagent solution the ferrous ions (Fe^{2+}) of hemoglobin are oxidized to the ferric (Fe^{3+}) state by potassium ferricyanide to form methemoglobin. Methemoglobin subsequently reacts with the cyanide ions provided by potassium cyanide to form cyanmethemoglobin. The amount of cyanmethemoglobin can be measured spectrophotometrically and compared to known hemoglobin standards in order to determine the hemoglobin concentration of the unknown sample. This procedure is applicable in diagnosing and monitoring therapy for hemoglobin deficiency anemia.

Specimen

Although specimens can be obtained using capillary blood, EDTA-anticoagulated whole blood obtained by venipuncture is recommended. Best results are obtained with blood drawn on the same day as testing; however, blood stored for up to 1 week at room temperature may be used. Hemolyzed specimens *cannot* be used.

Reagents, Supplies, and Equipment

1. Nonionic detergent in reagent-grade water: To prepare a working solution, pipette either 0.5 mL of Sterox SE Concentrated (Harleco) or 0.5 mL of Saponic 218 (Alcoac, Inc.) into a 1000-mL volumetric flask. Dilute to the calibration mark with reagent-grade water.

2. Potassium ferricyanide reagent: Prepare by weighing:
   500 mg of potassium cyanide (KCN)
   200 mg of potassium ferricyanide ($K_3FE[CN]_6$)
   140 mg of dihydrogen potassium phosphate (KH_2PO_4)
   Precaution: If any dry reagent is ingested, call a physician immediately. Wash hands immediately after handling the chemicals and do not allow food or drink in the area. Fill a clean 1000-mL volumetric flask approximately half-full with a working solution of nonionic detergent. Add each of the three dry chemicals to the flask and mix. Dilute to the calibration mark with nonionic detergent. Check the pH. The pH should be between 7.0 and 7.4. Transfer to a stoppered brown bottle and label with name of solution, date, and the name of the person who prepared the solution. This clear, pale-yellow solution is stable for several months at room temperature. *Do not allow to freeze. Precaution:* The amount of potassium cyanide present in 1 L of reagent is more than the minimum lethal dose for a human adult. Dispose of the solution carefully. Discard used reagents and samples in running water in the sink and do not allow them to come in contact with acid. Hydrogen cyanide is liberated by acidification of the reagent. Do not breathe fumes. Flush any surface areas of the body that come in contact with the reagent and get medical attention if the eyes are involved.

3. Pipettes: Microliter or Sahli-type pipettes ($20 \pm 0.1\ \mu L$); 5.0-mL graduated pipettes and a safety bulb or an autodilutor; plus variously sized pipettes, if the standard curve is being run concurrently

Note: The Unopette system can be used to replace the reagent and equipment in steps 2 and 3.

4. Spectrophotometer and curvettes
   Calibration: The spectrophotometer is calibrated with a secondary hemiglobincyanide (HiCN) calibrator material. The absorbance of HiCN at 540 nm is proportional to its concentration (Beer's law).

Preparation of a Standard Curve Using a 20-gm/dL Standard

A standard curve *must* be constructed each time new potassium ferricyanide reagent is prepared. A commercially prepared standard concentrate containing 80 mg/dL of cyanmethemoglobin can be used. It is equivalent to 20 gm/dL of hemoglobin. This standard is diluted to various concentrations for the preparation of a standard curve. This curve is appropriate as a reference, if 20 μL of whole blood and 5.0 mL of reagent are used. Prepare the dilutions in duplicate.

Concentration (gm/dL)	Volume of Reagent (mL)	Volume of Standard (mL)
Blank	6.0	0
5	4.5	1.5
10	3.0	3.0
15	1.5	4.5
20	0	6.0

Solutions should be transferred to matched cuvettes and read at 540 nm. The blank solution should be adjusted to read 0 absorbance or 100% transmission before reading the standard curve dilutions. If a digital readout photometer is available, record the absorbance (OD) values directly. If a digital readout photometer is not available, record the percent transmittance (%T) and use a conversion table to convert the readings to absorbance. Refer to the Calculations section of this procedure for details on constructing a standard curve.

Quality Control

Known commercial hemoglobin controls should be used. These standards should reflect at least two levels of hemoglobin values, normal and abnormal. The results must be within 2 standard deviations (SD) of the mean value as stated in the package insert.

Procedure

1. Dispense 5.0 mL of reagent into clean 16 × 100-mm test tubes. One tube is required for each test or control. An additional tube is needed as the **reagent blank.**

2. Draw a sample of well-mixed anticoagulated or capillary blood into a 20-μL pipette. Wipe the outside of the pipette with a clean gauze square to remove excess blood; however, *do not touch* the bore of the pipette with the gauze. Carefully adjust the amount of blood in the pipette to the calibration mark.

3. Lower the tip of the pipette into the reagent just below the meniscus. Gently expel the blood into the reagent. Rinse the pipette 8 to 10 times.
   Note: Specimens and dilutions must *not* be pipetted by mouth.

4. Cover the test tube and mix by inversion 5 to 6 times. Allow the tube to stand at room temperature for at least 5 minutes. Once the blood sample and reagent are mixed, the resulting HiCN solution is stable; however, it should be kept out of direct sunlight. If the test cannot be read within a reasonable period of time, it may be stored for periods ex-

(continued)

BASIC PROCEDURES (continued)

ceeding 6 hours if refrigerated, in the dark, and covered. Repeat this procedure for each test specimen and the controls.

5. Solutions should be transferred to matched cuvettes and read at 540 nm. If a digital readout photometer is available, record the absorbance (OD) values directly. Record the %T results if a digital readout photometer is not available, and use a conversion table to convert to absorbance (OD). The patient and control results can be obtained directly from the standard curve or calculated from the absorbance of the unknown and a known standard. Carefully dispose of the test dilutions and reagent blank. Refer to the reagent preparation section for precautions.

Calculations
Use the absorbance reading from a digital spectrophotometer or convert the %T to absorbance (OD) to plot absorbance versus concentration on regular graph paper. If semilog paper is used, the %T versus concentration can be plotted. Patient or control results can be read directly from the standard curve.

Alternative Calculation
Concentration of hemoglobin in the sample in

$$gm/dL = \frac{\text{absorbance of sample}}{\text{absorbance of standard}} \times \text{concentration of standard}$$

Reporting Results
Reference values: Males—13.5 to 18.0 gm/dL or 2.09 to 2.79 mmol/L (SI units); females—12.0 to 16.0 gm/dL or 1.86 to 2.48 mmol/L (SI units).

Procedure Notes
The addition of a nonionic detergent enhances erythrocyte lysis and minimizes turbidity caused by lipoprotein precipitation. Dihydrogen potassium phosphate is substituted for sodium bicarbonate in the classic Drabkin's reagent, which shortens the time needed for full color from more than 15 minutes to 3 minutes. Smokers' blood takes longer to convert.

Sources of Error
Lipemia or excessively increased leukocyte concentrations may falsely elevate the hemoglobin value up to 30 gm/dL because of turbidity. In lipemia, centrifugation can clear the specimen and the supernatant reading will be accurate.

Clinical Applications
Hemoglobin determination is used either for diagnosis or to monitor therapy in anemic individuals.

References
Henry, John B. (ed.). *Clinical Diagnosis and Management by Laboratory Methods* (17th edition). Philadelphia: Saunders, 1984, p. 1444.

Huseby, Rolf M. *Reference Procedure for the Quantitative Determination of Hemoglobin in Blood.* Vol. 4, No. 3. Villanova, PA: National Committee for Clinical Laboratory Standards, 1984.

Turgeon, Mary L. and J. L Bender. *Hematology and Coagulation Laboratory Manual.* Corning, NY: Corning Community College Press, 1985.

Leukocyte Differential Count

Principle
A stained smear is examined in order to determine the percentage of each type of leukocyte present and assess the erythrocyte and platelet morphology. Increases in any of the normal leukocyte types or the presence of immature leukocytes or erythrocytes in peripheral blood are important diagnostically in a wide variety of inflammatory disorders and leukemia. Erythrocyte abnormalities are clinically important in various anemias. Platelet size irregularities are suggestive of particular thrombocyte disorders.

Specimen
Peripheral blood, bone marrow, or body fluid sediments, such as spinal fluid, are appropriate specimens. Whole blood smears may be made from EDTA-anticoagulated blood or prepared from free-flowing capillary blood. Smears should be made within 1 hour of blood collection from EDTA specimens stored at room temperature to avoid distortion of cell morphology. Unstained smears can be stored for indefinite periods, but stained smears gradually fade.

Reagents, Supplies, and Equipment
1. A manual cell counter designed for differential counts
2. Microscope, immersion oil, and lens paper

Quality Control
Training and experience in examining immature and abnormal cell morphology are essential. A set of reference slides with established parameters should be established to assess the competence of an individual to perform differential and morphological identification of leukocytes and erythrocytes. Participation in a quality assurance program continues to document the expertise of the hematologist in microscopy. Questionable or abnormal smears should be referred to a supervisor for verification.

Procedure
1. Begin the slide examination with a correctly prepared and stained smear (see Chapter 2 for specimen preparation).
2. Focus the microscope on the 10× objective (low power). Scan the smear to check for cell distribution, clumping, and abnormal cells. Add a drop of immersion oil, and switch to the 100× (oil immersion) objective. Begin the count by determining a suitable area (Fig. 24.4). Extend the examination from the area where approximately half of the erythrocytes are barely overlapping to an area where the erythrocytes touch each other. *It is important to examine cellular morphology and to count leukocytes in areas that are neither too thick nor too thin.* In areas that are too thick, cellular details such as nuclear chromatin patterns are difficult to examine. In areas that are too thin, distortion of cells makes it risky to identify a cell type.

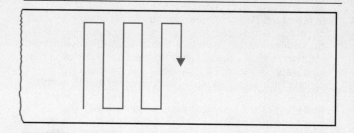

FIGURE 24.4 The method of slide examination in the leukocyte differential count.

(continued)

TABLE 24.1	A Comparison of Normal Leukocytes in Peripheral Blood					
	Segmented Neutrophil	**Band Neutrophil**	**Lymphocyte**	**Monocyte**	**Eosinophil**	**Basophil**
Nuclear shape	Lobulated	Curved	Round	Indented or twisted	Lobulated	Lobulated
Chromatin	Very clumped	Moderately clumped	Smooth	Lacy	Very clumped	Very clumped
Cytoplasmic color	Pink	Blue, pink	Light blue	Gray-blue	Granulated	Granulated
Granules	Many	Many	Few or absent	Many	Many	Many
Color of granules	Pink, a few blue	Pink	Red	Dusty blue	Orange	Dark blue
Average percentage	56%	3%	34%	4%	2.7%	0.3%

3. Count the leukocytes using a tracking pattern (see Fig. 24.4). Each cell identified should be immediately tallied as a neutrophil (band), neutrophil (segmented), or polymorphonuclear neutrophil (PMN); lymphocyte; monocyte; eosinophil; or basophil. A brief leukocyte morphology reference is included (Table 24.1); however, refer to specific chapters in the text for a complete discussion of leukocyte and erythrocyte cellular morphology.
4. Abnormalities of leukocytes, erythrocytes, and platelets should be noted. Nucleated erythrocytes are *not* included in the total count but are noted per 100 WBCs. A total of at least 100 leukocytes should be counted. Express the results as a percentage of total leukocytes counted.

Reporting Results
Reference values (see Table 24.1), particularly the band neutrophil percentage, may vary. Values for children differ from adult reference values. See Chapters 14 and 16 for a full discussion of reference values.

Procedure Notes
A well-made and well-stained smear is essential to the accuracy of the differential count. The knowledge and ability of the cell morphologist is critical to high-quality results.

A minimum of 300 leukocytes must be within the acceptable working area, when the total leukocyte count is no less than 4×10^9/L. The neutrophils, monocytes, and lymphocytes should appear evenly distributed in the usable fields of the film. Less than 2% of the leukocytes should be disrupted or nonidentifiable forms except in certain forms associated with pathological states. If a disrupted cell is clearly identifiable, include it in the differential count. Classify nonidentifiable disrupted cells (smudges or baskets) as "other" and note them on the report if more than a few are observed.

The blood smear preparation techniques described in Chapter 2 are commonly used in the laboratory for the preparation of blood smears. In certain circumstances, the preparation of a buffy coat peripheral blood smear increases the accuracy of the leukocyte differential count.

Preparation of Buffy Coat Smears
Principle
An anticoagulated specimen of whole blood is centrifuged to physically separate the blood into three layers: plasma, leukocytes and platelets, and erythrocytes. The interface layer between the plasma and erythrocytes is referred to as the buffy coat. If this layer of concentrated cells is removed by pipetting, push-wedge–type smears can subsequently be prepared and stained for microscopic examination. This technique is useful in the performance of leukocyte differential counts on patients with extremely low total leukocyte counts or in special testing procedures.

Specimen
A freshly drawn specimen of EDTA-anticoagulated whole blood is needed.

Procedure
1. Centrifuge the specimen of whole anticoagulated blood for at least 5 minutes at 2000 to 2500 rpm.
2. With a Pasteur pipette, remove most of the top plasma layer and discard.
3. The interface layer along with a small amount of plasma and a small volume of erythrocytes can then be removed using a Pasteur pipette.
4. A drop of this suspension can be placed on a microscope slide and a push-wedge smear prepared. Air-dry and stain.

Alternative Technique
A refinement of the classic buffy coat technique has been developed for use with automated blood smear equipment. In this technique saline solution and 22% albumin are added to the interface layer. This enhancement produces better cell separation on the peripheral smear and minimizes the spreading artifact during centrifugation. To add this enhancement to the basic technique:

1. Proceed from step 3 above by transferring the interface layer to a disposable Wintrobe (ESR) tube. This tube is placed into a 16 × 100-mm test tube and centrifuged for a minimum of 5 minutes at 2000 rpm.
2. After centrifugation, the top plasma layer is removed with a Pasteur pipette and discarded. Remove about 0.03 mL of the interface layer and a small volume of erythrocytes and transfer to a 20-mL test tube or plastic vial. Add enough isotonic (0.85%) saline solution to the test tube or vial to prepare a 1 to 2% suspension of cells.
3. Add 22% albumin to the suspension at the rate of 3 drops of albumin for each 10 mL of resulting cell suspension. If the amount of albumin is too great, the cells will appear too dark and may have pseudopods.
4. This preparation can then be transferred to the sample holder and treated according to the instrument manufacturer's directions.

(continued)

BASIC PROCEDURES (continued)

Clinical Applications
Selected Disorders Associated With Increases in Normal Leukocyte Types

Neutrophils

Bacterial infections
Inflammation
Stress
Chronic leukemia

Lymphocytes

Viral infections
Whooping cough
Chronic leukemia

Monocytes

Tuberculosis
Rheumatoid arthritis
Fever of unknown origin

Eosinophils

Active allergies
Invasive parasites

Basophils

Ulcerative colitis
Hyperlipidemia

References

DeNunzio, Jeanne. "Preparation of Buffy Coats from Blood Samples With Extremely Low White Cell Count." *Lab. Med.,* Vol. 16, No. 8, August, 1985, p. 497.
Henry, John B. (ed.). *Clinical Diagnosis and Management by Laboratory Methods* (17th edition). Philadelphia: Saunders, 1984, p. 1445.
Koepke, John A. *Leukocyte Differential Counting,* Vol. 4, No. 11. Villanova, PA: National Committee for Clinical Laboratory Standards, 1984.

··

Leukocyte Count

Principle

A specimen containing formed cellular elements, such as leukocytes and erythrocytes, is mixed with a weak concentration of either hydrochloric acid or acetic acid in specified volumes. These acids will lyse erythrocytes and darken leukocytes to facilitate enumeration. The manual enumeration of WBCs is important in cases where the counts are very low.

Specimen

EDTA-anticoagulated or capillary blood is preferred.

Reagents, Supplies, and Equipment

1. The leukocyte diluting fluid is either 1% (vol/vol) solution of hydrochloric acid or 2% (vol/vol) solution of acetic acid. To prepare either of these solutions:
   A. 1% hydrochloric acid: Fill a 100-mL volumetric flask approximately half-full with distilled water. Under a *safety hood* and wearing protective *safety glasses,* pipette 1 mL of concentrated hydrochloric acid into the flask with a rubber *safety bulb.* Dilute to the 100-mL calibration mark with distilled water. Mix. Transfer to a stoppered container and label.
   B. 2% acetic acid: Fill a 100-mL volumetric flask approximately half-full with distilled water. Under a *safety hood* and wearing protective *safety glasses,* pipette 2 mL of concentrated acetic acid into the flask with a rubber *safety bulb.* Dilute to the 100-mL calibration mark with distilled water. Mix. Transfer to a stoppered container and label.
2. Thoma WBC pipettes and appropriate aspirator equipment
3. Neubauer hemocytometer, coverslip, alcohol wipe, and lens paper. The improved Neubauer hemocytometer consists of two raised counting chambers. A specifically weighted coverslip for the hemocytometer is placed over these chambers for cell counting. Each chamber has nine large squares. Each square has a count; four large squares are counted with a total volume of 0.4 μL.
   Note: The Unopette system can be substituted for the reagents and equipment in steps 2 and 3.
4. Hand-held cell counter (optional)
5. Conventional microscope and lens paper

Quality Control

A normal control specimen should be counted.

Procedure

1. The specimen is gently mixed by inversion. If the specimen is whole blood, the best mixing is achieved with a mechanical rocking mixer.
2. Place a few milliliters of the diluting fluid into a small test tube or container.
3. Using a WBC pipette, the specimen is drawn up to the 0.5 mark with an aspiration device. *Do not pipette by mouth.* This produces a 1:20 dilution of blood in the pipette bulb. This must be an exact measurement. Wipe the pipette with a disposable wipe.
4. Carefully transfer the tip of the pipette to the diluent container. Slowly draw the diluent up into the pipette, until it reaches the 11 calibration mark. By slightly turning the pipette as the fluid is being drawn into it, the small glass bead in the bulb of the pipette will be kept from blocking the entrance to the bulb. Avoid introducing air bubbles into the pipette. Using a second WBC pipette, prepare a duplicate sample.
5. Remove the aspirating tube, label, and place the pipettes on a pipette shaker for a minimum of 5 to 10 minutes to ensure proper mixing and lysis of erythrocytes.
6. Clean the Neubauer hemocytometer and coverslip.
7. Remove the pipette from the shaker and discard the first 4 or 5 drops of diluting fluid. Load one side of the counting chamber with the first pipette. Repeat this procedure using the second pipette and load the opposite side of the hemocytometer. Do not allow any of the dilution to run over into the grooved area of the chamber and exercise care to avoid introducing air bubbles. Label the sample.
8. Allow the hemocytometer to sit for several minutes. During this time, the leukocytes will settle in the chamber.
9. Place the hemocytometer on the microscope stage and focus with the 10× objective (low power). The entire ruled area of the counting chamber includes nine 1-mm² areas. The leukocytes are counted in the four corner squares (see Fig. 24.2). These squares are further ruled into 16 smaller squares.

(continued)

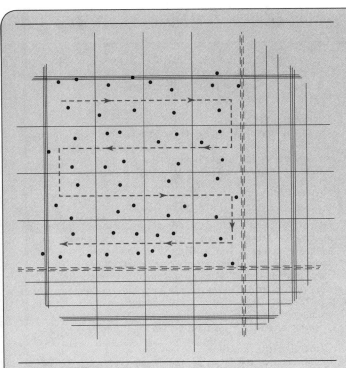

FIGURE 24.5 WBC counting square.

10. Begin counting in the upper left-hand square and count the leukocytes, which appear as round dark particles. Continue to count in the remaining three squares. Refer to Figure 24.5 for details on which cells to count. The variation in the number of cells counted in the four squares should not be more than 5 to 10 cells. Count the leukocytes on the other side of the hemocytometer; this total should be within 10 cells of the other side. The total leukocytes counted on each side are added together and divided by 2 to obtain the average. It is important to note that the distribution of cells should be roughly equivalent throughout the count and that no clumps of cells should be seen. If clumping is noted, another dilution must be made.

Calculations

$$
\begin{array}{l}
\text{Total leukocyte count} \\
= \begin{array}{ccc} \text{average} & \text{dilutional} & \text{volume} \\ \text{total} & \times \text{ factor} & + \text{correction} \\ \text{leukocytes} & & \text{factor} \end{array}
\end{array}
$$

1. The number of total leukocytes is the *average* of the two sides of the hemocytometer.
2. The dilutional factor is 20 based on the dilution of 1:20 (refer to step 4 under Procedure).
3. The volume correction factor is 2.5. This represents the volume desired (1.0 μL) divided by the volume counted (0.4 μL) (refer to the description of the Neubauer chamber in the Reagents, Supplies, and Equipment section of this procedure).

Example: If the average total of leukocytes counted was 180, the total leukocyte count would be:

$$180 \times 20 \times 2.5 = 9000$$
$$or\ 9.0 \times 10^3/\mu L$$
$$or\ 9.0 \times 10^9/L\ (SI\ units)$$

A simplification of this formula is to use a factor of 50 × the total average leukocyte count. The factor of 50 represents the dilutional factor of 20 times the volume correction factor of 2.5. *Example:* 180 total leukocytes counted × 50 = 9.0 × 10^9/L.

Reporting Results
Reference value: 4.5 to 11.0 × 10^3/μL or 4.5 to 11.0 × 10^9/L.

Procedure Notes

Sources of Error
Erroneous results can be due to contaminated diluting fluid, incorrect diluting or loading of the hemocytometer, and an uneven distribution of leukocytes in the counting chamber. Clean, dry pipettes and prompt counting of cells are important to the accuracy of the count.

Clinical Applications
In most cases, leukocyte counts are only performed manually when there are extremely low total leukocyte counts from whole blood or body fluid specimens. The total leukocyte count in whole blood specimens can be decreased or increased due to a variety of disorders.

Selected Quantitative Leukocytic Disorders

Decreased Leukocytes (Leukopenia)	Increased Leukocytes (Leukocytosis)
Viral disorders	Bacterial infections
Radiation- or chemotherapy-induced leukopenia	Inflammation
Aplastic anemia	Leukemias
Megaloblastic anemia	

Limitations of Procedure
If a WBC count is high (over 30,000), use a Thoma RBC pipette to obtain a 1:100 dilution. If the count is low, draw the blood to the 1.0 mark on a WBC pipette, which produces a 1:10 dilution. In each case, the dilutional factor must be *substituted* in the formula for calculating the total count.

Total Leukocyte Correction for Nucleated Erythrocytes
If more than 10 nucleated erythrocytes are seen on a differential blood smear, the total leukocyte count should be corrected.

$$\text{Corrected WBC} = \frac{\text{average total leukocyte count} \times 100}{100 + \text{no. of nucleated RBCs}/100 \text{ WBCs in the differential count}}$$

References
Henry, John B. (ed.). *Clinical Diagnosis and Management by Laboratory Methods.* Philadelphia: Saunders, 1984, p. 1444.
Seivard, Charles E. *Hematology for Medical Technologists.* Philadelphia: Lea & Febiger, 1972, p. 132.
Turgeon, Mary L. and J. Bender. *Hematology and Coagulation Laboratory Manual.* Corning, NY: Corning Community College Press, 1985.

Packed Cell Volume of Whole Blood: Microhematocrit Method

Principle
The packed cell volume (PCV) is a measurement of the ratio of the volume occupied by the RBCs to the volume of whole blood

(continued)

BASIC PROCEDURES (continued)

in a sample of capillary or venous blood. Following centrifugation, this ratio is measured and expressed as a percent or decimal fraction. Clinically, the PCV is used to detect anemia, polycythemia, hemodilution, or hemoconcentration. In conjunction with an erythrocyte count, the PCV is used to calculate the mean corpuscular volume (MCV). The PCV is also used in conjunction with the hemoglobin concentration to calculate the mean corpuscular hemoglobin concentration (MCHC).

Specimen
Venous blood anticoagulated with EDTA or capillary blood collected directly into heparinized capillary tubes can be used. Specimens should be centrifuged within 6 hours of collecting. Hemolyzed samples cannot be used for testing.

Reagents, Supplies, and Equipment
1. Capillary tubes (75-mm long with an ID of 1.155 mm). Blue-banded tubes contain no anticoagulant and are used with EDTA-anticoagulated blood. Red-banded tubes are heparinized for use with capillary blood.
2. Clay-type tube sealant
3. Microhematocrit centrifuge and reading device

Calibration
The calibration of the centrifuge should be checked regularly for timer accuracy, speed, and maximal packing of cells. Use a stopwatch for accuracy, a tachometer for speed, and a time-versus-constant-volume method to check packing of erythrocytes. Check the capillary tube reading device against another reader periodically.

Quality Control
Commercially available whole blood can be used to check the accuracy of normal and abnormal levels.

Procedure
1. Well-mixed anticoagulant blood should be drawn into two microhematocrit tubes by capillary action. The tubes should be filled to about three fourths of their length. Wipe off the outside of the tubes with gauze or wipes. Free-flowing capillary samples should be collected in the same manner.
2. Seal one end of each tube with a small amount of clay-like material. Place the dry end of the tube into the sealant, holding the index finger over the opposite end to prevent blood from leaking out of the tube onto the sealant.
3. Place the filled and sealed capillary tubes into the centrifuge. The sealed ends should point toward the outside of the centrifuge. The duplicate samples should be placed opposite each other in order to balance the centrifuge. Record the position number of each specimen.
4. Securely fasten the flat lid on top of the capillary tubes. Close the centrifuge top and secure the latch. Set the timer for 5 minutes. The fixed speed of centrifugation should be 10,000 to 15,000 rpm.
5. After the centrifuge has stopped, open the top and remove the cover plate. Promptly read the PCV on an appropriate piece of equipment or specially designed card. Measure the PCV by adjusting the top of the clay sealant to the 0 mark and reading the top of the red cell column. A reader with an ocular that has cross-markings produces the most accurate reading.
   Note: When taking readings, be sure that the bottom of the packed cell column is lined up correctly to the zero mark. Do not include the buffy coat in reading the packed erythro-

cyte column. *Do not* allow the tubes to remain in the centrifuge for more than 10 minutes because the interface between the plasma and the cells will become slanted and an inaccurate reading will result.

Reporting Results
The PCV is preferentially expressed as a decimal fraction, such as 0.45 L/L, rather than as 45%. In current practice, the percentage expression is commonly used. Reference values: Males—0.47 L/L ± 0.07; females—0.42 L/L ± 0.05.

Procedure Notes
Sources of Error
Erroneous results can be due to inclusion of the buffy coat in reading the packed column, hemolysis of the specimen, and inadequate mixing. If the centrifugation time is too short or the speed is too low, an increase in trapped plasma (1 to 3%) will occur in normal blood. Increased amounts of trapped plasma can produce errors in cases where an erythrocyte abnormality exists, such as sickle cell anemia. Other sources of error include prolonged tourniquet stasis and excess EDTA, which causes cells to shrink and pack more tightly than they should.

Clinical Applications
The PCV is used for detecting anemia, polycythemia, hemodilution, or hemoconcentration.

References
Turgeon, Mary L. and J. Bender. *Hematology and Coagulation Laboratory Manual.* Corning, NY: Corning Community College Press, 1985.
van Assendelft, Onno W. et al. *Procedure for Determining Packed Cell Volume by the Microhematocrit Method,* Vol. 5, No. 5. Villanova, PA: National Committee for Clinical Laboratory Standards, 1985.

Platelet Count: Brecker-Cronkite Manual Method

Principle
Whole blood is diluted with ammonium oxalate, which completely hemolyzes the erythrocytes. Platelets can then be counted, preferably using a phase hemocytometer and phase microscope. Enumeration of platelets is performed to detect either decreased states (thrombocytopenia) or increased states (thrombocytosis).

Specimen
EDTA-anticoagulated whole blood is preferred. Capillary blood may be used if venous blood is not available. The assay should be performed within 5 hours of the time that the blood specimen is collected or within 24 hours, if the specimen is refrigerated.

Reagents, Supplies, and Equipment
1. Ammonium oxalate, 1% (wt/vol): This solution is prepared as follows:
   A. Weigh out 1 gm of analytical-grade ammonium oxalate.
   B. Transfer the ammonium oxalate to a 100-mL volumetric flask and add distilled water to the calibration mark.
   C. Mix well and transfer to a permanent closed container. Label with the solution name, date of preparation, and name of the person who prepared the solution.

(continued)

D. *Store under refrigeration.* Discard if turbid.

E. *Filter* the solution prior to use.

2. Two RBC pipettes and an appropriate aspiration tube

   Note: The Unopette system can be used to replace the reagents and equipment in steps 1 and 2.

3. Pipette shaker

4. Phase hemocytometer and coverslip. This type of hemocytometer has a flat bottom rather than the concave type used for counting other cellular elements.

5. Petri dish with a piece of moistened filter paper inserted in the bottom

6. Phase contrast microscope and lens paper

7. Microscope slides and Wright-Giemsa stain. This is an optional but recommended quality control procedure.

Quality Control

Quantitative results should be checked against a well-made, stained peripheral smear.

Procedure

1. Thoroughly mix the blood sample. The use of a blood-mixing rocker for 5 minutes is preferred to inverting the sample by hand.

2. In an RBC pipette, draw the blood sample exactly up to the 0.5 calibration on the pipette. Carefully wipe off the outside of the pipette without touching the tip of the pipette. Transfer the tip of the pipette (with the blood in it) to the test tube containing the freshly *filtered* ammonium oxalate solution. Draw the oxalate solution up to the 101 calibration mark on the pipette. This produces a 1:200 dilution in the bulb. Repeat this procedure for the second pipette. This dilution should proceed to the next step as soon as possible; however, the dilution is stable for at least 8 hours.

3. Place the pipettes on a pipette shaker for 10 to 15 minutes to ensure proper mixing and the lysing of erythrocytes.

4. Prepare the hemocytometer and coverslip by wiping them with alcohol. Lens paper can be used to remove any dust or lint.

5. Remove the first pipette from the shaker and proceed with this step *promptly.* If more than 10 seconds elapse, the pipette must be remixed on the shaker. To load or charge the counting chamber, the first few drops of dilution left in the bore of the pipette should first be expelled. Fill one side of the counting chamber with the platelet–ammonium oxalate mixture, being careful not to let any of the solution run over the edges into the surrounding grooves. Repeat this procedure, using the second RBC pipette, and fill the opposite side of the counting chamber.

6. Place the hemocytometer into a Petri dish with moistened filter paper on the bottom and allow to stand for 15 to 30 minutes. Patient identification should be included on the Petri dish. The platelets will settle in the counting chamber and loss of moisture will be prevented by covering the hemocytometer.

7. Carefully wipe off any moisture that may have accumulated on the bottom of the hemocytometer before placing it on the microscope stage. Using the 10× objective (low power), focus the microscope on the large middle square of the counter chamber. The background should appear dark, while the platelets, leukocytes, fine debris, and markings of the hemocytometer appear illuminated.

8. Switch to the 43 to 44× objective (high power) and refocus, if necessary, with *only* the fine adjustment. The platelets should appear round or oval in shape and have a faintly purple-orchid appearance. Any extraneous debris will appear to be refractile when the depth of focus is altered using the fine adjustment.

9. Five squares (the same as an erythrocyte count) are counted on each side of the hemocytometer. Both sides of the chamber must be counted. The total number of platelets counted on each side should be within 10 of each other. Add the total number of platelets counted on each side together and divide by 2. This number represents the average number of platelets counted in five squares.

Calculations

The number of platelets per microliter is:

$$\text{Platelets}/\mu L = \begin{array}{c}\text{total average} \\ \text{no. of platelets} \\ \text{in 5 squares}\end{array} \times \begin{array}{c}\text{dilution} \\ \text{correction} \\ \text{factor}\end{array} \times \begin{array}{c}\text{volume} \\ \text{correction} \\ \text{factor}\end{array}$$

The dilution and volume correction factors are derived in the same manner as for the erythrocyte count.

Example: If the average total of platelets counted in five squares is 20, the platelet count per microliter is:

$$20 \times 200 \times 50 = 200,000/\mu L \text{ or}$$
$$200 \times 10^9/L \text{ (SI units)}$$

Reporting Results

The reference value is 150,000 to 400,000/μL or 150 to 400 $\times$ 10^9/L (SI units).

Procedure Notes

Sources of Error

A variety of technical errors can produce incorrect results. These include the age of the specimen, clumping of platelets, debris in the diluting fluid, platelet adherence to glass, and incorrectly diluting the specimen.

An even distribution of platelets through the counting area is critical. Clumping of platelets results from inadequate mixing or poor technique. If clumps are seen, the sample must be rediluted and recounted.

In cases of thrombocytopenia, the dilution may have to be increased to 1:100 in an RBC pipette or 1:20 in a WBC pipette. The new dilution factor must be included in the calculation formula.

Clinical Applications

The enumeration of platelets has now become a routine component of the complete blood cell count (CBC) because of automation. In cases of severe thrombocytopenia or whenever cellular abnormalities may be spuriously affecting the automated count, a manual phase contrast count should be performed.

Selected Quantitative Disorders of Platelets

Increased Platelets (Thrombocytosis)	Decreased Platelets (Thrombocytopenia)
Postsplenectomy	Aplastic anemia
Polycythemia vera	Idiopathic thrombocytopenia
Chronic myelogenous leukemia	Acute leukemias

References

Brecker, G. and E. P. Cronkite. "Morphology and Enumeration of Human Blood Platelets." *J. Appl. Physiol.*, Vol. 3, 1950, p. 365.

Henry, John B. (ed.). *Clinical Diagnosis and Management by Laboratory Methods* (17th edition). Philadelphia: Saunders, 1984, p. 1445.

(continued)

BASIC PROCEDURES (continued)

Seivard, Charles E. *Hematology for Medical Technologists* (4th edition). Philadelphia: Lea & Febiger, 1972, pp. 429–432.

Red Blood Cell Indices

The erythrocyte indices are used to mathematically define cell size and the concentration of hemoglobin within the cell. They are:

1. Mean corpuscular volume (MCV)
2. Mean corpuscular hemoglobin (MCH)
3. Mean corpuscular hemoglobin concentration (MCHC)

Mean Corpuscular Volume

Principle
The MCV expresses the average volume of an erythrocyte.

Calculations

$$MCV = \frac{\text{patient's PCV or hematocrit (L/L)}}{\text{erythrocyte count } (\times 10^{12}/L)} = fL$$

Example: If the patient's hematocrit is 35%, or 0.35 L/L, and the erythrocyte count is $4.0 \times 10^{12}/L$, the MCV is determined thus:

$$MCV = \frac{0.35 \text{ L/L}}{4.0 \times 10^{12}/L} = 87.5 \times 10^{-15} L = 87.5 \text{ fL*}$$

Reporting Results
Reference value: 80 to 96 fL.

Mean Corpuscular Hemoglobin

Principle
The MCH expresses the average weight (content) of hemoglobin in an average erythrocyte. It is directly proportional to the amount of hemoglobin and the size of the erythrocyte.

Calculations

$$MCH = \frac{\text{hemoglobin } (\times 10 \text{ gm/dL})}{\text{erythrocyte count } (\times 10^{12}/L)} = pg$$

Example: If the patient's hemoglobin is 14 gm/dL and the erythrocyte count is $4 \times 10^{12}/L$, the MCH would equal:

$$MCH = \frac{140 \text{ gm/dL}}{4 \times 10^{12}/L} = 35 \times 10^{-12} \text{ gm} = 35 \text{ pg†}$$

Reporting Results
Reference value: 27 to 32 pg.

Mean Corpuscular Hemoglobin Concentration

Principle
The MCHC expresses the average concentration of hemoglobin per unit volume of erythrocytes. It is also defined as the ratio of the weight of hemoglobin to the volume of erythrocytes.

---

*One femtoliter (fL) = 10^{-15} L = 1 cubic micrometer (μm^3).

†One picogram (pg) = 10^{-12} gm = 1 micromicrogram ($\mu\mu g$).

Calculations

$$MCHC = \frac{\text{hemoglobin (gm/dL)}}{\text{PCV or hematocrit (L/L)}} = gm/dL$$

Example: If the patient's hemoglobin is 14 gm/dL and the hematocrit is 0.45 L/L, the MCHC would equal:

$$MCHC = \frac{14 \text{ gm/dL}}{0.45 \text{ L/L}} = 31 \text{ gm/dL} = 31\%$$

Reporting Results
Reference value: 32 to 36%.

Reticulocyte Count: New Methylene Blue Method

Principle
Supravital stains, such as new methylene blue N or brilliant cresyl blue, bind, neutralize, and cross-link RNA. These stains cause the ribosomal and residual RNA to coprecipitate with the few remaining mitochondria and ferritin masses in living young erythrocytes to form microscopically visible dark-blue clusters and filaments (reticulum). An erythrocyte still possessing RNA is referred to as a **reticulocyte** (see Plate 6). The enumeration of reticulocytes is important in assessing the status of erythrocyte production in the bone marrow (erythropoiesis).

Specimen
Whole blood that is anticoagulated with either EDTA or heparin is suitable. Capillary blood drawn into heparinized tubes or immediately mixed with stain may also be used. The test should be performed promptly after blood collection. Stained smears retain their color for a prolonged period of time.

Reagents, Supplies, and Equipment
Reagent
New methylene blue solution: This solution is prepared as follows:

1. Weigh out 0.5 gm of new methylene blue N, 1.4 gm of potassium oxalate, and 0.8 gm of sodium chloride. Place these chemicals in a 100-mL volumetric flask and dilute to the calibration mark with distilled water.
2. Mix well. Place in a clean brown bottle that is properly labeled with the name of the reagent, date of preparation, and name of the individual who prepared the solution.
3. *Filter* solution daily or immediately before use to remove any precipitate.

Supplies and Equipment
1. WBC pipettes and appropriate aspiration equipment
2. Glass slides
3. Wright or Wright-Giemsa stain
4. Microscope, lens paper, and immersion oil
5. Miller ocular disc (optional)

Procedure
1. Using a WBC pipette, draw the filtered stain to the 1 mark on the pipette. Wipe off excess stain from the outside of the pipette.

(continued)

2. With the stain in the pipette, place the pipette tip into the well-mixed blood specimen and draw the blood up to the 1 mark. Do not pipette by mouth.
3. Draw both the stain and blood up into the pipette bulb (the bulb will not be full). Mix by rotating the pipette by hand. Label with the patient's name.
4. Allow this mixture to stand for at least 10 minutes.
5. Gently remix and expel small drops of the stain–blood mixture onto several microscope slides and prepare smears.
6. Air-dry.
7. Two or three dried slides may be counterstained with Wright stain (see procedure for staining blood smears).
8. Using the 10× microscope objective, focus the smear. Add a drop of oil to the slide and move to the oil immersion (100×) objective. The appropriate counting area is the portion of the smear where the erythrocytes are evenly distributed and not overlapping. Before beginning the count, scan the slide to check that reticulocytes can be located on that slide.
9. To count the reticulocytes, a minimum of 1000 (both reticulin-containing and nonreticulated) erythrocytes must be counted. Normally, 500 erythrocytes will be counted on each of two slides. If the number of reticulocytes on these two slides do not agree within 20%, a third slide of 500 erythrocytes must be counted. Be sure to count all cells that contain a blue-staining filament, fragment, or granule of reticulum in the erythrocyte. The counting field can be reduced by using paper hole reinforcers or small pieces of paper cut to fit the oculars with a small hole cut out in the middle of each. This makes counting easier than viewing the entire field.

Note: A Miller ocular disc (Fig. 24.6) can be used to facilitate counting the number of reticulocytes and total RBCs.

Calculations

If 47 reticulocytes are found when 1000 erythrocytes are examined (47 reticulocytes and 953 mature erythrocytes), the reticulocyte count is calculated as follows:

$$\frac{47}{1000} = 100 = 4.7\% \text{ reticulocytes (uncorrected)}$$

Reporting Results

Reference values: 0.5 to 1.5%; neonates—2.5 to 6.5%. Some laboratories express the reticulocyte count in absolute rather than proportional terms (see Chapter 5). Reporting in absolute terms is becoming the preferred method of reporting. The correction for anemia is additionally helpful for clinical interpretation of the reticulocyte count (see Chapter 5).

Alternative Procedure
Capillary Tube Technique

Steps 1 through 3 above may be replaced by using a capillary tube instead of a WBC pipette. Using this technique, one third of the capillary tube is filled with well-mixed blood. An equal amount of filtered stain is then drawn into the tube. The tube is rotated back and forth by hand and then allowed to stand for staining to take place. Continue as in the procedure above beginning with step 4. Another method is to mix 2 drops of blood and 2 drops of stain.

Miller Ocular Disc

Principle A Miller ocular disc inserted into the eyepiece of the microscope permits a rapid survey of erythrocytes. This disc (see Fig. 24.6) imposes two squares (one 9 times the area of the other) onto the field of view.

Procedure: Reticulocytes are counted in the large square and erythrocytes in the small square in successive microscopic fields until at least 300 RBCs are counted. This allows for an estimate of reticulocytes among a minimum population of 2700 erythrocytes. The **absolute reticulocyte count** can be determined by multiplying the reticulocyte percentage by the RBC count.

Calculations:

$$\text{Reticulocytes (expressed in percentage)} = \frac{\text{no. of reticulocytes in large squares}}{\text{no. of RBCs in small squares} \times 9} \times 100$$

Example: Given that there are 50 reticulocytes in the large squares and 300 red blood cells in the small squares:

$$\text{Reticulocytes (expressed in percentage)} = \frac{50}{300 \times 9} \times 100 = 1.86$$

Note: Reticulocytes may also be counted by automated methods. See Chapter 25 for more information.

Sources of Error

A refractile appearance of erythrocytes should not be confused with reticulocytes. Refractile bodies are due to poor drying owing to moisture in the air. Filtration of the stain is essential because precipitate can resemble a reticulocyte.

Erythrocyte inclusions should not be mistaken for reticulocytes. Howell-Jolly bodies appear as one or sometimes two, deep-purple, dense structures. Heinz bodies stain a light blue-green and are usually present at the edge of the erythrocyte. Pappenheimer bodies are more often confused with reticulocytes and are the most difficult to distinguish. These purple-staining iron deposits generally appear as several granules in a small cluster. If Pappenheimer bodies are suspected, stain with Wright-Giemsa to verify their presence.

Falsely decreased reticulocyte counts can result from understaining the blood with new methylene blue. High glucose levels can also cause reticulocytes to stain poorly.

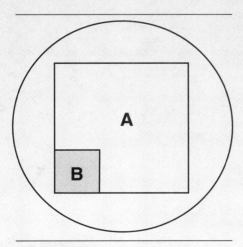

FIGURE 24.6 Miller ocular disc. Square A is nine times the area of square B. Reticulocytes are counted in square A; erythrocytes are counted in square B in successive microscopic fields until at least 300 RBCs are counted.

(continued)

BASIC PROCEDURES (continued)

Clinical Applications
Selected Disorders Associated With Abnormal Results

Decreased Reticulocytes	Increased Reticulocytes
Aplastic anemia	Blood loss
Aplastic crises of hemolytic anemia	Crisis associated with hemolytic anemia
Chemotherapeutic or radiation-induced hypoproliferation	Subsequent to treatment of pernicious anemia, folic acid deficiency, or iron deficiency
Pernicious anemia	
Decreased erythropoiesis	

References
Brecher, J. W. and M. Schneiderman. "A Time-Saving Device for the Counting of Reticulocytes." *Am. J. Clin Pathol.* Vol. 20, 1950, p. 1079.

Jandl, J. H. *Blood.* Boston: Little, Brown & Co., 1987, pp. 33, 51.

Method for Reticulocyte Counting. Proposed Standard H16-P. Villanova, PA: National Committee for Clinical Laboratory Standards, 1985.

Sedimentation Rate of Erythrocytes: Westergren Method

The Westergren method has been selected as the method of choice by the NCCLS.

Principle
The erythrocyte sedimentation rate (ESR), also called the sed rate, measures the rate of settling of erythrocytes in diluted human plasma. This phenomenon depends on an interrelationship of variables, such as the plasma protein composition, the concentration of erythrocytes, and the shape of the erythrocytes. The ESR value is determined by measuring the distance from the surface meniscus to the top of the erythrocyte sedimented in a special tube that is placed perpendicular in a rack for 1 hour. The clinical value of this procedure is in the diagnosis and monitoring of inflammatory or infectious states.

Specimen
Fresh anticoagulated blood collected in either sodium citrate or EDTA may be used. Sodium citrate is the preferred anticoagulant and the specimen must fill the entire tube, if an evacuated tube is used, in order to achieve the correct ratio of blood to anticoagulant. The ratio is 4 vol of blood to 1 vol of sodium citrate. If EDTA anticoagulant is used, it *must* be diluted to the ratio of 4 vol of blood to 1 vol of 0.9% sodium chloride.

Blood should be at *room temperature for testing* and should be no more than 2 hours old. If anticoagulated blood is refrigerated, the test must be set up within 6 hours. Hemolyzed specimens *cannot* be used.

Reagent, Supplies, and Equipment
1. Westergren pipettes
2. Vertical rack: This special rack is equipped with a leveling bubble device to ensure that the tubes are held in a vertical position within 1 degree. The fittings on the rack should be clean and uncracked to prevent leakage of the diluted blood.

Procedure
1. Mix the blood citrate or blood-EDTA-saline mixture thoroughly.
2. Aspirate a bubble-free specimen into a clean and dry Westergren pipette. Fill to the 0 mark. *Do not pipette by mouth.*
3. Place the pipette into the vertical rack at 20° to 25°C in an area free from vibrations, drafts, and direct sunlight.
4. After 60 minutes, read the distance in millimeters from the bottom of the plasma meniscus to the top of the sedimented erythrocytes.
5. Record the value as millimeters in 1 hour.

Reporting Results
The reference value of this test varies depending on age. In persons under 50 years old, the average reference values are up to 10 mm/hr in males and 13 mm/hr in females. For persons over 50 years old, average reference values are up to 13 mm/hr in males and up to 20 mm/hr in females.

Procedure Notes

Sources of Error
Numerous sources of error have been cited for the ESR procedure. The age of the specimen is important, the test should be performed at 20° to 25°C, and the blood should be at room temperature. Other sources of error include incorrect ratios of blood and anticoagulant, bubbles in the Westergren tube, and tilting of the ESR tube. Tilting of the tube accelerates the fall of erythrocytes and an angle of even 3 degrees from the vertical can accelerate sedimentation by as much as 30%.

Clinical Applications
The ESR is directly proportional to the weight of the cell aggregate and inversely proportional to the surface area. Microcytes sediment more slowly than macrocytes. Erythrocytes with abnormal or irregular shapes, such as sickle cells or spherocytes, hinder rouleaux formation and lower the ESR. The removal of fibrinogen by defibrination also produces a decreased ESR.

An increased ESR value can be seen due to various abnormal blood conditions: rouleaux, increased fibrinogen levels, a relative increase of plasma globulins due to the loss of plasma albumin, and an absolute increase of plasma globulins. Clinical conditions associated with increased ESR values include anemia; infections; inflammation; tissue necrosis, such as myocardial infarction; pregnancy; and some types of hemolytic anemia.

Reference
Koepke, John A. *Standardized Method for the Human Erythrocyte Sedimentation Rate (E.S.R.) Test.* Villanova, PA: National Committee for Clinical Laboratory Standards, 1978.

Sedimentation Rate of Erythrocytes: Wintrobe Method

Principle
See Principle at the Westergren Method (above) for details.

Specimen
Fresh blood collected in EDTA anticoagulant may be used. A minimum of 2 mL of whole blood is needed. The specimen must be

(continued)

well-mixed and the procedure must be performed within 2 hours of blood collection.

Reagent, Supplies, and Equipment

1. Wintrobe Sedrate tubes: These tubes are available in either reusable glass or disposable form. Depending on the type of Wintrobe rack used, the choice of tube includes graduated or plain.
2. Wintrobe sedimentation rack (graduated or plain)
3. Pasteur pipette (long-tipped) and rubber pipette bulb

Procedure

1. Gently and thoroughly mix the anticoagulated blood.
2. Draw as much blood as possible into the Pasteur pipette with the attached pipette bulb.
3. Place the tip of the pipette (filled with blood) into the Wintrobe tube until the tip touches the bottom of the tube.
4. Gently begin to press the pipette bulb and slowly move the pipette tip up from the bottom of the tube. *Continuous pressure must be kept on the pipette bulb while the pipette tip is moved up from the bottom of the tube.* The pipette tip must be in continuous motion in order to avoid introducing air bubbles into the column of blood.
5. The Wintrobe tube must be filled to the 0 mark.
6. Place the tube into a Wintrobe tube holder that has been adjusted to a perfectly level position.
7. Allow the tube to stand for 1 hour at room temperature in a draft-free room.
8. Read the tube from the bottom of the plasma meniscus to the top of the sedimented erythrocytes. Each line on the tube represents 1 mm.

Reporting Results

The patient's value is reported in millimeters per hour. The reference value for women is 0 to 20 mm/hr and for men it is 0 to 9 mm/hr.

Procedure Notes

One of the major drawbacks of this procedure is that the 100-mm tube length and the narrow bore of the tube limit readings in excess of 60 mm/hr. Care must be taken to avoid introducing air bubbles into the column and to fill the tube to the 0 mark.

Sources of Error

Falsely *increased* results can be produced by:

1. Positioning the tube at an incline rather than in a vertical position
2. Allowing the tube to stand for longer than 1 hour
3. A room temperature above normal

Falsely *decreased* results can be produced by:

1. An improper concentration of anticoagulant–whole blood ratio
2. Anticoagulated blood that is more than 2 hours old
3. Allowing the tube to stand for less than 1 hour
4. Refrigerated blood or a decreased room temperature

Clinical Applications

Refer to the Westergren Method above.

Reference

Seivard, Charles E. *Hematology for Medical Technologists*. Philadelphia: Lea & Febiger, 1972, pp. 308–313.

SPECIAL HEMATOLOGY PROCEDURES

Acidified Serum Lysis Test: Ham Method

Principle

Erythrocytes are incubated with fresh and heated serum in order to test for hemolysis. Weak acid is used in specific serum cell mixtures to maximize hemolytic activity. The presence of hemolysis, depending on the test conditions, may be observed in cases of antibody-sensitized coated erythrocytes, spherocytes, or paroxysmal nocturnal hemoglobinuria (PNH).

Specimen

Obtain 10 mL of fresh, defibrinated whole blood from both the patient and a normal control. The normal control must be ABO blood group–compatible with the patient. Hemolysis of the specimen during venipuncture must be avoided.

Reagents, Supplies, and Equipment

1. 0.2 N hydrochloric acid: Place approximately 40 mL of distilled water into a 100-mL volumetric flask. Add 20 mL of 1 N hydrochloric acid and dilute to the calibration mark with distilled water. Mix. Prepare prior to use.
2. 0.85% sodium chloride (isotonic saline solution) in a wash bottle
3. Drabkin's solution: Weigh 50 mg of potassium cyanide and 200 mg of potassium ferricyanide. Transfer to a 1-L volumetric flask and dilute to the calibration mark with distilled water. Mix and transfer to a labeled, stoppered, brown bottle.
4. Glassware: 10-mL test tubes, 10 to 20 glass beads, graduated conical centrifuge tubes
5. 1-mL and 5-mL graduated serological pipettes and safety bulb, six 12 × 75-mm or equivalent test tubes, Pasteur pipettes, and rubber bulb
6. 56°C water bath or heat block; 37°C water bath or heat block
7. Parafilm, tissue wipes, and waterproof marking pen
8. Centrifuge, spectrophotometer, and 12 × 75-mm cuvettes

Quality Control

A normal control specimen must be run concurrently with the patient specimen. The normal control must be ABO-compatible with the patient. A positive control can be added to the procedure to assess the complement activity of the donor serum by testing it with known PNH (positive) cells or with AET cells. AET cells are normal erythrocytes rendered PNH-like by treatment with *S*-2-aminoethylisothiuronium bromide.

Procedure

1. Place 10 mL of fresh, unclotted blood into a test tube with 8 to 10 glass beads. Rotate the test tube until the noise of the beads is no longer heard (about 10 minutes). Repeat, using the control.

(continued)

SPECIAL HEMATOLOGY PROCEDURES (continued)

TABLE 24.2 Acidified Serum Lysis Test (Ham Method): Procedural Setup

Constituents	Test Tubes (in mL)					
	1	2	3	4	5	6
Fresh normal serum	0.5	0.5	—	—	0.5	0.5
Patient's fresh serum	—	—	0.5	—	—	—
Heated normal serum	—	—	—	0.5	—	—
0.2N hydrochloric acid	0.05	—	0.05	0.05	—	0.05
50% patient's cells	0.05	0.05	0.05	0.05	—	—
50% normal cells	—	—	—	—	0.05	0.05

2. Centrifuge the specimens. Separate the serum using a Pasteur pipette and place in clean, labeled test tubes. Wash the cells remaining in the original tube 2 to 3 times with saline solution. After the final wash, add an equivalent amount of 0.85% sodium chloride (NaCl) to prepare a 50% cell suspension. Cover and mix by inversion.
3. Place 2 to 3 mL of the normal control serum at 56°C for 30 minutes. This heat processing destroys complement.
4. Label six 12 × 75-mm test tubes and add constituents as shown in Table 24.2.
5. Mix each tube and incubate at 37°C for 1 hour. Following incubation, centrifuge and visually observe for hemolysis.

Reporting Results
Normal patients and the normal control should exhibit no hemolysis of erythrocytes.

Alternate Measurement
If hemolysis is observed, an optional procedure is to determine the percentage of hemolysis. This can be performed as follows:

1. Zero blank: Add 0.5 mL of the normal serum to 0.85 mL of NaCl.
2. 100% hemolysis: Add 0.05 mL of the normal erythrocyte suspension to 0.9 mL of Drabkin's solution.
3. Add 0.5 mL of the supernatant from each of the tubes 1 through 6. Add 5 mL of Drabkin's solution to each. Mix and transfer each to a 12 × 75-mm cuvette.
4. Set a prewarmed spectrophotometer to 540 nm. Insert the zero blank cuvette and adjust to 100%T.
5. Read the %T of tubes 1 through 6 and the 100% hemolysis tube. Record. Using a conversion tube, convert the %T readings to OD.

Calculations

$$\% \text{ Hemolysis} = \frac{\text{OD of tubes 1-6}}{\text{OD of 100\% hemolysis tube}} \times 100$$

Reporting Results
A positive test exhibits 10 to 50% in the test tubes, with a range from 5% to 80%.

Procedure Notes

Sources of Error
Normal serum must be ABO-compatible with the patient's erythrocytes. A pH of 5.6 must be maintained in the acidified mix-

tures. The most important consideration is the PNH hemolytic activity of the normal serum. If the complement activity in the normal serum is low, a false-negative reaction may result. Less lysis occurs in PNH patients who recently received a blood transfusion because of the presence of normal circulating erythrocytes from the transfusion.

Clinical Applications
In a positive case of PNH, the typical visually graded hemolysis in the six test tubes should be:

Test Tube	Results
1	3+
2	Trace
3	1+
4	Negative
5	Negative
6	Negative

This pattern reflects the typical effect of complement found in fresh serum on PNH erythrocytes. Acidification of the mixture of fresh complement containing serum and PNH erythrocytes enhances hemolysis. PNH erythrocytes are unusually sensitive to the complement which, when activated, binds to erythrocytes and lyses abnormal erythrocytes. The patient's own serum may or may not produce hemolysis, depending on the amount of residual complement in the serum. A supporting positive result on a sucrose hemolysis test is also found in PNH.

If hemolysis occurs in the tube containing heated (complement-inactivated) serum (tube 4), the test result is not positive for PNH. In this case, spherocytes or antibody-sensitized cells may be responsible.

Limitations
A positive acidified serum test result also occurs in congenital dyserythropoietic anemia; however, hemolysis does not occur with the patient's own fresh serum. Additional testing in these cases, such as the sucrose hemolysis test, reveals negative results in congenital dyserythropoietic anemia.

Reference
Bauer, John D. (ed.). *Clinical Laboratory Methods* (9th edition). St. Louis: Mosby, 1982, p. 219.

(continued)

Bone Marrow Examination

Principle
A bone marrow aspiration is performed by a physician in order to examine the cellular activities of the marrow. Properly prepared specimens are usually stained with a Wright-Giemsa stain and special stains, such as Prussian blue, and cytochemical stains for various enzymes. A specimen of the marrow is also examined histologically using a hematoxylin-eosin (H and E) stain.

Bone marrow examination is of value in the diagnosis of disorders specifically involving the marrow, such as multiple myeloma, and in the study of leukemias and some types of anemia. In most cases, the bone marrow presents the early developmental events that produce the blood picture seen in peripheral blood or evidence of an underlying systemic disease.

Specimen
Refer to Chapter 2 for details on specimen collection and Wright-Giemsa staining. For details on special stains, refer to the specific staining procedure in this section. A peripheral blood smear should also be collected on the same day as the bone marrow aspiration.

Procedure
Examination of Bone Marrow Slides
1. Using the 10× objective, the smear is scanned for any apparent overall cellular abnormalities. An estimation of cellularity can also be appraised. Semiquantitative assessments of cellularity in aspirates can be classified into hypoplastic, normal, and hyperplastic levels. Cellularity varies with a patient's age and the site of the bone marrow aspiration. Marrow cellularity is expressed as the ratio of the volume of hematopoietic cells to the total volume of the marrow space (cells plus fat as well as other stromal elements).
2. Using the 100× (oil) immersion objective, a differential count of at least 200 cells is performed. Any abnormalities in distribution will be apparent by this examination. Erythrocyte maturational and morphological abnormalities and megakaryocyte morphology should be examined during cell differentiation. Nonhematopoietic cells of normal bone marrow may also be seen. These cells are reticulum cells (marrow macrophages), osteoblasts and osteoclasts, and mast cells. Reticulum cells are peaceful macrophages that represent the skeletal and structural components of the marrow sinuses. Osteoblasts and osteoclasts are uncommon in marrow aspirates because they are not involved in hematopoiesis. The function of osteoblasts and osteoclasts is formation and remodeling of bone. Mast cells are connective tissue cells with no defined ancestral relationship to the blood basophil or its precursors. Mast cells along with plasma cells are characteristic of marrow damage or depletion. Clusters of metastatic neoplastic cells may also be observed in bone marrow smears.
3. Using duplicate bone marrow smears, any special stains (e.g., iron) should be promptly performed and examined.
4. The peripheral blood smear should be simultaneously examined.

Reporting Results
The technologist usually refers the slides and slide examination report to a pathologist for comparison with the hematoxylin-eosin preparation. The cellularity of the specimen is usually determined from the histological specimen and the myeloid-erythroid (M/E) ratio is determined from the bone marrow aspiration slides. The pathologist will then assign a diagnosis to the case and suggest supplementary tests, if necessary.

Normal Distribution of Bone Marrow Cells in an Adult

Cell Type	Mean %
Rubricytic series	21.5%
Rubriblasts	0.6%
Prorubricytes	2.0%
Rubricytes	12.4%
Metarubricytes	6.5%
Neutrophil series	56.0%
Blasts	1.0%
Promyelocytes	3.4%
Myelocytes	11.9%
Metamyelocytes	18.0%
Bands	11.0%
PMNs	10.7%
Eosinophil series	3.2%
Basophils	<0.1%
Lymphocytes	15.8%
Monocytes	1.8%
Megakaryocytes	<0.1%
Reticulum cells	0.3%
Plasma cells	1.8%
M/E ratio	2.5:1

Reference
Jandl, James H. *Blood*. Boston: Little, Brown & Co., 1987, p. 27.

Donath-Landsteiner Screening Test

Principle
The Donath-Landsteiner antibody test is used to demonstrate the presence of this extremely potent hemolysin. This antibody requires cold incubation in order to exhibit hemolysis in the patient's serum. A positive result is diagnostic of paroxysmal cold hemoglobinuria (PCH), the rarest form of autoimmune hemolytic anemia.

Specimen
Fresh venous blood. Care must be taken to avoid hemolyzing the specimen during venipuncture.

Reagents, Supplies, and Equipment
1. 16 × 100-mm test tubes
2. Crushed ice water bath (4°C)
3. 37°C water bath or heat block

Quality Control
A normal patient control specimen is run concurrently with the patient's test specimen.

Procedure
1. Place two test tubes in a 37°C water bath or heat block. Warm a 10-mL syringe by holding it in the palm of the hand for a few minutes.
2. Draw 10 mL of blood and transfer 5 mL to each test tube. Label one tube "control" and immediately place at 37°C. Label the other tube "test" and place in an ice water bath at 4°C. Incubate both tubes for 1 hour. At the end of 1 hour, move the test sample to the 37°C water bath for an additional 30 minutes.

(continued)

SPECIAL HEMATOLOGY PROCEDURES (continued)

3. At the end of 90 minutes, carefully remove the tubes and examine for hemolysis.

Reporting Results

If the serum in both tubes is free of hemolysis, the test result is negative. If a pink or red color is present in the serum of the test sample and the control sample is free of hemolysis, the test result is positive. Normal blood will exhibit no hemolysis in either tube.

Procedure Notes

A positive result is diagnostic of PCH. This disease is caused by a cold autoantibody with several unique characteristics. It is a complement-dependent, IgG cold antibody; hemolysis occurs only after warming, even though complement activation may initially occur in the cold. The causative antibody, the **Donath-Landsteiner antibody,** is extremely lytic and is one of the most potent hemolysins known.

References

Bauer, John D. *Clinical Laboratory Methods* (9th edition). St. Louis: Mosby, 1982, pp. 426–427.
Seivard, Charles E. *Hematology for Medical Technologists.* Philadelphia: Lea & Febiger, 1972, p. 553.

....

Glucose-6-Phosphate Dehydrogenase Activity in Erythrocytes: Visual Fluorescent Screening Test

Principle

The enzyme glucose-6-phosphate dehydrogenase (G6PD) catalyzes the following reaction:

$$\text{Glucose-6-phosphate}$$
$$\text{(not fluorescent)}$$
$$+ \text{ NADP} \xrightarrow{\text{G6PD}} \text{6-phosphogluconate} + \text{NADPH}$$
$$\text{(fluorescent)}$$

The reaction mixture containing glucose-6-phosphate, nicotinamide adenine dinucleotide phosphate (NADP), and blood is incubated, and at timed intervals drops of the mixture are applied to filter paper. The fluorescence of reduced nucleotides, when activated with long-wave (340 to 370 nm) ultraviolet (UV) light, is used for visual examination of G6PD activity. The observed rate of the appearance of bright fluorescence is proportional to the blood G6PD activity. G6PD deficiency is one of the most prevalent hereditary erythrocyte enzyme deficiencies. A deficiency of this enzyme can produce drug- or stress-induced hemolytic anemia in afflicted persons.

Specimen

Anticoagulated blood or blood samples collected on filter paper and subsequently eluted can be used. The anticoagulants that can be used include heparin, EDTA, citrate phosphate dextrose (CPD), or acid citrate dextrose (ACD). Blood that has been anticoagulated with ACD can be used after several weeks of storage at 4°C. The screening test is recommended for detecting deficiencies.

Reagents, Supplies, and Equipment

1. 0.075 M phosphate buffer (pH 7.4) (Sigma Diagnostics No. 202)

2. G6PD screening substrate containing the following active ingredients: glucose-6-phosphate and NADP (Sigma Diagnostics No. 202). The vial of screening substrate needs to be reconstituted with 2.0 mL of 0.075 M phosphate buffer (reagent 1). After addition of the buffer, the vial should stand for 1 to 2 minutes. Mix carefully. *Use as soon as possible.* The reconstituted substrate is stable for approximately 2 weeks, if stored at 0°C.
3. A long-wave UV light in a viewing box or darkened room: Lamps that emit light between 320 and 400 nm are satisfactory. Short-wave UV light is not acceptable.
4. Pipettes: 10 μL and 2.0 mL
5. Glass or plastic test tubes (12 × 75 mm)
6. Pasteur pipettes
7. No. 1 filter paper
8. Heat block or water bath incubator at 37°C

Quality Control

Two commercial products are available for use as controls: a G6PD-deficient control (Sigma No. G 5888) and a normal G6PD control (Sigma No. G 6888). These controls are run in conjunction with patient tests. False-positive results have not been observed when proper controls are run.

Procedure

1. Label the patient and control test tubes. One tube is needed for each assay. Pipette 0.2 mL of the G6PD reagent substrate into each of the tubes.
2. Into the normal control tube, pipette 10 μL of normal blood and mix.
3. Promptly transfer a drop of this mixture onto a labeled filter paper and identify as "zero-time control." Place this tube at 37°C.
4. Repeat the procedure in step 3 for each of the respective patient samples or the G6PD-deficient control blood, except the labeling should be "zero-time test." Place each of the tubes at 37°C.
5. Transfer a drop of blood from each of the tubes to their respective filter papers at 5 minutes and 10 minutes following the zero-time test. The time needs to be approximate.
6. Allow the filter paper to air-dry and visually inspect with a long-wave UV light. Examine the spots for fluorescence *only* after drying and within 24 hours after the specimen has been applied.

Reporting Results

In normal samples, the zero-time control spot *should not* fluoresce or fluoresce only slightly. The samples from incubated G6PD normal samples should fluoresce brightly. Enzyme-deficient samples either fail to fluoresce or show only very dull fluorescence.

Procedure Notes

Sources of Error

If the (PCV) hematocrit exceeds 0.50 L/L, use only half as much blood because quenching of fluorescence occurs in the presence of high concentrations of hemoglobin. If the hematocrit is less than 0.20 L/L, a larger amount of blood may be necessary.

Clinical Applications

This assay is used in diagnosing G6PD deficiency, an X-linked disorder that can result in anemia. G6PD deficiency is the most

(continued)

prevalent hereditary erythrocyte enzyme deficiency. The enzyme is decreased in 13% of American black men. Although only 3% of American black women demonstrate an enzyme deficiency, 20% are carriers. Some other ethnic groups, such as Greeks, are also afflicted with the disorder. A decrease in G6PD may be associated with at least four clinical syndromes:

1. Some drug-induced acute hemolytic anemias (e.g., primaquine and sulfonamides)
2. Favism
3. Nonimmunological hemolytic disease of the newborn
4. Some cases of congenital nonspherocytic hemolytic anemia

An increase in G6PD is seen in conditions such as pernicious anemia and other megaloblastic anemias, hepatic coma, and chronic blood loss, as well as in the first week following a myocardial infarction.

References

"Glucose-6-Phosphate Dehydrogenase (G-6-PDH)." *Sigma Product Bull.*, Vol. 6. St. Louis: Sigma Diagnostics, 1983, p. 15.

Tanakada, Kouichi R. *Screening Red Blood Cell Glucose 6-Phosphate Dehydrogenase Activity* (Approved Standard), Vol. 4. No. 15. Villanova, PA: National Committee for Clinical Laboratory Standards, 1984.

Wallach, Jacques. *Interpretation of Diagnostic Tests* (5th edition). Boston: Little, Brown & Co., 1991.

··

Hemoglobin Electrophoresis: Cellulose Acetate Method

Principle

Electrophoresis may be defined as the movement of charged particles on various media under the influence of an electric current. Particles move at different speeds because of their weight and electric charge.

In hemoglobin electrophoresis, a hemolysate prepared from intact erythrocytes is placed on a medium such as cellulose acetate. The strips of cellulose acetate are placed in an alkaline buffer (pH 8.0 to 8.6) and electrical charge is applied. The strips are stained in order to see the hemoglobin fractions. A comparison of the unknown hemolysate with hemolysates from known hemoglobin types is made. Hemoglobin electrophoresis by cellulose acetate is useful in identifying and quantifying hemoglobin variants and abnormal quantities of hemoglobin fractions.

Specimen

Blood for hemolysate preparation may be capillary or venous blood. If venous blood is used, it can be anticoagulated with either EDTA or heparin. Venous blood drawn into EDTA anticoagulant can be stored under refrigeration for no longer than 2 weeks. Hemolysates can be refrigerated or frozen for future use.

Reagents, Supplies, and Equipment

1. Supre-Heme buffer, pH 8.4: *Working solution:* Dissolve one packet of buffer concentrate in 980 mL of distilled water.
2. Ponceau stain: Weigh out 0.5 gm, transfer to a 100-mL volumetric flask, and dilute to the calibration mark with 5% trichloracetic acid (TCA).
3. Disposable wicks and electrophoresis chamber
4. New Titan III H cellulose acetate strips with Mylar backing
5. Sample applicator, sample plate, and aligning base
   Note: The items listed in 1 through 5 are available from Helena Laboratories (Beaumont, Texas).
6. 5% acetic acid
7. 20% glacial acetic acid in absolute methanol
8. Absolute methanol
9. Filter or blotting paper, test tubes, and pipettes

Quality Control

Known samples are tested with patient samples.

Procedure

1. Prepare hemolysates for the patient and controls (see Preparation of a Hemolysate under Hemoglobin F Determination by Alkaline Denaturation) or the alternative macromethod:

   Alternative Macromethod
   A. Centrifuge approximately 5 mL of anticoagulated blood for 15 to 20 minutes at 2500 rpm in a graduated conical centrifuge tube. Remove the plasma.
   B. Wash the packed erythrocytes 3 to 4 times with saline solution. Mix by inversion after each wash. The final supernatant should be colorless. Remove this supernatant with a Pasteur pipette.
   C. Measure the packed erythrocytes, add 1.4 mL of distilled water for each 1 mL of cells, mix, and place in the freezer for 15 to 20 minutes. Remove from the freezer and allow to come to room temperature. Add 0.4 mL of toluene for each 1 mL of the original PCV. Cover and shake for 5 minutes.
   D. Centrifuge at 2500 to 3000 rpm for 15 to 20 minutes.
   E. Remove the toluene with a cotton tip swab. Insert a Pasteur pipette into the clear hemoglobin solution. Transfer to a clean test tube. Label. This hemolysate solution can be stored for several weeks, if frozen or refrigerated.
2. The hemolysate needs to be diluted to a 1:6 dilution with 1 vol of hemolysate and 5 vol of distilled water.
3. Pour buffer into the outer chamber of the electrophoresis chamber, soak the wicks, and properly position them. Identify the specimens on the Mylar side of the strips, lower the rack of plates slowly into the buffer, and soak in buffer for at least 5 minutes. Quickly blot the plates between two pieces of filter paper to remove excess moisture.
4. Apply the diluted hemolysate to the cellulose acetate side of the plate about 3 cm from the cathode using a microdispenser.
5. Place the plate, cellulose acetate side down, into the chamber with the application site near the cathode, and place a glass slide on the plate to establish good contact.
6. Cover the chamber and apply 350 V for 15 minutes at room temperature.
7. Remove the plates from the chamber and stain for 3 minutes with Ponceau S stain. Remove the plates from the stain.
8. Place in three consecutive 2-minute washes of 5% acetic acid until the background is white. Fix the plate in absolute methanol for 3 to 5 minutes. Clear the plate in 20% glacial acetic acid in absolute methanol for 10 minutes. Air-dry.

Reporting Results

Identify the hemoglobin types in the patient sample by comparing the migration distances with known controls. The slow types of hemoglobin, such as Hb A_2 and C, are found near the cathode end and the fast types, such as Hb H, are found near the anode end. The variants that are located about halfway include Hb F. The mobilities of various hemoglobins are illustrated in Figure 5.9. Quantitative results can be determined by scanning with a densitometer; however, Hb A_2 and F should not be quantitated because the results do not conform to those of other quantitative methods.

(continued)

SPECIAL HEMATOLOGY PROCEDURES (continued)

Procedure Notes

Sources of Error
Faulty technique is the major source of error in this procedure.

Clinical Applications
Hemoglobin electrophoresis is useful as part of a hematology profile in the diagnosis of hemoglobinopathies such as sickle cell disease and hereditary persistence of fetal hemoglobin.

Limitations
Some of the normal and abnormal hemoglobins migrate at the same speed. For example, Hb H and I are the same, Hb S and D are the same, and Hb F and G are the same. Hemoglobins with identical mobilities can be differentiated by supplementing electrophoresis with other procedures, such as Hb F or Hb S procedures, and by performing a citrate agar electrophoresis confirmatory identification of hemoglobins.

Reference
Bauer, John D. *Clinical Laboratory Methods* (9th edition). St. Louis: Mosby, 1982, pp. 67–69.

....

Hemoglobin F Determination by Alkaline Denaturation: Method of Pembrey

Principle
Alkali denaturation of Hb F (fetal hemoglobin) consists of preparing and diluting a hemolysate from whole blood. The resulting hemoglobin is converted to cyanmethemoglobin, with a quantitative assay resulting.

Although the determination of fetal hemoglobin by the alkali denaturation method of Singer, Chernoff, and Singer has been widely used, it is inaccurate for fetal hemoglobin levels below about 5%. This characteristic makes the Singer method unsuitable for the determination of small amounts of Hb F in adults. The Pembrey method is accurate for very low levels of Hb F but may also be used for levels up to 50%.

Specimen
Fresh whole blood collected either in heparinized capillary tubes or on filter paper is needed. If capillary blood is used, fill two heparinized microhematocrit tubes and seal one end of each with an appropriate clay sealant. Capillary tube specimens are stable for 1 week, if refrigerated.

An alternative procedure is to cut a piece of No. 3 Whatman paper into 1×3-in. strips. Draw two 12-mm circles, one next to the other at one end. The opposite end is for patient identification. Completely fill the circles with blood by bringing a drop of blood into contact with the undersurface of the filter paper. Allow the blood filling the circles to dry completely.

Reagents, Supplies, and Equipment
Reagents
1. 1.2 M sodium hydroxide (NaOH): Prepare a *fresh* solution prior to performing the test by weighing out 4.8 gm of NaOH pellets. Transfer to a 100-mL volumetric flask and dilute to the calibration mark with distilled water. Mix.

    A stock solution of 6 M NaOH may be prepared by dissolving 24 gm/100 mL. This solution is *stable* if kept in a tightly stoppered brown bottle and refrigerated. As needed, the work-ing 1.2 M solution can be prepared by diluting 1 mL of 6 M stock solution with 4 mL of distilled water.
2. Drabkin's reagent: Weigh and transfer 50 mg of potassium cyanide and 200 mg of potassium ferricyanide to a 1-L volumetric flask. Dilute to the calibration mark with distilled water.
3. Saturated ammonium sulfate: Weigh and transfer 100 gm of ammonium sulfate to a 100-mL volumetric flask. Dilute with distilled water to the calibration mark. Allow to stand, with occasional vigorous shaking to saturate the solution. The solution can be transferred to a tightly capped brown bottle for storage.
4. Saponin lysing reagent stock solution: Weigh out 1 gm of saponin powder. Transfer to a 100-mL volumetric flask and dilute with distilled water to the calibration mark.
5. 3% potassium cyanide (KCN). Prepare by weighing out 3 gm of KCN into a 100-mL volumetric flask and diluting to the calibration mark with distilled water.
6. Working saponin lysing solution: Combine 10 mL of the saponin lysing reagent stock solution, 90 mL of distilled water, and 2 mL of 3% KCN. Prepare *immediately* before use.

Supplies and Equipment
1. Pipettes: 1 mL and 10 mL graduated serological; safety bulb
2. Test tubes: 12×75 mm and 16×100 mm
3. Filter paper (No. 6 Whatman) and funnels
4. Stopwatch and timer
5. Conventional and microhematocrit centrifuges
6. Spectrophotometer and cuvettes

Quality Control
A normal adult blood specimen as well as a neonatal specimen should be tested in conjunction with the patient's sample.

Preparation of a Hemolysate: Micromethod
1. Centrifuge two heparinized capillary tubes for 5 minutes in a microhematocrit centrifuge. Score each tube slightly above the upper level of the sealing clay and snap the tube apart. Drop the packed cell column into a test tube containing 6 drops of the working solution.
2. Cover the tube and shake vigorously for 15 minutes to remove the blood from the tube and to hemolyze it. Repeat this procedure for the control specimens. Half a capillary tube of whole blood has a volume of about 0.04 mL and contains 3 to 6 mg of hemoglobin.

Alternate Method for Preparation of Hemolysate: Filter Paper
1. Use a paper hole punch to punch out two discs from the dried blood on the filter paper. Place the discs into two separate test tubes, each containing 3 drops of saponin hemolyzing reagent. Repeat this procedure for the control samples.
2. Invert the tubes to mix and allow to stand for 45 minutes at room temperature. Remove the filter paper with a pair of forceps and press against the wall of the test tube before removing. Use this specimen *immediately* or *freeze*. One full drop of whole blood collected on No. 3 filter paper contains 3 to 6 mg of hemoglobin.

Procedure
For each patient specimen and the controls:
1. Place 0.6 mL of hemolysate from each specimen into a 16×100-mm test tube. Add 10 mL of Drabkin's solution to each sample and mix well.

(continued)

2. Pipette 5.6 mL of this diluted hemolysate into a second test tube. Quickly add 0.4 mL of 1.2 M NaOH. Start a stopwatch and mix at once.
3. After *exactly* 2 minutes, pipette 4.0 mL of saturated ammonium sulfate and mix well. Allow this solution to stand for approximately 15 minutes.
4. Filter through No. 6 Whatman filter paper. If the initial filtrate is cloudy, refilter. The final filtrate must be perfectly clear.
5. To prepare a *total hemoglobin* sample for each test specimen, mix 1.4 mL of diluted hemolysate, 1.6 mL of distilled water, and 2 mL of saturated ammonium sulfate. Mix. Transfer 1 mL of this mixture to a test tube and add 9 mL of distilled water. This 1:10 dilution is the *total hemoglobin* solution.
6. Transfer each filtrate and its corresponding total hemoglobin solution to matched cuvettes. Set the spectrophotometer to 415 nm and adjust to 100%T (0 absorbance or OD) with distilled water. Read the absorbance of the filtrate and total hemoglobin directly if a digital spectrophotometer is used. If a conventional spectrophotometer is used, read the %T and use a conversion table to convert %T to absorbance (OD).

Calculations

$$\% \text{ Hb F} = \frac{\text{OD of filtrate}}{\text{OD of total hemoglobin}} \times 5$$

The factor of 5 equals 100 (to convert to percentage) divided by the ratio of the dilutions of the filtrate and total hemoglobin.

Reporting Results
Reference values: Adult—0.9%; infants over 1 year old—2%; neonates—70 to 90%.

Procedure Notes
Maternal hemoglobin can reach 10% to 15% of total hemoglobin.

Sources of Error
Improper technique can produce errors.

Clinical Applications
A variety of conditions are associated with high and low Hb F values.

Examples of Disorders Associated With Elevated Hemoglobin F
1. Up to 50%—beta thalassemia, Ph[1]-negative leukemia
2. Up to 25%—paroxysmal nocturnal hemoglobinuria
3. 10% to 20%—homozygous Hb S disease
4. 2% to 5%—acquired and congenital anemias

Reference
Bauer, John D. (ed.). *Clinical Laboratory Methods* (9th edition). St. Louis: Mosby, 1982, pp. 51–52.

....

Hemoglobin S Screening Test: Qualitative Differential Solubility Test

Principle
This is a biphasic system consisting of an upper organic phase of toluene and a lower, aqueous phase containing phosphate buffer, saponin, and reducing agents. Erythrocytes are lysed by toluene and saponin, with the released hemoglobin being reduced by sodium hydrosulfite. The resulting colors of the aqueous phase and the interface phase allow for the differentiation of hemoglobin types AA, AS, and SS.

Detection of the abnormal Hb S is diagnostic of sickle cell disease. Hb S, if inherited in the homozygous state (SS), results in sickle cell anemia. Inheritance of the heterozygous state (AS) produces a benign and asymptomatic condition, except under conditions of reduced oxygen levels. The detection of this heterozygous state is important to diagnose in individuals who are involved in strenuous physical sports, such as long-distance runners, or in individuals whose occupations have the potential for reduced oxygen levels, such as test pilots.

Specimen
Either fresh or anticoagulated blood may be used. Any of the following anticoagulants may be used: ACD, sodium citrate, heparin, or EDTA; however, EDTA is the anticoagulant of choice. Fresh blood should be tested immediately, prior to clotting.

Reagents, Supplies, and Equipment
1. Sicklequik reagent: The prepackaged test tubes contain enough reagent for one test. Each tube contains 0.5 mL toluene; 2.0 mL aqueous, buffered reducing and lysing reagents (active ingredients: 9 gm/L sodium hydrosulfite, 9 gm/L saponin, and a stabilizer); a stabilizer; and a phosphate buffer (pH 6.4 ± 0.2). If crystals are seen on the bottom of the tube due to loosening of the cap, the test vial cannot be used. This reagent is ready to use. If stored at 20 to 30°C, the reagent is stable until the expiration date shown on the label (12 months from date of manufacture). *Caution:* Toluene is flammable. It must not be used near an open flame or stored in direct sunlight, near room-heating devices, or near any heat-producing appliance.
2. Pipettes, disposable, 100 μL (0.1 mL), and pipette wipes or Pasteur pipettes and rubber bulbs
3. Clinical centrifuge
4. Vortex mixer (optional)
5. Positive hemoglobin (AS and SS), and negative (AA) blood controls

Quality Control
Positive blood controls for Hb AS and SS as well as a normal (negative) Hb AA control should be tested with each test run. These controls evaluate test performance and familiarize the technologist with the end points of the procedure. Commercial specimens or known patients can be used as positive and negative controls; however, commercially available hemolysates intended for hemoglobin electrophoresis are not suitable.

Procedure
1. Label the reagent tubes with the patient's name or, if a control, either AA, AS, or SS. One tube is required for each test.
2. Add 100 μL (0.1 mL) or 2 drops of the patient's whole blood or known control blood to their respective reagent tubes.
3. Recap the reagent tube tightly and shake it vigorously for at least 10 seconds or mix with a vortex mixer for 10 seconds.
4. Allow to stand for 5 minutes for hemoglobin reduction.
5. Centrifuge the mixture for 5 minutes at approximately 3400 rpm. Centrifuge speed is not critical to the test procedure. If the end point is not completely clear, recentrifugation may be required.
    or
    Allow the mixture to stand in a vertical position for at least 2 hours. The end point is stable for at least 72 hours; however, do not allow the mixture to stand for more than 72 hours before reading the results.

(continued)

SPECIAL HEMATOLOGY PROCEDURES (*continued*)

Reporting Results

Following centrifugation or after 2 hours of standing, several layers will form. Only the interface layer and the lower aqueous phase are significant to the interpretation of the test. The normal (AA) hemoglobin tube should have a dark-red lower aqueous phase and a gray-pink interface layer. In the AS or heterozygous types of hemoglobin, the lower aqueous phase can be various shades of red and the interface is a purple-red color. In SS-type hemoglobin, the lower aqueous phase is a straw-yellow to amber color and the interface is purple-red.

Hb SS types are detected at all levels. Although the Hb S content in AS samples varies from 25% to 40%, 7-gm/dL AS samples should contain sufficient Hb S to distinguish them from normal AA hemoglobin types by reading the interface layer as well as the lower aqueous phase. The sample size may be doubled if difficulty is encountered in interpreting the test results.

Procedure Notes

Sources of Error

1. Recently transfused patients with potentially abnormal hemoglobin types may produce heterozygous or negative results.
2. Due to interference from fetal hemoglobin (Hb F), samples from patients under 6 months old should not be tested. Hereditary persistence of fetal hemoglobin may also cause false-negative results.

Limitations of Procedure

In sickle cell variants, the same results will be obtained as in sickle cell trait. Heterozygous S results should be tested further using electrophoresis methods.

Clinical Applications

This procedure differentiates normal type AA hemoglobin from heterozygous and homozygous SS hemoglobins.

Reference

Sicklequik product insert. General Diagnostics, Division of Warner-Lambert Co., Morris Plains, NJ (Organon Teknika, Durham, NC).

Malarial Smears

Principle

Thick and thin blood smears are prepared, stained, and examined microscopically for the presence of one of four malaria types. Detection and correct identification of the species of malaria (*Plasmodium malariae, P. vivax, P. falciparum,* or *P. ovale*) are important to ensure proper treatment.

Specimen

Smears of capillary or EDTA-anticoagulated blood are prepared as described in the section on specimen preparation in Chapter 2.

Reagents, Supplies, and Equipment

1. ACS (American Chemical Society) grade methanol
2. ACS-grade glycerol
3. Buffer (pH 6.4 or 6.8)

   Solution A: Prepare by placing 9.47 gm of anhydrous secondary sodium phosphate (Na_2HPO_4) or 11.87 gm of hydrated sodium phosphate ($Na_2HPO_4 \cdot 2H_2O$) into a 1-L volumetric flask. Dilute to the calibration mark with deionized water. Mix.

   Solution B: Weigh and transfer 9.080 gm of primary potassium phosphate (KH_2PO_4) into a 1-L volumetric flask. Dilute to the calibration mark with deionized water. Mix.

   Solutions A and B can be mixed in various proportions to achieve a different pH. Buffer (6.4 pH). Mix 26.7 mL of solution A and 73.3 mL of solution B. Buffer (6.8 pH). Mix 49.6 mL of solution A and 50.4 mL of solution B. *Refrigerate all solutions to store.*
4. Giemsa stock stain: Prepare by adding 5 gm of powdered Giemsa stain to 330 mL of reagent grade glycerol. Mix. Place in a 60° C oven for 2 hours. Allow to cool. Mix. With constant stirring slowly add 330 mL of methanol. Transfer to a stoppered brown bottle and shake for a few minutes. Label. Filter *before use.*

   Working Giemsa stain: Prepare by adding 10 mL of filtered Giemsa stock stain to 90 mL of buffer solution. Mix.
5. Coplin or other type of staining jar and slide holder
6. Microscope, immersion oil, and lens paper

Quality Control

A reference slide set should be maintained in order to validate the ability of microscopists to identify various malarial species. Participation in a quality assurance program such as the College of American Pathologists (CAP) program is important in maintaining expertise in this area, particularly in laboratories that infrequently encounter positive results.

Procedure

1. Following blood smear preparation, allow the smears to air-dry for about 30 minutes. Fix the thin smears in methanol for a few seconds. Do not fix the thick smears.
2. Place the smears in a Coplin jar containing Giemsa staining solution for 30 minutes. Rinse the smears in running tap water and allow to air-dry.
3. Examine the smears using the oil immersion objective. The erythrocytes on the thick, unfixed smears will be destroyed, making examination easier. The thick smear is used as a screening test to establish the presence of the parasite. The thin smear, which allows for careful examination of cellular morphology, permits identification of the species of malaria.

Reporting Results

The diagnosis of malaria is based on the demonstration of the *Plasmodium* species in the blood. Refer to Plate 25 for illustrations of the typical appearance of various species. A brief morphological description is given in Table 24.3. For a complete discussion of each of the *Plasmodium* species, as well as other factors related to malaria, see Chapter 6.

Procedure Notes

Sources of Error

Malarial parasites can be confused with platelets. It is important to distinguish between malarial parasites *in* the erythrocyte compared to platelets that are superimposed on the erythrocyte. Malarial parasites are never seen in the spaces between erythrocytes.

Clinical Applications

It is important to recognize and distinguish between the various types of malaria in order to treat the patient properly. Treatment is important because plasmodia infect and destroy erythrocytes.

(continued)

TABLE 24.3 **Morphological Comparison of *Plasmodium* sp.**

Species	RBC Appearance		Parasitic Appearance	
	size	inclusions	cytoplasm	merozoites
P. vivax	Enlarged	Schüffner's dots	Blue discs with red nucleus Accolé forms Signet ring forms	12–24
P. falciparum	Normal	Maurer's dots	Minute rings Two chromatin dots Accolé forms Gametes: crescent-shaped	6–32
P. malariae	Normal	Ziemann's dots	One ring with one dot	6–12
P. ovale	Enlarged	Schüffner's dots	One ring form	6–14

Limitations

The procedure is tedious and it is frequently very difficult to locate infected erythrocytes.

References

Bauer, John L. *Clinical Laboratory Methods* (9th edition). St. Louis: Mosby, 1982, p. 976.

Markell, Edward K. et al. *Medical Parasitology* (6th edition). Philadelphia: Saunders, 1986, pp. 79–85.

Seivard, Charles E. *Hematology for Medical Technologists* (4th edition). Philadelphia: Lea & Febiger, 1972, pp. 284, 545, 546.

Monospot Test (Ortho Diagnostics, Raritan, NJ)

Principle

This procedure is based on agglutination of horse erythrocytes by heterophile antibody present in infectious mononucleosis. Because horse RBCs exhibit antigens directed against both Forssman and infectious mononucleosis antibodies, a differential absorption of the patient's serum is necessary to distinguish the specific heterophile antibody from those of the Forssman type. The basic principle of the absorption steps in this procedure is comparable to that originally described by Davidsohn in his sheep agglutinin test. Serum or plasma is absorbed with both guinea pig kidney and beef erythrocyte stroma. Guinea pig kidney contains only the Forssman antigen and beef erythrocytes contain only the antigen associated with infectious mononucleosis. Guinea pig kidney will absorb only heterophile antibodies of the Forssman type and beef erythrocytes will absorb only the heterophile antibody of infectious mononucleosis. Agglutination of horse RBCs by the absorbed patient specimen is indicative of a positive reaction for heterophile antibody.

Specimen Collection and Preparation

No special preparation of the patient is required prior to specimen collection. The patient must be positively identified when the specimen is collected. The specimen is labeled at the bedside and includes the patient's full name, the date the specimen is collected, and the patient's hospital identification number. The phlebotomist's initials should also appear on the label.

Blood should be drawn by an aseptic technique. The required specimen is a minimum of 2 mL of whole blood. Serum or plasma mixed with anticoagulants, including EDTA, sodium oxalate, potassium oxalate, sodium citrate, acid citrate dextrose (ACD) solution, and heparin, may be used.

Centrifuge the tube of blood and remove an aliquot of serum. Serum or plasma samples should be clear and particle-free. The presence of hemolysis makes the specimen unsuitable for testing. Inactivation of the serum is not necessary; however, inactivated serum may be used. Serum or plasma may be stored at 2° to 8°C for several days following collection before testing. If prolonged storage is desired, the serum or plasma may be frozen.

Capillary Specimens

Note: Refer to Chapter 2 for the proper technique for the collection of capillary blood.

1. With a standard heparinized or nonheparinized capillary pipette (75-mm length, 1.1 to 1.2-mm ID, 85-μL volume), obtain a minimum of four full capillary tubes of blood from a finger puncture. The required 0.05 mL of serum or plasma can be recovered by this procedure, if the patient's hematocrit is less than 50%. If the hematocrit is greater than 50% (e.g., in newborn infants or patients with polycythemia), additional tubes must be filled.
2. Seal the dry end of each capillary tube and centrifuge for 5 minutes in a microhematocrit centrifuge.
3. Break the capillary tubes at the interface between the serum or plasma and cells.
4. Use the serum or plasma from two tubes as the patient sample for each side of the slide according to the directions for use.

Reagents, Supplies, and Equipment

1. All of the following required materials are provided in the Monospot kit:
   A. Guinea pig antigen. A suspension of guinea pig kidney antigen preserved with 1% sodium azide. Store at 2° to 8°C. Do not freeze. If properly stored, the reagent is stable until the expiration date.
   B. Beef erythrocyte stroma. A suspension of beef erythrocyte stroma antigen preserved with 1% sodium azide. Store at 2° to 8°C. Do not freeze. If properly stored, the reagent is stable until the expiration date.
   C. Horse erythrocytes. A suspension of stabilized horse RBCs preserved with (1:3000) chloramphenicol and (1:10,000) neomycin sulfate. Store at 2° to 8°C. Do not freeze. If

(continued)

SPECIAL HEMATOLOGY PROCEDURES (continued)

properly stored, the reagent is stable until the expiration date.

Hemolysis will indicate that the cells are deteriorating but proper reactivity may be verified by use of the positive control serum.

Warning: The reagents and controls contain sodium azide as a preservative. Sodium azide may react with lead and copper plumbing to form highly explosive metal azides. On disposal, flush with a large volume of water to prevent azide buildup.

D. Glass slide
E. Microcapillary pipettes (20 M) for indicator cells
F. Rubber bulbs
G. Plastic pipettes for delivery of serum or plasma samples
H. Wooden applicator sticks

2. Additional required equipment: stopwatch or laboratory timer

Quality Control

Positive control serum (human) is a human serum containing the heterophile antibody of infectious mononucleosis, preserved with 0.1% sodium azide.

Negative control serum (human) is a human serum not containing the heterophile antibody of infectious mononucleosis, preserved with 0.1% sodium azide.

The control sera should be checked when the kit arrives and periodically during the dating period.

Caution: Because the control sera are derived from human sources, they should be handled in the same manner as clinical serum specimens (see section on universal blood and body fluid precautions in Chapter 1).

Procedure

Note: All of the reagent cells should be shaken well to provide a homogeneous suspension before testing. Reagents should be at room temperature.

Qualitative Method

1. Place the slide on a flat surface under a direct light source.
2. Invert the vial containing horse (indicator) erythrocytes to resuspend the cells. Using a clean microcapillary tube, place 10 M of cells on one corner of both squares on the slide.

To use the microcapillary tube, insert the end of the pipette marked with a heavy black line 1/4 in. into the neck of the rubber tube. Hold the rubber bulb between the thumb and third finger. Tilt the vial of cells and insert the pipette. Allow the pipette to fill by capillary action to the top (20-M) mark. *Do not draw the cells into the bulb.*

To deliver 10 M of cells to the slide, place the index finger over the hole in the top of the bulb and squeeze gently until the level of cells in the pipette reaches the first mark. Touch the pipette tip to a corner of square I to release the cells. Repeat the process to deliver the remaining 10 M of cells to the corner of square II.

3. Put 1 drop of thoroughly mixed guinea pig antigen (reagent I) in square I.
4. Put 1 drop of thoroughly mixed beef erythrocyte stroma (reagent II) in square II.
5. Using a disposable plastic pipette, add 1 drop of the patient serum or plasma to the center of each square on the slide.
6. Mix the serum or plasma and the guinea pig antigen in square I at least 10 times with a clean wooden applicator stick. *Avoid the horse erythrocytes.*

7. Mix the serum or plasma and the beef erythrocyte stroma in square II at least 10 times with a clean wooden applicator stick. *Avoid the horse erythrocytes.*
8. Blend the horse (indicator) erythrocytes over the entire surface of each square. *Use a clean wooden applicator for each side and use no more than 10 stirring motions to blend.*
9. Start a timer on completion of the final mixing. *Do not move or pick up the slide during the reaction period.*
10. Observe for agglutination for no longer than 1 minute after the final mixing.

Reporting Results
Qualitative Method

If the agglutination pattern is stronger on the left side (square I), the test result is positive. If the agglutination pattern is stronger on the right side (square II), the test result is negative. If no agglutination appears on either side (I or II) of the slide, or if agglutination is equal on both squares of the slide, the test result is negative.

Procedure Notes

If a positive qualitative result is demonstrated, a titration procedure may be performed to provide a semiquantitative indication of the level of heterophile antibody.

Titration Procedure for Semiquantitative Method

1. Serial dilutions of serum (Table 24.4) can be prepared by pipetting 0.5 mL of 0.85% saline solution into each of the desired number of tubes. Pipette 0.5 mL of patient serum into the first tube, mix, and transfer 0.5 mL of the diluted serum to the second tube. Repeat this process until the final tube is reached. Discard 0.5 mL of the diluted serum from the last tube.
2. Place a titration slide on a flat surface under a direct light source. Treat each of the dilutions as if they were individual sera and follow the steps for the qualitative procedure for each of the appropriately labeled squares. *Omit the use of beef stroma and only use guinea pig antigen.*
3. The highest dilution in which visible agglutination occurs is the end point. If agglutination is present in all of the dilutions, extend the serial dilutions. Record the titration value.

Note: The titer with Monospot cannot be compared with titration values obtained with other slide or tube test proce-

TABLE 24.4 Serial Dilutions of Serum for Titration Procedure

Tube	Dilution
1	1:2
2	1:4
3	1:8
4	1:16
5	1:32
6	1:64

Source: M. L. Turgeon, *Immunology and Serology in Laboratory Medicine.* St. Louis: Mosby, 1990, p. 209.

(continued)

dures since there are significant variations in sensitivity. Fresh, stabilized horse erythrocytes have been shown to be more sensitive than sheep erythrocytes or formalinized horse erythrocytes.

The relative value of titers performed on specimens with different techniques is proportional to the concentration of heterophile antibody present. Although the titration value is not indicative of the severity of the disease, sequential examinations may provide information of value to the clinician.

Sources of Error

To obtain accurate results, only clear, particle-free serum or plasma specimens should be used.

False-positive results can be caused by:

1. Observing agglutination that appears after the 1-minute observation time.
2. Misinterpreting agglutination that occurs because the slide is moved or rocked.
3. Other factors. Simultaneous occurrence of infectious mononucleosis and hepatitis has been reported. A result that is interpreted as false-positive may be due to residual heterophile antibody present after clinical symptoms have subsided.

Clinical Applications

Infectious diseases such as influenza, rubella, and hepatitis may cause clinical symptoms that mimic infectious mononucleosis and present problems in diagnosis. Although the final diagnosis of infectious mononucleosis depends on clinical, hematological, and serological findings, a positive test result is indicative of the presence of the heterophile antibody specific for infectious mononucleosis.

Limitations

Because the clinical symptoms of infectious mononucleosis are similar to those of many other diseases, it is often difficult to disprove the theoretical possibility of a concomitant infection. In addition, seronegative infectious mononucleosis has been reported. Because of a delayed heterophile antibody response, it is possible that clinical and hematological symptoms of infectious mononucleosis will appear before serological confirmation is possible.

Reference

Monospot product brochures. Raritan, NJ: Ortho Diagnostics, May 1984.

....

Osmotic Fragility of Erythrocytes: Dacie's Method

Principle

In the osmotic fragility test, whole blood is added to varying concentrations of sodium chloride solution and allowed to incubate at room temperature. The amount of hemolysis is then determined by examining the supernatant fluid either visually or with a spectrophotometer.

If erythrocytes are placed in an isotonic solution (0.85%) of sodium chloride, water molecules will pass in and out of the membrane in equal amounts. In hypotonic solutions, erythrocytes will hemolyze because more water molecules enter into the cell than leave. This net influx of water molecules eventually ruptures the cell membrane.

The main factor in this procedure is the shape of the erythrocyte, which is dependent on the volume, surface area, and functional state of the erythrocytic membrane. A spherocytic erythro-

cyte ruptures much more quickly than normal erythrocytes or erythrocytes that have a large surface area per volume, such as target or sickle cells. The fragility of erythrocytes is increased when the rate of hemolysis is increased. If the rate of hemolysis is decreased, the erythrocytic fragility is considered to be decreased. The clinical value of the procedure is in differentiating various types of anemia.

Specimen

Fresh defibrinated or heparinized whole blood may be used.

Reagents, Supplies, and Equipment

1. Stock buffered sodium chloride solution. Prepare by weighing out 90 gm of sodium chloride, 13.65 gm of dibasic sodium phosphate (Na_2HPO_4), and 2.43 gm of monobasic sodium phosphate ($NaH_2PO_4 \cdot 2H_2O$). Place in a 1-L volumetric flask and dilute to the calibration mark with deionized water. Mix. Transfer to a stoppered stock bottle and label. This solution is stable at room temperature for several months, if tightly closed.
2. 1% buffered sodium chloride. Prepare by mixing 20 mL of stock buffered sodium chloride with 180 mL of distilled water.
3. Test tubes (16 × 100 mm); Parafilm covering
4. Pipette, graduated 1 mL and 10 mL, and safety bulb
5. Centrifuge
6. Spectrophotometer and cuvettes

Quality Control

A normal control sample should be tested simultaneously.

Procedure

1. Prepare dilutions of buffered sodium chloride and place in labeled test tubes (Table 24.5). *Caution:* Do not pipette by mouth.
2. Cover the tubes and mix by inversion. Transfer 5 mL of each dilution to a second set of tubes. This set is for the control.

TABLE 24.5 Osmotic Fragility of Erythrocytes (Dacie's Method): Preparation of Dilutions

Test Tube	1% NaCl (mL)	Distilled Water (mL)	Final Concentration (%)
1	10	0.0	1.00
2	8.5	1.5	0.85
3	7.5	2.5	0.75
4	6.5	3.5	0.65
5	6.0	4.0	0.60
6	5.5	4.5	0.55
7	5.0	5.0	0.50
8	4.5	5.5	0.45
9	4.0	6.0	0.40
10	3.5	6.5	0.35
11	3.0	7.0	0.30
12	2.0	8.0	0.20
13	1.0	9.0	0.10
14	0.0	10.0	0.00

(continued)

SPECIAL HEMATOLOGY PROCEDURES (continued)

3. Mix blood. Add 0.05 mL of blood to each of 14 test tubes. Repeat for control blood. Mix by gentle inversion.
4. Allow tubes to stand at room temperature for 30 minutes. Remix gently and centrifuge at 2500 rpm for 5 minutes.
5. Transfer supernatant to cuvettes and read on spectrophotometer at 550 nm. If the spectrophotometer is digital, set the absorbance at 0 with the supernatant in tube 1, 0% hemolysis, and read the absorbance (OD) of all the tubes. If the spectrophotometer is a conventional type, read the percentage transmittance (%T) of all the tubes and use a conversion table to obtain the absorbance (OD).

Visual Reading

Note the tubes in which hemolysis is complete. The tube with the highest concentration of sodium chloride is the end point.

Calculations

$$\% \text{ Hemolysis for each tube} = \frac{\text{OD of supernatant}}{\text{OD of 100\% hemolysis (tube 14)}} \times 100$$

Reporting Results

In normal blood, hemolysis should end at 0.30% sodium chloride and beginning hemolysis should not occur in a concentration over 0.45% (Table 24.6). Patient and normal control results may be reported in graphic form (Fig. 24.7).

Procedure Notes

Sources of Error

Buffered saline solution must be used.

Clinical Applications

The osmotic fragility test is of value in the diagnosis of different types of anemia and conditions in which the physical properties of the erythrocytic membrane are altered. The fragility of erythrocytes is increased in anemias in which the erythrocytes

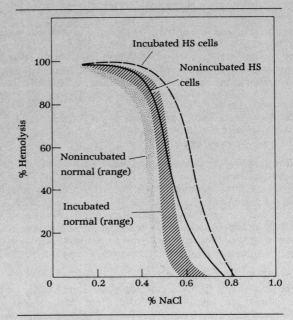

FIGURE 24.7 Osmotic fragility curves, preincubation and postincubation, normal and abnormal. HS = hereditary spherocytosis. (From P. R. Reich, *Hematology* [2nd edition]. Boston: Little, Brown & Co., 1984.)

are spherocytic rather than disc-shaped, such as in hereditary spherocytic anemia or hereditary spherocytosis. Fragility is also increased in the hemolytic anemias. The fragility of erythrocytes is decreased in anemias in which the erythrocytes are partially empty, thin, or sickle-shaped. Anemias such as severe iron deficiency anemia and sickle cell anemia are examples. The presence of target cells, as in thalassemia major, also demonstrates decreased fragility. Other conditions in which decreased erythrocyte fragility can be detected are hepatic disease and polycythemia vera. Decreased erythrocyte fragility also can be detected following splenectomy.

Erythrocyte Fragility in Selected Disorders

Decreased Fragility	Increased Fragility
Hb C disease	Acquired autoimmune hemolytic
Iron deficiency anemia	anemia
(severe)	Burns
Sickle cell anemia	Chemical poisons
Thalassemia major	Hemolytic disease of the newborn
Polycythemia vera	Hereditary spherocytosis

Limitations

This procedure must be part of a hematological profile in order to establish a definitive diagnosis.

Reference

Dacie, J. V. and S. M. Lewis. *Practical Hematology* (5th edition). New York: Churchill-Livingstone, 1975.

TABLE 24.6 **Normal Ranges for Osmotic Fragility**

Test Tube	Concentration of NaCl (%)	Hemolysis (%)
1	1.00	0
2	0.85	0
3	0.75	0
4	0.65	0
5	0.60	0
6	0.55	0
7	0.50	0–5
8	0.45	0–45
9	0.40	50–90
10	0.35	90–99
11	0.30	97–100
12	0.20	100
13	0.10	100
14	0.00	100

(continued)

Sucrose Hemolysis Test

Principle
Erythrocytes in PNH lyse when exposed to serum solutions of low ionic strength containing complement. This test demonstrates the sensitivity of erythrocytes to the protein, complement. Normal erythrocytes under similar circumstances do not lyse.

Specimen
Whole blood anticoagulated in sodium citrate is preferred.

Reagents, Supplies, and Equipment
1. Aqueous sucrose: Weigh out and transfer 9.24 gm of sucrose to a 100-mL volumetric flask. Dilute to the calibration mark with deionized water.
2. Fresh serum that is ABO blood group–compatible with the patient's erythrocytes
3. A 50% suspension of patient's erythrocytes: Prepare by placing 3 to 4 mL of anticoagulated blood in a graduated conical centrifuge tube. Fill with saline solution, mix, and centrifuge. Remove and discard the supernatant. Repeat this procedure 3 times. After the final wash, add a volume of saline solution equal to the quantity of packed erythrocytes and mix.
4. Spectrophotometer and cuvettes

Quality Control
A normal specimen should be run concurrently.

Procedure
1. Label two small test tubes: (1) test and (2) control.

Reagents	Test Tubes 1	Test Tubes 2
Fresh serum	0.05 mL	0.05 mL
Sucrose solution	0.85 mL	—
Saline solution	—	0.85 mL
50% suspension of patient's erythrocytes	0.1 mL	0.1 mL

2. Mix and incubate at 37° C for 30 minutes.
3. Centrifuge tubes and examine for gross hemolysis. If indicated, examine spectrophotometrically at 540 nm.

   Zero blank: add 0.05 mL of ABO-compatible serum to 0.85 mL of isotonic saline solution.

   100% hemolysis: Add 0.1 mL of red cell suspension to 0.9 mL of Drabkin's solution.

   Patient's hemolysis: Add 0.5 mL of supernatant from tube 1 to 5 mL of Drabkin's solution.

Calculations

$$\frac{\text{OD of patient's hemolysis}}{\text{OD of 100\% hemolysis}} \times 100 = \text{\% sucrose hemolysis}$$

Reporting Results
Less than 10% hemolysis should be considered to be a negative result.

Clinical Applications
The erythrocytes of some patients with leukemia or myelosclerosis may produce small amounts of lysis. Hemolysis in PNH varies from 10% to 80%.

Limitations
Erythrocytes from patients with congenital dyserythropoietic anemia associated with a positive acidified serum test result give a negative result on the sucrose lysis test. This procedure should be run in conjunction with acid serum hemolysis (Ham test).

Reference
Hartman, R. C. et al. "Diagnostic Specificity of Sucrose Hemolysis Test for Paroxysmal Nocturnal Hemoglobinuria." *Blood*, Vol. 35, 1970, p. 462.

SPECIAL STAINS

Acid Phosphatase in Leukocytes: Cytochemical Staining Method With and Without Tartrate

Principle
Peripheral blood or bone marrow smears are fixed and incubated in a solution of naphthol AS-BI phosphoric acid and fast garnet GBC salt. Naphthol AS-BI, released by enzymatic hydrolysis, couples immediately at acid pH with fast garnet GBC to form an insoluble maroon dye deposit at sites of activity. This is the reaction that occurs at the cellular sites of acid phosphatase activity (see Plate 66).

Naphthol AS-BI phosphate–acid phosphatase → naphthol AS-BI

Naphthol AS-BI + fast garnet GBC → insoluble maroon pigment

Duplicate blood or bone marrow smears are incubated in a solution that also contains l-(+)tartrate-containing substrate. Cells containing tartaric acid-sensitive acid phosphatase do not exhibit any dye deposits, while those mononuclear cells containing tartaric acid-resistant acid phosphatase are not affected by such treatment.

Most leukocytes exhibit a positive acid phosphatase reaction to varying degrees. Lymphocytes display less activity than other leukocytes. Most of the acid phosphatase isoenzyme is inhibited by l-tartaric acid. The cells of hairy cell leukemia, Sezary syndrome, and some T cell acute lymphoblastic leukemias are tartrate-resistant.

Specimen
Blood, bone marrow films, tissue touch preparations, and cytocentrifuge preparations may be used. Either EDTA or heparin an-

(continued)

SPECIAL STAINS (continued)

ticoagulant can be used. Smears must be promptly prepared and *fixed* in a solution of citrate-acetone (refer to Reagent, Supplies, and Equipment section for preparation). Blood and bone marrow smears may be stored at 18°–26°C for several weeks or fixed smears may be stored for several weeks without appreciable change.

Slide Fixation
Place thoroughly dried smears in a room-temperature citrate-acetone solution for 30 seconds. Rinse carefully in deionized water and air-dry for at least 15 minutes before staining.

Reagents, Supplies, and Equipment
1. Citrate concentrate, pH 5.4: Store at 2° to 6°C and discard if turbidity develops. *Dilute* citrate solution is prepared by adding 2.0 mL of citrate concentrate to 18 mL of deionized water.
2. *United States Pharmacopeia (USP)*–grade acetone.
3. Fixative solution: Prepare by mixing 20 mL of *dilute* citrate solution and 30 mL of acetone. This solution must be prepared *daily* and be kept in a tightly capped bottle when not in use.
4. Tartrate solution: Store at 2° to 6°C and discard if turbidity develops.
5. Acetate solution: Store at 2° to 6°C and discard if turbidity develops.
6. Naphthol AS-BI phosphoric acid: Store at 2° to 6°C. Reagent label bears expiration date. *Caution:* Avoid contact with skin.
7. Fast garnet GBC salt: Store at 2° to 6°C. Reagent label bears expiration date. *Caution:* Possible carcinogen. Minimize contact with skin. Do not inhale dust.
8. Acid hematoxylin solution: Store at room temperature. May be returned to original container after use. Discard when staining time exceeds the time recommended in the procedure for more than 5 minutes.
9. Coplin staining jars or staining dishes, and a slide holder
10. Graduated cylinders, beakers, pipettes, and deionized water
11. Microscope and immersion oil

Quality Control
A normal control blood should be included.

Procedure
1. Label two 100-mL beakers and add:
   Beaker A—46 mL of distilled water, 2.0 mL of naphthol AS-BI phosphoric acid solution, 2.0 mL of acetate solution
   Beaker B—44 mL of distilled water, 2.0 mL of naphthol AS-BI phosphoric acid solution, 2.0 mL of acetate solution, 2.0 mL of tartrate solution
2. Add contents of one capsule of fast garnet GBC to each beaker. Stir on magnetic mixer for 30 to 60 seconds.
3. Filter each solution through No. 54 Whatman filter paper into separate staining jars labeled A and B.
4. Place at least two duplicate fixed blood films in each jar containing the filtered solution.
5. Incubate slides for 1 hour at 37°C in the dark.
6. Remove slides and wash in deionized water for 3 minutes.
7. Stain in acid hematoxylin for 5 minutes.
8. Rinse slides in deionized water for 3 minutes and air-dry.
9. Examine microscopically using the oil immersion (100×) objective.

Reporting Results
In the absence of tartaric acid, all leukocytes demonstrate granular sites of enzyme activity. When incubated with tartrate, an occasional granule may be observed in lymphocytes and some specialized macrophages, e.g., Gaucher cells and hairy cells. In blood smears, a positive reaction is denoted by the presence of more than two cells with diffuse and intense activity, i.e., more than 40 granules. To evaluate Golgi staining, characteristics of thymus-derived lymphocytes (T cells), Sigma procedure #181 is recommended.

Procedure Notes

Sources of Error
Improperly stored or old reagents and old or improperly fixed blood specimens.

Clinical Applications
This procedure distinguishes lymphocytes from other types of mononuclear cells. Because the cells of hairy cell leukemia are among the few abnormal cell types that are tartrate-resistant, it is considered to be a significant marker in this disease.
   Caution: Refer to Material Safety Data Sheets for any updated risk, hazard, or safety information.

Reference
"Acid Phosphatase, Leukocyte." Procedure No. 386. *Sigma Product Bull.*, Vol. 6. St. Louis: Sigma Diagnostics, 1996.

Alkaline Phosphatase in Leukocytes: Cytochemical Staining Method

Principle
Peripheral blood or bone marrow smears are fixed and incubated in an alkaline-dye solution of naphthol AS-MX phosphate and fast blue RR salt or fast violet B salt. As the result of phosphatase activity, naphthol AS-MX is liberated and immediately coupled with a diazonium salt, forming an insoluble, visible pigment at the sites of phosphatase activity. The following reactions occur at cellular sites of alkaline phosphatase activity:

Naphthol AS-MX phosphate–alkaline phosphatase
→ naphthol AS-MX

Naphthol AS-MX + fast blue RR salt → blue pigment

or

Naphthol AS-MX + fast violet B salt → violet pigment

Leukocyte alkaline phosphatase activity can be increased, normal, or decreased in a variety of conditions. This procedure is frequently used to distinguish between leukemoid reactions and chronic granulocytic (myelogenous) leukemia.

Specimen
Capillary blood is preferred to anticoagulated whole blood. If anticoagulated whole blood must be used, heparin is preferred. EDTA must be avoided. Blood smears should be stained within 8 hours after preparation. However, if this is not possible, gradual loss of alkaline phosphatase activity may be delayed by fixation and storage overnight in the freezer. Smears should be dried at

(continued)

least 1 hour before fixation, and 3 hours post-fixation, before freezing.

Reagents, Supplies, and Equipment

Reagents: Sigma Diagnostics Kit No. 85, fast blue RR salt, fast violet B salt, Napthol AS-MX Phosphate Alkaline Solution, and Mayer's Hematoxylin Solution—are provided ready for use in the procedure. Store fast blue RR salt and fast violet B salt below 0°C. Store Napthol AS-MX Phosphate Alkaline Solution at 2°–8°C. Reagents are stable until expiration date. Store Mayer's Hematoxylin Solution tightly capped at 18°–26°C. Do not return to original container after use in Coplin jar. Citrate concentrate is not included in the 85 kit.

1. Discard when the time required for a suitable stain exceeds the time recommended in the procedure by 5 minutes.
   Note: Mayer's Hematoxylin Solution is harmful by inhalation, in contact with skin, and if swallowed.
2. Citrate concentrate: Store at room temperature. Suitable for use if no turbidity (microbial growth) is observed.
   Citrate working solution: Prepare by pipetting 2 mL of citrate concentrate into a 100-mL volumetric flask. Dilute to the calibration mark with deionized water. Store at 2° to 6°C. Suitable for use if turbidity (microbial growth) is absent.
3. Acetone (ACS- or USP-grade).
4. Fixative solution: Prepare by adding 2 vol of *room-temperature citrate working solution* to 3 vol of acetone. Stir constantly. Discard after use.
5. (optional) Reagent: Scott's tap water substitute concentrate. Store at room temperature. If a small quantity of crystals form, they will not affect reagent performance.
6. Coplin jars or staining dishes, and slide holder
7. 100-mL Erlenmeyer flask
8. Microscope, immersion oil, and lens paper

Quality Control

A negative control can be prepared by immersing a normal fixed blood smear into boiling water for 1 minute in order to inactivate the enzyme. Blood from women who are either in their third trimester of pregnancy or within 2 days postpartum provides a highly positive control. A blood sample from a healthy adult provides a suitable normal control.

Procedure

Fixation of Blood Smears

1. Allow smears to dry for at least 1 hour prior to fixation.
2. Immerse smears in room-temperature fixative for 30 seconds.
3. Rinse thoroughly but gently for 45 seconds in deionized water. Do not allow slides to dry.

Staining and Counterstaining Procedure

1. Prepare stains *immediately* before use. Into an Erlenmeyer flask, place 48 mL of distilled water. Add the contents of a fast blue RR salt capsule or fast violet B salt capsule. Mix thoroughly. A magnetic stirrer is helpful. Add 2 mL of naphthol AS-MX phosphate alkaline solution. Mix. Use immediately and discard after use.
2. Immediately immerse slides in this fresh mixture and incubate at 23° to 26°C for 30 minutes away from direct light.
3. Remove slides and wash gently with deionized water for 2 minutes. Do not allow slides to dry.
4. Place in Mayer's Hematoxylin Solution for 10 minutes to counterstain.
5. If fast blue RR salt was used, rinse counterstained slides for 3 minutes in deionized water. This produces a red-violet nu-

TABLE 24.7 Leukocyte Alkaline Phosphatase Cytochemical Stain Scoring Characteristics

Cell Rating	Amount (%)*	Size of Granule	Stain Intensity
0	None	—	None
1+	50	Small	Faint to moderate
2+	50–80	Small	Moderate to strong
3+	80–100	Medium to large	Strong
4+	100	Medium to large	Brilliant

*Percent volume of cytoplasm occupied by dye precipitate.

clear staining. If fast violet B salt was used, rinse slides in tap water (if alkaline) or immerse in Scott's tap water substitute for 2 minutes. This will produce a blue nuclear stain.
6. Air-dry and examine as unmounted slides. Unmounted stained slides usually remain unchanged for years.

Calculations

The deposits of blue or violet pigment viewed microscopically reflect the sites of granulocytic alkaline phosphatase activity. The granulocyte population is rated on the basis of the number of cells stained and the intensity of the pigment deposits.

Scan the smear using the oil immersion (100×) objective and select a thin area where erythrocytes are barely touching. Select 100 consecutive band and segmented neutrophilic granulocytes. Rate on a scale of 0 to 4+ on the basis of quantity and intensity of precipitated dye within the cytoplasm of cells (Table 24.7).

The percentage represents the proportion of total cytoplasmic volume occupied by the dye precipitate.

Obtaining Results

To obtain the leukocyte alkaline phosphatase activity (LAP) score, the number of cells counted in each category (0 to 4+) is multiplied by the value for that category. These scores are summed for the cumulative total.

Example:

50 cells with a 4+ rating =	200
30 cells with a 3+ rating =	90
20 cells with a 2+ rating =	40
Total 100 cells	330 LAP score

Reporting Results

The normal range depends on the type of azo dye used. If fast blue RR is used, the normal range is 32 to 182. If fast violet B is used, the normal range is 12 to 180.

Procedure Notes

Sources of Error

Certain drugs and the age of the specimen are known to influence circulating alkaline phosphatase activity. Oral contraceptives, cortisol, and stress may result in elevated leukocyte alkaline phosphatase scores. Occasionally, weak staining lymphocytes may be observed. Bone marrow osteoblasts and endothelial cells stain strongly.

(continued)

SPECIAL STAINS (continued)

Clinical Applications

This test is clinically most useful in differentiating chronic my-elogenous leukemia from leukemoid reactions. Leukemoid reactions may result from infections, toxic conditions, and neoplasms as well as miscellaneous conditions such as the treatment of megaloblastic anemia, acute hemorrhage, and acute hemolysis.

Alkaline phosphatase activity can be associated with various conditions and disorders. Postsurgical patients experience a rise in activity with a peak 2 to 3 days postoperatively and a gradual return to normal values within 1 week. Persisting elevation of the LAP score is strong evidence of an active inflammatory process. LAP scores are useful in diagnosing ectopic pregnancy and an anovulatory menstrual cycle. The LAP score is also useful in differentiating choriocarcinoma from hydatidiform mole because the test score is normal in choriocarcinoma and high in cases of hydatidiform mole.

Limitations

This procedure depends on the subjective rating of stained cells. This can result in a wide variation of ratings.

LAP Scores and Some Related Conditions

Increased	Usually Normal	Usually Decreased
Leukemoid reactions	Infectious mono-nucleosis	Chronic myeloge-nous leukemia
Bacterial infections	Viral hepatitis	Paroxysmal noc-turnal hemoglo-binuria
Chronic and acute lym-phatic leukemia	Relative polycy-themia	
Multiple myeloma		Hereditary hypo-phosphatasia
Polycythemia vera		
Hodgkin's disease		
Lymphoma		
Pregnancy and immedi-ately postpartum		
Trisomy 21 (Down syn-drome)		

References

"Alkaline Phosphatase." Procedure No. 85. *Sigma Product Bull.*, Vol. 6. St. Louis: Sigma Diagnostics, 1995.

Wallach, Jacques. *Interpretation of Diagnostic Tests* (5th edition). Boston: Little, Brown & Co., 1991.

Esterase (Alpha-Naphthyl Acetate Esterase) in Leukocytes: Cytochemical Staining Method

Principle

Esterases are ubiquitous in nature and encompass a variety of different enzymes acting on selective substrates. In this procedure, blood or bone marrow smears or touch preparations are incubated with alpha-naphthyl acetate in the presence of a stable diazonium salt. Enzymatic hydrolysis of ester linkages liberates free naphthol compounds. These naphthol compounds then couple with diazonium salt, forming highly colored deposits at the sites of enzyme activity (see Plate 65). Under defined condi-tions, this method provides a means to distinguish cells of the granulocytic series from cells of the monocytic series. This is particularly useful in the differentiation of leukemias.

Specimen

Fresh blood specimens collected in EDTA or heparin are needed. Blood or bone marrow smears may be stored *unfixed for several days* or for several weeks if fixed at 18°–26°C. Frozen tissue sections can also be used. Do not ship whole blood. Send either unfixed or fixed smears. Slides should be kept cool during transit. Allow smears to dry for at least 1 hour before fixation.

Fixation of Specimens

Blood or bone marrow smears may be stored *fixed* at room temperature for several weeks. All smears *must be fixed* prior to performing the procedure in citrate-acetone-methanol fixative. To prepare the fixative:

1. Prepare *dilute citrate solution* by mixing 1 part of *citrate concentrate* (Sigma Diagnostics kit No. 386-1 or included with kit No. 90-A1) with 9 parts of deionized water. This solution is stable for *1 week*, if stored tightly capped at room temperature (18° to 26°C).
2. Mix 18 mL of *dilute citrate solution* with 27 mL of ACS-grade acetone and 5 mL of absolute methanol. Store tightly capped at room temperature. This solution is stable for *8 hours*.

Reagents, Supplies, and Equipment
Reagents

1. Fast blue RR salt capsules: Store at 0°C, labeled with expiration date.
2. Trizma 7.6 buffer concentrate (200 mmol/L): Store at room temperature. Suitable for use in the absence of visible microbial growth. Contains chloroform, which may cause cancer or heritable genetic damage. Toxic by inhalation, in contact with skin, and if swallowed.

   The *dilute buffer solution* should be prepared prior to testing by mixing 1 part of the *buffer concentrate* with 9 parts of deionized water. The pH should be 6.3 at 25°C. *Use once and then discard.*
3. Alpha-naphthyl acetate capsules: Store below 0°C, with expiration date labeled. Remove from freezer, as needed. *Avoid contact with skin. Do not breathe dust.*

   Prepare the alpha-naphthyl acetate solution by dissolving the contents of one capsule in 2 mL of ethylene glycol monomethyl ether. Prepare *immediately prior to use. Avoid contact with skin.*
4. Ethylene glycol monomethyl ether: Store at room temperature. Discard if colored or turbid.
5. Mayer's hematoxylin: Store tightly capped at room temperature. *Filter before use.* Discard if the time required for staining exceeds the time in the procedure by more than 5 minutes. Harmful if swallowed, inhaled, or absorbed through skin.
6. Beaker and glass stirring rod
7. 37°C incubator
8. Coplin staining jars or larger staining dishes and slide holder
9. Coverslips and mounting media
10. Microscope, immersion oil, and lens paper

(continued)

Quality Control
A normal blood specimen should be run concurrently with the patient specimen.

Procedure
1. Fix slides for 1 minute in citrate-acetone-methanol fixative at room temperature; dip or rinse thoroughly using deionized water, and air-dry for at least 20 minutes..
2. To 50 mL of Trizma 7.6 dilute buffer solution, *prewarmed* to 37°C, add, with constant stirring, one capsule of fast blue RR salt.
3. When the salt is completely dissolved in the buffer, add 2 mL of alpha-naphthyl acetate solution. This solution will be yellow and slightly turbid. Continue stirring for 15 to 20 seconds. Transfer this solution to the staining jar or dish *without filtering*.
4. Place specimens in staining solution and incubate at 37°C for 30 minutes. *Protect the solution from light.*
5. At the end of 30 minutes, remove the slides from the staining solution. Wash the slides in running water for 3 minutes. Discard this staining solution.
6. If desired, counterstain for 5 to 10 minutes in Mayer's hematoxylin solution and wash in tap water.
7. Air-dry coverslip with mounting media, and examine microscopically.

Reporting Results
Alpha-naphthyl acetate esterase enzyme is detected primarily in monocytes, macrophages, and histiocytes and is almost absent in granulocytes. Monocytes should demonstrate black granulation. Lymphocytes may occasionally exhibit some activity. A full discussion of cytochemical staining is presented in Chapter 19.

Procedure Notes
Blood or bone marrow smears must be fixed properly. All reagents must be stored and prepared as directed. *Caution:* Refer to Material Safety Data Sheets.

....

Double Staining Esterase

1. Perform alpha-naphthyl acetate esterase test as described in procedure. Do not counterstain.
2. Rinse slides 5 minutes in deionized water.
3. Perform naphthol AS-D chloroacetate esterase test as described in the procedure, beginning with step #3.

Reporting Results
Specimens taken through the double staining procedure will demonstrate the granulocytes with red granulation, and monocytes with black granulation.

....

Alpha-Naphthyl Acetate Esterase With Fluoride Inhibition

To differentiate positive reacting cells conclusively from monocytes, sodium fluoride is incorporated with the incubation system. The monocyte enzyme is inactivated in the presence of this compound. The following procedure may be used to perform the fluoride inhibition test.

1. Fix slides in citrate-acetone-methanol fixative for 1 minute at room temperature (18°–26°C).

2. Wash thoroughly in deionized water and air dry at least 20 minutes.
3. Label two beakers (A and B), and add the following:

	Beaker A	Beaker B
Prewarmed 37°C TRIZMAL™	50 mL	50mL
Add with constant stirring, Fast Blue RR	1 capsule	1 capsule
Alpha-naphthyl acetate solution	2 mL	2 mL
Sodium fluoride (2 g/dL) stored at room temperature (18°–26°C)	—	2 mL

4. Mix well and pour into Coplin jars labeled A and B.
5. Proceed as described in steps 6–9 of alpha-naphthyl acetate esterase procedure.

Reporting Results
All cells of monocytic origin will be negative for enzyme activity, with the exception of differentiated histiocytes or specialized macrophages in tissue, which may also be resistant to sodium fluoride.

Clinical Applications
Esterase reactions may be used in the classification of acute nonlymphoblastic leukemia. The staining characteristics are: M0 and M1 = negative; M2 and M3 = NCAE-positive, NAE-negative; M4 = variable reactions with NCAE and NAE; M5a = NCAE-negative, NAE-variable; M5b = NCAE-negative, NAE-positive; M6 NCAE-negative, NAE-variable; M7-NCAE-negative, NAE-variable. NCAE = naphthol AS-D chloroacetate esterase; NAE = alpha-naphthyl acetate esterase.

Reference
"Naphthol AS-D and Chloroacetate Esterase and Alpha-Naphthyl Acetate Esterase." Procedure No. 90. *Sigma Product Bull.*, Vol. 6. St. Louis: Sigma Diagnostics, 1991.

....

Esterase (Naphthol AS-D Chloroacetate Esterase) in Leukocytes: Cytochemical Staining Method

Principle
(See Alpha-Naphthyl Acetate Esterase.) In this procedure, blood or bone marrow smears are incubated with naphthol AS-D chloroacetate in the presence of a stable diazonium salt. Naphthol compounds are coupled with diazonium salt, forming highly colored deposits at the sites of enzyme activity (see Plate 64).

Specimen
Fresh blood specimens collected in EDTA or heparin are needed. Blood or bone marrow smears may be stored *unfixed for several days* without a marked change in enzyme activity. Slides may be refrigerated if stored in tightly sealed envelopes containing desiccant. Do not ship whole blood for this assay to other laboratories. Send either unfixed or fixed smears. Slides should be kept cool during transit.

Fixation of Specimens
Blood or bone marrow smears may be stored *fixed* at room temperature for several weeks. All smears *must be fixed* prior to per-

(continued)

SPECIAL STAINS (continued)

forming the procedure in citrate-acetone-methanol fixative. To prepare the fixative:

1. Prepare dilute citrate solution by mixing 1 part of *citrate concentrate* (Sigma Diagnostics No. 386-1 or included with kit No. 90-A1) with 9 parts of deionized water. This solution is stable for *1 week,* if stored tightly capped at room temperature (18° to 26°C).
2. Mix 18 mL of *dilute citrate solution* with 27 mL of ACS-grade acetone and 5 mL of absolute methanol. Store tightly capped at room temperature. This solution is stable for *8 hours.*

Reagents, Supplies, and Equipment
Reagents (Sigma No. 90-C2)
1. Fast Corinth V salt: Store under refrigeration. Label with expiration date. *Caution:* Possible carcinogen. *Avoid contact with skin. Do not breathe dust.*
2. Trizma 6.3 dilute buffer solution (200 mmol/L): Store at room temperature. Suitable for use in the absence of visible microbial growth. The *dilute buffer solution* should be prepared prior to testing by mixing 1 part of the *buffer concentrate* with 9 parts of deionized water. The pH should be 6.3 at 25°C. *Use once and then discard.*
3. Naphthol AS-D chloroacetate: Store below 0°C. Label with expiration date. Remove one capsule from the freezer as needed. Naphthol AS-D chloroacetate solution is prepared by dissolving the contents of one capsule in 2 mL of dimethylformamide. *Prepare immediately prior to use. Avoid contact with the skin.*
4. Dimethylformamide: Store at room temperature. Discard if colored or turbid. Avoid contact with skin. Do not breathe fumes.
5. Acid hematoxylin: This is a solution of Mayer's hematoxylin, pH 3.3. *Filter before use.* Store at room temperature. Solution may be returned to container after use. Discard when the time required for staining exceeds the recommended time by more than 5 minutes.
6. Beaker and glass stirring rod
7. 37°C incubator
8. Coplin staining jars or larger staining dishes and slide holder
9. Coverslips and mounting media
10. Microscope, immersion oil, and lens paper

Quality Control
A normal specimen should be run concurrently with the patient's specimen.

Procedure
1. Fix slides for 2 minutes in citrate-acetone-methanol fixative at room temperature. Dip or wash thoroughly in deionized water and air-dry.
2. To 50 mL of Trizma 6.3 dilute buffer solution *prewarmed* to 37°C, add, with constant stirring, one capsule of fast Corinth V salt.
3. When salt is completely dissolved in buffer, add 2 mL of naphthol AS-D chloroacetate solution. The solution will appear quite turbid. Continue stirring for 15 to 30 seconds. Transfer to a Coplin jar or staining dish *without filtering.*
4. Place specimens in staining solution and incubate at 37°C for 5 minutes. *Protect from light.* Wash slides in running water for 3 minutes. Discard staining solution.

5. If desired, counterstain in acid hematoxylin solution for 5 to 10 minutes; wash in tap water.
6. Air-dry, mount coverslip, and examine microscopically.

Method of Scoring
Scan the smear and select a thin area with few erythrocytes. Sites of naphthol AS-D chloroacetate esterase activity will appear as bright red granulation; alpha-naphthyl acetate esterase as black granulation. Rate from 0–4+ on the basis of quantity and intensity of individual dyes within the cytoplasm of the respective cell types. Characteristics of scoring are based somewhat on subjective interpretation. A suggested format with conclusions centered on the relative presence or absence of staining is:

Cell Rating	Intensity of Staining	Interpretation
0	None	Negative
1+	Faint to Moderate	+/−
2+	Moderate to Strong	+
3+	Strong	+
4+	Brilliant	+

Reporting Results
Naphthol AS-D chloroacetate esterase enzyme is usually considered specific for cells of granulocytic lineage. They should show red granulation. Activity is weak or absent in monocytes and lymphocytes. A full discussion of cytochemical staining is presented in Chapter 19.

Procedure Notes
Blood or bone marrow smears must be fixed properly. All reagents must be stored and prepared as directed. *Caution:* Refer to Material Safety Data Sheets.

Reference
"Naphthol AS-D and Chloroacetate Esterase and Alpha-Naphthyl Acetate Esterase." Procedure No. 90. *Sigma Product Bull.,* Vol. 6. St. Louis: Sigma Diagnostics, 1985.

··

Heinz Bodies

Principle
Whole blood is mixed with crystal violet stain and allowed to incubate. Moist preparations of the blood and stain mixture are examined for the presence of Heinz bodies in the erythrocytes. Heinz bodies represent unstable types of hemoglobin which are denatured by dyes, such as crystal violet or brilliant cresyl blue, and appear as intraerythrocytic stained bodies (see Plate 21).

Specimen
Whole blood collected in EDTA or heparin anticoagulants.

Reagents, Supplies, and Equipment
1. 0.85% sodium chloride (NaCl)
2. 1% brilliant cresyl blue
   Working solution: Weigh out 1.0 gm of dye. Transfer to a 100-mL volumetric flask and dilute to the calibration mark with 100 mL of NaCl. Mix and filter the stain through No. 42 Whatman paper before use.
3. Test tubes (12 × 75 mm)

(continued)

Quality Control

A normal control blood must be run simultaneously with the patient's blood. The control must demonstrate a low percentage of Heinz bodies.

Procedure

1. Place 1.0 mL of well-mixed whole blood into a test tube.
2. Add 0.5 mL of the brilliant cresyl blue solution.
3. Mix and allow to incubate at 37°C for a maximum of 2 hours.
4. At intervals of 30 minutes, 1 hour, and 2 hours, prepare specimens for examination. This procedure consists of remixing the blood and stain solution and placing a small drop of the mixture onto a glass slide. Place a coverslip over this preparation.
5. Examine the unstained slides immediately after preparation, using the oil immersion (100×) objective.

Reporting Results

Heinz bodies appear as blue, refractile, intracytoplasmic inclusions. They are irregularly shaped bodies of varying sizes, up to 2 μm in diameter, and are found close to the cellular membrane. There may be more than one Heinz body present in an erythrocyte. The test detects in vivo precipitated Heinz bodies.

Procedure Notes

Heinz bodies are detectable in wet preparations and by using supravital stains such as brilliant cresyl blue, new methylene blue N, methyl violet, and crystal violet. Heinz bodies are *not* seen when stained with Wright or Wright-Giemsa stain. In patients whose erythrocytes have defective reducing systems, many (45% to 92%) of the erythrocytes may contain five or more Heinz bodies.

Clinical Applications

Heinz bodies are formed when the glycolytic enzymes in the erythrocytes are unable to prevent the oxidation of hemoglobin. As a result, the hemoglobin is eventually denatured and precipitated to form Heinz bodies. Erythrocytic enzyme systems decrease as the cell ages; therefore, occasional Heinz bodies will be observed in normal blood.

Increased numbers of Heinz bodies represent unstable forms of hemoglobin that are present in a number of hemolytic disorders. Heinz bodies occur in disorders such as G6PD or glutathione deficiencies, secondary to the action of certain oxidant drugs, and in the presence of unstable hemoglobins such as Hb Zurich and Hb H.

Caution: Refer to Material Safety Data Sheets.

Reference

Bauer, John D. *Clinical Laboratory Methods* (9th edition). St. Louis: Mosby, 1982, pp. 67–69.

Hemoglobin F Determination by Acid Elution: Kleihauer and Betke Method Modified by Shepard, Weatherall, and Conley

Principle

After blood smears are fixed with ethyl alcohol, a citric acid–phosphate buffer solution removes (*elutes*) hemoglobin other than Hb F from erythrocytes. The Hb F (fetal hemoglobin)–containing erythrocytes are visibly identifiable on microscopic examination when appropriately stained. Shortly after birth, the amount of Hb F in humans decreases to low levels. Increased amounts of Hb F are found in various hemoglobinopathies such as hereditary persistence of fetal hemoglobin, sickle cell anemia, and the thalassemias.

Specimen

Capillary or EDTA-anticoagulated blood are appropriate for this procedure. Smears made from fresh blood give the best results. Whole blood drawn into EDTA anticoagulant can be stored under refrigeration for no longer than 2 weeks. However, *as soon as the blood smears are made, the test must be performed.*

Reagents, Supplies, and Equipment

1. Ethyl alcohol, 80% (vol/vol)
2. Citric acid–phosphate buffer

Stock Solutions

A. 0.2 M dibasic sodium phosphate (Na_2HPO_4). Weigh 2.84 gm of dibasic sodium phosphate and transfer to a 100-mL volumetric flask. Dilute to the 100-mL calibration mark with distilled water. Transfer to a dark-brown bottle. Label the container with the reagent name and date. *Refrigerate this stock solution.*

B. 0.1 M citric acid. Weigh 2.1 gm of citric acid. Transfer to a 100-mL volumetric flask and dilute to the 100-mL calibration mark with distilled water. Transfer to a dark-brown bottle. Label the container with the reagent name and date. *Refrigerate this stock solution.*

Working Solution

Prior to use, prepare the citric acid–phosphate buffer by mixing 13.3 mL of 0.2 M dibasic sodium phosphate and 36.7 mL of 0.1 M citric acid. A pH of 3.2 to 3.3 is critical; check using a pH meter.

3. An aqueous solution of 0.1% erythrosine B. Weigh 0.2 gm of erythrosine B and transfer to a 200-mL volumetric flask. Add approximately 170 mL of distilled water. Add 2 to 3 drops of glacial acetic acid. Dilute to the 200-mL calibration mark with distilled water. Mix and filter through No. 42 Whatman filter paper. Transfer to a labeled brown bottle. Store at room temperature and filter prior to use.
4. Mayer's hematoxylin. To prepare this solution, add 1 gm of hematoxylin (color index No. 75290) to an Erlenmeyer flask containing 500 mL of distilled water. Heat just to boiling on a hot plate and add another 500 mL of distilled water. Mix. Add 0.2 gm of sodium iodate. Mix. Add 50 gm of aluminum potassium sulfate · 12 H_2O. Mix. Transfer to a large stoppered bottle and shake for 1 minute. Filter. Transfer to a brown bottle, label with reagent name and date. This solution should be stored at room temperature and keeps indefinitely.
5. Six staining containers with covers and a timer
6. Microscope, immersion oil, and lens paper

Quality Control

Control tests using a normal adult blood sample as well as blood from a neonatal infant should be performed simultaneously with a patient specimen. The adult blood should have only a rare cell containing Hb F, while the newborn infant sample should have a high percentage of acid-resistant cells per microscopic field.

Procedure

1. Make four thin blood smears from each specimen: patient, normal control, and neonatal control. Label.
2. Allow these smears to air-dry for 10 to 60 minutes.
3. Prepare the working citric acid–phosphate buffer solution. Transfer to a staining jar and cover. Incubate at 37°C for 30 minutes.

(continued)

SPECIAL STAINS (continued)

4. The solutions needed for steps 5 through 9 should be prepared and filtered (if needed), and dispensed into labeled containers before proceeding with the next step.
5. Place the dry slides into 80% ethyl alcohol for about 5 minutes. At the end of this time, gently rinse or dip the smears in distilled water and allow to air-dry.
6. After the smears are completely dry, place the slides in the prewarmed citric acid–phosphate buffer solution for 5 minutes. At the end of 1 minute, dip the slides up and down. Repeat again at 3 minutes.
7. After 5 minutes, remove the slides from the citric acid–phosphate buffer solution and rinse with distilled water. Air-dry.
8. After the smears are completely dry, stain in Mayer's hematoxylin for 3 minutes. Rinse with distilled water.
9. Place the slides in erythrosine B for 4 minutes. Rinse with distilled water and allow to air-dry.
10. Examine with the (100×) oil immersion objective for Hb F. Cells containing Hb F stain a dark red-orange color depending on the concentration of Hb F. Normal adult erythrocytes appear as ghost cells. The neonatal blood sample should have many dense-appearing erythrocytes per field.

Calculations
The percentage of Hb F–containing cells can be determined by counting the number of dense-staining cells and the number of ghost cells per field (see Case 3, Ch. 5). Using the high-power dry (43 to 44×) objective, count 500 ghost cells and record the number of dense Hb F–containing cells seen during the count.

Reporting Results
An adult specimen should have approximately the same number of dense Hb F–containing cells as the normal adult blood. These cells should appear rarely. The results are expressed as a percentage. Normal adults have less than 1% Hb F–containing cells. Infant values are higher, with newborn infants having 70 to 90% Hb F–containing cells.

Procedure Notes

Sources of Error
False-positive results may be obtained if anticoagulated blood is allowed to stand overnight or if a patient has a very high percentage of reticulocytes. Reticulocytes may resist elution and give the appearance of cells containing Hb F. To cross-check high concentrations of Hb F, a reticulocyte count can be performed.

In hemoglobinopathies such as sickle cell disease, the amount of Hb F varies, producing inconsistent staining results. Cells containing small amounts of Hb F stain lightly.

Clinical Applications
Increased amounts of Hb F are found in various hemoglobinopathies such as hereditary persistence of fetal hemoglobin, sickle cell anemia, and the thalassemias. Refer to a previous section, Hemoglobin F Determination by Alkaline Denaturation, for additional special examples of disorders in which Hb F is increased.

Limitations
This procedure is a semiquantitative method.

Reference
Shepard, M. K. et al. "Semiquantitative Estimation of the Distribution of Fetal Hemoglobin in Red Cell Populations." *Bull. John Hopkins Hosp.*, Vol. 110, 1962, p. 293.

Lymphocyte Enzyme Stains: Alpha-Naphthyl Butyrate Esterase and Beta-Glucuronidase

Background and Principle
Dissection of normal T cell maturation into discrete stages by the use of enzyme cytochemistry and monoclonal antibodies has shown that T cell malignancies mirror the same ontogenetic diversity. These findings, for the most part, support the conclusion that T cell neoplasias reflect maturation arrest during normal development.

The OKT series (Ortho Diagnostic Systems, Raritan, NJ) of monoclonal antibodies recognizing T cell surface antigens, delineates prothymocytes/thymocytes and lymphatic tissue when stained by enzymes such as acid phosphatase, beta-glucuronidase, and alpha-naphthyl butyrate esterase, and display characteristic, age-related cytochemical profiles. Acid phosphatase is acquired by early fetal thymocytes and is retained throughout T cell differentiation. Beta-glucuronidase, appearing later in development, is found in postgestational thymocytes. A maturation scheme differentiating T cell progress proposes that the markers progress from acid phosphatase–positive to beta-glucuronidase–negative; alpha-naphthyl butyrate esterase–positive to negative; and finally acid phosphatase–positive, beta-glucuronidase–positive, and alpha-naphthyl butyrate esterase–positive.

The majority of mature T cells, as defined by sheep RBC rosetting, display a distinct focal (dot) pattern when stained for acid phosphatase, beta-glucuronidase, and alpha-naphthyl butyrate esterase, and express surface receptors for IgM (T, Tμ, Fcr). Those characterized by a diffuse/granular stain express Fc receptors for IgG (Tδ, δFcr). Discordant data concerning this relationship have been reported. At present, it appears that enzyme phenotypes assist primarily in determining the stage of maturation arrest in T cell malignancies, and allow differentiation between T, B, and non-T/non-B lymphoproliferative disorders.

The described procedures allow dissection of the T cell compartment into three discrete phases of development. These techniques do not obviate the use of monoclonal antibodies for phenotypic analysis, but when used in concert, may supply added information concerning the nature of T cell lymphoproliferative disorders.

According to Sigma Diagnostics techniques, cytocentrifuge preparations or films are fixed in a citrate-acetone-formaldehyde solution. Alpha-naphthyl butyrate esterase and beta-glucuronidase are then visualized by the following simultaneous capture principles.

Alpha-Naphthyl Butyrate Esterase

Alpha-naphthyl naphthyl butyrate–alpha-naphthyl butyrate/ hexazotized pararosaniline (HPR)
→ insoluble-chromogenic alpha-HPR complex (red-brown)

Beta-glucuronidase

Alpha-naphthol AS-BI beta-D-glucuronide–beta-glucuronidase/ hexazotized pararosaniline
→ insoluble-chromogenic naphthol AS-BI-HPR complex (red)

Specimen Collection and Storage
Samples may be collected in either EDTA or heparin. After fixation, slides may be stored at room temperature for at least 2

(continued)

weeks. If mononuclear cells are to be isolated using HISTO-PAQUE-1077, separation should be performed within 4 hours, although fair recovery has been noted after 24 hours. Blood films, particularly from leukopenic individuals, are not recommended for these procedures since evaluation of this material is quite time-consuming. Cytocentrifuge or buffy coat preparations should be employed. Bone marrow films and tissue touch preparations pose no problems with respect to microscopic evaluation.

Reagents, Supplies, and Equipment

Provided reagents (for research use only; not for use in diagnostic procedures)

1. Alpha-naphthyl butyrate solution: Alpha-naphthyl butyrate, 2.4 gm/L, in methanol solution with solubilizers. See hazard statement below. Store in freezer below 0° C. Warm to 37°C and mix well prior to use. Discard if reagent turns yellow or if precipitate forms.
2. Naphthol AS-BI phosphoric acid solution: Naphthol AS-BI phosphoric acid, 4 gm/L, in methanol solution with solubilizers. See hazard statement below. Store in freezer below 0°C. Warm to 37°C and mix well prior to use. Discard if reagent turns yellow.
3. Naphthol AS-BI beta-D-glucuronic acid solution: Naphthol AS-BI beta-D-glucuronic acid, 2.5 gm/L, in methanol solution with solubilizers. See hazard statement below. Store in freezer below 0°C. Warm to 37°C and mix well prior to use. Discard if reagent turns yellow.

    Danger: Poison, flammable. Catalog Nos. 180-1, 180-2, and 180-3 contain methanol. *May be fatal or cause blindness if swallowed. Vapor is harmful.* Keep away from heat, sparks, and open flame. Do not pipette by mouth. Cannot be made nonpoisonous.
4. Pararosaniline solution: Pararosaniline, 40 gm/L, in 2 mol/L of hydrochloric acid. Store at room temperature protected from light. Discard if solution does not turn amber after the addition of sodium nitrite solution. *Danger: Causes burns;* do not get in eyes, on skin, or on clothing; avoid breathing vapor; wash thoroughly after handling.
5. Fast garnet GBC base solution: Fast garnet GBC base, 7.0 mg/mL, in 0.4 mol/L of hydrochloric acid and stabilizer. Store in refrigerator (2° to 6°C). The reagent label bears expiration date. *Danger: causes burns, is a carcinogen.* Avoid all contact. Wear gloves and mask.
6. Sodium nitrite solution: Sodium nitrite, 0.1 mol/L. Store in refrigerator (2° to 6°C). Suitable for use in the absence of microbial growth.
7. Sodium nitrite tablets: Sodium nitrite, 250 mg/tablet. Store at room temperature.

    Sodium nitrite tablet solution, 4 gm/dL, is prepared by dissolving the bottle contents (10 tablets) in 62.5 mL of deionized water. Store this solution tightly stoppered at 2° to 6°C. Warm to room temperature before use. Discard if turbidity develops.
8. Citrate solution: Citric acid, 18 mmol/L, sodium citrate, 9 mmol/L, sodium chloride, 12 mmol/L, and surfactant. Store in refrigerator (2° to 6°C). Suitable for use in the absence of microbial growth. The pH should be 3.6 ± 0.1.
9. Acetate solution: Acetate buffer, 2.5 mol/L, pH 5.2. Store in refrigerator (2° to 6°C). Discard if turbidity develops.
10. Phosphate buffer: Sodium and potassium phosphates. Store at room temperature.

    Phosphate buffer solution is prepared by dissolving contents of phosphate buffer in 500 mL of deionized water.

Buffer has a concentration of 0.067 mol/L, pH 7.7, at 25°C. Store in refrigerator (2° to 6°C). Discard if microbial growth is evident.

Note: Microbial growth may be retarded by filtration through a 0.22-μ filter unit.
11. Methylene blue solution: Methylene blue, 1.4% (wt/vol) in 95% ethanol. Store tightly capped at room temperature. *Danger: Flammable.* Keep away from heat, sparks, and open flame. Keep container closed. Use with adequate ventilation.

    Methylene blue counterstain is prepared by adding 5 mL of methylene blue solution to 45 mL of deionized water. Mix well. Prepare fresh daily.

Reagents Required but Not Provided

12. Acetone, reagent-grade
13. Formaldehyde: Formaldehyde, 37%, solution in 10% to 15% methyl alcohol
14. Citrate-acetone-formaldehyde fixative: To 25 mL of citrate solution add 65 mL of acetone and 8 mL of 37% formaldehyde. Place in glass bottle and cap tightly. Store in refrigerator (2° to 6°C). Warm to 23° to 26°C prior to use. Stable if stored tightly capped in refrigerator.

Optional Reagent, for Isolation of Mononuclear Cells

15. HISTOPAQUE-1077: Ficoll (type 400), 5.7 gm/dL, and sodium diatrizoate, 9 gm/dL. Aseptically filtered solution. Density 1.077.

Instruments

1. Microscope
2. Centrifuge
3. Shandon Cytospin II, if cytocentrifuge preparations are desired

Materials

1. Microscope slides or coverslips
2. Coplin jars or staining dishes
3. Oven or water bath capable of maintaining 37°C shielded from light
4. Appropriate micropipettes or macropipettes and safety pipetting devices

Quality Control

Cells from healthy donors should be included with each test. Cells isolated on Ficoll–sodium diatrizoate gradients may be stored in liquid nitrogen for control purposes. To accomplish this, 1×10^7 to 10^8 cells are frozen in a medium containing 50% fetal calf serum, 40% RPMI-1640 (or other appropriate tissue culture fluids), and 10% dimethylsulfoxide (DMSO). They may be stored in either the liquid or vapor phase of liquid nitrogen.

Procedures

Alpha-Naphthyl Butyrate Esterase Procedure

1. Prewarm phosphate buffer solution to 37°C.
2. Immediately prior to fixation, add 1.5 mL of sodium nitrite table solution to 1.5 mL of pararosaniline solution. Mix gently by inversion, let stand at least 5 minutes, and then add to 40 mL of prewarmed phosphate buffer solution.
3. Add 5 mL of alpha-naphthyl butyrate solution.
4. Mix well and pour into a Coplin jar. The solution will be amber. The formation of precipitate indicates reagent deterioration.
5. Fix slides for 10 seconds in citrate-acetone-formaldehyde fixative at room temperature. Rinse in deionized water for 45 seconds. Do not allow slides to dry.

(continued)

— S P E C I A L   S T A I N S   (c o n t i n u e d)

6. Immediately after rinsing, place slides into the solution from step 4 and incubate 1 hour at 37°C. *Note:* If slides are not placed in incubation solution after fixation, they must be allowed to air-dry for at least 45 minutes.
7. After 1 hour, remove the slides from the Coplin jar and rinse 2 to 3 minutes in running tap water. Discard the staining solution.
8. Allow slides to air-dry at least 15 minutes before counterstaining.
9. Counterstain for 5 minutes in methylene blue counterstain.
10. Rinse in deionized water.

Beta-Glucuronidase Procedure
1. Prewarm enough deionized water for a day's use to 37°C.
2. Immediately prior to fixation, add 0.5 mL of sodium nitrite tablet solution to 0.5 mL of pararosaniline solution. Mix gently by inversion, let stand for 5 minutes, and then add to 38 mL of prewarmed deionized water.
3. Add 5 mL of acetate solution.
4. Add 5 mL of naphthol AS-BI beta-D-glucuronic acid solution.
5. Mix well and pour into a Coplin jar. The solution will be amber. The formation of precipitate indicates reagent deterioration.
6. Fix slides for 30 seconds in citrate-acetone-formaldehyde fixative at room temperature. Rinse in deionized water for 45 seconds. Do not allow the slides to dry.
7. Immediately after rinsing, place the slides into the solution from step 5 and incubate for 90 minutes at 37°C protected from light. *Note:* If the slides are not placed in the incubation solution after fixation, they must be allowed to air-dry for at least 45 minutes.
8. After 90 minutes, remove the slides from the Coplin jar and rinse for 2 to 3 minutes in running tap water. Discard the staining solution.
9. Allow the slides to air-dry for at least 15 minutes before counterstaining.
10. Counterstain for 3 minutes in methylene blue counterstain.
11. Rinse in deionized water.

Results
Note: Slides should be evaluated using 1000× magnification. Dydimium filters may enhance color, particularly of the diffuse staining alpha-naphthyl butyrate esterase.

Alpha-Naphthyl Butyrate Esterase
The focal (dot) staining pattern observed in some lymphocytes is associated with mature T cells bearing Fc receptors for IgM. This subset overlaps the helper T cell population to some extent but is not an accurate measure of helper function. The diffuse or granular staining lymphocytes bear receptors to the Fc portion of IgG and overlap to some extent the suppressor T cell population. Monocytes display an intense, diffuse red-orange stain.

Beta-Glucuronidase
Positive staining appears associated with mature thymocytes, circulating T cells, and a subpopulation of immature B cells. The focal (dot) and diffuse granular patterns mark in a fashion analogous to alpha-naphthyl butyrate esterase. Monocytes and granulocytes are usually negative (unstained). *Caution:* Refer to Material Safety Data Sheets.

Reference
"Lymphocyte Enzymes." *Sigma Products Bull.* St. Louis: Sigma Diagnostics, 1987.

....

Periodic Acid–Schiff (PAS) in Leukocytes: Cytochemical or Histochemical Staining Method

Principle
When treated with periodic acid, glycols are oxidized to aldehydes. After reaction with Schiff's reagent (a mixture of pararosanilin and sodium metabisulfite) a pararosaniline adduct is released that stains the glyco-containing cellular elements (see Plate 63). Clinically, the PAS stain is helpful in recognizing some cases of erythroleukemia and acute lymphoblastic leukemia.

Specimen
Fresh anticoagulated blood or bone marrow can be used. Either EDTA or heparin can be used as anticoagulants. Smears should be fixed as soon as possible.

Reagents, Supplies, and Equipment
1. Formaldehyde (37%)
2. Ethanol (95%)
3. Fixative solution: To prepare, mix 5 mL of formaldehyde with 5 mL of 95% ethanol. This solution must be prepared *fresh daily*.

The following reagents (4 through 7) are available in Sigma Diagnostics kit No. 395A.

4. Periodic acid solution: Store at 2° to 6°C. The reagent label bears an expiration date. *Caution:* Avoid contact with skin and clothing. Bring to room temperature *prior to use*.
5. Schiff's reagent: Store at 2° to 6°C. Bring to room temperature and filter if precipitate is present. Reagent label bears expiration date. *Caution:* Corrosive. Avoid contact with skin and clothing.
6. Hematoxylin solution, Gill No. 3: Store at room temperature and protect from light. Reagent label bears expiration date. Solution may be returned to container after use but should be discarded, if solution turns brown or purple. *Filter* before use.
7. Coplin staining jars or staining dishes and slide holder

Quality Control
A normal blood specimen should be tested concurrently with the patient specimen.

Standard Procedure
Fixation of Smears
1. Place dried blood smears in fixative solution for 1 minute at room temperature.
2. Rinse slides for 1 minute in slowly running tap water.

Staining Procedure
1. Immerse slides in periodic acid solution for 5 minutes at room temperature.
2. Rinse slides in several changes of distilled water.

(continued)

3. Immerse slides in Schiff's reagent for 5 minutes at room temperature. *Note:* Immediately after use, cap Schiff's reagent and return to refrigerator (2° to 6°C).
4. Wash slides in running tap water for 5 minutes.
5. Counterstain slides in freshly filtered hematoxylin solution Gill no. 3 for 90 seconds.
6. Rinse slides in running tap water for 15 to 30 seconds, air-dry, and examine microscopically under oil immersion lens. Slides may be mounted in xylene-base mounting media.

Alternate Techniques
Consult package insert for blood and bone marrow microwave procedure and tissue sections technique.

Reporting Results
Polymorphonuclear leukocytes will show an intense red cytoplasmic stain.

Procedure Notes

Sources of Error
Directions must follow manufacturer's specifications.

Clinical Applications
In normal bone marrow the earliest myeloid precursors do not stain, but diffuse and granular staining increases as a function of maturation along myeloid pathways. Erythrocytic precursors do not stain but megakaryocytes and platelets stain intensely. Monocytes stain faintly and may display granules.

In acute lymphoblastic leukemia, PAS activity is highly variable. In most cases, some precursor cells show coarse granules or block-like positivity. In acute granulocytic leukemia, myeloblasts are usually negative, although a faint diffuse reaction product may occasionally be observed. In erythroleukemia, intense cytoplasmic granular PAS staining may be observed in early erythroid precursors. Diffuse staining may be present in more mature nucleated erythrocytes. A full discussion of cytochemical staining is included in Chapter 19. *Caution:* Refer to Material Safety Data Sheets.

Reference
"Periodic Acid–Schiff (PAS) Staining System." Procedure No. 395. *Sigma Products Bull.*, Vol. 6, St. Louis: Sigma Diagnostics, 1986.

....

Peroxidase (Myeloperoxidase) in Leukocytes: Cytochemical Staining Method

Principle
Myeloperoxidase (MP) is detected by means of the enzyme's interaction with diaminobenzidine (DAB), a benzidine substitute. The brown reaction product is first intensified with copper salts followed by Gill's modified Papanicolaou stain, which results in intense gray-black granules at sites of neutrophil and monocyte myeloperoxidase activity (see Plate 62). The reaction can be illustrated as:

$$DAB + H_2O_2 - MP \rightarrow \text{oxidized DAB (light brown pigment)}$$
$$\text{Oxidized DAB} + Cu(NO_3)_2 \rightarrow \text{gray–black pigment}$$

This procedure differentiates cells of lymphoid origin from granulocytes and their precursors and monocytes.

Specimen
Whole blood anticoagulated with heparin or EDTA, bone marrow aspirates, or buffy coat preparations may be used. If samples are stored at room temperature and protected from light, no loss of activity will occur for several months.

Reagents, Supplies, and Equipment
Reagents: Sigma No. 390A
1. Glutaraldehyde stock solution: Store *under refrigeration*. Reagent label bears expiration date. Discard if turbidity develops.
   Glutaraldehyde fixative solution: Prepare by adding 25 mL of reagent-grade acetone to 75 mL of glutaraldehyde stock solution. This solution is stable for several months if stored under *refrigeration* in a tightly capped bottle. pH must remain at 7.6 ± 0.4.
2. Hematoxylin solution, Gill No. 3: Store at room temperature. Protect from light. Reagent label bears expiration date. *Filter before use.* Discard if solution turns brown or purple.
3. Copper nitrate: Store at room temperature. Reagent label bears expiration date. *Danger:* Strong oxidizer, causes irritation; contact with other material may cause fire.
   Copper nitrate solution: Prepare by dissolving contents of 1 vial of copper nitrate in 250 mL of deionized water. Store at room temperature. Discard if turbidity develops.
4. Trizma buffer concentrate: Store at room temperature. Discard if turbidity develops.
   Trizma working solution is prepared by diluting 1 vol of Trizma buffer concentrate with 9 vol of deionized water. Store under *refrigeration*. Discard if turbidity develops.
5. Diaminobenzidine: Store under *refrigeration*. Reagent label bears expiration date. *Caution:* Possibly carcinogenic. Avoid contact with skin. Do not breathe dust.
   Diaminobenzidine staining solution is prepared by dissolving the contents of 1 diaminobenzidine vial in 50 mL of Trizma working solution. *Prepare immediately before use.*
6. Gill modified EA solution: Store tightly stoppered at room temperature. Reagent label bears expiration date. *Danger:* Poison, flammable, may be fatal or cause blindness if swallowed; vapor is harmful; cannot be made nonpoisonous. Keep away from heat, sparks, and open flame.
7. Scott's tap water substitute concentrate: Store at room temperature. Discard if turbidity develops.
   Scott's tap water substitute working solution is prepared by diluting 1 vol of Scott's tap water substitute concentrate with 9 vol of deionized water. Store covered at room temperature.
8. 15 Coplin staining jars or staining dishes and slide holder
9. Stopwatch or second-hand timer
10. Coverslips and mounting medium
11. Microscope, lens paper, and immersion oil

Quality Control
A normal control specimen should be run concurrently with the patient's specimen.

Procedure
Preparation Prior to Staining
Label and fill each staining jar with one of the following:
1. Glutaraldehyde-acetone fixative solution at 4° to 8°C
2. Diaminobenzidine working solution
3. Copper nitrate solution
4. Hematoxylin solution, Gill No. 3
5. Scott's tap water substitute
6. Gill modified EA solution
   A. G_1 and G_2—two jars with 95% ethanol
   B. H_1 and H_2—three jars with absolute ethanol

(continued)

SPECIAL STAINS (continued)

C. I_1, I_2, and I_3—three jars with xylene
D. Deionized water and several staining jars

Staining Procedure

Before beginning, read the staining procedure. This staining sequence must *not* stop once it is started:

1. Add 0.5 mL of 1% H_2O_2 to staining jar B: diaminobenzidine working solution. Mix well.
2. Fix slides at 4° to 8° C in fixative solution (jar A) for 1 minute.
3. Rinse for 30 seconds in deionized water.
4. Incubate for 45 seconds in diaminobenzidine-peroxide (jar B).
5. Rinse for 30 seconds in deionized water.
6. Immerse in copper nitrate solution (jar C) for 2 minutes with gentle agitation.
7. Rinse for 30 seconds in deionized water.
8. Dip 4 times (8 seconds) in hematoxylin solution (jar D).
9. Rinse in two changes of deionized water for 5 seconds with agitation.
10. Immerse for 12 seconds (six dips) in Scott's working solution (jar E).
11. Rinse in two jars of deionized water.
12. Immerse in Gill modified EA stain (jar F) for 1 minute.
13. Rinse in two changes of 95% ethanol for 3 seconds each (jars G_1 and G_2).
14. Rinse in two changes of absolute ethanol for 3 seconds each (jars H_1, H_2).
15. Rinse in three changes of xylene for 3 seconds each (jars I_1, I_2, and I_3).
16. Coverslip with mounting medium and examine microscopically. Color will fade if the slides are not mounted.

Reporting Results

Neutrophils and their precursors show gray-black intracellular granulation. Monocytes stain less intensely. Eosinophils stain red-orange. Basophils stain blue. Lymphocytes do not show peroxidase activity.

Procedure Notes

Sources of Error

Weak or contaminated solutions can produce false-negative results. Some types of chemotherapy and defects, either hereditary or acquired, in myeloperoxidase can produce false-negative test results.

Clinical Applications

The most probable results to be expected with peroxidase staining procedures in cases of acute nonlymphocytic leukemia (ANLL) are: M1 = 5% to 15% of blasts may be positive; M2 and M3 = positive; M4 = positive (usually a mixed population of cells); M5a = may be positive; M5b = a fine granular deposit may be observed in more mature cells; M6 and M7 = myelocytic cells are positive; ALL = negative (L1, L2, and L3).

A complete discussion of the clinical applications of this test can be found in Chapter 19.

Limitations

Although myeloperoxidase is generally considered a marker for cells of myelocytic lineage, it is imperative to recognize that monocytoid cells may also display weak peroxidase activity. A negative peroxidase reaction should never be considered to be diagnostic of acute nonmyelogenous leukemia. Other cytochemical reactions such as naphthol AS-D chloroacetate esterase, α-naphthyl acetate esterase or α-naphthyl butyrate esterase and Sudan Black B, should be performed. Only when a complete cytochemical profile is available and is used in conjunction with a clinical history should a presumptive diagnosis be made. *Caution:* Refer to Material Safety Data Sheets.

Reference

"Leukocyte Peroxidase (Myeloperoxidase)." Procedure No. 391. *Sigma Products Bull.*, Vol. 6. St. Louis: Sigma Diagnostics, 1994.

....

Siderocyte Stain: Prussian Blue Staining Method

Principle

The Prussian blue reaction precipitates free iron into small blue or blue-green granules in erythrocytes (see Plate 23). Free iron is not identifiable on Wright- or Wright-Giemsa–stained blood smears. An immature or mature erythrocyte containing free iron is referred to as a sideroblast or siderocyte, respectively. Increased numbers of siderocytes are seen in disorders such as thalassemia major or in patients after a splenectomy. If the iron granules encircle the nucleus of the erythrocyte, it is referred to as a **ringed sideroblast.** Although alcoholism is the most common cause of ringed sideroblasts, they may also be seen in cases of lead poisoning or anemia.

Specimen

Whole anticoagulated blood or capillary blood.

Reagents, Supplies, and Equipment

1. Absolute methyl alcohol
2. 2% potassium ferrocyanide: Prepare by weighing 1 gm of potassium ferrocyanide and transferring to a 50-mL volumetric flask. Dilute to the calibration mark with distilled water. Mix. Transfer to a labeled and dated stoppered brown bottle. This solution is stable for *1 month.*
3. 2% hydrochloric acid (HCl) (vol/vol): Prepare by filling a 100-mL volumetric flask about half-full with distilled water. Using a safety bulb, pipette 2 mL of concentrated HCl into the flask. Dilute to the calibration mark with distilled water. This dilute solution is stable for a short period of time.
4. 0.1% aqueous eosin: Weigh out 0.1 gm of eosin dye and transfer to a 100-mL volumetric flask. Mix and *filter* before use.
5. Prussian blue reagent: Prepare this solution *immediately* before use by mixing 50 mL of 2% potassium ferrocyanide and 50 mL of 2% HCl in a flask. Mix.
6. 5 Coplin staining jars or staining dishes and holders
7. Microscope and immersion oil

Procedure

1. Prepare the blood smears and allow to dry thoroughly.
2. Place the smears in absolute methyl alcohol for 10 minutes. Remove and air-dry the slides.
3. Immerse the smears in Prussian blue reagent for 15 minutes.
4. Rinse or dip the slides thoroughly in distilled water.
5. Immerse the slides in 0.1% aqueous solution of eosin for 1 minute.
6. Rinse or dip the slides in distilled water. Allow to air-dry.
7. Examine the smears using the oil (100×) immersion objective. Examine a thin area. Siderocytes are erythrocytes con-

(continued)

taining blue or blue-green granules. Count 1000 erythrocytes and record the number of erythrocytes containing granules.

Calculations

$$\% \text{ Siderocytes} = \frac{\text{no. of erythrocytes containing granules}}{\substack{100 \text{ erythrocytes} \\ (\text{erythrocytes} + \text{siderocytes}) \times 100}}$$

Reporting Results

Reference values range from 0 to 1% of mature erythrocytes. In the bone marrow 30% to 50% of metarubricytes are sideroblasts.

Procedure Notes

Sources of Error

Outdated reagents or improperly stored reagents can produce false-negative results. Iron contamination from glassware or water can produce false-positive results.

Clinical Applications

An increase in sideroblasts is associated with thalassemia major or minor and with the sideroblastic anemias. The sideroblastic anemias are a miscellaneous group of diseases due to drugs or chemicals, and various disorders, and are of hereditary or idiopathic origin. Siderocytes are uncommon in peripheral blood but may be seen after a splenectomy. *Caution:* Refer to Material Safety Data Sheets.

References

Seivard, Charles E. *Hematology for Medical Technologists* (4th edition). Philadelphia: Lea & Febiger, 1972, pp. 529–532.

Wallach, Jacques. *Interpretation of Diagnostic Tests* (5th edition). Boston: Little, Brown & Co., 1991.

••

Sudan Black B Stain: Cytochemical Staining Method

Principle

Following fixation, blood or bone marrow films are immersed in a buffered Sudan black B solution. After rinsing, slides are counterstained with Mayer's hematoxylin. Cells are examined microscopically for the presence of blue-black discrete granulation (see Plate 61). Cells committed to the lymphoid pathway display negative staining reactions, while myeloid and monocytoid forms display characteristic positive reactions. The Sudan black B staining pattern usually parallels the myeloperoxidase stain and is useful in the identification of myelogenous and myelomonocytic leukemias.

Specimen

Fresh whole or anticoagulated blood or bone marrow smears may be used. The slides must be *fixed* as soon as possible.

Reagents, Supplies, and Equipment

Reagents: Sigma Kit No. 380-A

1. Sudan black B staining reagent: Store at room temperature. Reagent label bears expiration date. *Danger:* Poison, flammable, and corrosive. Do not pipette by mouth. Avoid contact with eyes, skin, and clothing.
2. Hematoxylin solution, Gill No. 3: Store at room temperature. Protect from light. Reagent label bears expiration date. *Filter before use.* Discard if solution turns brown or purple.
3. Glutaraldehyde stock solution: Store *under refrigeration*. Reagent label bears expiration date. Discard if turbidity develops.

Glutaraldehyde fixative solution: Prepare by adding 25 mL of reagent-grade acetone to 75 mL of glutaraldehyde stock solution. Stable for several months if stored under *refrigeration* in a tightly capped bottle.

4. 70% ethanol
5. Coplin staining jars or staining dishes, and a slide holder
6. Microscope, immersion oil, and lens paper
7. Coverslip and mounting medium optional

Quality Control

Blood from a normal person should be run concurrently with the patient's specimen.

Procedure

1. Cool the fixative solution in the refrigerator.
2. Place blood smears into the cool fixative for 1 minute. Gently agitate during this minute. Rinse or dip in deionized water.
3. Immerse in Sudan black B stain for 5 minutes. Gently agitate.
4. Rinse or dip in 70% ethanol until no more dye washes out.
5. Rinse thoroughly in distilled water.
6. Immerse in hematoxylin solution for 5 minutes. Rinse thoroughly in tap water.
7. Air-dry and examine slides microscopically using oil (100×) immersion objective.

Reporting Results

Neutrophils and their precursors show blue-black intracellular granulation. Monocytes stain less intensely and lymphocytes do not stain with Sudan black B.

Procedure Notes

Sources of Error

Fresh specimens that are promptly fixed are important to avoid false-negative results. All solutions must be stored and prepared as directed. Weak or contaminated solutions can produce false-negative results.

Clinical Applications

This cytochemical stain in conjunction with other testing is useful in the identification of myelogenous and myelomonocytic leukemias. Refer to Chapter 19 for a full discussion of cytochemical staining and the FAB classification of acute leukemias.

Limitations

A negative Sudan black B reaction alone should never be considered diagnostic of acute nonmyelocytic leukemia. Other cytochemical stains should be performed. Only when a complete cytochemical profile is available and is used in conjunction with a clinical history should a presumptive diagnosis be made. *Caution:* Refer to Material Safety Data Sheets.

Reference

"Sudan Black B Staining System." *Sigma Product Bull.*, Vol. 6. St. Louis: Sigma Diagnostics, 1984.

••

Terminal Deoxynucleotidyl Transferase Test

Principle

Terminal deoxynucleotidyl transferase (TdT) is a non–template-directed DNA polymerase that catalyzes the irreversible addition of deoxynucleotides to the 3'-hydroxy groups on the end of

(continued)

SPECIAL STAINS (continued)

DNA. The primary methods of detection are immunofluorescence and immunoperoxidase using a monoclonal antibody.

TdT is a cell marker found on immature and neoplastic cells frequently seen in leukemic states.

Specimen

Storage conditions for the preservation of nuclear TdT are not yet well established. Therefore, it is recommended that cytocentrifuged preparations and blood or bone marrow smears be examined for TdT as soon as possible. If immediate evaluation cannot be performed, store slides dessicated at −70°C until ready for use.

Reagents, Supplies, and Equipment

Reagents

1. Methanol, absolute (acetone-free)
2. Hydrogen peroxide, 30%
   Working solution: Hydrogen peroxide, 3%, in phosphate-buffered saline (PBS) solution is prepared by adding 1 part hydrogen peroxide, 30%, to 9 parts PBS solution. Prepare fresh, as needed.
3. Sheep serum, normal (10% vol/vol) in PBS solution with preservative
4. Monoclonal anti-TdT (1%) in PBS solution with bovine serum albumin
5. Sheep anti-mouse IgG-biotin (10 μg/mL) in PBS solution with bovine serum albumin, 1.5% with preservative
6. Peroxidase reagent: Extravidin-conjugated peroxidase in PBS solution with preservative
7. Acetate buffer, 2.5 mol/L, pH 5.0
8. 3-Amino-9-ethylcarbazole (AEC) chromogen in *N,N*-dimethylformamide
   or
9. Diaminobenzidine (DAB) tablets, 10 mg with additives: May be used as an alternative to the AEC chromogen. Dissolve 1 tablet in 10 mL of PBS solution. Add 1 drop of 3% hydrogen peroxide. Prepare just prior to use. If less intense staining is desired, dissolve 1 tablet in 25 mL of PBS, with 1 drop of 3% hydrogen peroxide. Transfer 4 mL to vial 6 for use in staining.
   PBS solution: A dry mixture of sodium chloride, 120 mmol, potassium chloride, 2.7 mmol, and phosphate buffer salts, 10 mmol.
   Working PBS solution (pH 7.4) at 25°C: Prepare by dissolving the contents of the PBS package in 1 L of deionized water. Discard if turbidity develops.
10. Mayer's hematoxylin solution, 1 gm/L, with stabilizers. Store at room temperature.
    Precautions: Acetate buffer, Mayer's hematoxylin solution, and diaminobenzidine tablets are *harmful* if inhaled, in contact with skin, and if swallowed. They are irritating to the eyes, respiratory system, and skin. In case of contact with the eyes, rinse immediately with plenty of water and seek medical advice. Wear suitable protective clothing.
    AEC chromogen is *harmful* if inhaled, if in contact with the skin, and if swallowed. It is irritating to the eyes, respiratory system, and skin. Do not breathe dust—it is toxic and may act as a carcinogen. Use suitable protective clothing and equipment. The container must be kept tightly closed in a cool, well-ventilated place. *Combustible.*
    Diaminobenzidine tablets have a possible risk of irreversible effects; it is a possible carcinogen. Do not breathe dust.

Supplies and Equipment

1. Light microscope
2. Cytocentrifuge
3. Microscope slides and diamond pencil
4. Humid chamber
5. Laboratory wash bottle

Quality Control

Negative control: Dilute normal mouse serum in PBS solution.

Positive control: Human leukemia or normal peripheral blood cells fixed in methanol on glass slides. Store desiccated and frozen at −70°C until use.

Positive and negative control slides are commercially available.

Procedure

All rinses are with PBS, pH 7.4. Following incubations, slides should be washed gently with PBS from a wash bottle. *Avoid letting the stream directly hit the area of cells.* Carefully wipe around the cells on each slide to remove excess fluid before application of the next reagent. Be certain to apply sufficient reagent to cover the cells. *Do not* allow slides to dry out at any time during the procedure. It is recommended that incubations be performed in a humid chamber. All incubations are at room temperature unless otherwise specified. Wash steps can include placing slides in a PBS bath for 2 minutes.

1. Circle the area of cells with a diamond pencil. Fix the slides in methanol at 4°C for 5 minutes.
2. Wash the slides with deionized water.
3. Cover the circled area with hydrogen peroxide, 3%, in PBS for 5 minutes to quench endogenous peroxidase. Rinse briefly with PBS solution.
4. Block the nonspecific binding sites by applying sufficient sheep serum to cover the cells. Let stand for 5 minutes. Wipe off excess reagent but do not wash the slides.
5. Apply 1 drop of monoclonal anti-TdT or negative control to cover the cells. Incubate the slides for 30 minutes at room temperature in a humid chamber.
6. Rinse slides briefly with PBS solution from the wash bottle.
7. Apply 1 drop of sheep anti–mouse IgG-biotin to cover the cells. Incubate the slides for 30 minutes at room temperature in a humid chamber.
8. Rinse the slides as in step 6.
9. Apply 1 drop of peroxidase reagent to cover the cells. Incubate the slides for 30 minutes at room temperature in a humid chamber.
10. Rinse the slides as in step 6.
11. Prepare the substrate reagent in a mixing vial: 4 mL of deionized water, 2 drops of acetate buffer, 1 drop of AEC chromogen, and 1 drop of 3% hydrogen peroxide. Mix well. Alternatively, prepare the diaminobenzidine substrate as specified in the Reagents section. Transfer 4 mL to the mixing vial. Mix well.
12. Apply enough substrate reagent to cover the cells completely. Incubate for up to 15 minutes at room temperature in a humid chamber protected from light. Check microscopically for color development.
13. Rinse the slides in deionized water. Apply sufficient Mayer's hematoxylin solution to cover the cells and incubate for up to 1 minute. *Note:* Examination of the cells prior to counterstaining with hematoxylin may be helpful in interpreting the final result.

14. Coverslip with an aqueous mounting medium and examine the slides under light microscope. *Note: Do not* use xylene- or toluene-based mount media when using AEC.

Reporting Results

When using AEC chromogen, specific sites of TdT activity exhibit red to brownish-red nuclear staining against a pale-blue counterstained nucleus. Diaminobenzidine will result in light- to dark-brown nuclear staining. Negative cells show only pale-blue nuclei. The enzyme TdT has been demonstrated in cytoplasmic as well as nuclear sites.

Procedure Notes

Except where noted, TdT reagents should be stored refrigerated (2° to 6°C). Reagents are stable until the expiration date on the label.

Sources of Error

Cytoplasmic staining may also occur if endogenous peroxidase is not completely quenched.

Clinical Applications

This procedure is useful in identifying lymphoblastic cells on peripheral blood and/or bone marrow smears.

Limitations

TdT reagents are for "research use only." They are not for diagnostic purposes.

Reference

"Terminal Deoxynucleotidyl Transferase (TdT)." *Sigma Product Bull.*, Vol. 6. St. Louis: Sigma Diagnostics, 1991.

COAGULATION PROCEDURES

In coagulation testing, replicate analysis is frequently performed. However, in a study of replicate testing it was concluded that repeat testing does *not* enhance the precision or the accuracy of coagulation tests. Accuracy and precision are controlled by quality assurance procedures, such as frequent calibration checks and multilevel commercial controls, as well as the practices described below.

Specimen Quality

All coagulation testing critically depends on the quality of the specimen. Minimum tissue trauma and the avoidance of hemolysis are essential. Proper phlebotomy techniques described in Chapter 2 must be strictly followed.

Special Collection Techniques

In order to reduce the possibility of introducing tissue thromboplastin into a whole blood sample and the subsequent utilization of certain factors with clot formation, certain techniques should be followed. Specimens collected for coagulation studies are normally drawn last, if multiple samples are collected. If a single sample is collected using an evacuated tube, a small amount of blood should be allowed to enter the plastic needle holder prior to collecting blood in the tube. Nonwettable evacuated tubes should be used to prevent activation of factors XII and VII by the glass walls of the container.

If a sample is collected using the syringe technique, two syringes are used. About 1 mL of venous blood is collected in the first tube, and this syringe is disconnected from the needle hub. Immediately, a second syringe is connected to the hub of the needle and the specimen is collected in this syringe.

Anticoagulants

For most procedures, sodium citrate (3.2%) is the anticoagulant of choice (see Chapter 2). EDTA is *not* satisfactory. Variations exist in the composition of the additives used, such as antimicrobial agents, buffers, and stopper components. These variations may produce differences in coagulation test results between laboratories and make it important for each laboratory to establish its own normal ranges.

Because of the importance of the ratio of blood to anticoagulant, the proper vacuum in an evacuated tube must be maintained. The expiration date on the tube container needs to be monitored. If tubes are stored in sealed metal containers, precautions should be taken to monitor the premature loss of the tubes' vacuum. Tubes are stored best in open containers in an upright position.

The ratio of 9:1 in a specimen anticoagulated with sodium citrate is achieved with a properly collected specimen if a patient's packed cell volume is between 0.20 and 0.60 L/L. However, in polycythemic or grossly anemic patients a correction in the amount of anticoagulant or the amount of blood drawn must be made.

To determine the *amount of anticoagulant* in extreme cases, the following correction formula is used:

$$0.00185 \times \text{volume of blood (mL)} \times (100 - \text{patient's packed cell volume})$$

To determine the *amount of whole blood* needed:

$$\frac{60}{100 - \text{patient's packed cell volume}} \times 4.5$$

Specimen Handling

Once a sample is in vitro, changes begin to occur and labile factors, such as factor VIII, begin to deteriorate quickly. The NCCLS recommends that after the blood specimen is drawn, the plasma should be separated within 60 minutes and stored on melting ice in plastic tubes (to prevent contact activation of procoagulants). It is important to keep the tubes *stoppered* during centrifugation and until the plasma is separated for testing. If plasma is to be frozen, it should be rapidly frozen to −20°C. To use a frozen specimen, it should be rapidly thawed at 37°C to prevent denaturation of fibrinogen.

Specimen Preparation

Platelet-poor plasma is needed for many coagulation procedures, such as the activated partial thromboplastin time (APTT) and prothrombin time (PT). This is prepared by centrifuging the whole blood specimen for a minimum of 20 minutes at 2500 rpm.

Specialized testing for coagulation factors may require *adsorbed plasma* or *aged serum*. Plasma can be adsorbed using either barium sulfate or aluminum hydroxide. After adsorption, the resulting adsorbed plasma should contain factors V, VIII, XI, and XII. Aged serum should contain factors VII, IX, X, XI, and XII. Refer to the factor substitution studies procedure in this section for the technique.

Barium sulfate adsorption: To 1 mL of plasma add 50 mg of barium sulfate. Incubate at 37°C for 15 minutes with frequent mixing. Centrifuge at 2000 rpm to obtain a clear supernatant fluid. Use immediately after preparation.

Aluminum hydroxide adsorption: An aluminum hydroxide suspension is prepared by adding 1 gm of aluminum hydroxide to 4 mL of distilled water. Add 1 vol of the suspension to 9 vol of citrated plasma. Mix well and incubate for 5 minutes at 37° C. Centrifuge at 2500 rpm to obtain a clear supernatant.

Aged serum: A specimen of nonanticoagulated whole blood should be allowed to clot. This specimen should be incubated at 37°C for 3 hours. Add 0.1 M sodium citrate in the ratio of 1 vol of 0.1 M sodium citrate to 9 vol of whole blood to the specimen tube. Allow the tube to incubate at 37°C for an additional 2 hours. Centrifuge for 10 minutes and remove the serum. Serum should be used immediately or stored at −20°C. Prior to use, dilute the aged serum with 0.85% sodium chloride using a ratio of 1 vol of serum to 4 vol of sodium chloride.

General Sources of Error

Glassware must be clean. Disposable glassware is preferred to reusable equipment because detergent residues and scratched glassware can produce erroneous results. All procedural directions must be strictly followed because variations in pH, reagent concentration, and temperature are major sources of error.

Quality Control

Water baths and heat blocks must be continually monitored for accurate temperatures. Refrigerators and freezers should also be monitored to ensure the stability of specimens and test reagents. Reagents must not be beyond their stated expiration date.

Procedural technique must be consistent and appropriate. Most clotting procedures may be performed manually using a nichrome wire or a tilt-tube technique. Automated instruments employing an electromechanical principle may be used; however, instruments that are based on optical measurements of clot formation may not be suitable unless otherwise specified by the manufacturer.

REFERENCES

Poulsen, Keila D. "Controlling Preanalytical Variables in Coagulation Testing." *J. Med. Technol.,* Vol. 3, No. 11, November, 1986, pp. 561–565.

Sage-El, Adrienne, Edward Burns, and Barry Wenz. "The Unwarranted Use of Replicate Analysis in Routine Coagulation Studies." *Am. J. Clin. Pathol.,* Vol. 84, No. 6, December, 1985, pp. 81–83.

Tentative Guideline H21-T. Standardized Collection, Transport, and Preparation of Blood Specimens for Coagulation Testing. Villanova, PA: National Commission on Clinical Laboratory Standards, 1984.

COAGULATION PROCEDURES

Activated Partial Thromboplastin Time

Principle
The APTT procedure measures the time required to generate thrombin and fibrin polymers via the intrinsic pathway. Although a partial thromboplastin time test can be performed, contact factors can be activated more thoroughly by the addition of substances such as kaolin in the activated form of this assay.

In the APTT, calcium ions and phospholipids that substitute for platelet phospholipids are added to blood plasma. The generation of fibrin is the end point. Clinically, the APTT is used to identify and quantitate deficiencies in the intrinsic clotting system and to control anticoagulant therapy.

(continued)

Specimen

Fresh plasma from citrated whole blood is needed. Centrifuge unopened whole blood specimens at 2500 rpm for 20 minutes. Promptly transfer the plasma to a labeled plastic tube and place in an ice bath until tested. Specimens should be tested within 2 hours of collection.

Reagents, Supplies, and Equipment

1. Partial thromboplastin substrate containing an activator (such as platelin plus activator or automated APTT from Organon Teknika Corp. or equivalent)
2. 0.025 M calcium chloride
3. Ice bath
4. (If manually performed) Stopwatch, 12 × 75-mm test tubes, nichrome loop, 0.1-mL pipettes, and a 37°C water bath or heat block

Quality Control

The routine testing of control materials is essential. Both normal and abnormal controls should be tested simultaneously with patient specimens. Results within and outside of the normal range are equally important to monitor.

Commercial normal and abnormal control plasmas should be used for a comprehensive quality control program. To prepare these controls, reconstitute normal and abnormal plasma with the *exact* amount of reagent-grade water specified on the label. Allow to stand for 30 minutes at room temperature. Swirl gently to ensure complete rehydration. Mix gently prior to use. Store rehydrated vials at 2° to 8°C and use within 24 hours. Unopened vials should be stored at 2° to 8°C and used before the expiration date on the label.

Procedure

1. Place an aliquot of 0.025 M calcium chloride in a test tube and incubate at 37°C for a minimum of 5 minutes and a maximum of 60 minutes.
2. Pipette 0.1 mL of the partial thromboplastin substrate into a test tube and incubate for 2 minutes.
3. Pipette 0.1 mL of patient or control plasma into the substrate. Shake briskly to mix. Begin timing for *exactly 5 minutes.*
4. After 5 minutes of activation, transfer 0.1 mL of prewarmed calcium chloride to the mixture. *Immediately* begin to time with a stopwatch. Insert nichrome loop and sweep it across the bottom of the tube at the rate of 2 times/sec.
5. At the first appearance of fibrin, stop the stopwatch. Record the number of seconds. Repeat this procedure (steps 2 through 5) for each assay.
   Note: Performance of this test by automated methods is described in Chapter 25.

Reporting Results

Reference values are dependent on the activator and phospholipid reagents used; however, 20 to 35 seconds is typically normal. In some laboratories ranges may be from 28 to 42 seconds, with 42 to 46 seconds being marginal.

Procedure Notes

Sources of Error

Various sources of error include poor specimen collection or storage, improper reconstitution and storage of reagents, reaction temperature, timing, and clot detection.

Clinical Applications

The APTT is widely advocated as the test of choice for the control of heparin therapy. It is also important in the screening pro-file of prekallikrein; high-molecular-weight kininogen; factors XII, XI, IX, VIII, X, V, II, and I; and inhibitors against these factors.

References

Henry, John B. (ed.). *Clinical Diagnosis and Management by Laboratory Methods* (17th edition). Philadelphia: Saunders, 1984, p. 1444.

Lenahan, Jane G. and K. Smith. *Hemostasis* (17th edition). Durham, NC: Organon Teknika, 1985, p. 17.

Proctor, R. R. and S. I. Rapaport. "The Partial Thromboplastin Time with Kaolin." *Am. J. Clin. Pathol.*, Vol. 36, 1961, p. 212.

Antithrombin III: Clotting Assay Method

Principle

In the presence of heparin, thrombin is neutralized at a rate that is proportional to the antithrombin (AT III) concentration. Following defibrination, plasma is assayed in a two-stage procedure that utilizes standardized amounts of heparin, fibrinogen, and thrombin. The resulting clotting time is interpreted using a calibration curve. Clinically, the AT III assay is useful prior to and subsequent to treatment with heparin in cases of disseminated intravascular coagulation (DIC).

Specimen

A 4.5-mL sample of whole blood should be mixed with 0.5 mL of 3.8% sodium citrate solution immediately prior to testing. The specimen should be centrifuged at 2500 rpm for 15 minutes. The plasma needs to be transferred to a plastic tube within 30 minutes of collection and stored at 2° to 6°C for up to 2 hours before defibrination. If frozen, plasma can be stored for several weeks before testing. Frozen samples should be thawed at 37°C for 5 minutes before testing.

Reagents, Supplies, and Equipment

Reagents 1 through 5 are available in kit No. 855-B from Sigma Diagnostics, St. Louis, MO.

1. Atroxin: Store at 2° to 6°C. Reagent label bears expiration date. Atroxin solution is prepared by reconstituting one vial with 1.0 mL of deionized water. Swirl to mix. Stable for up to 1 month if kept at 2° to 6°C.
2. Fibrinogen (human): Store at 2° to 6°C. Reagent label bears expiration date. Fibrinogen solution is prepared by reconstituting one vial with 4.0 mL of deionized water. Place at 37°C and swirl to dissolve. *Do not shake.* Store at room temperature prior to testing. Stable for 8 hours.
3. Thrombin: Store at 2° to 6°C. Reagent label bears expiration date and thrombin content. Thrombin solution is prepared by reconstituting one vial with deionized water. Volume required is stated on reagent label. Store in ice bath during assay. Stable for 8 hours.
4. Heparin reagent: Store at 2° to 6°C. Reagent label bears expiration date. Withdraw solution as required through the rubber stopper with a sterile syringe. Discard if turbidity develops.
5. Citrated plasma control: Store at 2° to 6°C. Reagent label bears expiration date. Plasma control solution is prepared by reconstituting one vial with 1.5 mL of deionized water. Store in ice bath during assay. Stable for 8 hours.
6. Pipettors: 0.2, 0.1, and 0.01 mL
7. Serological pipettes: 0.5, 5.0, and 10 mL

(continued)

COAGULATION PROCEDURES (continued)

8. Disposable plastic test tubes, 12 × 75 mm
9. Stopwatch
10. Wooden applicator sticks
11. 37°C water bath or heat block
12. Ice bath
13. Centrifuge

Calibration

A calibration curve prepared from a normal plasma pool from donors not receiving medication or oral contraceptives or donors not suffering from liver disease needs to be prepared by each laboratory. This plasma is defibrinated according to the technique outlined in the Procedure section. Dilutions of defibrinated plasma in heparin reagent are prepared as follows:

Plasma	Heparin Reagent	Dilution	At III activity (%)
0.1	2.9	1:30	100
0.1	3.9	1:40	75
0.1	5.9	1:60	50
0.1	11.9	1:120	25
—	0.5	—	0

Follow the instructions in the Procedure section to determine the clotting time for each dilution. Plot the clotting times (in seconds—y axis) versus AT III activity (x axis) in percentages on *semilog* graph paper.

Quality Control

All tests should be performed in duplicate. A citrated normal human plasma sample should be tested simultaneously.

Procedure

Defibrination of Plasma

1. Label two plastic test tubes for each specimen to be tested.
2. Add 0.5 mL of patient or control plasma to the labeled tubes.
3. Add 0.01 mL of Atroxin solution to each tube. Mix and incubate for 15 minutes at 37°C.
4. After incubation, rim the clot with a wooden applicator and centrifuge for 10 minutes at 2500 rpm.
5. Transfer the clear plasma to a second labeled plastic tube for each specimen and place in an ice bath until assayed.

Clotting Time Measurement

1. Pipette 0.2 mL of fibrinogen solution into labeled plastic tubes for assay to be performed. Place tubes in a 37°C water bath for 3 to 5 minutes.
2. Dilute the defibrinated plasma by pipetting 0.1 mL of plasma into 2.9 mL of heparin reagent in a clean, labeled plastic tube.
3. Pipette 0.5 mL of each defibrinated dilution into a correspondingly labeled plastic tube. Place these tubes into a 37°C water bath for 3 to 5 minutes.
4. After the appropriate incubation time, pipette 0.1 mL of thrombin solution into one tube containing the 0.5 mL of plasma dilution. Start the stopwatch and mix well.
5. *Exactly* 30 seconds after the addition of the thrombin, remove 0.1 mL of this mixture and pipette it into a tube containing the 0.2 mL of fibrinogen solution. Observe for clotting and record the time. Repeat steps 4 and 5 for patient and control assays. If many assays are to be performed, begin with step 1 in order to avoid excessive incubation of the fibrinogen solution.

Calculations

Convert the clotting time of the assay to percent AT III activity using the calibration curve described in the Calibration section of this procedure.

Reporting Results

The normal plasma control activity of AT III should range from 80% to 100%. If the activity is less than 80% or greater than 100%, a new calibration curve should be constructed. The adult normal mean value for AT III is 107% (±19%). Normal values should be established in each laboratory.

Procedure Notes

If the assay demonstrates AT III activity greater than 100% (clotting time longer than 100%), the assay can be repeated using 0.1 mL of plasma and 5.0 mL of heparin reagent. This is twice the dilution of the sample used for assay. Multiply the result obtained from the calibration curve by 2.

Reference

"Anti-Thrombin III (AT-III)." Procedure No. 855. *Sigma Products Bull.*, Vol. 6. St. Louis: Sigma Diagnostics, 1984.

Bleeding Time: Standardized Ivy Method

Principle

The bleeding time test is an in vivo measurement of platelet adhesion and aggregation on locally injured vascular subendothelium. This test provides an estimate of the integrity of the platelet plug and thereby measures the interaction between the capillaries and platelets. The bleeding time reflects this aspect of platelet function by measuring the length of time two standardized punctures of the ventral forearm take to stop bleeding. Clinically, the bleeding time is prolonged in thrombocytopenia, qualitative platelet disorders such as von Willebrand's disease, aspirin ingestion, or the presence of vascular problems.

Specimen

Free-flowing blood is needed.

Reagents, Supplies, and Equipment

1. Blood pressure cuff
2. Sterile, disposable blood lancet and alcohol wipes
3. Whatman No. 1 filter paper
4. Stopwatch

Procedure

1. Select a site approximately 2 in. below the elbow on the ventral surface of the forearm. Cleanse with an alcohol wipe and allow to air-dry for at least 30 seconds. If a patient has marked hair, lightly shave the area.
2. Adjust a blood pressure cuff to 40 mm Hg.
3. Firmly grasp the underside of the arm. The incision must be made consistently either parallel or perpendicular to the fold of the elbow. Make two punctures 1 mm wide and 3 mm deep. *Caution:* Avoid subcutaneous veins.
4. Start a stopwatch. Blot each puncture with separate pieces of filter paper (being careful not to touch the skin) every 30 seconds.

(continued)

5. When bleeding ceases, stop the watch and release the blood pressure cuff. Record the time for each puncture.

Calculations
Average the bleeding time in minutes and seconds.

Reporting Results
Normal bleeding time is 1 to 7 minutes, with a reading of 7 to 11 minutes being borderline.

Procedure Notes
If bleeding continues for more than 15 minutes, discontinue the test. Release the blood pressure cuff and apply pressure to the wounds. If the test results are above or below the normal limits, repeat the test, except in excessively prolonged tests.

Other Methods
The Duke bleeding time method is not recommended because it is not closely reproducible and it has a wide range of normal values. Two other methods, the Mielke method (a modification of the Ivy bleeding time) and the Simplate method (a modification of the Mielke method with equipment manufactured by General Diagnostics), are in use. These methods are currently popular because of their reproducibility.

Simplate Method
Supplies and Equipment
The same as for the Ivy procedure, except that the Simplate Bleeding Device is substituted for a lancet.

Procedure
Similar to the Ivy time, except that the incision is made with the Simplate device.

Normal Values
The normal values are similar to the Mielke method: 2 to 8 minutes. Normal values for the Simplate method are 2.3 to 9.5 minutes.

Clinical Applications
As the platelet count drops below 100×10^9/L, the bleeding time progressively increases from normal. A prolonged bleeding time in a patient with a platelet count above 100×10^9/L indicates either impaired platelet function or a defect of subendothelial factor VIII:vWF multimers.

Aspirin Tolerance Test
The aspirin tolerance test is often useful and is repeated 2 hours after aspirin challenge. Aspirin has a powerful effect. In hyperresponders, profuse bleeding can result from the ingestion of aspirin, particularly in surgical patients.

Procedure
Measure the bleeding time, have patient ingest 2 tablets (10 grains) of aspirin, and repeat the bleeding time in 2 hours.

Reference Values
In 92% to 95% of normal patients, the bleeding time is doubled 2 hours after ingesting two aspirin tablets.

Clinical Applications
In 5% to 8% of patients who are sensitive to aspirin, the bleeding time is increased 3 to 10 times the preaspirin ingestion value. The bleeding time has been found to be prolonged in 25% of patients with von Willebrand's disease, especially 2 hours after the ingestion of 300 mg of aspirin.

References
Deykin, Daniel and J. B. Miale. "Clinical Importance of Bleeding Time Test," in *New Directions in Hematology*. Morris Plains, NJ: General Diagnostics, 1982.

Henry, John B. (ed.). *Clinical Diagnosis and Management by Laboratory Methods* (17th edition). Philadelphia: Saunders, 1984, p. 1444.

Ivy, A. C. et al. "The Standardization of Certain Factors in the Cutaneous Venostasis Bleeding Time Technique." *Clin. Med.*, Vol. 26, 1940, p. 1812.

Seivard, Charles B. *Hematology for Medical Technologists* (4th edition). Philadelphia: Lea & Febiger, 1972, pp. 399–400.

Simplate package insert. General Diagnostics Division of Warner-Lambert Co., Morris Plains, NJ, 1985.

Wallach, Jacques. *Interpretation of Diagnostic Tests* (5th edition). Boston: Little, Brown & Co., 1991.

Circulating Anticoagulants

Principle
Some coagulation deficiencies are caused by inhibitors to specific factors rather than the lack of a factor. These inhibitors are sometimes referred to as circulating anticoagulants. In order to detect a circulating anticoagulant, the APTT and/or the prothrombin time (PT) that were originally abnormal are repeated using various dilutions of patient plasma and normal plasma. The dilutions are incubated at 37°C and tested after 10, 30, 60, and 120 minutes of incubation. If the abnormality is a deficiency, 10% normal plasma will correct the test result to close to the normal range, as will the addition of 50% normal plasma. If the abnormality is caused by a circulating anticoagulant, more correction will usually be shown as the ratio of normal plasma increases in the mixture. The detection of an inhibitor may show up immediately or may require incubation of the normal plasma in the presence of the inhibitor. Differentiation between a coagulation factor deficiency and a circulating anticoagulant is important in the correct treatment of a patient.

Specimen
Refer to the APTT procedure for treatment of the original specimen.

Reagents, Supplies, and Equipment
Refer to the APTT procedure.

Quality Control
A normal patient plasma should be tested at the same time as the unknown patient.

Procedure
1. Using fresh plasma, prepare the following dilutions:

Patient Plasma	Normal Plasma
9 parts	1 part
5 parts	5 parts
1 part	9 parts

2. Incubate the control and patient specimens and mixtures at 37°C, and perform an APTT or PT assay on each plasma, control, and plasma-control mixture after 10, 30, and 60 minutes.

Reporting Results
If the abnormality is that of a deficiency, a normal plasma sample will correct the assay results to a reference value. If the abnormality is caused by a circulating anticoagulant (inhibitor), a greater correction is demonstrated as the ratio of normal plasma increases in the mixture.

(continued)

COAGULATION PROCEDURES (continued)

Patient	Normal	Deficiency	Inhibitor
9 parts	1 part	Significant correction	No significant correction
5 parts	5 parts	Significant correction	Some correction
1 part	9 parts	Significant correction	More correction

Note: It is important to incubate the test specimens for 60 minutes because some inhibitors act progressively, and it may take time for the APTT and/or PT results of the patient plasma and patient plasma–normal control mixtures to show the effects of the inhibitor (a prolonged clotting time). To interpret the results, the end point of the normal control has to be compared to the patient–normal plasma mixtures. As the specimens incubate, a slight increase in the end points will be observed due to the loss of labile clotting factors. The degree of prolongation in the patient and patient-control mixtures must be greater than the normal control plasma.

Clinical Applications
Various types of anticoagulants may interfere with coagulation at different stages, especially factor VIII, heparin-like activity, and antithromboplastins. Most acquired anticoagulants are autoantibodies (usually IgG, sometimes IgM) directed against specific coagulation factors. Below is a list of circulating anticoagulants associated with clinical disorders.

Factor	Disorder
II	Myeloma, systemic lupus erythematosus (SLE)
V	Streptomycin administration, idiopathic
VIII	SLE, rheumatoid arthritis, drug reaction, asthma, inflammatory bowel disease, postpartum
VIII, IX	Following replacement therapy for hereditary deficiency
IX	SLE-rare
X	Amyloidosis
X, V	SLE—common
XI	SLE—very rare
XIII	Isoniazid administration, idiopathic

About 5% to 10% of patients with SLE, many patients on phenothiazine therapy, patients taking a variety of medications, and patients with lymphoproliferative disorders may demonstrate inhibitors known as **lupus-like anticoagulants.**

In addition to testing for circulating anticoagulants to specific coagulation factors, the platelet neutralization procedure (PNP) and the tissue thromboplastin inhibition test (TTIT) may be of value. The PNP test separates lupus-like inhibitors from factor VIII, X, and V inhibitors but does not distinguish the presence of heparin from an acquired inhibitor. The TTIT procedure is less specific than the PNP but screens for lupus-like anticoagulant with inhibitory activity against tissue thromboplastin. Details of the PNP and TTIT procedures can be found in Lenahan and Smith (1985, pp. 38–39).

References
Hardisty, R. M. and C. I. C. Ingram. *Bleeding Disorders: Investigation and Management.* Oxford: Blackwell Scientific, 1965.

Henry, John B. (ed.). *Clinical Diagnosis and Management.* Philadelphia: Saunders, 1984, pp. 780–781.

Jandl, James H. *Blood.* Boston: Little, Brown & Co., 1987, p. 1128.

Lenahan, Jane G. and K. Smith. *Hemostasis* (17th edition). Durham, NC: Organon Teknika, 1985, pp. 37–39.

Wallach, Jacques. *Interpretation of Diagnostic Tests* (5th edition). Boston: Little, Brown & Co., 1991.

....

Clot Retraction: Single-Tube Method

Principle
When platelets are activated, the process can be visibly observed as clot retraction. When clot dissolution (fibrinolysis) is very active, the fibrin clot may be dissolved almost as quickly as it is formed, and clot retraction will be impaired. Clinically, this procedure is useful as a gross screening test of platelet quantity and function, and fibrinolysis.

Specimen
Fresh, whole blood without anticoagulant or a clot from the whole blood clotting time procedure is needed.

Quality Control
A normal blood specimen should be tested simultaneously.

Reagents, Supplies, and Equipment
1. Specimen of fresh, clotted blood
2. 37°C water bath

Procedure
Place a test tube of whole fresh blood in a 37°C water bath. Examine at 1, 2, 4, and 24 hours for clot retraction (pulling away of the clot from the sides of the tube).

Reporting Results
At 37°C, normal clot retraction should begin within 1 hour and be complete by 24 hours.

Procedure Notes
Clot retraction reflects the number and quality of platelets. The degree of clot retraction is directly proportional to the number of platelets and inversely proportional to the hematocrit and the level of the blood coagulation factor, fibrinogen. A decreased platelet count produces a prolonged clot retraction time.

Clinical Applications
Clot retraction is a supplementary test in hemorrhagic disorders, such as in thrombocytopenia purpura.

Alternate Procedure: MacFarlane Serum Method
Procedure
Place 5 mL of freshly drawn, nonanticoagulated blood in a 10-mL graduated centrifuge tube. Place the tube in a 37°C water bath for several hours. Carefully remove the clot and read the remaining volume of serum.

Calculation

$$\% \text{ Serum} = \frac{\text{volume of serum}}{\text{volume of whole blood}}$$

Reporting Results
Normal value of serum: 44% to 64%.

(continued)

References

Lenahan, Jane G. and K. Smith. *Hemostasis*. Durham, NC: Organon Teknika, 1985, p. 37.

Seiverd, Charles B. *Hematology for Medical Technologists* (4th edition).
Philadelphia: Lea & Febiger, 1972, pp. 433–436.

Clot Lysis

Principle

Excessive fibrinolysis produces rapid clot dissolution or in some
cases the formation of a small clot initially. Clinically, the observation of clot lysis is useful in cases of excessive fibrinolysis, as
in DIC.

Specimen

Refer to Clot Retraction.

Reagents, Supplies, and Equipment

Refer to Clot Retraction.

Quality Control

A normal blood specimen should be tested simultaneously.

Procedure

The blood clot used for clot retraction should be kept at 37°C
for 12 to 24 hours. Examine at the end of 2, 12, and 24 hours
for lysis.

Reporting Results

Normally, no clot lysis is observed before 48 hours.

Procedure Notes

This technique is insensitive to mild fibrinolysis. False normals
can result from the inactivation of plasmin by antiplasmin or
the depletion of plasminogen. This procedure has been replaced
in the clinical laboratory by the euglobulin lysis time.

Reference

Bauer, John D. *Clinical Laboratory Methods* (9th edition). St. Louis:
Mosby, 1982, p. 292.

Ethanol Gelation Test: Breen and Tullis Method

Principle

The ethanol gelation test is designed to detect the presence of
fibrin monomers in the plasma. This screening procedure aids
with the diagnosis of primary fibrinolysis or DIC. The fibrin
monomer is precipitated from platelet-poor plasma by ethyl
alcohol and forms a gel-type precipitate.

Specimen

Whole blood should be collected in a plastic syringe. Mix 9
parts of whole blood with 1 part of buffered citrate anticoagulant. Collect a normal control blood at the same time. Centrifuge at 2500 rpm for 20 minutes to obtain platelet-poor plasma.
Perform the test within 1 hour of blood collection.

Reagents, Supplies, and Equipment

1. 50% ethyl alcohol: Prepare prior to use by diluting 5.3 mL of
   95% ethyl alcohol with 4.7 mL of distilled water.
2. Test tubes (12 × 75 mm) and 1-mL graduated pipettes

Quality Control

A fresh normal platelet-poor plasma should be tested at the
same time as the patient sample.

Procedure

1. Pipette 0.5 mL of plasma into a small test tube.
2. Add 0.15 mL of ethyl alcohol. Mix gently and allow to sit un-
   disturbed for *exactly* 10 minutes.
3. Examine for gel formation by tilting the tube.

Reporting Results

Normal plasma will have no clumping.

Procedure Notes

Sources of Error

Fibrin strands or granular formation in this test is considered to
be a negative or doubtful reaction. False-negative results can be
seen in severe hypofibrinogenemia. False-positive results can occur due to a dysproteinemia or hyperfibrinogenemia.

Clinical Applications

Gel formation is indicative of DIC.

Reference

Breen, F. A. and J. L. Tullis. "Ethanol Gelation: A Rapid Screening Test
for Intravascular Coagulation." *Ann. Intern. Med.*, Vol. 69, 1968, p.
1197.

Euglobulin Lysis Time

Principle

The euglobulin fraction of plasma contains plasminogen, fibrinogen, and activators with the potential for transforming plasminogen to plasmin. This fraction is precipitated with 1% acetic
acid and resuspended in a borate solution. The euglobulins are
then clotted by the addition of thrombin. The clot is incubated
and the time of lysis is reported. Clinically, the euglobulin lysis
test is a screening procedure for fibrinolytic activity.

Specimen

Oxalated plasma from fresh whole blood in a mixture of 1 part
of 0.1 M sodium oxalate to 9 parts of whole blood is used. Citrated plasma should not be used because the presence of citrate tends to increase fibrinolytic activity.

Collect blood with a plastic syringe, and *immediately* mix
with anticoagulant and place on ice. Centrifuge at 2500 rpm for
10 minutes and immediately proceed with the test. This procedure must be carried out within 20 minutes of blood collection.

Reagents, Supplies, and Equipment

1. Thrombin (5 units/mL): Dilute according to manufacturer's directions. Place an aliquot in a plastic test tube and incubate
   at 37°C.
2. 1% acetic acid: Pipette 1 mL of glacial acetic acid into a
   100-mL volumetric flask and dilute to the calibration mark
   with distilled water. Prepare fresh.
3. Borate solution, pH 9.0: Prepare by adding 9.0 gm of sodium
   chloride and 1.0 gm of sodium borate to 100 mL of water.
4. 37°C water bath
5. 16 × 100-mm test tubes
6. Stopwatch or timer

(continued)

COAGULATION PROCEDURES (continued)

Quality Control
Collect and test a normal control plasma simultaneously.

Procedure
1. Pipette 9.0 mL of distilled water, 0.5 mL of patient's plasma, and 0.1 mL of 1% acetic acid into a 16 × 100-mm test tube. Refrigerate the mixture for 30 minutes at 4°C to allow euglobulin precipitation.
2. Centrifuge at 2500 rpm for 5 minutes at 4°C. Pour off the supernatant and invert the tube on filter paper to drain.
3. Add 0.5 mL of borate solution and place at 37°C. Mix gently.
4. Add 0.5 mL of thrombin solution, mix, and start the stopwatch.
5. Continue to incubate the test tube at 37°C and periodically check for lysis. When lysis begins, check the tube every 5 minutes until lysis is complete. Report the results as the length of time from clot formation to complete clot lysis.

Reporting Results
Normal clot lysis does not occur in less than 2 hours but is usually complete within 4 hours.

Procedure Notes
A falsely decreased time will be produced by a decrease in fibrinogen. A decrease in plasminogen activator or plasminogen will produce a falsely prolonged time.

The euglobulin lysis test is more sensitive than the *clot lysis time*. Normally occurring inhibitors are not present in this fraction of plasma. Once a clot is formed, clot lysis occurs more quickly than in whole blood.

Clinical Applications
Clot lysis in less than 2 hours is indicative of abnormal fibrinolytic activity.

References
Bauer, John D. *Clinical Laboratory Methods* (9th edition). St. Louis: Mosby, 1982, pp. 310–311.

Seiverd, Charles B. *Hematology for Medical Technologists* (4th edition). Philadelphia: Lea & Febiger, 1972, pp. 310–311.

Substitution Studies and Factor Assays

Substitution studies and factor assays can be used to identify specific coagulation factor deficiencies.

Substitution Studies
Principle
Substitution studies may be performed using adsorbed plasma and aged serum with the APTT to identify deficiencies of blood coagulation. Substitution studies may also be performed using adsorbed plasma with the PT to identify a factor VII deficiency.

Specimen
Prepare the necessary specimens as described in Special Collection Techniques at the beginning of this section.

Reagents, Equipment, and Supplies
Refer to the APTT and PT procedures.

Procedure: Partial Thromboplastin Substitution Test
1. An APTT procedure is performed on the patient's undiluted plasma, a normal undiluted control plasma, the patient's plasma diluted 1:1 with 0.85% sodium chloride, and a 1:1 dilution of the normal control plasma. Both of the control samples (undiluted and diluted) must be within normal test result ranges.
2. If either of the patient's test results are *abnormal*, the patient's plasma and normal control plasma (diluted in a ratio of 1:1) should be tested. If the results of this test are normal, the APTT procedure should be performed on the following 1:1 dilutions:
   A. Patient plasma plus adsorbed plasma
   B. Normal control plasma plus adsorbed plasma
   C. Patient plasma plus aged serum
   D. Normal control plus aged serum

Procedure: Prothrombin Substitution Test
A PT procedure is performed on the patient's undiluted plasma and an undiluted normal control plasma. The control value should be normal. If the patient's results are prolonged (abnormal), the PT procedure should be performed on the following 1:1 dilutions:

1. Patient plasma plus 0.85% sodium chloride
2. Normal control plasma plus 0.85% sodium chloride
3. Patient plasma plus normal control plasma
4. Patient plasma plus adsorbed plasma
5. Patient plasma plus aged serum
6. Normal control plasma plus aged serum

Clinical Interpretation
Table 24.8 gives the factors that may be deficient in these screening procedures.

TABLE 24.8 Probable Coagulation Deficiencies Based on Activated Partial Thromboplastin Time (APTT) and Prothrombin Time (PT) Test Results

Test	Deficient Factor					
	V	VII	VIII	IX	X	XI or XII
PT	Abnormal	Abnormal	Normal	Normal	Abnormal	Normal
APTT	Abnormal	Normal	Abnormal	Abnormal	Abnormal	Abnormal
Adsorbed plasma	Corrects	No change	Corrects	No change	No change	Corrects
Aged serum	No change	Corrects	No change	Corrects	Corrects	Corrects

(continued)

Specific Factor Assays
Principle
Factor assays are based on the ability of the plasma in question to correct a factor-deficient substrate, such as factor VIII. The actual assay is the same as the APTT with the exception of the factor-deficient substrate. Identification of specific factor deficiencies is of value in both the diagnosis and the treatment of patients.

Specimen
A fresh whole blood specimen anticoagulated with sodium citrate is used. The specimen must be placed on ice because of the labile nature of some factors, such as factor VIII. Centrifuge immediately, transfer plasma into a clean plastic tube, and keep chilled until assay. The assay for factor VIII *must be performed promptly.*

Reagents, Supplies, and Equipment
All reagents must be kept at 4°C unless otherwise stated.
1. Factor VIII-deficient plasma: Reconstitute according to manufacturer's directions.
2. Platelin Plus Activator or Automated APTT (General Diagnostics, Warner-Lambert) or equivalent
3. 0.025 M calcium chloride
4. Other equipment and supplies (refer to the APTT procedure)

Calibration
A normal plasma activity curve must be prepared (Table 24.9). This curve is prepared with known dilutions of normal plasma. Ten percent is arbitrarily defined as 100% activity. These dilutions are tested in the same manner as test samples.

Quality Control
Normal and abnormal controls should be used.

Procedure
1. Dilute patient and control plasmas to 10% with buffered saline. Prepare the buffered saline by mixing 3.4 gm of imidazole, 5.85 gm of NaCl, and 186 mL of 0.1 N HCl; dilute to 1 L with water. The pH of this buffer is 7.3.
2. Place dilutions in crushed ice.
3. Pipette 0.2 mL of calcium chloride into tubes containing 0.1 mL of Platelin Plus Activator. Incubate at 37°C for 2 minutes.
4. After incubation, pipette 0.1 mL of factor VIII–deficient substrate and 0.1 mL of diluted patient plasma into the tube containing the Platelin. Mix well and incubate for 5 minutes.

TABLE 24.9 **Preparation of Activity Curve**

Tube	Plasma	Buffered Saline	Factor VIII Activity (%)
1	0.1	0.9	100
2	0.5 from tube 1	0.5	50
3	0.5 from tube 2	0.5	25
4	0.5 from tube 3	0.5	12.5
5	0.5 from tube 4	0.5	6.25
6	0.5 from tube 5	0.5	3.125
7	0.5 from tube 6	0.5	1.6
8	0.5 from tube 7	0.5	0.8
9	0.5 from tube 8	0.5	0

5. At exactly 5 minutes, pipette 0.1 mL of calcium chloride into the mixture. Start the stopwatch. Observe for clot formation. Record the time.

Calculations
The calibration curve is graphed. The known percent activity is plotted on the horizontal axis and the time in seconds from testing on the vertical axis of a 2 × 3–cycle log paper. Draw the best straight line. The patient and unknown assay times in seconds are converted to percent activity by reading from the normal curve.

Reporting Results
The reference range for factor VIII is 50% to 150%.

Procedure Notes
Other factor assays are performed in the same way as this factor VIII assay; however, the factor-deficient substrate is specific for the factor in question.

Reference
Lenahan, Jane G. and Kathleen Smith. *Hemostasis* (17th edition). Durham, NC: Organon Teknika, 1985, pp. 26–27.

Fibrin Split Products: Thrombo-Wellcotest Method

Principle
Whole blood is added to thrombin (to ensure complete clotting) and soya bean enzyme inhibitors (to prevent any breakdown of fibrin). After incubation, the patient's serum is diluted and mixed with latex particles that have been coated with antifibrin split products. If fibrin split products are present, agglutination will occur. If these products are present in increased amounts with normal hepatic and renal function, it is assumed that a recent fibrinolytic event has taken place or is taking place. Clinically, elevated results demonstrate that the activation of plasmin has occurred or is occurring, such as in primary fibrinolysis and DIC with secondary fibrinolysis.

Specimen
Fresh whole blood is used. Either 2.0 mL of blood can be drawn into a syringe and transferred immediately to the sample collection tube provided in the kit or the tubes can be used directly as evacuated tubes that will draw 2 mL of blood. Mix by inversion. Place the specimen at 37°C for 20 minutes followed by centrifugation for 5 minutes at 2000 rpm. Remove serum and place in labeled tubes.

Reagents, Supplies, and Equipment
Available from Wellcome Reagents Division, Burroughs Wellcome Company, Research Triangle Park, NC.

1. Sample collection tube (containing thrombin)
2. Glycine saline buffer
3. Latex suspension
4. Positive and negative controls
5. Glass slide, droppers, and mixing rods

Quality Control
A positive and negative control should be tested simultaneously with the patient specimen.

(continued)

COAGULATION PROCEDURES (continued)

Procedure

1. Label two tubes for each test specimen (1:5 and 1:10).
2. Using a dropper from the kit, place 0.75 mL of glycine buffer into the 1:5 tube. Add 5 drops of patient's serum. Mix and transfer 4 drops of this diluted serum into the 1:10 tube.
3. Place 1 drop of each control in an appropriate ring. Place 1 drop of the 1:5 dilution and 1 drop of the 1:10 dilution into their respective rings. Do not touch the dropper on the glass slide.
4. Mix the latex suspension, and add 1 drop to each ring. Stir with a separate applicator stick and spread over the entire area of the ring. Rotate for exactly 2 minutes. Examine for agglutination.

Reporting Results

Reference value in adults is less than 8 to 10 μg/mL. If agglutination occurs in the 1:5 dilution, the concentration is between 10 and 20 μg/mL. If agglutination occurs in the 1:10 dilution, report as greater than 20 μg/mL.

Procedure Notes

Further serial dilutions can be made to determine quantitative results. Follow the procedure above to prepare 1:20, 1:40, 1:80, and 1:160 dilutions. If agglutination occurs in these dilutions, the respective concentrations are greater than 40, greater than 80, greater than 160, and greater than 320 μg/mL.

Sources of Error

False-positive results can be seen after 2 minutes of rotation due to drying. Graininess should not be interpreted as agglutination. Patients with rheumatoid arthritis may have false-positive results if their serum is also positive for the rheumatoid factor.

Reference

Detection of Fibrinogen Degradation Products and Fibrinogen. Research Triangle Park, NC: Wellcome Reagents Division, Burroughs Wellcome Co., 1973.

Fibrin-Stabilizing Factor: Urea Solubility

Principle

Factor XIII (fibrin-stabilizing factor, or FSF) is responsible for converting the fibrin clot to a more stable form.

Fibrin—factor XIII → stable fibrin clot

In this procedure, test plasma is clotted with calcium chloride and urea is added to the clot. When factor XIII is present, the fibrin clot formed is insoluble in 5 M urea and should not dissolve in the urea when left standing for 24 hours. Clinically a deficiency of factor XIII is rare.

Specimen

Citrated plasma from anticoagulated whole blood.

Reagents, Equipment, and Supplies

1. 5 M urea: Prepare by weighing and transferring 30.1 gm of desiccator-dried, reagent-grade urea to a 100-mL volumetric flask. Add deionized water to the calibration mark. Mix. Stable at room temperature for several months.
2. 0.025 M calcium chloride: Can be prepared by weighing and transferring 0.276 gm of anhydrous calcium chloride to a 100-mL volumetric flask. Dilute to the calibration mark with deionized water and mix. Refrigerate at 4° to 6°C. This product is also available commercially.
3. 16 × 100-mm test tubes
4. 5-mL graduated pipettes
5. Applicator sticks
6. 37°C water bath

Quality Control

A normal control specimen must be collected at the same time as the patient (test) specimen. A positive control (a clot that will dissolve in 5 M urea) can be prepared by adding 0.5 mL of 20 NIH units/mL of thrombin to 0.5 mL of EDTA plasma. Place clot in 5.0 mL of 5 M urea. This clot should dissolve within 24 hours due to the lack of calcium, which is necessary for activating factor XIII.

Procedure

1. Pipette 0.2 mL of plasma from the patient and normal control into each of two test tubes. Add 0.2 mL of 0.025 M calcium chloride to each tube. Incubate at 37°C for 30 minutes.
2. Loosen the clots by tapping the sides of the tube gently. Transfer one of the clots from each assay (one patient clot and one normal control clot) to 5 mL of 5 M urea. Transfer a second clot from the patient and the normal control to a third test tube with 5 mL of urea.
3. Allow the mixture to stand at room temperature and examine at 1, 2, 3, and 24 hours. Check for dissolution of the clot. In the absence of factor XIII, the clot usually dissolves within 2 to 3 hours.

Reporting Results

Report the length of time for clot dissolution or report that the clot was insoluble after 24 hours. Reference: no dissolution in 24 hours.

Procedure Notes

If factor XIII is not present in the plasma, the clot is dissolved in less than 24 hours by the urea. The mixed clot of patient and normal control plasma should also remain intact. If the mixture dissolves, it may be due to fibrinolysis, rather than to factor XIII deficiency.

Reference

Losowsky, M. S. et al. "Congenital Deficiency of Fibrin-Stabilizing Factor." *Lancet,* Vol. 2, 1965, p. 156.

Fibrinogen Assay: Method Clotting Assay

Principle

Fibrinogen—thrombin factor II → fibrin

When plasma is diluted and clotted with excess thrombin, the fibrinogen concentration is inversely proportional to the clotting time, yielding a linear relationship when plotted on log-log paper. Fibrinogen assays are useful in detecting deficiencies of fibrinogen and in detecting an alteration in the conversion of fibrinogen to fibrin.

Specimen

Plasma from citrated whole blood.

(continued)

Reagents, Supplies, and Equipment

Items 1 through 3 are available as kit No. 880A from Sigma Diagnostics, St. Louis.

1. Fibrinogen reference
2. Thrombin, bovine
3. Barbital buffer with albumin
4. (Optional) Citric acid and oxalic acid

Calibration

A calibration curve prepared from serial dilutions (e.g., 1:10, 1:20) of a fibrinogen reference is used to determine the fibrinogen concentration in the test sample. Fibrinogen concentration is inversely proportional to the clotting time, yielding a linear relationship when plotted on log-log paper.

Quality Control

A commercial control can be used as an abnormal control in quantitative assays of clottable fibrinogen and for screening tests for fibrinogen concentrations. Unopened, controls are stable until the labeled expiration date. Store reconstituted vials between 2° and 8°C and use within 3 days. Prepare by reconstituting the vial with the exact amount of reagent-grade water specified on the vial. Swirl gently and allow to stand for 30 minutes at room temperature for complete rehydration. Test in the same manner as the patient specimen.

Procedure

1. Prepare a 1:10 dilution of plasma to be tested with buffer diluent (0.1 mL of plasma plus 0.9 mL of buffer).
2. Place dilutions in an ice bath. Dilutions are stable for up to 4 hours.
3. Perform duplicate clotting time determinations for each sample as follows: Transfer duplicate 0.2 mL of dilutions to reaction vessel and incubate at 37° C for at least 1 minute but no longer than 5 minutes. Rapidly add 0.1 mL of thrombin solution and measure the clotting time at 37°C. Record the times.

Calculations

Average the duplicate times obtained for each dilution. Determine the fibrinogen concentration from a calibration curve.

Reporting Results

The normal titer of fibrinogen is 1:128 to 1:256. A titer below 1:64 is abnormal.

Procedure Notes

The normal quantitative value of fibrinogen is 200 to 400 mg/dL. The titer and quantitative values may be decreased as a result of liver disease or consumption of fibrinogen due to accelerated intravascular clotting.

References

General Diagnostics, Morris Plains, NJ, 1984.
"Fibrinogen." *Sigma Product Bull.*, Vol. 6. St. Louis: Sigma Diagnostics, 1983, p. 18.

··

Platelet Aggregation

See Chapter 25.

··

Protamine Sulfate Assay

Principle

Protamine is used to neutralize the effects of heparin. If protamine is administered in excess therapeutically, it is capable of

TABLE 24.10 Protamine Sulfate Assay: Preparation of Dilutions

Dilution	Protamine Sulfate Dilutions (mL)	0.85% NaCl (mL)	Final Concentration of Protamine Sulfate (μg)
1	0.1	0.9	10.0
2	0.5 of tube 1	0.5	5.0
3	0.5 of tube 2	0.5	2.5
4	0.5 of tube 3	0.5	1.25
5	0.5 of tube 4	0.5	0.625
6	0.5 of tube 5	0.5	0.3125

interfering with factor IX activity and thromboplastin generation. A positive result indicates the inappropriate presence of intravascular fibrin monomers. (See Chapter 25 for more information on platelet aggregation.)

Specimen

Plasma from whole blood anticoagulated with citrate (1 part of 3.1% sodium citrate to 9 parts of whole blood).

Reagents, Supplies, and Equipment

Protamine sulfate, 100 μg in 100 mL of 0.85% saline: Dilute the protamine sulfate solution as shown in Table 24.10.

Quality Control

A normal plasma should be tested at the same time as the unknown patient specimen.

Procedure

1. Add 0.05 mL from each dilution to 0.2 mL of test plasma.
2. Perform an APTT test.
3. Select the dilution that gives the shortest APTT.
4. Pipette 1.0 mL of plasma into a tube, and incubate at 37°C for 5 minutes. Add 0.1 mL of 1% protamine sulfate. Mix by tilting.
5. Return to 37°C water bath and incubate for 15 minutes.
6. At the end of the incubation period, examine for thin, white fibrin threads by gently tilting the test tube.

Reporting Results

The presence of fibrin threads is positive for fibrinogen degradation products. If positive, the quantity as expressed in the tube dilution used can be reported. An opalescent appearance of the plasma is interpreted as negative.

Procedure Notes

False-negative results will be produced by unnecessary mixing of the solution, which causes the breakup of fibrin threads.

··

Prothrombin Time

Principle

This basic procedure involves adding plasma to an excess of extrinsic thromboplastin-calcium substrate. Thromboplastin is derived from tissues that supply phospholipoprotein, such as ani-

(continued)

COAGULATION PROCEDURES *(continued)*

mal brain. The length of time required to form a fibrin clot is measured in seconds.

Clinically, this procedure is used to monitor oral anticoagulant therapy, as a screening test in the diagnosis of coagulation deficiencies, and as a component of a liver profile assessment. Prolonged results can indicate a deficiency of one or more factors in the extrinsic pathway: factors VII, X, and V, and factor II or I. The presence of an inhibitor will also produce prolonged values.

Specimen
Fresh plasma from citrated whole blood is preferred, although oxalated plasma may be used. The sample should be centrifuged promptly after collection, with the plasma removed from the erythrocytes. Plasma may be stored for several hours at 2° to 6°C prior to testing.

Reagents, Supplies, and Equipment
1. Thromboplastin
2. 12 × 75-mm test tubes
3. Pipettes: 0.1 mL (100 μL)
4. 37°C water bath or heat block
5. Stopwatch
6. Nichrome loop

Quality Control
Normal and abnormal citrated or oxalated test plasma should be run with each patient assay or test batch.

Procedure
This procedure is commonly performed using automated equipment. However, in some cases a manual procedure may be desired.
1. Prewarm plasma at 37°C for a minimum of 2 minutes and a maximum of 10 minutes.
2. Prewarm thromboplastin at 37°C for a minimum of 2 minutes and a maximum of 60 minutes.
3. Add 0.1 mL of plasma to 0.2 mL of thromboplastin. If performing this procedure manually, pipette quickly. Start a stopwatch simultaneously.
4. Using the nichrome loop technique, the loop is swept through the mixture at 2 sweeps/sec until the first strand of fibrin appears. The tube may also be tilted using a magnifier to observe clot formation.
5. Repeat this procedure in duplicate for all specimens, including controls. The duplicate results should be within 1 second of one another.

Reporting Results
Reference values range from 10 to 15 seconds. Report both the patient and control specimens in seconds. An older alternative method of reporting is to express the percentage of patient activity. This is calculated as:

$$\frac{\text{Control time (seconds)}}{\text{Patient's time (seconds)}} \times 100 = \% \text{ activity of patient}$$

Procedure Notes

Clinical Applications
This test depends on the activity of factors VII, V, X, II, and I. A deficiency of any of these may produce a 3- to 4-second prolongation in the test.

References
Turgeon, Mary L. and J. Bender. *Procedure Manual for Hematology and Coagulation.* Corning, NY: Corning Community College Press, 1985.
Quick, A. J. *Bleeding Problems in Clinical Medicine.* Philadelphia: Saunders, 1970.

Thrombin Time

Principle
The thrombin time test determines the rate of thrombin-induced cleavage of fibrinogen to fibrin monomers and the subsequent polymerization of hydrogen-bonded fibrin polymers. Clinically, extremely low fibrinogen levels, abnormal fibrinogen thrombin inhibitors, and high concentrations of immunoglobulin (e.g., myeloma proteins) will produce abnormal results. The presence of heparin and high concentrations of fibrin-fibrinogen degradation products will also prolong the time. This procedure is particularly useful if other parameters, such as the APTT and PT, are prolonged.

Specimen
Fresh citrated plasma is needed.

Reagents, Supplies, and Equipment
1. Thrombin solution: Reconstitute 1 vial of 50-unit human thrombin with 1 mL of reagent-grade water. Allow it to sit at room temperature for 5 minutes. Mix gently. Remove the entire contents of the vial and add 9 mL of 0.1 M calcium chloride to produce a *working solution* of thrombin-calcium. Rinse the vial with the mixture to ensure that all the thrombin has been removed. Store at 4°C. Make fresh daily.
2. 0.1 M calcium chloride: Make an accurate 1:10 dilution of 1 M calcium chloride, which is kept as a stock.
3. 37°C water bath

Quality Control
A normal control should be assayed simultaneously.

Procedure
1. The thrombin-calcium mixture should be prewarmed to 37°C, using an aliquot of working solution.
2. Warm 0.2 mL of plasma for 3 minutes in a 37°C water bath.
3. Add 0.1 mL of the thrombin-calcium solution and *immediately* start a stopwatch.
4. Observe for clot formation. Test each plasma in duplicate.

Reporting Results
The reference value is less than 20 seconds, with an average of 8 to 10 seconds. The normal range depends on the method and choice of reagents.

Procedure Notes
Prolonged results will be seen if the fibrinogen concentration is less than 100 mg/dL. Abnormal results will also be encountered in the presence of thrombin inhibitors such as heparin, fibrin split products, or high concentrations of immunoglobulins that interfere with fibrin monomer polymerization, such as in cases of multiple myeloma.

Reference
Lenahan, Jane G. and K. Smith. *Hemostasis* (17th edition). Durham, NC: Organon Teknika, 1985, p. 39.

REVIEW QUESTIONS

Basic Procedures

Questions 1 and 2: match the appropriate procedure and reagent.

1. ___ Leukocyte count.
2. ___ Reticulocyte count.

A. New methylene blue.

B. Phyloxine B.

C. Solution lyses erythrocytes and darkens the cells to be counted.

Questions 3 through 5: match the appropriate procedure and characteristic.

3. ___ Hemoglobin assay.
4. ___ Leukocyte count.
5. ___ Westergren method.

A. The diluting solution lyses erythrocytes with propylene glycol and contains sodium carbonate and water.

B. The procedure measures the rate of erythrocyte settling.

C. Ferrous ions are oxidized to the ferric state.

D. The diluting solution is either 1% hydrochloric acid or 2% acetic acid.

Questions 6 through 8: match the procedure and the source of error that will have the greatest effect on the test result.

6. ___ Erythrocyte count.
7. ___ Leukocyte count.
8. ___ Packed cell volume (hematocrit).

A. Incorrect dilution of blood and diluent.

B. Hemolysis of whole blood specimen.

C. Excessive anticoagulant will produce shrinkage of cells.

Questions 9 and 10: match the procedure and the source of error that will have the greatest effect on the test result.

9. ___ Platelet count.
10. ___ Reticulocyte count.

A. Refractile bodies can produce a false-positive observation.

B. Specimens stored at room temperature for more than 5 hours will produce inaccurate results.

Questions 11 through 13: match the procedure and correct reference value.

11. ___ Erythrocyte count (adult male).
12. ___ Hemoglobin assay (adult female).
13. ___ Lymphocytes (adult average).

A. 0.15 to 0.3 × 10^9/L.

B. 12.0 to 16.0 gm/dL.

C. 4.6 to 6.2 × 10^{12}/L.

D. 34%.

Questions 14 through 18: match the procedure and reference value.

14. ___ Total leukocyte count.
15. ___ Packed cell volume.
16. ___ Direct platelet count.
17. ___ Reticulocyte count (newborn infant).
18. ___ Westergren ESR method (adult male):

A. Up to 10 mm/hr.

B. 2.5 to 6.5%.

C. 150 to 400 × 10^9/L.

D. 0.42 ± 0.05 L/L.

E. 4.5 to 11 × 10^9/L.

Questions 19 and 20: match the following procedures with a clinical or specimen condition that will produce an *increased* test result.

19. ___ Hemoglobin assay.
20. ___ Total leukocyte count.

A. Active allergies.

B. Immediate hypersensitivity reactions.

C. Inflammation.

D. A lipemic blood specimen.

Questions 21 through 24: match the following procedures with a clinical or specimen condition that will produce an *increased* test result.

21. ___ Packed cell volume.
22. ___ Platelet count.
23. ___ Reticulocyte count.
24. ___ Westergren ESR method.

A. Splenectomy.

B. Rouleaux formation.

C. Polycythemia.

D. Crisis associated with hemolytic anemia.

Questions 25 through 28: match the following leukocyte types with a clinical condition that will produce an *increased* value.

25. ___ Neutrophils.
26. ___ Lymphocytes.
27. ___ Monocytes.
28. ___ Eosinophils.

A. Invasive parasites.

B. Bacterial infections.

C. Viral infections.

D. Tuberculosis.

Questions 29 through 31: match the following procedure with a clinical condition that will produce a *decreased* value.

29. ___ Platelet count.
30. ___ Reticulocyte count.
31. ___ Westergren ESR.

A. Polycythemia vera.

B. Acute leukemias.

C. Megaloblastic anemia.

32. If a hemoglobin standard with an assay value of 20 gm/dL has an optical density (absorbance) of 0.40 and a patient's specimen diluted according to the procedure has an optical density of 0.35, what is the patient's hemoglobin concentration?

A. 13.0 gm/dL.

B. 15.0 gm/dL.

C. 16.5 gm/dL.

D. 17.5 gm/dL.

33. A normal blood smear should have no more than about ___ (maximum) number of platelets per oil immersion field in an area where the erythrocytes are just touching each other.
    A. 10.
    C. 20.
    B. 15.
    D. 25.

34. If you made an appropriate WBC dilution and subsequently counted a total of 250 cells in the four leukocyte counting areas on an appropriate hemocytometer, what is the patient's total leukocyte count?
    A. $5.0 \times 10^9/L$.
    C. $12.5 \times 10^9/L$.
    B. $10.0 \times 10^9/L$.
    D. $15.0 \times 10^9/L$.

35. What is the corrected total leukocyte count, if 10 nucleated erythrocytes were noted per 100 leukocytes on the leukocyte differential count? The initial total leukocyte count was $20 \times 10^9/L$.
    A. $15.5 \times 10^9/L$.
    C. $17.3 \times 10^9/L$.
    B. $16.5 \times 10^9/L$.
    D. $18.2 \times 10^9/L$.

36. The packed cell volume procedure can be affected by the:
    A. Speed of the centrifuge.
    B. Length of time of centrifugation.
    C. Ratio of anticoagulant to whole blood.
    D. All of the above.

37. Which of the following erythrocytic inclusions contain RNA and can be observed by staining with new methylene blue?
    A. Howell-Jolly bodies.
    B. Heinz bodies.
    C. Pappenheimer bodies.
    D. Reticulocytes.

38. The sedimentation rate of erythrocytes can be affected by the:
    A. Ratio of anticoagulant to whole blood.
    B. Position of the tube.
    C. Temperature of the specimen or laboratory.
    D. All of the above.

Special Hematology Procedures and Special Stains

Questions 39 through 42: match the following procedures with the appropriate test reaction.

39. ___ Acidified serum lysis test (Ham's test).
40. ___ Donath-Landsteiner test.
41. ___ Alpha-naphthyl acetate esterase.
42. ___ Naphthol AS-D chloroacetate esterase.

A. Positive in monocytes.
B. Measures an extremely potent hemolysin at 4°C.
C. Positive in cell of granulocytic lineage.
D. Measures hemolysis.

Questions 43 through 46: match the following procedures with the appropriate test reactions. Use an answer only *once*.

43. ___ Glucose-6-phosphate dehydrogenase (G6PD) activity.
44. ___ Heinz bodies.
45. ___ Kleihauer-Betke test.
46. ___ Hemoglobin S screening test.

A. Erythrocytes lysed by toluene and saponin with the released product being reduced by sodium hydrosulfite.
B. Fetal hemoglobin is not eluted.
C. Denatured by crystal violet.
D. Screens for one of the most prevalent hereditary enzyme deficiencies.

Questions 47 through 50: match the following procedures with the appropriate test reactions.

47. ___ Osmotic fragility.
48. ___ Periodic acid–Schiff.
49. ___ Peroxidase stain.
50. ___ Prussian blue stain.

A. Precipitates free iron into blue or blue-green granules.
B. Observation of hemolysis in varying sodium chloride dilutions.
C. Lymphocytes stain negative.
D. Intense cytoplasmic granular staining in erythroleukemia.

Questions 51 through 54: match the procedure with a possible source of error.

51. ___ Acidified serum lysis test (Ham's test).
52. ___ Donath-Landsteiner test.
53. ___ G6PD assay.
54. ___ Hemoglobin electrophoresis.

A. Identical mobilities.
B. Use of ABO-incompatible test serum.
C. Quenched by PCVs over 0.50 L/L.
D. Hemolyzed specimen.

Questions 55 through 58: match the procedure with a possible source of error.

55. ___ Hemoglobin S screening test.
56. ___ Malaria preparation.
57. ___ Sickle cell screening.
58. ___ Sudan black B.

A. Superimposed platelets may produce a *false-positive* result.
B. Blood specimen from a recently transfused patient may produce a *false-negative* result.
C. Old blood specimen will produce a *false-negative* result.
D. Test reagent more than 1 day old will produce a *false-negative* result.

Questions 59 through 62: match the procedure with the appropriate reference value or positive test result.

59. ___ Acidified serum lysis test (Ham's test).

60. ___ Leukocyte alkaline phosphatase.

61. ___ G6PD assay.

62. ___ Kleihauer-Betke test.

A. Normal range: 32 to 182 with fast blue RR dye.

B. Positive test: 10 to 50% hemolysis.

C. Normal: less than 1% Hb F in adults.

D. Zero time control should not fluoresce or fluoresce only slightly.

Questions 63 through 65: match the procedure with the appropriate reference value or positive test result.

63. ___ Alkaline denaturation.

64. ___ Prussian blue stain.

65. ___ Sucrose hemolysis test (sugar water test).

A. Negative: less than 10%.

B. Newborn normal: 70 to 90%.

C. Normal: 0 to 1% of mature erythrocytes.

Questions 66 through 68: match the procedure with a disorder that can be recognized through the use of the test.

66. ___ Acid serum lysis test (Ham's test).

67. ___ Leukocyte alkaline phosphatase stain.

68. ___ Donath-Landsteiner test.

A. Positive in paroxysmal cold hemoglobinuria.

B. Diagnostic for paroxysmal nocturnal hemoglobinuria.

C. Increased in hereditary spherocytosis.

D. Increased in a leukemoid reaction.

Questions 69 through 71: match the procedure with a disorder that can be recognized through the use of the test.

69. ___ Heinz bodies.

70. ___ Kleihauer-Betke test.

71. ___ Osmotic fragility test.

A. Detects physical alterations in the erythrocyte membrane.

B. Positive result if unstable hemoglobins are present.

C. Increased in cord blood samples.

72. Which of the following procedures is used to detect the complement-sensitive cells in paroxysmal nocturnal hemoglobinuria?

A. Sucrose lysis test.
B. Donath-Landsteiner test.
C. Acidified serum lysis (Ham's test).
D. Both A and C.

73. Leukocytes that demonstrate a positive reaction in the tartrate-resistant acid phosphatase cytochemical stain are the lymphocytes seen in:

A. Infectious lymphocytosis.
B. Malignant lymphoma.
C. Acute lymphoblastic leukemia (non-T type).
D. Hairy-cell leukemia.

74. A decreased leukocyte alkaline phosphatase (LAP) score is seen in:

A. Polycythemia vera.
B. Chronic myelogenous leukemia.
C. Leukemoid reactions.
D. Acute myelogenous leukemia.

Questions 75 through 77: steps in leukocyte alkaline phosphatase scoring, in sequence, are (75) ___, (76) ___, and (77) ___.

A. Adding the scores for the 100 neutrophils counted.
B. Grading the neutrophils using a 0 to 4+ scale.
C. Averaging the scores for all neutrophils counted.
D. Multiplying the number of neutrophils in each category by their respective scores.

78. In the leukocyte alkaline phosphatase procedure, blood smears should be stained:

A. Within 8 hours of specimen collection.
B. Within 48 hours of specimen collection.
C. Within 72 hours of specimen collection.
D. Within 5 days of specimen collection.

Questions 79 and 80: the alpha-naphthyl acetate esterase stain is detected primarily in (79) ___ and is almost absent in (80) ___.

A. Megakaryocytes.
B. Monocytes.
C. Granulocytes.
D. Erythrocytes.

81. If many dense and dark-staining cells are seen in the Kleihauer-Betke test, the specimen could be from a patient with:

A. Beta thalassemia.
B. Hereditary persistence of fetal hemoglobin.
C. Sickle cell anemia.
D. All of the above.

Questions 82 through 86: indicate whether the osmotic fragility is increased or decreased in each of the following disorders:

82. ___ Hemolytic disease of the newborn.

83. ___ Hereditary spherocytosis.

84. ___ Severe iron deficiency anemia.

85. ___ Polycythemia vera.

86. ___ Sickle cell anemia.

A. Increased osmotic fragility.

B. Decreased osmotic fragility.

87. The reagent used in the traditional sickle cell screening test is:

A. Sodium chloride.
B. Sodium citrate.
C. Sodium metabisulphite.
D. Sodium-potassium oxalate.

88. Which of the following is a nucleated erythrocyte with diffuse iron in the cytoplasm?

A. Ringed sideroblast.
B. Sideroblast.
C. Pappenheimer bodies.
D. Siderocyte.

89. An increased number of siderocytes can be seen:
    A. In chronic lymphocytic leukemia.
    B. In lead poisoning.
    C. Post splenectomy.
    D. Both B and C.

Coagulation Procedures

Questions 90 through 93: match the following procedures with the appropriate principle or description of the test.

90. ___ Activated partial thromboplastin time (APTT).
91. ___ Antithrombin III assay.
92. ___ Bleeding time.
93. ___ Circulating anticoagulant assay.

A. In the presence of heparin, thrombin is neutralized at a rate proportional to ___.
B. Measures the time required to generate thrombin and fibrin polymers via the intrinsic pathway.
C. Measures inhibitors of specific factors.
D. An in vivo measurement of platelet adhesion and aggregation on locally injured vascular subendothelium.

Questions 94 through 98: match the following procedures with the appropriate principle or description of the test.

94. ___ Clot retraction.
95. ___ Clot lysis.
96. ___ Ethanol gelation test.
97. ___ Euglobulin lysis.
98. ___ Factor assay.

A. Based on the ability of the questionable substance in the plasma to correct a deficient substrate.
B. Gross screening test of platelet quantity and function, and fibrinolysis.
C. Use to detect fibrin monomers in plasma.
D. An observation of excessive fibrinolysis.
E. Plasminogen, fibrinogen, and activators are clotted with thrombin and the clot produced is observed.

Questions 99 and 100: match the following procedures with the appropriate principle or description of the test.

99. ___ Fibrin split products.
100. ___ Fibrin-stabilizing factor.

A. Measures the adherence to glass.
B. Patient's serum is mixed with latex particles that have been coated with anti-fibrinogen and observed for agglutination.
C. Based on the reaction

Fibrin $-$ XIII factor $\rightarrow$ fibrin

this procedure tests the stability of the end product in 5 M urea.

Questions 101 through 105: match the following procedures with the appropriate reference value or diagnostic characteristic.

101. ___ APTT.
102. ___ Antithrombin III.
103. ___ Ivy bleeding time.
104. ___ Aspirin tolerance test.
105. ___ Circulating anticoagulant.

A. Positive result: increased ratio of normal plasma to patient plasma.
B. Normal: 2 to 8 minutes.
C. Normal: 20 to 35 seconds (28 to 42 seconds), the range depending on the activator and phospholipid reagents.
D. Increased twofold in 92 to 95% of patients after ingesting two tablets of salicylate.
E. Normal: 80 to 100% (range is 107 ± 19%).

Questions 106 through 109: match the following procedures with the appropriate reference value or diagnostic characteristic.

106. ___ Factor deficiency assay.
107. ___ Clot lysis.
108. ___ Ethanol gel test.
109. ___ Euglobulin lysis time.

A. 5 to 15 minutes.
B. No breaking up of clot before 48 hours.
C. Normal plasma exhibits no clumping.
D. Normal: breaking up of clot does not occur in less than 2 hours but is usually complete within 4 hours.
E. Corrected by normal plasma.

Questions 110 through 113: match the following procedures with the appropriate reference value.

110. ___ Factor VIII assay.
111. ___ Fibrin split products.
112. ___ Fibrin-stabilizing factor.
113. ___ Fibrinogen assay.

A. Normal: no dissolution of the clot at 24 hours.
B. Normal: less than 8 to 10 μg/mL.
C. Normal: 50 to 150%.
D. Normal: 200 to 400 mg/dL or a titer of 1:123 to 1:256.

Questions 114 and 115: match the following procedures with the appropriate reference value or diagnostic characteristic.

114. ___ Protamine sulfate assay.
115. ___ Prothrombin time.

A. Normal: 10 to 15 seconds.
B. Normal: over 20 seconds.
C. Positive: presence of fibrin threads.
D. Normal: 75% to 97% retention.

Questions 116 through 119: match each of the following procedures with the appropriate clinical application.

116. ___ APTT.

117. ___ Antithrombin III.

118. ___ Bleeding time.

119. ___ Clot retraction.

A. Increased time, if platelet count is decreased.

B. The test of choice for the control of heparin therapy.

C. Useful prior to and subsequent to treatment with heparin in disseminated intravascular coagulation (DIC).

D. If platelet count is normal, an increase suggests either impaired platelet function or a defect of subendothelial factor VIII:vWF multimers.

Questions 120 through 123: match each of the following procedures with the appropriate clinical application.

120. ___ APTT.

121. ___ Euglobulin lysis.

122. ___ Fibrin-stabilizing factor.

123. ___ Fibrinogen assay.

A. Abnormal results indicate fibrinolytic activity.

B. Screens for a lack of factor XIII.

C. Abnormal in cases of severe liver disease.

D. Detects prekallikrein, high-molecular-weight kininogen, factors XII, XI, IX, VIII, X, V, II, and I, and inhibitors against these factors.

Questions 124 and 125: match each of the following procedures with the appropriate clinical application.

124. ___ Ethanol gelation test.

125. ___ Prothrombin time.

A. Monitors oral anticoagulant therapy and screens for one or more deficiencies in the *extrinsic pathway*.

B. An abnormal result is diagnostic of DIC and primary fibrinolysis with DIC.

C. Is increased in factor deficiencies, in the presence of circulating anticoagulants, and with decreased platelets.

Questions 126 through 129: match the procedures with the appropriate source of error.

126. ___ Clot lysis.

127. ___ Ethanol gelation test.

128. ___ Factor VIII assay.

129. ___ Fibrin split product screening test.

A. A *false-normal* can result from the inactivation of plasmin by antiplasmin or the depletion of plasminogen.

B. Observing for agglutination after 2 minutes of rotation can produce a *false-positive* reaction.

C. Conducting the test at less than 37°C will produce a prolonged whole blood coagulation time.

D. Severe hypofibrinogenemia can produce a *false-negative* result.

E. A very fresh specimen is needed because of *rapid* deterioration of this plasma constituent.

Questions 130 through 132: match the procedures with the appropriate source of error.

130. ___ Euglobulin lysis test.

131. ___ Protamine sulfate test.

132. ___ Prothrombin time.

A. Unnecessary mixing of the solution can break up fibrin threads and produce a *false-negative* result.

B. *False-normal* results if deficiencies are present in more than one factor.

C. Severe hypofibrinogenemia produces a *falsely* decreased time.

D. Plasma needs to be promptly removed from erythrocytes.

133. Which of the following is a source of error that can affect *most* coagulation procedures?

A. Improper specimen storage.
B. Improperly reconstituting and storing test reagents.
C. Improper temperature of reaction.
D. All of the above.

134. Which of the factors is *not* important to the accuracy of *most* coagulation tests?

A. Use of sodium citrate as an anticoagulant, if plasma is required.
B. A proper ratio of anticoagulant to whole blood, if plasma is required.
C. The use of 3.2% sodium citrate, if plasma is required.
D. Immediately placing all specimens on ice after collection.

135. In the Ivy bleeding time method, the usual puncture site is the:

A. Finger.
B. Forearm.
C. Heel.
D. Ear lobe.

136. Adsorbed plasma corrects a deficiency of:

    A. Factor V.
    B. Factor VIII.
    C. Factors XI and XII.
    D. All of the above.

137. Aged serum corrects a deficiency of:

    A. Factor VII.
    B. Factor IX.
    C. Factors X, XI, and XII.
    D. All of the above.

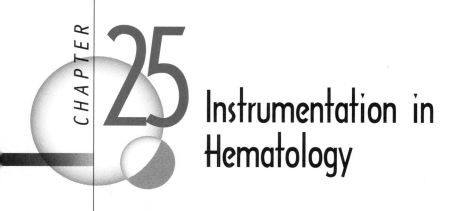

25 Instrumentation in Hematology

OBJECTIVES

Instrumental principles
- Describe the basic theory of the electrical impedance principle of cell counting and sizing.
- Describe the basic theory of the optical detection principle of cell counting and sizing.
- Explain the fundamental concepts of laser technology.
- Describe the principles of flow-cell cytometry and two basic uses of this technology in hematology.

Whole blood cell analyzers
- Define the terms **parameter** and **sample.**
- List the parameters measured by basic bench-top hematology analyzers.
- Describe the methods used to measure the parameters named in the preceding objective.
- Name the parameters measured by total cell counting systems.
- Define the abbreviation **RDW.**
- Describe the process and output of total cell and histogram electrical impedance systems.
- Describe the process and output of a laser scatter technology system.
- Compare the process and output of the continuous flow system to the other two types of total cell and differential cell counters.
- Describe the general characteristics of histograms.

Analysis of electrical impedance instrumental data output
- Describe the appearance of microcytic and macrocytic erythrocytes on a histogram.

- Name two conditions that would contribute to a bimodal cellular distribution on an erythrocyte histogram.
- Explain how the RDW is calculated and give the normal range.
- Describe the relationship of the RDW to the MCV.
- Name the six classifications of erythrocytes based on the RDW and MCV.
- Explain how the RCMI is calculated and give the normal value.
- Describe the appearance of a leukocyte histogram generated by the electrical impedance method.
- Describe the appearance of a leukocyte histogram generated by the optical detection method.
- Describe the construction of a platelet histogram.
- Explain how the MPV is calculated.
- Compare the relationship between MPV and the platelet count.
- Name at least four disorders in which the MPV is abnormal.
- Explain the purpose of the PDW and its normal value.

Laser technology
- Describe the generation, by laser technology, of a histogram for RBCs.
- Explain how a platelet histogram is generated.
- Describe the analysis and interpretation of the peroxidase analysis.

- Explain the output of the basophil/lobularity channel.
- Describe the process of lymphocyte subtyping.

Case studies

- Analyze and discuss the significance of the erythrocyte and leukocyte histograms and the nomogram presented in the six case studies.

Applications of flow cytometry

- Describe the general functions that flow cytometry analysis can provide.
- Name the three factors that have contributed to the rapid advance of the technology of flow cytometry.
- Name and discuss three hematological applications of flow cytometry.
- Name and discuss three other cellular applications of flow cytometry.

Single-purpose cell counting and analyzing instruments

- Explain the principles of a pattern recognition leukocyte differential analyzer.

Instruments in coagulation studies

- Describe the two most common types of instruments used in the clinical laboratory for the detection of fibrin clots.
- Explain the principles of electromechanical and optical detection systems.
- Describe the methodological principle of platelet aggregation.

*I*nstrumentation and the automation of procedures continue to increase in the clinical hematology laboratory. Since the first Coulter Cell Counter Model A (Coulter Electronics, Hialeah, Fla.) was introduced in the 1950s, the types of automated equipment and instrumental capabilities of this equipment have become more diverse and sophisticated. Microprocessor applications have increased instrument programming capabilities and data output in ways that were unimagined a decade ago.

Some equipment, such as blood smear preparation and slide staining instruments, simplifies work in the laboratory. Larger instruments not only count and differentiate cellular elements of the blood but additionally generate data that were previously not available by instrumental methods. Sample procedural protocols for various instruments are included in this chapter.

INSTRUMENTAL PRINCIPLES

Basic Cell Counting Principles

The counting of the cellular elements of the blood (erythrocytes, leukocytes, and platelets) is based on one of two classic methods:

1. Electrical impedance
2. Optical detection

The Electrical Impedance Principle

This method of cell counting was originally developed by Coulter Electronics and is referred to as the Coulter principle. Cell counting and sizing is based on the detection and measurement of changes in electrical impedance (resistance) produced by a particle as it passes through a small aperture. Particles such as blood cells are nonconductive but are suspended in an electrically conductive diluent. As a dilute suspension of cells is drawn through the aperture, the passage of each individual cell momentarily increases the impedance (resistance) of the electrical path between two submerged electrodes that are located on each side of the aperture (Fig. 25.1). The number of pulses generated during a specific period of time is proportional to the number of particles or cells. The amplitude (magnitude) of the electrical pulse produced indicates the cell's volume (Fig. 25.2). The output histogram is a display of the distribution of cell volume and frequency. Each pulse on the x axis represents size in femtoliters (fL); the y axis represents the relative number of cells.

The Optical Detection Principle

In the optical or hydrodynamic focusing method of cell counting and cell sizing, laser light is used. A diluted blood specimen passes in a steady stream through which a beam of laser light is focused. As each cell passes through the sensing zone of the flow cell, it scatters the focused light. Scattered light is detected by a photodetector and converted to an electrical pulse. The number of pulses generated is directly proportional to the number of cells passing through the sensing zone in a specific period of time.

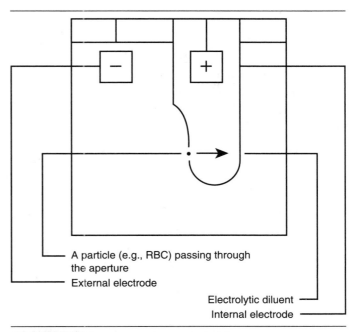

A particle (e.g., RBC) passing through the aperture
External electrode
Electrolytic diluent
Internal electrode

FIGURE 25.1 Coulter aperture: electronic impedance principle. When the aperture of an electronic particle counter is immersed in a dilution of whole blood in an electrolyte solution, changes in electrical resistance can be measured. The passage of each cell increases the resistance of the electrical path between two electrodes that are located on each side of the aperture. (Adapted from *Significant Advances in Hematology.* Hialeah, FL: Coulter Electronics, 1985, p. 6.)

The application of light scatter means that as a single cell passes across a laser light beam, the light will be reflected and scattered. The patterns of scatter are measured at various angles (forward scatter 180 degrees, and right angle 90 degrees). Scattered light provides information about cell structure, shape, and reflectivity. These characteristics can be used to differentiate the various types of white blood cells and to produce scatter plots with a five-part differential.

Characteristics of Light Scatter
Optical Light Scatter

In this category, light amplification is generated by stimulated emission of radiation. Three independent processes are operational. These are:

1. Diffraction—the bending of light around corners with the use of small angles
2. Refraction—the bending of light because of a change in speed with the use of intermediate angles
3. Reflection—light rays turned back by the surface or an obstruction with the use of large angles

Angles of Light Scatter

Various angles of light scatter can aid in cellular analysis. These are:

1. Forward light scatter 0 degrees. This is diffracted light, which relates to the volume of the cell.
2. Forward low angle light scatter 2–3 degrees. This characteristic can relate to size or volume.

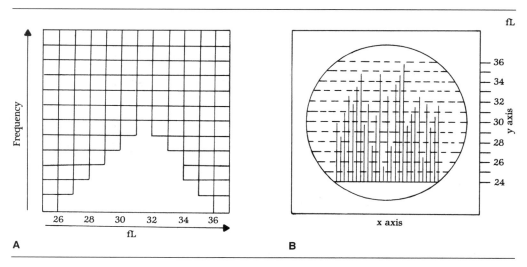

FIGURE 25.2 Cell counting: impedance principles. The number of pulses on the oscilloscope screen indicates the number of particles passing through the aperture. The height (amplitude) of each pulse reflects the volume of each cell. **A.** Histogram distribution of normal erythrocytes. **B.** Oscilloscope appearance as erythrocytes pass through the cell counting aperture and produce an electrical resistance. (Adapted from R. Pierre, *Seminars and Case Studies: The Automated Differential.* Hialeah, FL: Coulter Electronics, 1985, p. 4.)

3. Forward high angle 5–15 degrees. This type of measurement allows for description of the refractive index of cellular components.
4. Orthogonal light scatter 90 degrees. The result of this application of light scatter is the production of data based on reflection and refraction of internal components, which correlates with internal complexity.

Radio Frequency (RF)

In this method, high-voltage electromagnetic current is used to detect cell size, based on the cellular density. The RF pulse is directly proportional to the nuclear size and density of a cell. RF or conductivity is related to the nuclear:cytoplasmic ratio, nuclear density, and cytoplasmic granulation.

The Fundamentals of Laser Technology

In 1917, Einstein speculated that under certain conditions atoms or molecules could absorb light or other radiation and then be stimulated to shed this gained energy. In the 1950s, physicists theorized how this borrowed energy could be multiplied and emitted in high quantities. A decade later, new lasers were developed and used in medical and industrial applications.

The electromagnetic spectrum ranges from long radio waves to short, powerful gamma rays (Fig. 25.3). Within this spectrum is a narrow band of visible or white light which is composed of red, orange, yellow, green, blue, and violet light. Laser (*light amplified by stimulated emission of radiation*) light ranges from the ultraviolet and infrared spectrum through all of the colors of the rainbow.

In contrast to other diffuse forms of radiation, laser light is concentrated. Laser light is almost exclusively of one wavelength or color and its parallel waves travel in one direction. Through the use of fluorescent dyes, laser light can occur in numerous wavelengths. The types of laser include glass-filled tubes of helium and neon lasers; the YAG type (*yttrium, aluminum, garnet*), an imitation diamond; argon; or krypton.

Lasers sort the energy in atoms and molecules, concen-

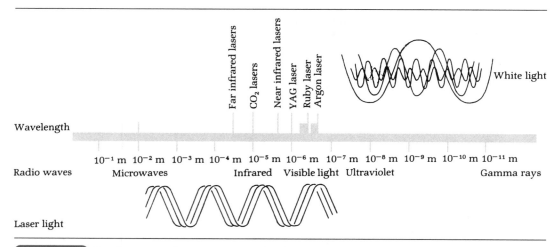

FIGURE 25.3 The electromagnetic spectrum ranges from long radio waves (10^{-1} m) to short gamma rays (10^{-11} m). The narrow band of the electromagnetic spectrum that constitutes white or visible light is composed of red, orange, yellow, green, blue, and violet light. A comparison of white light and laser light demonstrates that visible or white light as well as all radiation waves are diffused and jumbled. Laser light by comparison is organized and concentrated. YAG = yttrium, aluminum, garnet.

trate it, and release it in powerful waves. In most lasers a medium of gas, liquid, or crystal is energized by high-intensity light, an electrical discharge, or even nuclear radiation. When an atom extends beyond the orbits of its electrons or when a molecule vibrates or changes its shape, they instantly snap back, shedding energy in the form of a **photon.** The photon is the basic unit of all radiation. When a photon reaches an atom of the medium, the energy exchange stimulates the emission of another photon in the same wavelength and direction. This process continues until a cascade of growing energy sweeps through the medium.

Photons travel the length of the laser and bounce off mirrors. First a few and eventually countless photons synchronize themselves, until an avalanche of light streaks between the mirrors. In some gas lasers, transparent discs, referred to as Brewster windows, are slanted at a precise angle, which polarizes the laser's light. The photons, which are reflected back and forth, finally gain so much energy that they exit as a powerful beam. The power of lasers to pass on energy and information is rated in watts.

Principles of Flow Cytometry

The principle of flow cytometry is based on the fact that cells are stained in suspension with an appropriate fluorochrome, which may be either an immunological reagent, a dye that stains a specific component, or some other marker with specified reactivity. Fluorescent dyes used in flow cytometry must bind or react specifically with the cellular component of interest, such as reticulocytes, peroxidase enzyme, or DNA content. Fluorescent dyes include acridine orange, thioflavin T, pyronin Y, fluorescein isothiocyanate (FITC), and phycoerythrin (PE). FITC and PE are used when dual color analysis is desired.

Laser light is the most common light source used in flow cytometers because of the properties of intensity, stability, and monochromatism. Argon is preferred for FITC labeling. Krypton is often used as a second laser in dual analysis systems and serves as a better light source for compounds labeled by tetramethylrhodamine isothiocya-

nate (TRITC) and tetra-m cyclopropylrhodamine isothiocyanate (XRITC).

A suspension of stained cells is pressurized using gas and transported through plastic tubing to a flow chamber (Fig. 25.4) within the instrument. In the flow chamber, the specimen is injected through a needle into a stream of physiological saline solution called the sheath. The sheath and specimen both exit the flow chamber through a 75-μm orifice. This laminar flow design confines the cells to the very center of the saline sheath with the cells moving in single file.

The stained cells next pass through the laser beam. The laser activates the dye and the cell fluoresces. Although the fluorescence is emitted throughout a 360-degree circle, it is usually collected via optical sensors located at 90 degrees relative to the laser beam. The fluorescence information is then transmitted to a computer. Flow cytometry performs fluorescence analysis on single cells at rates up to 50,000 cells/min.

The computer is the heart of the instrument; it controls all decisions regarding data collection, analysis, and cell sorting. The major applications of this technology are as follows:

1. Identification of cells
2. Cell sorting prior to further analysis

The Basis of Cellular Identification

One of the major advantages of flow cytometry is that more than one measurement can be made on every cell during the few milliseconds that the cell spends passing through the laser beam. Each cell can be optically measured for the intensity of scattered light. Measurements include cell size, the number of lobules comprising the cellular nuclei, and the distribution of dye within the cell. This capability allows for the counting of the types of cells in a sample or the measurement of certain components, such as DNA, inside a cell.

The cellular light scatter patterns can be used to identify cells. The scattered light passes through a variety of filters and lenses and is then measured by photomultiplier tubes,

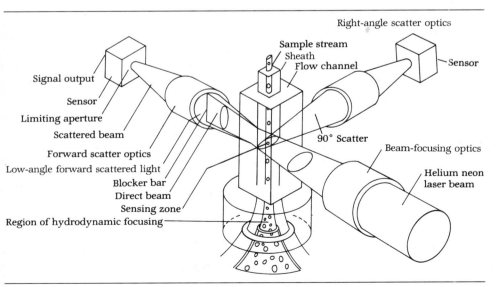

FIGURE 25.4 Laser flow cytometry. The optical detection of forward- and right-angle light scatter using a laser light source is accomplished by using a sensor as the cells pass through the beam under conditions of laminar flow. (Courtesy of Ortho Diagnostic Systems, Westwood, MA, 1985.)

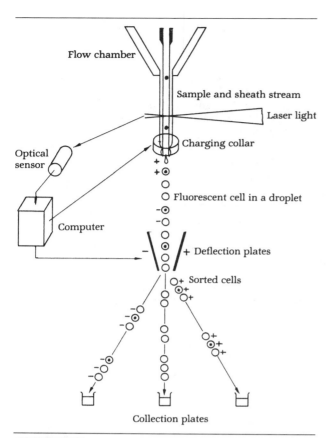

FIGURE 25.5 Laser and cell-sorting schematic. In a flow cytometry system, stained cells flow through a sample tube. As the cells and a stream of saline solution leave the flow chamber, they move like a string of beads in the center of the sheath. The fluorescence of the cells is detected by a sensor. Cells can be appropriately charged as they move through a charging collar or deflection plates. Sorting of the cells is accomplished by deflecting charged cells depending on the charge (either positive or negative).

which convert the light signals into electronic signals for computer analysis. Data are plotted on histograms. If any two parameters are correlated, a three-dimensional histogram can be generated.

Cell Sorting

Using flow cytometry, cells can be sorted from the main cellular population into subpopulations for further analysis (Fig. 25.5). Sorting is accomplished using stored computer information.

WHOLE BLOOD CELL ANALYZERS

Small hematology analyzers are commonly used in stat labs, free-standing clinics, physicians' offices, and small hospital laboratories. Larger and more complex systems are used in larger clinical and research laboratories.

The degree of instrumental sophistication is frequently described by the number of parameters that the instrument generates. The term **parameter** is a statistical term that refers to any numerical value that describes an entire population.

Parameter should be clearly distinguished from the term **sample,** which is a subset of a population. Any numerical value describing a sample is called a **statistic.**

Types of Automation

The smaller hematology instruments measure erythrocytes (red blood cells, RBCs), leukocytes (white blood cells, WBCs) and platelets. Examples of whole blood samples for entry level eight hematology parameters (WBC, RBC, Hgb, Hct, MCV, MCH, MCHC, and platelets) are the Sysmex (K-800) and the Beckman-Coulter Ac.T 8 of the Ac.T series.

The computerized systems generally flag high or low patient results. These systems are automated from sample aspiration through result printout (Fig. 25.6).

Instruments with expanded capabilities produce more than the eight parameters previously cited. These additional parameters include erythrocyte morphology information expressed as either the red cell distribution width (RDW), mean platelet volume (MPV), and a leukocyte histogram differential. Other calculated output is expressed differently depending on the manufacturer (Table 25.1).

Types of Automated Cell Counting Instruments

Four major types of automation (Table 25.2) are representative of the ways that blood cells can be counted, leukocytes differentiated, and other components (e.g., MCH and MCHC) calculated. Hemoglobin is measured by the traditional cyanmethemoglobin flow-cell method at 525–546 nm, depending on the instrument manufacturer. Because models and features of instrumentation change rapidly, the reader is advised to refer to the respective manufacturers' web sites, listed below.

Summary of Automated Instruments

Abbott (http:www//abbott.com)

Cell-Dyn (1200) (3200). This system uses multiangle polarized scatter separation (MAPSS) flow cytometry with hydrodynamic focusing of the cell stream. It features dual leukocyte counting methods. The leukocyte differential is accomplished by light scatter with 0, 90, 10, 90 (depolarized) degrees and nuclear optical count by light scatter at 0 and 10 degrees. Erythrocytes and platelets are counted by light scatter at 0 and 10 degrees. A unique feature is cyanide-free hemoglobinometry.

Cell-Dyn (4000). This system features three independent measurements and focused flow impedance. Multidimensional light scatter and fluorescent detection are used as well.

Bayer Diagnostics (http:www//bayerdiag.com)

Two instruments in current use are the Advia 120 and Advia 60. This technology uses unifluidics, a darkfield optical method. Duel leukocyte methods of peroxidase staining and basophil lobularity are used. Erythrocytes and platelets are counted by flow cytometry. Hemoglobin has dual readings—colormetric or cynmethemoglobin and corpuscular hemoglobin concentration mean.

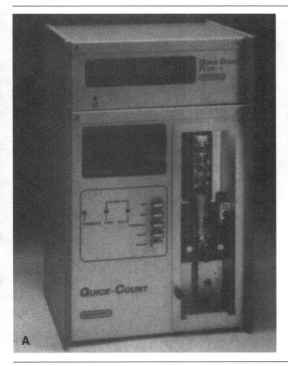

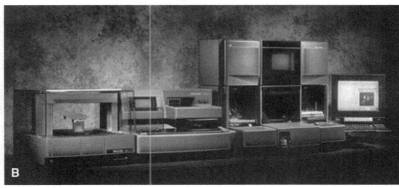

FIGURE 25.6 Basic cell counters. **A.** Seragen Quick-Count Plus-2. (Courtesy of Seragen Diagnostics, Indianapolis, IN.) **B.** Coulter Gen-S. (Courtesy of Coulter Electronics, Hialeah, FL.)

Beckman-Coulter (http://www.beckmancoulter.com)

STKS. This instrument uses electrical impedance to measure the volume of the cells by direct current. Radio frequency (RF) or conductivity is used to gather information related to cell size and internal structure. Scatter or laser light is used to obtain information about cellular granularity and cell surface structure. Opacity is monitored to delineate internal structure including nuclear size, density, and nuclear cyto-plasmic ratio. A three-dimensional analysis is the output.

Gen-S. The Gen-S features Intellikinetics, with the hardware and software to control fluctuations within the laboratory environment (e.g., temperature, reaction time, reagent deliv-

ery). This also improves separation of cell populations. Another feature is AccuGate Gating, a software tool that applies statistics for better separation of overlapping populations. It also allows for more accurate flagging of abnormalities, e.g., variant lymphocytes and monocytes and better abnormal cell detection.

Sysmex (http://www.Sysmex.com)

SE-Series. Erythrocytes and platelets are analyzed by hydro-dynamic focusing, direct current, and automatic discrimina-tion. The leukocyte count is analyzed by the direct current detection method and automatic discrimination. A five-part differential is produced for leukocytes by a differential detec-

TABLE 25.1 Calculated Output

Type	Hematocrit	RDW	MCV
Beckman-Coulter	RBC × MCV	CV% of RBC histogram	Mean of RBC size distribution histogram
Abbott	RBC × MCV	Relative value to CV	Mean of RBC size distribution histogram
Sysmex	Mean pulse	RDW-SD (fL)	HCT/RBC
Bayer	RBC × MCV	CV%	Mean of RBC volume histogram

CV = coefficient of variation, RDW = red cell distribution width.

TABLE 25.2 Types of Automated Cell Counting Instruments

Type	RBC Count	WBC Count	Platelet Count
Abbott (Cell-Dyn)	Impedance	Optical scatter	Impedance
Bayer (Advia)	Laser light and light scatter with a low angle and a high angle (cell volume and refractive index)	Peroxidase: light scatter and absorbance; Baso/Lobularity: forward light scatter and nuclear characteristics	Laser light and light scatter with a low angle and a high angle (cell volume and refractive index)
Beckman-Coulter STKS	Impedance	Impedance	Impedance
Sysmex	Hydrodynamic focusing, direct current (DC) detection	Radio frequency (RF), direct current (DC) detection, impedance	Hydrodynamic focusing, direct current (DC) detection

tor channel (analyzed by radio frequency and direct current). A differential scattergram and an IMI scattergram are produced.

Data Output

Different cell types are distinguished electronically by impedance by the pulses they generate. The pulses that are generated are sorted according to size. These individual pulses appear on the oscilloscope and are categorized by the computer. From the WBC histogram, the percent and absolute number of lymphocytes, mononuclear cells, and granulocytes are determined. Each channel on the x axis represents size increasing by 1 femtoliter (1 femtoliter [fL] = 1 μm^3) from left to right. Each division on the y axis represents one in that channel, providing the relative number of cells (Fig. 25.7).

Quality Control of Output Data. A variety of quality control methods are available via computerized programming. These include instrument checks that ensure that the background is acceptably low and confirm the calibration stability of the electronic system. Control specimen data can be monitored with the generation of a Levey-Jennings graph for each parameter.

Patient results can be monitored with continuous X$_B$ analysis (weighted moving averages), which uses the patient's own data to monitor population values and instrument performance. Batches of 20 samples are used to track MCV, MCH, and MCHC values. This method can be used to detect changes in sample handling, reagents, or instrument performance.

Delta checks are another quality control method for comparing a patient's own leukocyte, hemoglobin, MCV, and platelet values with previous results. If the difference between the two is greater than laboratory-set limits, the current result is immediately flagged for review.

General Histogram Characteristics

Histograms are graphic representations of cell frequencies versus sizes. In a homogeneous cell population, the curve assumes a symmetrical bell-shaped or **gaussian distribution.** A wide or more flattened curve is seen when the standard deviation from the mean is increased. Histograms not only provide information about erythrocyte, leukocyte, and platelet frequency and their distribution about the mean, but also depict the presence of subpopulations.

Histograms provide a means of comparing the sizes of a patient's cells with normal populations. Shifts in one direction or the other can be of diagnostic importance. The position of the curve on the x axis reflects cell size. In the Coulter system, the size (volume in femtoliters) is represented on the x axis.

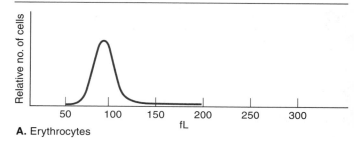

A. Erythrocytes

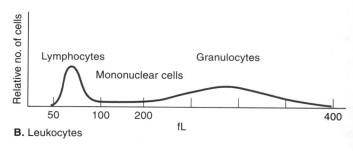

B. Leukocytes

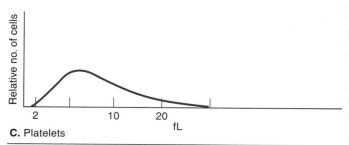

C. Platelets

FIGURE 25.7 Volume histogram. The output of the electrical impedance histogram displays three histograms: erythrocyte **(A)**, leukocyte **(B)**, and platelets **(C)**. fL, femtoliters. (Adapted from R. Pierre, *Seminars and Case Studies: The Automated Differential.* Hialeah, FL: Coulter Electronics, 1985, p. 39.)

ANALYSIS OF INSTRUMENTAL DATA OUTPUT

The Erythrocyte Histogram

The erythrocyte histogram reflects the native size of erythrocytes or any other particles in the erythrocyte size range. The erythrocyte histogram in the Coulter system displays cells as small as 24 fL, but only those greater than 36 fL are counted as erythrocytes. The extension of the lower end of the scale from 36 to 24 fL allows for the detection of erythrocyte fragments, leukocyte fragments, and large platelets.

Although normal quantities of leukocytes are present in the erythrocyte bath and are included in the erythrocyte count, they are *not* significant in the histogram. The system can be calibrated to compensate for 7.5×10^9/L leukocytes. If the leukocyte count is markedly elevated, the histogram will be affected.

If the cells are larger than normal, the histogram curve will be more to the right (Fig. 25.8), as in the megaloblastic anemias. If the cells are smaller than normal, the curve will be more to the left (Fig. 25.9), as in untreated iron deficiency anemia. After appropriate treatment of the underlying cause of an anemia, the curve should move toward the normal range.

If the normal unimodal distribution is altered, the early stages of an underlying disorder may be revealed. A histogram distribution that is bimodal can be seen in various situations, including cold agglutinin disease, after the transfusion of normal erythrocytes into a person with abnormally sized erythrocytes, in the presence of erythrocyte fragments, or with agglutination.

Quantitative Descriptors of Erythrocytes

Two expressions of erythrocyte size are available from two series of instruments: RDW in the Coulter series and RCMI in the Ortho series. Both terms refer to variation in erythrocyte size. Correlations between the RDW and the MCV exist

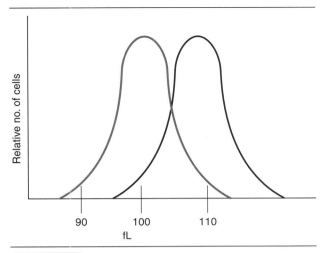

FIGURE 25.9 Erythrocyte histogram. An erythrocyte population that is smaller in size than normal is represented by a curve that is more to the left of the normal erythrocyte size distribution. fL, femtoliters. (Adapted from R. Pierre, *Seminars and Case Studies: The Automated Differential.* Hialeah, FL: Coulter Electronics, 1985.)

for various types of anemia. A classification of erythrocyte populations has been proposed based on the similarities or dissimilarities in the erythrocyte population and in the RDW and MCV.

Red Cell Distribution Width

A new parameter, the RDW, expresses the coefficient of variation of the erythrocyte volume distribution. It is calculated directly from the histogram. A portion of the curve (Fig. 25.10) at the extreme ends is excluded from the computation to exclude clumps of platelets, large platelets, or electrical interference on the left side of the curve. The portion of the right side of the curve that is excluded represents grouped or clumped erythrocytes.

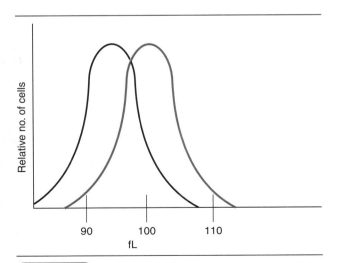

FIGURE 25.8 Erythrocyte histogram. An erythrocyte population that is larger in size than normal is represented by a curve that is more to the right of the normal erythrocyte size distribution. fL, femtoliters. (Adapted from R. Pierre, *Seminars and Case Studies: The Automated Differential.* Hialeah, FL: Coulter Electronics, 1985.)

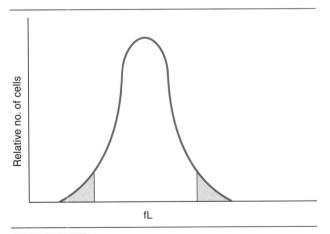

FIGURE 25.10 Red cell distribution width (RDW) calculation. The RDW is an expression of the coefficient of variation of the red cell volume distribution. Both the mean corpuscular volume (MCV) and RDW are calculated from the erythrocyte (RBC) histogram. The MCV is calculated from the entire area under the curve, but the RDW is calculated *only* on the basis of the trimmed histogram (*middle area*). (Adapted from R. Pierre, *Seminars and Case Studies: The Automated Differential.* Hialeah, FL: Coulter Electronics, 1985, p. 39.)

TABLE 25.3 Examples of the Relationship of Mean Corpuscular Volume (MCV) and Red Cell Distribution Width (RDW)

	MCV		
RDW	high	normal	low
High	Megaloblastic anemias	Anemic hemoglobinopathies	Iron deficiency anemia
Normal	Acquired aplastic anemia in adults	Reticulocytosis* due to compensated hemolytic anemias	Heterozygous thalassemias Anemias of chronic diseases

*The MCV and RDW are normal because the reticulocytes are only slightly larger than the cells into which they will mature. Their frequency distributions are similar.

Source: Adapted from Robert Pierre, *Seminar and Case Studies: The Automated Differential.* Hialeah, FL: Coulter Electronics, 1985.

The RDW is calculated by dividing the standard deviation (SD) by the mean of the red cell size distribution.

$$RDW = \frac{SD}{mean\ size} \times 100$$

The RDW is expressed numerically as the coefficient of variation percentage. The normal range is 11.5% to 14.5%. Abnormalities can be observed on the high side but no abnormalities have been noted on the low side. The RDW is increased above the normal limits in iron deficiency, vitamin B_{12} deficiency, and folic acid deficiency. In the hemoglobinopathies, the RDW is increased in proportion to the degree of anemia that accompanies the hemoglobin disorder.

Relationship of RDW and MCV

Quantitative descriptors of erythrocyte size include both the RDW and the conventional erythrocyte index, the MCV. The RDW is independent of high, low, or normal MCV and is an earlier sign of nutritional deficiency than the MCV. The relationship of the RDW and MCV can characterize various erythrocytic abnormalities (Table 25.3).

The MCV of a specimen is calculated using the entire area under the erythrocyte curve. Because the RDW is a mathematical ratio, patients with an increased MCV may have a wide or heterogeneous distribution curve and a normal RDW. Patients with a low MCV may have a distribution curve with a normal (homogeneous) width, which produces a high RDW. A particularly valuable distinction based on the RDW is one between iron deficiency (high RDW and either low or normal MCV) and anemia of chronic disease (normal RDW and normal or low MCV).

Classification of Erythrocytes Based on MCV and RDW

As long as the red cell volume distribution histogram is unimodal, erythrocyte size is described efficiently by the mean (MCV) and coefficient of variation (RDW). An increased RDW may occur with a low MCV even when the width of the curve is normal.

Erythrocytes with a normal RDW are homogeneous in character and would exhibit very little anisocytosis on a peripheral blood smear. Erythrocytes with an increased RDW are referred to as heterogeneous and would exhibit a high degree of anisocytosis on a peripheral blood smear. A classification of erythrocytes that includes the homogeneity

or heterogeneity of the erythrocytes in addition to the MCV and RDW values has been proposed (Table 25.4).

The Leukocyte Histogram

Size-referenced leukocyte histograms display the classification of leukocytes according to size following lysis. It does *not* display the native cell size. The lytic reagent causes a cytochemical reaction. As a result of the reaction, the cytoplasm collapses around the nucleus, producing differential shrinkage. Therefore the histogram of leukocyte subpopulations reflects the sorting of these cells by their relative size, which is primarily related to their nuclear size.

The Coulter Model S-Plus system classifies approximately 20,000 particles when the leukocyte count is at the 10.0 × 10^3 cells/μL level. As the leukocytes pass through the aperture in the electrical impedance system, they displace their volume in a conductive fluid, which causes a change in electrical resistance as each cell passes through the aperture. This change is proportional to the cell volume. The histogram generated by the Coulter principle provides size information.

Although the Coulter leukocyte histogram displays all cells as small as 30 fL, only those greater than 35 fL are counted as leukocytes. The histogram differentiates lymphocytes, mononuclear cells, and granulocytes (Fig. 25.11). Mononuclear cells include blasts or other immature cells, such as promyelocytes and myelocytes, and monocytes;

TABLE 25.4 Classification of Anemias Based on RDW and MCV

	MCV		
RDW	high	normal	low
High	Macro, hetero	Normo, hetero	Micro, hetero
Normal	Macro, homo	Normo, homo	Micro, homo

RDW = red cell distribution width; MCV = mean corpuscular volume; macro = macrocytic; normo = normocytic; micro = microcytic; hetero = heterogeneous; homo = homogeneous.

Source: Adapted from J. D. Bessman and P. R. Gilmer, "Improved Classification of Anemias by MCV and RDW." *Am. J. Clin. Pathol.,* Vol. 80, No. 3, 1983, pp. 322–326.

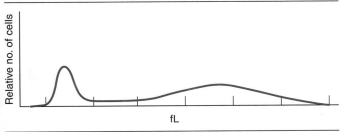

however, in a normal specimen, monocytes represent the mononuclear cells.

On the x axis of the histogram four regions are noted at approximately 35, 90, 160, and 450 fL. There are certain expected characteristics of the curves at these locations. A valley or depression should be seen between the lymphocytes and mononuclear cells and between the mononuclear cells and granulocytes.

The computer program uses these locations to determine the three populations; however, each differential analysis is individualized to determine the position of the populations in each specimen. Leukocytes normally occur at 35 fL or above; the region below 35 fL should be clear. Particles such as clumped or giant platelets, nucleated erythrocytes, and nonlysed erythrocytes might produce interference at or below 35 fL.

The instrument detects abnormal patterns. The types of alert signals include:

1. Cells below 35 fL.
2. Cells between the lymphocyte and mononuclear cell region. Lymphocytes that are larger than normal, such as variant lymphocytes, certain blast forms, plasma cells, or in some cases, eosinophilia and basophilia, can trigger an alert.
3. Cells between the mononuclear and granulocyte populations; an increase in immature granulocytes or other abnormal cell populations, such as certain types of blasts and eosinophils.
4. Cells to the far-right region of the curve, usually a high absolute granulocyte count.
5. An abnormality detected at exactly the 35-fL threshold.
6. A significant increase in the mononuclear population.
7. A multiple alert, when more than one of these regions is affected.

Platelet Histograms

Platelet counting and sizing in both the electrical impedance and optical systems reflect the native cell size. In the electrical impedance method, counting and sizing take place in the RBC aperture. In the optical system, forward light scatter pattern discrimination between erythrocytes and platelets

in the flow cell determines the platelet count and frequency distribution.

In the electrical impedance system, the analyzer's computer classifies particles that are greater than 2 fL or less than 20 fL as platelets. In optical systems, the cell pulse area is determined. The raw data from either the RBC aperture or forward light scatter are sorted. These raw data histograms are then smoothed and tested against mathematical criteria that eliminate nonplatelet particles, and finally fitted to a log-normal distribution curve in the impedance method. This distribution curve has a range of 0 to 70 fL. The final platelet count is derived from the integrated area under this "best-fit" log-normal curve (Fig. 25.12).

The expected cell coincidence error (more than one cell passing through the aperture at the same time) is corrected based on mathematical probability. In the Coulter Model S-Plus system, a minimum of 400 particles per aperture must be detected and evaluated. If an insufficient number of particles are present in the 2 to 20-fL range, a "no-fit" condition is reported. The data for the size distribution histogram are taken from three sensing channels in this system. This method additionally creates three curves and compares the counts. All three must agree statistically. If any inconsistency exists, an alert results. An alert is also generated if the results are not within the range of 3 to 15 fL.

Particles within the platelet size range can interfere with the platelet count and histogram. Small particles, such as bubbles or dust, can overlap at the low end of the histogram. Microcytic erythrocytes can interfere at the upper end. However, the curve-fitting process attempts to eliminate interference at the upper and lower ends to obtain a correct platelet count. If the histogram does not return to the baseline at both the right and left of the peak, either there is severe thrombocytopenia or nonplatelets are being counted. Either erythrocyte or leukocyte fragments may be responsible. In such cases, the platelet count and derived parameters of MPV and PDW are not reliable.

Derived Platelet Parameters

Platelet size has been measured for more than a decade by either micrometry or flow cytometry methods. However, sizing information from data obtained from whole blood specimens and the application of computer technology now makes it possible for additional parameters to be generated

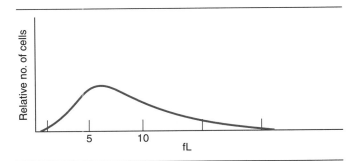

instrumentally. The Coulter Model S-Plus systems yield the additional parameters of MPV and PDW. These parameters are derived from the platelet histogram and allow for a size comparison between a patient's specimen and normal populations. Size comparisons are useful as an indicator of certain disorders.

Mean Platelet Volume Calculation

The MPV is a measure of the average volume of platelets in a sample. The MPV is analogous to the erythrocytic MCV. It is derived from the same data as the platelet count. In ethylenediaminetetraacetic acid (EDTA)—anti-coagulated blood, platelets undergo a change in shape. This alteration (swelling) causes the MPV to increase about 20% during the first hour. After this length of time the size is stable for at least 12 hours; however, MPV values should be based on specimens that are between 1 and 4 hours old.

In normal patients, there is an inverse relationship between platelet count and size (Fig. 25.13). The volume increases as the platelet count decreases. Because of this inverse relationship, the MPV and the platelet count must be considered together. This relationship between the platelet count and MPV is illustrated as a graph, the **MPV nomogram,** and is used to determine whether a patient's MPV is normal. The distribution of platelet size is generally a right-skewed, single peak.

No single normal range exists. Patients with a lower platelet count normally have a higher MPV and patients with a higher platelet count have a lower MPV. Analysis of a nomogram demonstrates that an MPV between 9.0 and 9.8 fL is in the normal range, if the platelet count is normal.

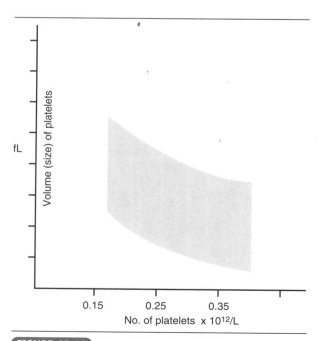

FIGURE 25.13 Mean platelet volume (MPV) nomogram. An inverse relationship between platelet size and platelet count exists and is expressed as the MPV nomogram. (Adapted from R. Pierre, *Seminars and Case Studies—The Automated Differential.* Hialeah, Fla.: Coulter Electronics, 1985.)

TABLE 25.5 Mean Platelet Volume (MPV) in Selected Disorders

Decreased MPV	Increased MPV
Aplastic anemia	Idiopathic thrombocytopenic purpura
Megaloblastic anemia	After splenectomy
Wiskott-Aldrich syndrome	Sickle cell anemia
After chemotherapy	

MPVs from 7.8 to 8.9 fL or from 9.9 to 12.0 fL may or may not be in the normal range, depending on the platelet count.

Disorders of Mean Platelet Volume

Various disorders are associated with altered MPV values (Table 25.5). The MPV is often decreased in aplastic anemia, in megaloblastic anemia, or as the result of chemotherapy. Hypersplenism is associated with an MPV that is inappropriately low for the platelet count. In septic thrombocytopenia, the nomogram varies as thrombocytopenia develops, with the MPV rising as the platelet count falls. Platelet destruction associated with disseminated intravascular coagulation causes an increase in the MPV proportional to the severity of thrombocytopenia. The MPV is often increased in patients with myeloproliferative disorders or heterozygous thalassemia.

Platelet Distribution Width

The PDW is a measure of the uniformity of platelet size in a blood specimen. This parameter serves as a validity check and monitors false results. A normal PDW is less than 20%.

The PDW can be increased in aplastic and megaloblastic anemias, in chronic myelogenous leukemia, and as the result of antileukemic chemotherapy. The causes of increased PDW are not known but are probably related to dysfunctional megakaryocytic development. Falsely elevated results can be caused by extraneous particles, such as erythrocyte fragments, which broaden the platelet volume distribution beyond that of actual platelets.

LASER TECHNOLOGY

Some systems utilize the principle of flow cytometry based on differential light-scattering and cytochemistry. Three distinct steps are involved in its function:

1. Cytochemical reactions prepare the blood cells for analysis.
2. A cytometer measures specific cell properties.
3. Algorithms convert these measurements into familiar results for cell classification, cell count, cell size, and hemoglobinization.

The instrument's sampling mechanism divides blood samples into aliquots that are treated in four separate reaction chambers:

1. Hemoglobin
2. Red cell/platelet

3. Peroxidase
4. Basophil/lobularity or "nuclear" channel

Red Blood Cells/Platelets

The red blood cell/platelet channel uses a laser-based optical assembly that is shared with the basophil/lobularity channel. A buffered reagent isovolumetrically spheres and fixes red blood cells and platelets. The light scattered at low and high angles simultaneously measures red blood cell volume (size) and optical density (hemoglobin concentration) of each cell. The signal pairs are transformed by a computer into a cytogram and two histograms (Fig. 25.14).

Additional parameters (see Chapter 5 for a full discussion of red blood cell parameters) obtained from the histograms are MCV and the RDW (reference range 10.2 to 11.8%). Based on the hemoglobin concentration of each cell, the cellular

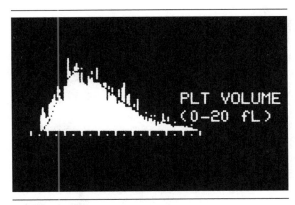

FIGURE 25.15 Platelet histogram. (From E. Simson et al. [eds.], *Atlas of Automated Cytochemical Hematology*. Tarrytown, NY: Technicon Instruments, 1991.)

hemoglobin concentration mean (CHCM) is determined. The hemoglobin distribution width (HDW) is determined. The hemoglobin distribution width (HDW) is the standard deviation of the hemoglobin concentration histogram. Hematocrit, MCH, and MCHC are calculated from the measured hemoglobin, RBC count, and MCV. The red cell cytogram enables simultaneous observation of cell volume and hemoglobin concentration.

The platelet histogram (Fig. 25.15) is derived from measurements made with the high angle detector. The mean platelet volume (MPV) is the mode of the measured platelet volumes.

Peroxidase

In this tungsten light–based optics channel, red blood cells are lysed and white blood cells are fixed and then stained. A dark precipitate forms in the primary granules of leukocytes containing peroxidase when a chromogen is added with hydrogen peroxide as the substrate. Eosinophils and neutrophils are strongly positive and monocytes are weakly positive. Peroxidase is not present in basophils, lymphocytes, blasts, or large unstained cells (LUCs).

Thousands of cells are characterized by a combination of their size (scatter) and peroxidase activity (absorbance) (Fig. 25.16). Scatter is plotted on the y-axis and absorption on the x-axis. Each cell is represented by a dot. The position of the dot is dependent on the combination of the light scattered and absorbed by each cell.

The clusters of dots that are generated are defined and analyzed, the number of cells in each is counted, and the cells are classified based on information stored in the computer. This information is used to generate the total white blood cell count and differential count, except for basophils. The relative percentages and absolute values of leukocytes are included. The parameter **mean peroxidase index** (MPXI), the index of the mean peroxidase activity of neutrophils as measured by their stain intensity, is generated. Increased myeloperoxidase activity may be associated with megaloblastic anemia, hyperproliferative granulopoiesis, or reactive states. Increased numbers of LUCs may indicate the presence

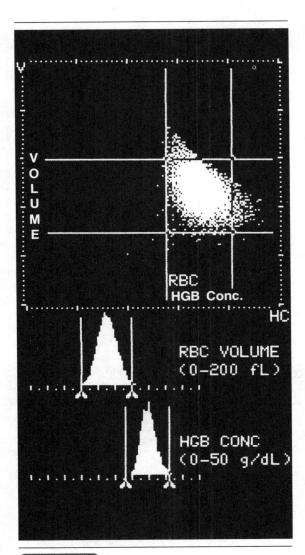

FIGURE 25.14 A cytogram and histogram for RBC volume and hemoglobin concentration. (From E. Simson et al. [eds.], *Atlas of Automated Cytochemical Hematology*. Tarrytown, NY: Technicon Instruments, 1991.)

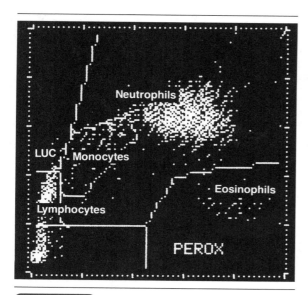

FIGURE 25.16 Peroxidase profile. (From E. Simson et al. [eds.], *Atlas of Automated Cytochemical Hematology*. Tarrytown, NY: Technicon Instruments, 1991.)

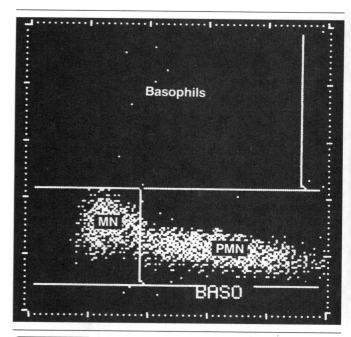

FIGURE 25.17 Basophil/lobularity channel. (From E. Simson et al. [eds.], *Atlas of Automated Cytochemical Hematology*. Tarrytown, NY: Technicon Instruments, 1991.)

of blasts or abnormal lymphocytes. The reference ranges of 0 to 3.7% for LUCs and 0 to 5.4% for HPX have been established.

Basophil/Lobularity (Nuclear) Channel

The nuclear channel is used to measure the conformation of the nucleus of white blood cells. The principle of the reaction in this channel is that when white cells are exposed to a surfactant at a low pH, the membranes and cytoplasm of specific leukocytes, neutrophils, eosinophils, lymphocytes, and monocytes disintegrate and only the bare nuclei remain.

The nuclear channel cytometer distinguishes leukocytes by differences in nuclear shape and counts basophils. This laser-based cytometer measures light scattering at two different angles, low (0 to 5°) and high (5 to 15°). Low-angle scatter measures size, and the low-angle scatter of intact basophils is much greater than the bare nuclei of other leukocytes. A fixed horizontal threshold separates basophils from the nuclei of other leukocytes (Fig. 25.17). High-angle scatter is responsive to the lobularity of nuclei. The more lobulated the nuclei, the larger the high-angle signal. On the cytogram, polymorphonuclear nuclei (PMN) appear on the right and mononuclear nuclei (MN) appear on the left with a valley between them. A vertical threshold separates the two clusters. The ratio of PMN:MN, the lobularity index (LI), is an index of the degree of PMN nuclear segmentation; a low value suggests a left shift. Blast cells appear to the left of the normal mononuclear cells on the x-axis and are counted for flagging purposes. (A system of flags for abnormal morphology alerts the instrument operator that additional work, such as microscopic examination of the blood, may be required.) Nucleated red blood cells, if present, appear within the PMN cluster.

Lymphocyte Subtyping

An immunoperoxidase reaction is employed for lymphocyte subtyping (Fig. 25.18). A specific monoclonal antibody is first reacted with whole blood. A second biotinylated antibody, which binds only to the monoclonal antibody, is added, followed by an avidin-peroxidase reagent. Peroxidase is then stained for, using a similar method to that of the peroxidase channel. Lymphocytes, which have been labeled by the immunoperoxidase reaction, appear between the unlabeled lymphocyte population and the monocytes. Cells with endogenous peroxidase such as neutrophils stain intensely and appear far to the right.

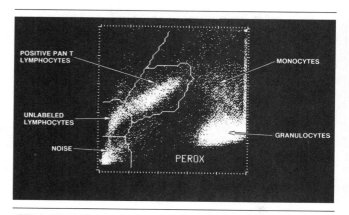

FIGURE 25.18 Lymphocyte subtyping. (From E. Simson et al. [eds.], *Atlas of Automated Cytochemical Hematology*. Tarrytown, NY: Technicon Instruments, 1991.)

C A S E   S T U D I E S

CASE 1

Laboratory Data

A 28-year-old white woman had the following erythrocyte results:

RBC count 3.2 × 10¹²/L
Hemoglobin 8.7 gm/dL
Hematocrit 0.26 L/L
MCV 81 fL
MCH 19 pg
MCHC 27.2%
RCMI 13.2

Her RBC histogram appears below. All of the other parameters were within normal ranges.

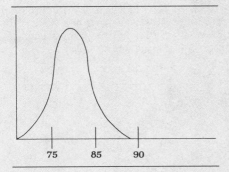

Questions

1. Do the histogram or other erythrocyte results demonstrate any abnormalities?
2. What type of disorder, if any, is suggested by the RBC results and histogram?
3. What further laboratory testing should be considered?

Discussion

1. The histogram demonstrates a nongaussian distribution and is shifted to the left. The hemoglobin, hematocrit, MCV, MCH, and RCMI are not within their respective normal ranges.
2. The data generated suggest a microcytic anemia of unknown cause.
3. A peripheral blood smear should be examined to further describe the morphology of the erythrocytes. Other tests could include serum iron and total iron-binding capacity because microcytic anemias are frequently due to an iron deficiency. See Chapter 10 for a full discussion of the anemias. In this case, further testing led to the diagnosis.

Diagnosis: Iron deficiency anemia

CASE 2

Laboratory Data

A 48-year-old black woman had the following RBC results:

RBC 2.36 × 10¹²/L
Hemoglobin 8.6 gm/dL
Hematocrit 0.27 L/L

MCV 114 fL
MCH 36.4 pg
MCHC 32%
RDW 28%

Her RBC histogram appears below. All of the additional parameters were within normal ranges.

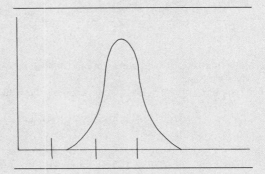

Questions

1. Do the histogram or other erythrocyte results demonstrate any abnormalities?
2. What type of disorder, if any, is suggested by the RBC results and histogram?
3. What further laboratory testing should be considered?

Discussion

1. All of the erythrocyte parameters, except the MCHC, are abnormal.
2. The RDW is indicative of a substantial amount of anisocytosis in this patient's specimen. The MCV and erythrocyte histogram demonstrate that the variation in cell size is in the macrocytic direction.
3. A peripheral blood smear should be examined to further evaluate the morphology of the erythrocytes. Macrocytic erythrocytes frequently reflect a deficiency of vitamin B₁₂ or folic acid. Additional tests should include assays for vitamin B₁₂ and folic acid. See Chapter 11 for a full discussion of the anemias. In this case, further testing led to the diagnosis.

Diagnosis: Megaloblastic anemia (pernicious anemia)

CASE 3

Laboratory Data

A 57-year-old white man with a total leukocyte count of 15 × 10⁹/L had a three-part leukocyte differential:

Lymphocytes 68%
Mononuclear cells 4%
Granulocytes 28%
Absolute lymphocyte value 10.2 × 10⁹/L
Absolute granulocyte value 4.2 × 10⁹/L

The WBC histogram appears below. All of the other parameters were within normal ranges.

(continued)

C A S E S T U D I E S (*continued*)

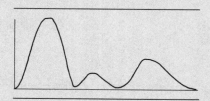

Questions
1. Do the histogram or other leukocyte results demonstrate any abnormalities?
2. What type of disorder, if any, is suggested by the WBC results and histogram?
3. What further laboratory testing should be considered?

Discussion
1. The WBC histogram demonstrates a reversal in the normal adult proportions of lymphocytes and granulocytes. Additionally, the percentage and absolute values for the lymphocytes are increased, while the percentage and absolute values for the granulocytes are decreased.
2. A condition of lymphocytosis is demonstrated by the data presented.
3. A peripheral blood smear should be examined to further evaluate the morphology of the lymphocytes. Other laboratory tests need to be conducted to determine the cause of this disorder and to establish a definitive diagnosis.

✐ Diagnosis: Chronic lymphocytic leukemia

CASE 4

Laboratory Data
A 14-year-old white girl with a total leukocyte count of 29×10^9/L had the following histogram results:

Lymphocytes 15%
Mononuclear cells 48%
Granulocytes 37%

Her WBC histogram appears below. The platelet count was decreased. All of the erythrocytic parameters were within normal ranges; however, the values tended to be in the low ends of the ranges.

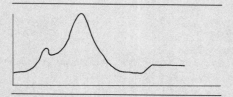

Questions
1. Do the histogram or other leukocyte results demonstrate any abnormalities?
2. What type of disorder, if any, is suggested by the WBC results and histogram?
3. What further laboratory testing should be considered?

Discussion
1. The histogram and percentage of mononuclear cells far exceed the normal distribution for this type of cell.
2. A variety of disorders may be revealed by this type of cellular distribution. Increases in mononuclear cells may result from the presence of immature cells or monocytes.
3. A peripheral blood smear should be examined to further evaluate the morphology of the mononuclear cells. Other laboratory tests need to be conducted to determine the nature of this disorder and to establish a definitive diagnosis.

✐ Diagnosis: Acute myelogenous leukemia (FAB M1)

CASE 5

Laboratory Data
A 12-year-old black boy had a total leukocyte count of 55.0×10^9/L. His histogram appears below. His platelet count was low, as were his erythrocyte parameters. Additionally, his platelet histogram was abnormal.

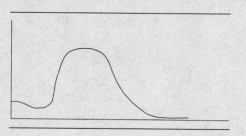

Questions
1. Do the histogram or other leukocyte results demonstrate any abnormalities?
2. What type of disorder, if any, is suggested by the WBC results and histogram?
3. What further laboratory testing should be considered?

Discussion
1. Although his total WBC count was extremely elevated, the histogram failed to separate the leukocyte subpopulations. From the appearance of the histogram an excessive number of mononuclear cells may be interfering with discrimination of the adjacent subpopulations.
2. The total WBC count reflects an extreme leukocytosis; however, the nature of the increase cannot be determined.
3. A peripheral blood smear should be reviewed to further evaluate the morphology of the leukocytes. Other laboratory tests need to be conducted to determine the nature of this disorder and to establish a definitive diagnosis.

✐ Diagnosis: Acute lymphoblastic leukemia

CASE 6

Laboratory Data
This 28-year-old white woman underwent a chemotherapeutic regimen for the treatment of leukemia. Her initial platelet

(*continued*)

count and MPV as well as successive platelet counts and MPVs, beginning on the 7th day after the termination of treatment, were assayed every other day and charted by the laboratory.

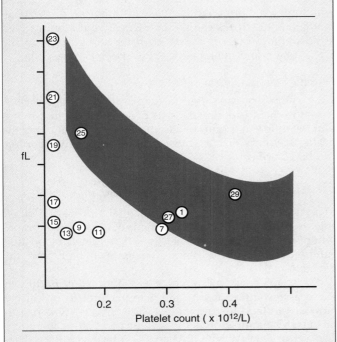

Questions
1. Did the patient have an initial abnormality?
2. Did the patient develop any abnormalities following treatment?
3. Did the patient's values return to normal?

Discussion
1. Initially, the patient's platelet count and MPV were within the normal range as demonstrated on the nomogram.
2. Subsequent to treatment, the patient's platelet count and MPV were decreased. As the recovery period began, the MPV began to rise before the total platelet count. The nomogram demonstrates that the relationship between the platelet count and MPV is not within the normal range.
3. On the 27th day after treatment both the platelet count and MPV returned to normal. The results remained within the normal range on the 29th day after treatment.

✏ **Diagnosis: Posttherapeutic platelet response in a case of acute leukemia**

APPLICATIONS OF FLOW CYTOMETRY

The introduction of the flow cytometer into the clinical laboratory is a major technological advance. Flow cytometry is a field that has evolved rapidly over the past 3 decades. Instruments based on the flow cytometry principle were initially designed to count and size cells. Later modifications were designed to perform differential leukocyte counts by identifying specific cytochemical reactions in the cells. The current type of flow cytometry–based instruments can analyze cells for many constituents as well as sort cells into subpopulations.

General Properties of Flow Cytometry

Most flow-cell instruments can simultaneously analyze multiple parameters at the rate of 5,000 to 10,000 cells/sec. The cellular analysis yields quantitative data about the chemical and physical properties of individual cells, and after analysis cells can be physically separated into subpopulations for further study at the rate of 5,000 cells/sec. The major advances in this technology are due to several factors:

1. The ability to produce monoclonal antibodies resulted in the subsequent development of specific surface markers for various subpopulations of cells.
2. The development of new fluorescent probes for DNA, RNA, and other cellular components increased the variety of possible applications at the molecular and cellular level.
3. The expansion of computer applications has improved the instrumentation technology, making it easier to operate and more practical for use in clinical as well as research laboratories.

Hematological Applications

Flow cytometry can be applied practically to several techniques in the clinical hematology laboratory. These applications include leukocyte differentiation, reticulocyte enumeration, and malarial parasite screening.

Types of Automated Differentials

Automated differentials can be based on a variety of principles. These include determination of cell volume by electrical impedance or forward light scatter, cytochemistry or peroxidase staining and VCS technology. Evaluation of internal cellular organelles and nuclear characteristics can be by:

- 90-degree laser scatter
- polarizing laser light
- radio frequency

Separate measurements can be made of individual measurements of volume, conductivity, and light scatter. An additional method is to integrate the three into VCS (volume, conductivity, and light scatter) technology into a three-dimensional leukocyte analysis. The volume aspect is by volumetric sizing by impedance and radio frequency (RF) opacity for internal composition. In addition, He Ne laser light scatter is applied so that laser light can produce scattering characteristics of each cell at different angles for granularity and nuclear structure.

In addition, different reagents can be used to lyse certain cells. Four different types of technology are used by instrument manufacturers to produce an automated leukocyte differential. These are:

Beckman-Coulter VCS: volume, conductivity, scatter
Abbott MAPPS: multiangle polarized scatter separation—0, 90, 10, 90 degrees depolarized

Sysmex RF: radio frequency; DC: direct current
Bayer: peroxidase staining; optical scatter and absorption;
basophils: differential lysis-laser scatter high and low

Reticulocytes

Reticulocytes can be counted by staining blood cells with fluorescent dyes such as acridine orange, thioflavin T, and pyronin Y. Because younger erythrocytes contain more RNA, they fluoresce more brightly than mature erythrocytes that lack RNA. Comparisons of this methodology with the traditional new methylene blue manual methods correlate well. The manual method is tedious and time-consuming and analyzes fewer erythrocytes than do flow cytometry systems. Newer instruments (e.g., Bayer's Technicon H-3 RTX system, Advia 120, and the Coulter STKS, feature an integrated reticulocyte channel. The Coulter system uses neo-methylene blue and sulfuric acid as reagents. The STKS normal reference range is 0.7%–2.8%.

Blood Parasites

Malarial parasites can be screened by flow cytometry methods. If erythrocytes are stained with acridine orange, the mature erythrocytes containing no DNA do not fluoresce with this stain. However, malarial erythrocytes contain DNA and so will fluoresce.

Other Cellular Applications

Flow cytometry applications are extended to various areas of cellular study. These applications include lymphocyte analysis of cell cycle kinetics and chromosome analysis.

Measuring T Cells for Acquired Immunodeficiency Syndrome (AIDS) Analysis

The quantitation of T and B cells using monoclonal surface markers can be performed using flow cytometry. With the flow cytometer 10,000 cells can be assayed into subsets in 1 minute with multiparameter analysis. Through the use of monoclonal antibodies, T and B cell populations can be divided into subpopulations with specific functions. For example, T cells are divided into two functional subpopulations, T helper (T_H) and T suppressor (T_S) cells. Normal individuals have a T_H/T_S ratio of 2 to 3:1. This ratio is inverted in certain disorders and diseases. These conditions include the acute phase of cytomegalovirus mononucleosis, subsequent to bone marrow transplantation, and acquired immunodeficiency syndrome (AIDS). The analysis of the T cell–B cell ratio is clinically useful in evaluating the immune system status of patients who may be at an increased risk of opportunistic infections. The Coulter STKS offers optional CD4/CD8 lymphocyte counting.

Cell Cycle Kinetics

Because approximately a 2-week lag exists between bone marrow activity and its resultant expression in the peripheral blood, it is important to assess the current status of the bone marrow cells under certain conditions. Flow cytometry allows for analysis of the bone marrow cell cycle parameters with no time lag.

Flow cytometry techniques with bone marrow cells are applicable to DNA cell cycle analysis, which quantitates the number of cells in various phases of the cell cycle (see Fig. 3.7). When the cells are stained with a fluorescent dye, such as propidium iodine, the amount of fluorescence is proportional to the DNA content of the cells. Cells in the G_2 phase will fluoresce more brightly than cells in the G_1 phase. Chemotherapeutic drugs can be more effective if administered at an optimal time. It is best to have normal cells in the G_0/G_1 phase and malignant cells in the S/G_2 phase.

Chromosomal Analysis

Flow cytometry can be used for karyotyping analysis. A chromosomal histogram consists of seven peaks that represent the different groups of chromosomes. By evaluating the peaks, disorders such as translocations or trisomy disorders can be identified.

SINGLE-PURPOSE INSTRUMENTS

Many laboratories are no longer manually preparing blood smears; therefore automated methods of blood smear preparation are included in this section. Automated blood film equipment is of two types: the spinner type and the wedge type.

The spinner-type instruments use either whole or diluted blood as recommended by the manufacturer to produce a monolayer blood film on a glass slide. Spinner-type instruments are manufactured by several companies including Geometric Data (Wayne, PA) and Coulter Electronics (Hialeah, FL). Geometric Data's Hemaspinner uses 0.2 mL of undiluted blood, and diluted blood is used by the Coulter instrument. The spun film produced is a monolayer dispersion of erythrocytes, leukocytes, and thrombocytes covering at least the center half of the glass slide. These monolayer slide preparations are suited for manual and automated leukocyte differential counts.

The Miniprep instrument manufactured by Geometric Data produces a wedge-type blood smear. This instrument produces two slides that are ready to be air-dried and stained. The Miniprep has an adjustment for smear length and thickness. To prepare the smear, two microscopic slides are loaded into appropriate slots on the instrument. A drop of blood is placed on each of the two slides and a lever is pulled down. The instrument automatically spreads the blood into a wedge-shaped configuration in a few seconds.

INSTRUMENTS IN COAGULATION STUDIES

The earliest instruments to detect blood clotting were developed between 1920 and 1940. Instruments were based primarily on detection of the formation of a fibrinogen clot by manual, electromechanical, clot elasticity, optical density, or fibrin adhesion methods. Manual methods were replaced by automated clot detection systems.

Clinical Blood Clotting Instruments

Electromechanical instruments were widespread by the mid-1960s, but have been replaced by photo-optical methods in most laboratories.

Electromechanical Methods

The principle of electromechanical methodology is the measurement of conduction or impedance of an electrical current by the formation of fibrin. An example of such a semiautomated instrument is the Fibrometer (Baltimore Biological Laboratory) (Fig. 25.19). This system consists of a 37°C heat block, an automatic pipette, and a mechanical mixer–timer block.

After the appropriate containers are filled and plasma samples and thromboplastin substrate are incubated, plasma is added to the substrate to initiate the timing mechanism. This timing mechanism triggers a digital readout time and the probe unit. The probe arm holds two electrodes. When in operation, it drops down and allows the electrodes to fall into place within the reaction well containing the plasma-thromboplastin mixture. The stationary probe *does not* move when the instrument is in operation but functions in conjunction with the moving electrode. This stationary electrode is responsible for creating an electrical potential between it and the moving electrode. The moving electrode is located in front of the stationary electrode in the probe arm. When a test is being performed, this electrode cycles through the plasma-thromboplastin mixture every half-second until a clot forms. A detection circuit is activated when a fibrin strand is formed between the two electrodes, thus completing the circuit. Circuit activation stops the timer and prevents further movement of the moving electrode.

Electromechanical methods, such as the Fibrometer, can be used for various coagulation assays. These include APTT, PT, and factor assays. The procedure for operating this instrument is presented in the next section on procedural protocols.

Photo-optical Methods

The principle of photo-optical measurement is that a change in light transmission measured as optical density (absorbance) versus time can be used to quantitatively determine the activity of various coagulation stages or factors. Photo-optical clot detection systems can be used for the determination of APTT, PT, fibrinogen levels, and thrombin time. Quantitative factor assays based on the APTT (factors VIII, IX, XI, and XII) and quantitative factors assays based on the PT (factors V, VII, and X) can be conducted.

These microprocessor-controlled instruments have separate detector cells with their own red light-emitting diode (LED) light source, which is driven by a constant current regulator to give each a noise-free light beam. The light beam passes through a cuvette, where it is altered by fibrin clot formation. The light beam then passes through a diffuser and falls on the sensor, which instantly converts the transmitted light into an electrical signal. An amplified signal is converted to a digital value for further processing. The computer-processed results are subsequently sent to the visual display monitor and printer.

A system is ready for operation when the temperature indicator reads 37 ± 1°C. The PT-APTT mode selects the test parameters for each test method, which determines the proper volumes of specimen and reagents. The appropriate amounts of reagents are placed in the specific reagent storage wells. Pressing the start button initiates the test cycle. In the test cycle, the dispenser pumps automatically deliver the reagents at predetermined intervals, the electrical clock is activated, and the electro-optical sensor is activated after a 9-second delay for PT and a 14-second delay for APTT. These delay times prevent premature end points caused by stratification of reagents or turbulence during mixing immediately following reagent delivery.

The optical density (absorbance) of the reaction mixture is then monitored until the rate of change exceeds a predetermined level for a defined period of time, indicating the presence of a fibrin clot end point. The time (in seconds) of the end point is stored and may be printed or displayed on demand at the end of each series of determinations.

Quality control in these systems includes automatic self-checking of the optical system and the storage of standard and assay curves. A coefficient of determination can be used to check precision. In addition to routine clot testing, newer systems (e.g., Beckman Coulter [ACL™]) offer chromogenic channel models to automate the growing range of specialized diagnostic tests in coagulation. Newer point-of-care analyzers for prothrombin time (PT) and activated partial thromboplastin time (APTT) optimize anticoagulant therapy. Examples of this type of equipment include the Thrombolytic Assessment System manufactured by Cardiovascular Diagnostics.

Platelet Agglutination

The ristocetin cofactor assay measures the ability of a patient's plasma to agglutinate formalin-fixed platelets in the presence of ristocetin. The rate of ristocetin-induced agglutination is related to the concentration of von Willebrand factor, and the percent normal activity can be obtained from the standard curve. Patient values are determined by comparison to a standard curve, allowing quantitation of % ristocetin cofactor activity.

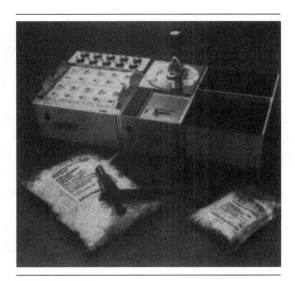

FIGURE 25.19 Fibrometer. (Courtesy of BBL Microbiology Systems, Cockeysville, MD.)

Platelet Aggregation

Most platelet aggregation procedures are based on some variation of Born's method. Agents such as ADP, collagen, epinephrine, snake venom, thrombin, and ristocetin can also be used to aggregate platelets.

The principle of the test is that platelet-rich plasma is treated with a known aggregating agent. If aggregated, cloudiness or turbidity patterns are determined by photo-metrically comparing the light transmitted through a suspension of aggregated platelets with that of a suspension of nonaggregated platelets using an aggregometer. The curve that is obtained can be used to assess platelet function.

Primary Response

Primary response is the reversible aggregation of platelets by the aggregating agent. The appearance of a biphasic reaction, showing both primary and secondary response, can occur for some agonists at low concentrations.

Secondary Response

Secondary response is the result of enhancement of the initial aggregation process due to release of endogenous ADP and the formation of thromboxane A_2. The secondary response is irreversible.

New Automation

The PFA-100™ In Vitro Diagnostic System, manufactured by Dade Behring, Miami, Florida (http:www//DadeBehring) is an automated system that incorporates a high shear flow system to simulate the in vivo hemodynamic conditions of platelet adhesion and aggregation as encountered at a vascular lesion. The system evaluates the ability of platelets to occlude an aperture in a biochemically active membrane. Results are reported as closure time (CT). This instrument offers several advantages over traditional aggregometry because it assesses multiple facets of primary hemostasis—adherence, activation, and aggregation.

═INSTRUMENTAL PROTOCOLS

Each piece of laboratory instrumentation is accompanied by a procedures manual that details the physical construction and electrical components of the instruments, the method of operation, preventative maintenance procedures, and troubleshooting guidelines. The following sample procedural protocols and supplementary information have been provided for the convenience of students in a simulated clinical laboratory situation. All of the available types of instrumentation have not been included because of the large number of instruments currently available. However, some of the more commonly used instruments in student laboratories have been included.

• •

Hematology Instruments

Small Coulter Counters (Models ABI, ZF, Fn, F, and A)

Startup and Operation
1. Locate the *On/Off* switch on the front panel and pull it to the *On* position.
2. Empty the waste flask. Check the diluent supply in the electrolyte reservoir flask and fill, if necessary.
3. Lower the sample stand and place a vial filled with diluent on the platform. Position the external electrode in the diluent so that it is not touching the aperture tube or vial.
4. Slowly raise the platform, immersing the aperture tube and external electrode, making sure there is 1/8-in. clearance between the bottom of the aperture tube and the vial.
5. Fill or flush the aperture tube with diluent as follows:
   A. Make sure that both stopcocks are *closed*.
   B. Open the *Auxiliary* stopcock located on the side.
   C. *Slowly* open the *Vacuum Control* stopcock in the front.
   D. Allow the diluent to fill the aperture tube completely. A

steady stream of diluent should be observed in the waste flask.
   E. Close the *Control* stopcock and then close the *Auxiliary* stopcock.
6. Adjust the aperture image in the debris monitor.
7. Open the *Control* stopcock and observe the mercury level in the manometer. The level should fall halfway between the top of the lower coalescing bulb and the start contact.
8. Inspect the baseline image on the oscilloscope. If necessary adjust the appropriate controls. *Do not* make the image any brighter than necessary. Close the *Control* stopcock and check the timing of the manometer from start of contact to stop of contact. For a 100-μm aperture it should be 13 ± 1 seconds.
9. Perform a background count by:
   A. Obtaining a fresh vial and filling with diluent. Use the same diluent that will be used to dilute the blood specimens.
   B. Lower the platform and place the vial on the sample stand. Immerse the aperture tube into the diluent by slowly raising the platform.
   C. Open the *Control* stopcock.
   D. When the particle pattern appears on the oscilloscope, *close* the *Control* stopcock.
   E. The maximum allowable background count is 50. If the background count is higher than 50, repeat the count.

Troubleshooting
High background count
1. Contaminated diluent
   Change diluent in vial and electrolyte reservoir flask and flush aperture tube.

(continued)

2. Bubbles in diluent
    Let diluent stand until bubbles settle out.
3. External electrode *not* submerged in diluent
    Add more diluent to vial or reposition electrode so that it hangs freely and does *not* touch the aperture tube.
4. Blocked aperture
    Gently wipe the aperture with a camel's-hair brush.
5. Electrical noise
    Remove or turn off the interference source. Be sure that instrument is plugged into a properly grounded outlet.

No operation
No lights, readout, etc.
    Blown fuse on the rear of the unit should be replaced after the unit is *turned off*.

---

10. Thoroughly mix and dilute normal and abnormal controls. Count the particles as outlined in step 9B to D. Two separate dilutions are prepared: one for the RBC count, and the other for the WBC count and hemoglobin assay.

Red Blood Cell Dilution
A 1:50,000 dilution is required. This ratio may be achieved by mixing 2 μL of whole blood with 100 mL of electrolyte diluent. A more common method is a two-step procedure:

1. Make a 1:500 dilution by mixing 20 μL of whole blood with 10 mL of diluent.
2. Take 0.1 mL of this dilution and mix with 10 mL of diluent.

White Blood Cell and Hemoglobin Dilution
A 1:500 dilution is required. This ratio can be achieved by mixing 20 μL of whole blood with 9.88 mL of diluent. Add 3 drops of a stromatolysing agent. Mix by inversion and perform the count *within* 30 minutes.

Troubleshooting
Low counts
1. Vacuum leak
    Repeat startup procedure.
2. Blocked aperture
    Wipe aperture with brush.

No reset or the instrument is slow to reset
1. Airlock between diluent in aperture and top of mercury
    Flush aperture tube by opening the *Auxiliary* stopcock and then slowly opening the *Vacuum Control* stopcock.
2. Vacuum leak
    Check tubing connections.
    Check stopper of waste flask.

Preventive Maintenance
Daily
1. Do not allow the aperture to remain immersed in a diluted blood specimen for an extended period of time. Remove a blood sample promptly and place a clean vial of diluent under the aperture and external electrode.
2. If the instrument will not be used for several hours, soak the aperture tube and external electrode in a vial filled with cleaning agent.
3. Before using the instrument or after multiple blood samples have been counted:
    A. Place the aperture tube and external electrode into a vial of clean diluent.

B. Open both stopcocks and allow the aperture tube to fill with diluent.
C. Close both stopcocks.

Daily Shutdown
At the end of each working day, flush the aperture with cleaning agent as follows:

1. Place vial filled with cleaning agent on the sample stand.
2. Replace diluent in electrolyte reservoir flask with cleaning agent.
3. Open the *Auxiliary* stopcock (lower left) a one-quarter turn in a clockwise direction to a vertical position. Open the *Control* stopcock (upper right) a one-quarter turn in a clockwise direction to a vertical position.
4. Allow the cleaning agent to fill the aperture tube completely. A steady stream of cleaning agent should enter the waste flask.
5. Close the *Control* stopcock by turning it to a horizontal position. Close the *Vacuum* stopcock by turning it to a horizontal position.
6. Turn off power to all instruments and empty the waste flask.

Weekly
The aperture should be thoroughly cleaned each week with a bleaching method.

Reference
Calibrating and Caring For Semiautomated Models of the Coulter Counter. Hialeah, FL: Coulter Electronics, September, 1982.

Coulter S-Plus Analyzer
Systems Check
1. The instrument should be filled with Isoterge.
2. Turn pneumatic power supply to *On* position.
3. Check gauge readings:
    A. Compressor pressure—over 45 psi
    B. 5 PSIG—5 psi (adjustable)
    C. 25 PSIG—25 psi (adjustable)
    D. Vacuum pump—15 to 20 in. of vacuum
4. Inspect the levels of all reagents:
    A. Isoton—cube sufficient
    B. Lyse S—bottle sufficient
5. Drain Isoterge from baths—*Drain* button.
6. Cycle Isoton as a sample four times through the instrument. While cycling, inspect for normal operation:
    A. Bubble rate should be sufficient.
    B. The baths should empty completely.
    C. The Lyse S reagent should enter the system.
    D. No air bubbles should be observed in the sampling valve lines.
7. Print form card on the fourth Isoton cycle. The *background count* should read less than:
    A. 0.4 for WBC count
    B. 0.02 for RBC count
        If the *background count* is higher than the acceptable values, check for dirty glassware and *repeat* cycling the Isoton until an acceptable background count is obtained.
8. Cycle an anticoagulated blood specimen through the instrument four times. During the operation of the cycle
    A. Inspect the instrument for normal operation as in step 6.
    B. Check the results of each of the four samplings for reproducibility with $\pm$ 2 standard deviations:
        (1) WBC $\pm$ 0.4 $\times$ 10^3 μL
        (2) RBC $\pm$ 0.07 $\times$ 10^6 μL

(continued)

INSTRUMENTAL PROTOCOLS (continued)

(3) Hemoglobin ± 0.2 gm/100 mL
(4) Hematocrit ± 1.0%
(5) MCV ± 2.0 μm^3
(6) MCH ± 0.7 pg
(7) MCHC ± 1.0%

9. Aspirate a normal and abnormal control. Check the results against the known values on the assay sheet. If the values exceed the allowable limits, aspirate the control again. If the controls continue to exceed the allowable control limits, check for dirty glassware, increased or decreased bubble patterns, dirty apertures, dirty blood sampling valves, and proper draining and rinsing.

10. If control values are acceptable, patient specimens may be aspirated and cycled through the instrument. The control values may be checked during the sample run. At the completion of testing, the instrument should be filled with Isoterge for storage.

Automated Blood Staining

Several automated microscopic slide stainers are available: the Midas II stainer (EM Diagnostic Systems, Gibbstown, NJ), the Hema-Tek II Slide Stainer (Ames Division of Miles Laboratories, Elkhart, IN), and the Hemastainer (Geometric Data, Wayne, PA).

The Midas II Automated Stainer

The Midas II stainer (Fig. 25.20) can be used for staining blood or other specimens with several procedures, including Wright stain, and it can also be used for microbiology staining. This instrument is microprocessor-controlled and has six user-definable programs, each containing up to 25 possible processing steps. Up to 20 slides can be stained in less than 4 minutes.

Reagents

Available from EM Diagnostic Systems: Wright stain, phosphate buffer pH 6.4 or 6.8, and Hemacolor fixative solution. A *working stain-buffer solution* must be prepared by mixing 50 mL of Wright stain, 30 mL of phosphate buffer (pH 6.8), and 220 mL of deionized water. Mix and allow to stand for 10 minutes prior to use. For a more eosinophilic stain, use buffer with a pH of 6.4.

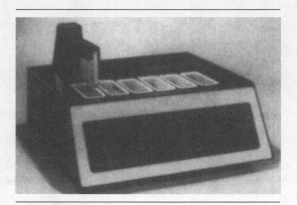

FIGURE 25.20 Midas II automated slide stainer. (Courtesy of EM Diagnostic Systems, Gibbstown, NJ.)

Procedure

A sample protocol for this instrument using Wright stain consists of adding the following solutions to the instrument:

Solution	Container No.	Time
Fixative	2	30 seconds
Wright stain	3	3 minutes
Stain-buffer	4	6 minutes
Deionized water	5	1.5 minutes
Drying stage	6	3 minutes

The slides are loaded into a removable slide carrier. The carrier is mounted onto the carrier arm. During operation, the slide carrier moves from station to station in a preprogrammed sequence. The carrier arm moves up and down automatically every 2 seconds in the staining vessel. If station No. 5 has been programmed, the autorinse turns the water on and off. If station No. 6 has been programmed, the slides are hot-air-dried. When the sequence is complete, the slide carrier moves back to the beginning of the sequence and alerts the operator.

Hema-Tek II Slide Stainer

This instrument allows continuous loading of slides in the Wright staining of smears for differential counting.

Reagents

Accustain Automated (Sigma Diagnostics, St. Louis, MO, No. WS HT) is a Romanowsky-based Wright stain designed for use with the Ames Hema-Tek automated stainer, although other products may be used. Accustain Automated consists of separate solutions of thiazine and xanthene dyes along with a special rinse. Reagent volumes are adjustable with the Hema-Tek.

Procedure

A conveyor system carries slides for staining face down at a preset speed from one station to the next across a platen. The slides are automatically stained, buffered, rinsed, and dried before being deposited in a collection drawer that has the capacity to hold 100 slides. After an initial warm-up, the rate of processing varies from one slide every 2 minutes to two slides per minute, depending on the selected staining time.

Hemastainer

The Hemastainer is sold as a component part of the Geometric Data automated differential system, the Hematrack Differential System. Reagents are available for several manufacturers. The design of the stainer accommodates up to 50 slides at one time. A complex Wright staining cycle takes about 7 to 9 minutes plus time for automatic drying. The staining times are adjustable.

Coagulation Instruments

Fibrometer

This system consists of three components: the fibrometer, a thermal heating block, and an automatic pipette. A digital readout gives the clotting time in seconds to 1/10th of a second. The probe arm consists of two electrodes. When the unit is in operation, it drops down and allows the electrodes to be placed within the reaction well containing the plasma-thromboplastin mixture. The stationary electrode does not move when the in-

(continued)

strument is in operation; however, the moving electrode sweeps back and forth through the reaction mixture every half-second until a fibrin clot is formed. When the clot is formed, an electronic circuit is triggered to stop the timer. The timing bar can be pushed manually, if the automatic pipette is not used.

Procedure

Coagulation procedures, such as the APTT and PT, are essentially the same as the manual procedures described in Chapter 24. Using the fibrometer, the electrical system and direct readout replace a visual end point. The following procedure is for the prothrombin time test.

1. Warm up the instrument by turning it on at least 10 minutes before use. When the fibrometer unit has reached 37°C, the indicator light will go on and remain on as long as the instrument is at 37°C. The light will go on and off depending on the heating demand.
2. When the instrument has reached 37°C, the appropriate number of reaction cups can be placed in the heating wells.
3. Check to be sure that the automatic pipette is securely plugged into the fibrometer and that the setting on the pipette is in the *Off* position. Insert a disposable tip firmly in the hole in the forward end of the automatic pipette. Turn the plunger of the pipette to the 0.2-mL setting.
4. Fully depress the plunger of the pipette and place the fibrometer tip in the thromboplastin mixture. Gently allow the plunger to retract completely.
5. Place the side of the tip near the inside edge of the reaction cup. *Do not* touch the inside wall of the cup. Depress the plunger to expel the 0.2 mL of thromboplastin.
6. Repeat steps 4 and 5 until the appropriate number of reaction cups have been filled. The minimum number of cups per test or controls should be two.
7. Place patient and control plasmas into appropriately labeled 12 × 75-mm test tubes. Insert the test tubes into the deep wells in the thermal block.

8. Incubate the reaction cups and plasmas for a *minimum* of 3 minutes. The testing should be conducted promptly after the reaction mixture has reached 37°C. Prolonged incubation will produce erroneous results due to evaporation of the thromboplastin.
9. After the plasmas and thromboplastin have reached the appropriate temperature, place one of the thromboplastin-containing reaction cups in the reaction well under the probe.
10. Place a clean tip on the automatic pipette and turn the plunger to the 0.1-mL position. Depress the plunger and draw up 0.1 mL of the prewarmed control plasma.
11. *Check to be sure that the digital readout is at zero* (000.0). Depress the digital readout button if it does not read zero. Move the pipette switch to the *On* position and carefully dispense the plasma into the reaction cup. Within 1.5 seconds the probe arm will drop into the mixture and the sweeping motion will begin. The timer will stop when a fibrin clot has formed.
12. Record the time and reset the digital readout back to zero.
13. Gently lift the probe arm to the resting position and carefully wipe the electrodes with a clean, lint-free tissue.
14. Reset the automatic pipette to the 0.2-mL setting and reset to the *Off* position.
15. Repeat steps 10 through 14 for all of the remaining plasmas. The duplicate results for each test should be within 0.5 second of each other if the results are within the normal range. Both the normal and abnormal plasmas must be within the range of the manufacturer's accepted assay values.

Sources of Error
1. Improper reaction temperature
2. Improper dilution or overincubation of the thromboplastin reagent
3. Overincubation of test plasmas

SUMMARY

Instrumental Principles

Various principles of cell counting are used in instrumentation. The impedance principle is based on the detection and measurement of changes in electrical resistance produced by a particle as it passes through a small aperture. In the optical principle, the degree of scatter and the amount of light reaching the sensor depend on the volume of the cell. The volume of each cell is proportional to the intensity of the forward scatter of light. In both systems, the number of pulses generated is directly proportional to the number of cells passing through the sensing zone in a specific period of time.

Based on the original ideas of Einstein and physical theories in the 1950s, laser (*l*ight *a*mplified by *s*timulated *e*mission of *r*adiation) light was applied to medical and scientific instrumentation. Lasers are able to sort the energy in atoms and molecules, concentrate it, and release it in powerful waves.

Flow-cell cytometry is another method that is applied in the study of cells. The principle of flow cytometry is based on the fact that cells can be stained specifically with a fluorescent dye in order to identify exact cell types. Laser light is combined with this method in state-of-the-art instrumentation for cell identification and sorting.

Automated instruments that count and/or identify blood cells range from small bench-top units to large sophisticated instruments. The values that an instrument generates are referred to as parameters. The simplest units count erythrocytes, leukocytes, and platelets. The most sophisticated instruments generate many additional parameters. Some instruments are based on a variety of principles including the electrical impedance principle, and the optical principle of laser scatter technology. In addition to numerical outputs, the larger instruments are capable of generating graphic displays of the frequency distributions of erythrocytes, leukocytes, platelets, and histograms. Quality control systems, such as Levey-Jennings charts, are also generated by the larger instruments.

Analysis of Electrical Impedance Instrumental Data Output

Erythrocyte histograms are valuable in determining the similarity of the population of RBCs being tested. Quantitative parameters that express variation in the erythrocyte population are either the RDW or the RCMI. The RDW and MCV can be correlated and classified in various disease categories.

The graphic display of leukocytes, the WBC histogram, classifies them into three categories: lymphocytes, mononuclear cells or monocytes, and granulocytes. Computer programming allows for the differentiation of leukocytes graphically, in terms of percentage and absolute values.

Platelet histograms, the MPV, and the DPW can be generated by computer-assisted instruments in addition to the platelet count. The MPV is an expression of the measure of the average volume of the platelets in the sample. No single normal value exists for the MPV; however, an inverse relationship exists between the MPV and the platelet count. This relationship is expressed graphically in a nomogram. The PDW is a measure of the uniformity of platelet size. A normal PDW is less than 20%. Increased or decreased values are associated with various categories of disease.

Laser Technology

Some systems are based on the principle of differential light-scattering cytochemistry. Cytochemical reactions prepare the blood cells for analysis, a cytometer measures specific cell properties, and algorithms convert these measurements into cell classification, cell count, cell size, and hemoglobinization.

Case Studies

Because the relationship of histogram or nomogram information is important to understanding the data output capabilities of modern instrumentation, specific examples become important in establishing a diagnosis and monitoring treatment of a patient. A knowledge and understanding of these newer sources of patient information is important to the clinical laboratory scientist. Each of the cases presented in this chapter represents a fairly typical example of a specific type of disorder.

Applications of Flow Cytometry

Instruments based on the flow-cell cytometry principle were initially designed to count and size cells; later modifications included leukocyte differential analysis. Today, the applications of the technology are highly diverse and include both cellular component identification as well as cell sorting capabilities.

Monoclonal antibodies and fluorescent probes have had a major impact on advances in flow cytometry applications. In the hematology laboratory, in addition to leukocyte differentiation, applications can include reticulocyte counting and screening for malarial parasites. Other cellular applications include analysis of the ratio of T cells to B cells in immunodeficiency states such as AIDS, the study of DNA in cell cycle kinetics, and the investigation of chromosomes.

Single-Purpose Instruments

Semiautomated instruments continue to be used in the clinical laboratory. These instruments include blood smear preparation and staining equipment.

Instruments in Coagulation Studies

Manual methods have been replaced in the clinical hematology laboratory by electromechanical and optical systems. In the electromechanical system, two electrodes work in conjunction with one another. When a fibrin strand forms in the plasma-thromboplastin mixture between these two electrodes, a complete circuit is formed. Completion of the circuit automatically stops the timer and the length of the reaction time is displayed.

In the optical system, a change in light transmission through the reaction mixture of plasma-thromboplastin-Ca^{2+} is measured as optical density versus time. Formation of a fibrin clot alters the light path, and after the data are processed by the on-board microprocessor, the time in seconds that the reaction took is displayed or printed.

Both methods can measure APTT, PT, factor levels, and various other parameters. The optical systems offer the advantage of internal quality control features. Chromogenic capabilities are also available.

Platelet aggregation procedures are used to test the qualitative response of platelets to various aggregating agents, such as collagen, thrombin, and ristocetin. Turbidity patterns are determined photometrically by comparing the patient's platelet activity with nonaggregated suspension and normal platelets. A curve is generated using a recording spectrophotometer.

BIBLIOGRAPHY

Albert, Nelson L. (ed.). "Blood Cell Counters With Three Population Diff." *Clin. Instrument Systems*, Vol. 6, Nos. 6 and 7, June/July, 1985, pp. 1–16.

Bessman, D., L. J. Williams, and P. R. Gilmer. "Mean Platelet Volume. The Inverse Relation of Platelet Size and Count in Normal Subjects and an Artifact of Other Particles." *Am. J. Clin. Pathol.*, Vol. 76, No. 3, 1981, p. 289.

Bessman, J. David. "New Parameters on Automated Hematology Instruments." *Lab. Med.*, Vol. 14, No. 8, August, 1983, pp. 488–491.

Bollinger, Pamela et al. "Evaluation of Whole-Blood Platelet Analyzers." *Lab. Med.*, Vol. 14, No. 8, August, 1983, pp. 492–502.

Boraiko, Allen A. "A Splendid Light—Lasers." *National Geographic*, March, 1984, pp. 335–341.

Burns, Edward R. et al. "Leukocyte Differential Analyzers: Pattern Recognition vs. Flow Cytometry." *Lab. Med.*, Vol. 17, No. 5, May, 1986, pp. 271–274.

Calibrating and Caring for Semiautomated Models of the Coulter Counter. Hialeah, FL: Coulter Electronics, 1982.

Coag-A-Mate 2001 Operator's Manual. Morris Plains, NJ: General Diagnostics, Division of Warner-Lambert Co., 1981.

Coag-A-Mate X2 Operator's Manual. Morris Plains, NJ: General Diagnostics, Division of Warner-Lambert Co., 1984.

Cornbleet, Joanne. "Automation in Hematology—An Overview." *Lab. Med.*, Vol. 14, No. 8, August, 1983, p. 482.

Coulter Counter Model Z_F Instruction Manual. Hialeah, FL: Coulter Electronics, 1972.

Coulter Electronics, Inc. "Platelet Counting in the '80s." 1982.

Coulter Electronics, Inc. "S-Plus Differential Information." 1983.

Coulter Electronics, Inc. "Expanding Information." 1983.

Coulter Electronics, Inc. "Significant Advances in Hematology." 1983 (slide-tape program).

Coulter Electronics, Inc. "Improved Classification of Anemias." 1985 (slide-tape program).

Coulter T660 Hematology System. Hialeah, FL: Coulter Electronics, 1985.

Dutcher, Thomas F. "Automated Leukocyte Differentials: A Review and Prospectus." *Lab. Med.,* Vol. 14, No. 8, August, 1983, pp. 483–487.

Gulati, Gene L. et al. "Hematology Instruments for Clinical Laboratories." *Lab. Med.,* Vol. 15, No. 6, June, 1984, pp. 395–401.

Horan, Paul K. "Single Cell Analysis Enters the Space Age." *Diagn. Med.* (Special Issue), Vol. 12, October, 1981, pp. 63–85.

Jones, A. Richardson. *Evaluation of the Coulter Histogram Differential: A Review of the Literature.* Hialeah, FL: Coulter Electronics, 1986.

Koepke, John A. et al. *Leukocyte Differential Counting (Tentative Standard),* Vol. 4, No. 11. Villanova, PA: National Committee for Clinical Laboratory Standards, 1984.

Midas II Automated Stainer Operator's Manual. Gibbstown, NJ: EM Diagnostic Systems, 1986.

Ortho ELT-15 Operator's Manual. Westwood, MA: Ortho Diagnostics Systems, May, 1986.

Ortho Histogram Training Manual. Westwood, MA: Ortho Diagnostics Systems, 1986.

Pierre, Robert. *Seminar and Case Studies: The Automated Differential.* Hialeah, FL: Coulter Electronics, 1985.

Roberts, Cheryl J. and Valerie E. Macdonald. "A New Automated Coagulation Instrument." *Am. Clin. Products Rev.,* Vol. 12, April, 1986, pp. 31–39.

Scheinin, Richard. "Images from the Medical Frontier." *The Philadelphia Inquirer Magazine,* March 10, 1985, p. 14.

Seragen Product Brochure. Indianapolis, IN.: Seragen Diagnostics, 1986.

Sigma Diagnostics Summary Technical News and Notes, Vols. 1 and 2. St. Louis, MO: Sigma Diagnostics, 1985.

Sigma Spectrum 1983 Additions. St. Louis: Sigma Chemical Co., 1983, p. 11.

Simson, E. "The Technicon H*1 System," in *Atlas of Automated Cytochemical Hematology.* E. Simson et al. (eds.). Tarrytown, NY: Technicon Instruments, 1988, pp. 9–12.

Tisdall, Philip A. "Evaluation of a Laser-Based Three-Part Leukocyte Differential Analyzer in Detection of Clinical Abnormalities." *Lab. Med.,* Vol. 16, No. 4, April, 1985, pp. 228–233.

Waller, Kathy V. and Diane B. Bruzzese. "Flow Cytometry in the Clinical Laboratory." *Lab. Med.,* Vol. 16, No. 8, August, 1985, pp. 480–484.

Walpole, Ronald E. *Elementary Statistical Concepts.* New York: Macmillan, 1976, p. 6.

Wardlaw, S. et al. "An Instrument for White Blood Cell Subclassification." *Am. Clin. Products Rev.,* Vol. 11, June, 1985, pp. 21–26.

REVIEW QUESTIONS

1. Which of the following is *not* a benefit of laboratory instrumentation to the hematology laboratory?

   A. Produces faster results from specimens.

   B. Reduced cost on rarely performed procedures.

   C. Less variation in technique from technologist to technologist.

   D. Increased accuracy because data are collected on more cells counted or analyzed.

Questions 2 and 3: match the following principles of cell counting instrumentation.

2. ___ Electrical impedance principle.

3. ___ Optical detection principle.

   A. The volume of each cell is proportional to the degree of light scatter.

   B. Each cell momentarily increases resistance.

4. The abbreviation *laser* stands for:

   A. Light-associated simulated emission of radiation.

   B. Largely amplified by simulated emission of radiation.

   C. Light amplified by stimulated emission of radiation.

   D. Liquid amplified by stimulated emission of radiation.

5. A *photon* is:

   A. A diffuse form of energy.

   B. A piece of equipment in a laser assembly.

   C. The basic unit of all radiation.

   D. Equivalent to an atom.

6. The major application of flow-cell cytometry is:

   A. Determination of cell size and granularity.

   B. Sorting of cells and cellular identification using monoclonal antibodies.

   C. Treatment of cancer cells and identification of specific virus types.

   D. Counting of leukocytes and platelets.

7. The term *parameter* means:

   A. A subset of a population.

   B. The mean value of a sample.

   C. Two standard deviations on either side of the mean value.

   D. Any numerical value that describes an entire population.

8. Data output from three-part differential counters include:

   A. An erythrocyte histogram.

   B. A leukocyte histogram.

   C. A platelet histogram.

   D. All of the above.

9. Which parameters are calculated rather than directly measured?

   A. Hematocrit and erythrocyte distribution width.

   B. Erythrocyte count and leukocyte count.

   C. Leukocyte count and hematocrit.

   D. Platelet count and platelet volume.

10. The *delta check* method of quality control:

   A. Uses the patient's own data to monitor population values.
   B. Uses batches of 20 samples to track MCV, MCH, and MCHC values.
   C. Compares patient's leukocyte and platelet counts with his or her previous results.
   D. Monitors the patient's values within 2 standard deviations of the mean.

11. Applying the optical principle of laser scatter technology to cell counting and analysis, discrimination between erythrocytes and platelets depends on the:

   A. Cellular volume.
   B. Cellular refractive index.
   C. Time of flight through the sensing zone.
   D. All of the above.

12. In an erythrocyte histogram, the erythrocytes that are *larger* than normal will be to the ___ of the normal distribution curve.

   A. Right.
   C. Middle.
   B. Left.

13. A bimodal histogram distribution is suggestive of:

   A. Cold agglutinin disease.
   B. Posttransfusion of normal red cells to a person with abnormally sized red cells.
   C. The presence of RBC fragments.
   D. All of the above.

Questions 14 and 15: match the appropriate formulas.

14. ___ Red cell distribution width.

15. ___ Red cell measurement index.

A. $\dfrac{\text{Patient RBC variation} - \text{average normal RBC variation}}{\text{SD of average normal RBC variation}}$

B. $\dfrac{\text{SD}}{\text{Mean}} \times 100$

16. The red cell distribution width (RDW) and mean corpuscular volume (MCV) are both quantitative descriptors of erythrocyte size. If both are increased, the most probable erythrocytic abnormality would be:

   A. Iron deficiency anemia.
   B. Acquired aplastic anemia.
   C. Megaloblastic anemia.
   D. Hemoglobinopathy.

17. If the RBC distribution on a histogram demonstrates a homogeneous pattern and a small standard deviation, the peripheral blood smear would probably exhibit:

   A. Extreme anisocytosis.
   B. Very little anisocytosis.
   C. A single population of spherocytes.
   D. A single population of macrocytes.

18. The ___ can be determined from a WBC histogram.

   A. Percent of lymphocytes.
   B. Absolute number of lymphocytes.
   C. Frequency distribution of granulocytes.
   D. All of the above.

Questions 19 and 20: the sorting of leukocyte subpopulations in the WBC histogram determined by electrical impedance reflects the *(19)* ___, which is primarily related to their *(20)* ___.

19.
   A. Overall size.
   C. Nuclear size.
   B. Relative size.
   D. Chromatin pattern.

20.
   A. Cytoplasmic size.
   B. Nuclear size.
   C. Concentration of granules.
   D. Cytoplasmic color.

21. The mononuclear cells in a WBC histogram can include:

   A. Blast cells.
   C. Monocytes.
   B. Promyelocytes.
   D. All of the above.

22. A combined scatter histogram measures:

   A. Overall size versus nuclear size.
   B. Cytoplasm-to-nucleus ratio.
   C. Cell size and granularity.
   D. Cell shape and cytoplasmic color.

23. The mean platelet volume (MPV) is:

   A. Analogous to the MCHC.
   B. A direct measure of the platelet count.
   C. A measurement of the average volume of platelets.
   D. A comparison of the patient's value to the normal value.

24. The MPV is often decreased:

   A. In sickle cell anemia.
   B. In megaloblastic anemia.
   C. In idiopathic thrombocytopenic purpura.
   D. After splenectomy.

25. A normal platelet distribution width is:

   A. Less than 5%.
   C. Less than 15%.
   B. Less than 10%.
   D. Less than 20%.

26. Which of the following can be an application of flow-cell cytometry?

   A. Screening erythrocytes for malaria.
   B. Counting of reticulocytes.
   C. Quantitation of T and B cells.
   D. All of the above.

27. The newer clinical instruments for measuring blood clotting are based on:

   A. Clot elasticity.
   B. Fibrin adhesion.
   C. Conduction of impedance of an electrical current by fibrin.
   D. Changes in optical density.

28. The fibrometer relies on the principle of:

   A. Clot elasticity.
   B. Fibrin adhesion.
   C. Conduction or impedance of an electrical current by fibrin.
   D. Changes in optical density

29. In the photo-optical method, the change in light transmission versus the ___ is used to determine the activity of coagulation factors or stages.

   A. The amount of patient's plasma.
   B. The amount of test reagent.
   C. Time.
   D. Temperature.

30. In measuring platelet aggregation, platelet-rich plasma can be treated with ___ to aggregate platelets.
    A. Saline.
    B. Collagen.
    C. Epinephrine.
    D. Both B and C.

31. With a particle counting instrument, a high background count can be due to:
    A. A partial obstruction of the aperture.
    B. Electrical line interference.
    C. Contaminated diluent.
    D. Bubbles in the diluent.

32. A source of error when using the fibrometer in coagulation studies can be:
    A. Improper reaction temperature.
    B. Overincubation of the substrate reagent.
    C. Overincubation of the test plasmas.
    D. All of the above.

26

Principles and Disorders of Hemostasis and Thrombosis

Principles of Hemostasis and Thrombosis

Blood vasculature: structure and function
Arteries and veins
Arterioles and venules
Capillaries
Vasculature physiology
The role of vasoconstriction in hemostasis
The role of endothelium
Maintenance of vascular integrity
The megakaryocytic cell series
General characteristics of megakaryocytic development
The developmental sequence of platelets

Cellular ultrastructure of a mature platelet
Platelet kinetics, life span, and normal values
Platelet function in hemostasis
The overall functions of platelets
Platelet adhesion
Platelet aggregation
Platelet plug consolidation and stabilization
Laboratory assessment of platelets
Blood coagulation factors
The basic concepts of blood coagulation
Common characteristics of coagulation factors

Characteristics of individual factors
The mechanism of coagulation
Fibrin formation
Laboratory assessment of blood coagulation factors
Normal protective mechanisms against thrombosis
The normal blood flow
Removal of activated clotting factors and particulate material
The natural anticoagulant systems
Cellular regulators
Summary
Bibliography
Review questions

OBJECTIVES

Blood vasculature: structure and function
- Describe and compare the histological features of the tissues of the arteries and veins.
- Name the blood vessels that constitute the microcirculation and compare their size and other features with those of arteries and veins.
- Define the term **vasoconstriction.**
- Explain how vasoconstriction participates in hemostasis.
- Describe the metabolic activity of the endothelium and its role in hemostasis.
- Outline the general process of hemostasis in small vessels that contributes to the maintenance of vascular integrity.

The megakaryocytic cell series
- Define the term **endoreduplication,** and relate this process to megakaryocytic development.
- List and explain the three functions of thrombopoietin or thrombopoietin-like cytokines.
- Describe the morphological features of the mature stages of development in the megakaryocyte series.

- Describe the process of formation of platelets from a megakaryocyte.
- List the ultrastructural components and cytoplasmic constituents of a mature platelet and describe the overall function of each.
- Explain the life span activities of a mature platelet.
- Explain the function of platelets in response to vascular damage.
- Define generally the terms **platelet adhesion** and **platelet aggregation.**
- Explain the events that take place during platelet adhesion, including the substances produced.
- Explain the events that take place during platelet aggregation.
- List substances that promote and substances that inhibit some aspect of platelet aggregation.
- Briefly describe the process of platelet plug consolidation and stabilization.

Blood coagulation factors
- Explain the procedure for naming the coagulation factors.
- List the principal coagulation factors.

- Name the three groupings of coagulation factors and describe their similarities.
- Describe the individual functional characteristics of each of the coagulation factors.
- Name the four basic phases of blood coagulation.
- Describe the sequence of events in the extrinsic pathway.
- Describe the sequence of events in the intrinsic pathway.
- Describe the sequence of events in the coagulation pathway.
- Name and explain the principles of the laboratory tests that are used in assessing blood coagulation factors.

Normal protective mechanisms against thrombosis

- Explain the effect of normal blood flow and the removal of substances from the circulation on protecting the body from thrombosis.
- Describe the activities of antithrombin III as a normal body defense mechanism.
- Name the two heparin-dependent thrombin inhibitors and describe their role as part of the natural anticoagulant system.
- Describe the functions of protein C and protein S.
- Explain the activities of the cellular proteases and the role of specific body cells in the production of coagulation factors and cofactors.
- Name and describe the assay techniques that can be used for the detection of fibrin split products.

*T*he maintenance of circulatory hemostasis is achieved through the process of balancing bleeding (hemorrhage) and clotting (thrombosis). Hemostasis, the arresting of bleeding, depends on several components. The four major components are the vascular system, platelets (thrombocytes), blood coagulation factors, and fibrinolysis and ultimate tissue repair. Three other, less important components are the complement and kinin systems, and serine protease inhibitors. Functionally, several processes are involved in hemostasis following injury to a small blood vessel: 1) Blood vessel spasm; 2) Formation of a platelet plug; 3) Contact between damaged blood vessel, blood platelet, and coagulation proteins; 4) Development of a blood clot around the injury; and 5) Fibrinolytic removal of excess hemostatic material to reestablish vascular integrity.

BLOOD VASCULATURE: STRUCTURE AND FUNCTION

Arteries and Veins

Arteries are the distributing vessels that leave the heart, and veins are the collecting vessels that return to the heart. Arteries have the thickest walls of the vascular system.

Although variations in the size (Fig. 26.1A) and type of vessel exist, the tissue (Fig. 26.1B) in a vessel wall is divided into three coats or tunics. These coats are the tunica intima, tunica media, and tunica adventitia. The tunica intima forms the smooth glistening surface of endothelium that lines the lumen (inner tubular cavity) of all blood and lymphatic vessels and the heart. The simple squamous epithelium that lines these vessels is referred to as endothelium. The tunica intima consists of a single layer of endothelial cells thickened by a subendothelial connective tissue layer containing elastic fibers. The tunica media, the thickest coat, is composed of smooth muscle and elastic fibers. The tunica adventitia consists of fibrous connective tissue that contains autonomic nerve endings and the vasa vasorum, small networks of blood vessels that supply nutrients to the tissues of the wall.

Veins are larger and have a more irregular lumen than the arteries. In comparison to arteries, veins are relatively thin-walled with a weaker middle coat. Elastin fibers are usually found only in larger veins, and there are fewer nerves distributed to the veins than to the arteries.

Arterioles and Venules

Arteries branch extensively to form a tree of ever-smaller vessels. Arterioles are the microscopic continuation of arteries that give off branches called metarterioles, which in turn join the capillaries. The walls become thinner as the arterioles approach the capillaries, with the wall of a very small arteriole consisting only of an endothelial lining and some smooth muscle surrounded by a small amount of connective tissue.

The microscopically sized veins are referred to as venules. Venules connect the capillaries to the veins.

Capillaries

The capillaries, arterioles, and venules constitute the major vessels of the microcirculation. As a unit, the microcirculation functions as the link between the arterial and venous circulation. Blood passes from the arterial to the venous system via the capillaries. Capillaries are the thinnest-walled and most numerous of the blood vessels. Sinusoids, which are specialized types of capillaries, are found in locations such as the bone marrow, spleen, and liver.

Capillaries are small structures consisting of a supportive basement membrane to which a single layer of endothelium is tightly anchored. The basement membrane, immediately adjacent to the endothelium, is composed of a diffuse network of small fibers that support the endothelium and act as a barrier against particulate material that may gain access to the extravascular space. Collagen bands also offer structural support to the microvascular unit. Unlike the vessels of the arterial and venous systems, capillaries are composed of only one cell layer of simple squamous epithelium, which permits a more rapid rate of transport of materials between blood and tissue.

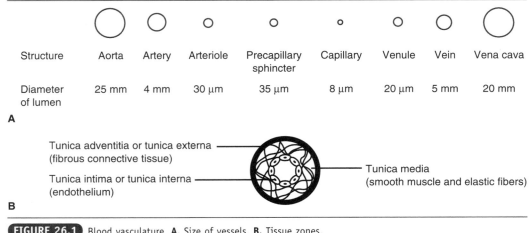

Structure	Aorta	Artery	Arteriole	Precapillary sphincter	Capillary	Venule	Vein	Vena cava
Diameter of lumen	25 mm	4 mm	30 μm	35 μm	8 μm	20 μm	5 mm	20 mm

A

Tunica adventitia or tunica externa (fibrous connective tissue)

Tunica intima or tunica interna (endothelium)

Tunica media (smooth muscle and elastic fibers)

B

FIGURE 26.1 Blood vasculature. **A.** Size of vessels. **B.** Tissue zones.

VASCULATURE PHYSIOLOGY

The Role of Vasoconstriction in Hemostasis

Vascular injury to a large or medium-size artery or vein requires rapid surgical intervention in order to prevent exsanguination. When a smaller vessel, such as an arteriole, venule, or capillary, is injured, contraction occurs in order to control bleeding. This contraction of the blood vessel wall is called **vasoconstriction.**

Vasoconstriction is a short-lived reflex reaction of the smooth muscle in the vessel wall produced by the sympathetic branches of the autonomic nervous system. This narrowing, or **stenosis,** of the lumen of the blood vessel decreases the flow of blood in the injured vessel and surrounding vascular bed, and may be sufficient to close severed capillaries.

The Role of the Endothelium

The endothelium is involved in the metabolism and clearance of molecules such as serotonin, angiotensin, and bradykinin that affect blood pressure regulation, the movement of fluid across the endothelium, and inflammation. With respect to blood coagulation, one of the basic characteristics of normal, intact endothelium is its nonreactivity with platelets and inability to initiate surface contact activation of clotting factor XII (Table 26.1).

In 1985, a family of peptides, named the endothelins, was isolated and identified. The three members of the family—endothelin-1, endothelin-2, and endothelin-3—are produced in a variety of tissues, where they act as modulators of vasomotor tone, cell proliferation, and hormone production.

Endothelin-1 is the only family member produced in endothelial cells, and it is also produced in vascular smooth-muscle cells. It is not stored in secretory granules within endothelial cells. Stimuli such as hypoxia, ischemia, or shear stress induce the mRNA and synthesis and secretion of endothelin-1 within minutes. The half-life is approximately 4 to 7 minutes.

Endothelin-2 is produced predominantly within the kidney and intestine, with smaller amounts produced in the myocardium, placenta, and uterus. The cells of origin are not clear. Endothelin-2 has no unique physiologic functions, as compared with endothelin-1.

Endothelin-3, like endothelin-1, circulates in the plasma, but its source is not known. Endothelin-3 has been found in high concentrations in the brain and may regulate

important functions, such as proliferation and development in neurons and astrocytes. It also is found throughout the gastrointestinal tract and in the lung and kidney.

All three endothelins bind to two types of receptors (A and B) on the cells of many mammalian species, including humans. Endothelin-A receptors are expressed abundantly on vascular smooth-muscle cells and cardiac myocytes. These receptors mediate the vasoconstrictor action of endothelin-1, although endothelin-B receptors may contribute to this action in some vascular beds. Type B receptors are expressed predominately on endothelial cells and to a much lesser extent on vascular smooth-muscle cells. Endothelin-B receptors bind endothelin-1 and endothelin-3 with similar affinity.

Function of Endothelium

The endothelium contains connective tissues such as collagen and elastin. This connective tissue matrix regulates the permeability of the inner vessel wall and provides the principal stimulus to thrombosis following injury to a blood vessel. The endothelium is highly active metabolically and is involved in the clotting process by producing or storing clotting components (discussed in detail in a later section of this chapter). It is also rich with plasminogen activator, which, if appropriately stimulated, is released and activates plasminogen, which ensures rapid lysis of fibrin clots. Additionally, the endothelium elaborates prostacyclin, which is synthesized by the endothelium from prostaglandin precursors and strongly inhibits platelet aggregation and adhesion.

Minimal interactions leading to platelet activation or clot formation occur between the circulating blood and intact endothelial surfaces. However, disrupted endothelial cells release thromboplastic substances that can initiate coagulation. Collagen, in particular, initiates contact activation of factor XII, thereby initiating blood coagulation.

The endothelium forms a biologic interface between circulating blood elements and all of the various tissues of the body. It is strategically situated to monitor systemic as well as locally generated stimuli and to adaptively alter its functional state. This adaptive process typically proceeds without notice, contributing to normal homeostasis. However, nonadaptive changes in endothelial structure and function, provoked by pathophysiologic stimuli, can result in localized, acute and chronic alterations in the interactions of endothelium with the cellular and macromolecular components of circulating blood and of the blood vessel wall. These alterations can include:

- Enhanced permeability to (and subsequent oxidative modification of) plasma lipoproteins
- Hyperadhesiveness for blood leukocytes
- Functional imbalances in local prothrombotic and antithrombotic factors, growth simulators and inhibitors, and vasoactive (dilator, constrictor) substances (Tables 26.2 and 26.3).

These manifestations, collectively termed *endothelial dysfunction,* play an important role in the initiation, progression, and clinical complications of various forms of inflammatory and degenerative vascular diseases. Various stimuli of endothelial dysfunction have been identified including immuno-

TABLE 26.1 Endothelial Functions

Angiogenesis	Synthesis of stromal components
Coagulation	Vascular-tone regulation
Inflammation	Special metabolic functions*
Immune responses	

*Transport of molecules from the vascular lumen to the subendothelium, production of angiotensin-converting enzyme and the binding of lipoproteins, high-density lipoproteins and low-density lipoproteins.

TABLE 26.2 Endothelial Prothrombotic-Antithrombotic Balance

Prothrombotic	Antithrombotic
Platelet-activating factor	Prostacyclin
Tissue factor	Thrombomodulin
von Willebrand factor	Tissue plasminogen activator (tPA)
Plasminogen activator	Urokinase
Inhibitor-1	Heparin-like molecules
Other coagulation factors: synthesis of factor V; binding of factors V, IXa, Xa; factor XII activation	

These various endothelial-associated factors and functions contribute to a dynamic physiological antagonism or "balance" that determines the status of local hemostatic/thrombotic activity.

regulatory substances such as tumor necrosis factor (TNF) and interleukin-1 (IL-1), viral infection and transformation, bacterial toxins, and cholesterol and oxidatively modified lipoproteins.

Disruption of the endothelium directly activates all four components of hemostasis. After this event, the following events take place:

1. Initially, rapid vasoconstriction for up to half an hour reduces blood flow and promotes contact activation of platelets and coagulation factors.
2. In the second phase, platelets adhere immediately to the exposed subendothelial connective tissue, particularly collagen. The aggregated platelets enhance sustained vasoconstriction by releasing thromboxane A_2 and vasoactive amines, including serotonin and epinephrine.
3. In the third phase, coagulation is initiated through both the **intrinsic** and **extrinsic** systems.
4. Finally, fibrinolysis occurs following the release of tissue plasminogen activators from the vascular wall. Fibrinolytic removal of excess hemostatic material is necessary to reestablish vascular integrity.

Maintenance of Vascular Integrity

Vascular integrity or the resistance to vessel disruption requires three essential factors. These factors are circulating

TABLE 26.3 Endothelial Vasoconstrictor-Vasodilator Balance

Constrictor	Dilator
Endothelin-1	Prostacyclin
Angiotensin-II	Nitric oxide
Vasoconstrictor	Other "EDRF-like" substances
Prostaglandins	

These various endothelial-generated substances contribute to the local regulation of vascular tone through their effects on smooth muscle contractility.

functional platelets, adrenocorticosteroids, and ascorbic acid. A lack of these factors produces fragility of the vessels, which makes them prone to disruption. Maintenance of vascular integrity through the hemostatic process depends on the events previously described. The importance of these reactions varies with vessel size; for example, capillaries seal easily due to vasoconstriction. The integrity of arterioles and venules depends on vasoconstriction, the formation of a plug of fused platelets over the injury, and the formation of a fibrin clot. Arteries, because of their thick walls, are the most resistant to bleeding; however, hemorrhage from these vessels is the most dangerous. Vasoconstriction is of ultimate importance in damaged arteries. Veins, which contain 70% of the blood volume, may rupture with a slight increase in hydrostatic pressure.

THE MEGAKARYOCYTIC CELL SERIES

Mature **platelets (thrombocytes),** metabolically active cell fragments, are the second critical component in the maintenance of hemostasis. These anuclear cells circulate in the peripheral blood after being produced from the cytoplasm of bone marrow **megakaryocytes,** the largest cells found in the bone marrow.

General Characteristics of Megakaryocytic Development

Bone marrow megakaryocytes are derived from pluripotential stem cells. The sequence of development from megakaryocytes to platelets is thought to progress from the proliferation of progenitors to polyploidization, that is, nuclear endoreduplication, and finally to cytoplasmic maturation and the formation of platelets.

There appears to be a complex relationship between the circulating platelet mass and the number, ploidy, and size of megakaryocytes, but the sensing mechanisms that regulate platelet production have not yet been identified. Recently, the gene for the human mpl protein was cloned and found to be expressed selectively in megakaryocytic cells. It was then found that antisense oligonucleotides that block the synthesis of human mpl protein inhibit the formation of megakaryocyte colonies but not of erythroid or granulocyte-macrophage colonies in vitro. This orphan receptor of unknown function might be the receptor for thrombopoietin. The protein may act synergistically with other growth factors during the proliferation state. It is not known whether further hormonal stimulation is needed for cytoplasmic maturation or platelet release.

Megakaryocytopoiesis proceeds initially through a phase characterized by mitotic division of a progenitor cell, followed by a wave of nuclear endoreduplication. **Endoreduplication** is the process in which chromosomal material (DNA) and the other events of mitosis occur *without* subsequent division of the cytoplasmic membrane into identical daughter cells. Recognizable megakaryocytes have ploidy values of $4n$, $8n$, $16n$, and $32n$. The maturation of megakaryocytes from immature, largely non–DNA-synthesizing cells to morphologically identifiable megakaryocytes involves processes such as the appearance of cytoplasmic organelles, the acquisition of membrane antigens and glycoproteins, and the release of platelets.

Thrombopoietin, the hormone thought to stimulate the production and maturation of megakaryocytes, which in turn produce platelets, has recently been purified and cloned. Thrombopoietin activity results from several different cytokines: erythropoietin, interleukin-3 (IL-3), and granulocyte-macrophage colony-stimulating factor (GM-CSF). These substances have been shown to be able to increase megakaryocyte size, maturational stage, and ploidy.

The Developmental Sequence of Platelets

Early Development

Two classes of progenitors have been identified: the burst-forming-unit megakaryocyte (BFU-M) and the colony-forming-unit megakaryocyte (CFU-M). The BFU-M is the most primitive progenitor cell committed to megakaryocyte lineage.

The next stage of megakaryocyte development is a small, mononuclear marrow cell that expresses platelet-specific phenotypic markers, but is not morphologically identifiable as a megakaryocyte (Plate 79). These transitional cells represent 5% of marrow megakaryocyte elements. Some transitional immature megakaryocyte cells may be capable of cellular division, but most are nonproliferating while actively undergoing endomitosis.

Megakaryocytes

The final stage of megakaryocyte development is the morphologically identifiable megakaryocyte (Plate 80). These cells are readily recognizable in the marrow because of their large size and lobulated nuclei. These cells are polyploid (Table 26.4).

Megakaryocytes are the largest bone marrow cells, ranging up to 160 μm in size. The nuclear-cytoplasmic (N:C) ratio can be as high as 1:12. Nucleoli are no longer visible. A distinctive feature of the megakaryocyte is that it is **multilobular,** not multinucleated. The fully mature lobes of the megakaryocyte shed platelets from the cytoplasm on completion of maturation. Platelet formation begins with the initial appearance of a pink color in the basophilic cytoplasm of the megakaryocyte and increased granularity.

Mature Platelets

Platelets (Plate 81) have an average diameter of 2 to 4 μm, with younger platelets being larger than older ones. In contrast to megakaryocytes, platelets have no nucleus. The cytoplasm is light blue, with evenly dispersed, fine red-purple granules. An inactive or unstimulated platelet circulates as a thin, smooth-surfaced disc. This discoid shape is maintained by the microtubular cytoskeleton beneath the cytoplasmic membrane.

Platelets circulate at the center of the flowing bloodstream through endothelium-lined blood vessels without interacting with other platelets or with the vessel wall. Platelets are extremely sensitive cells and may respond to minimal stimulation by forming pseudopods that spontaneously retract. Stronger stimulation causes platelets to become sticky without losing their discoid shape; however, changes in shape to an irregular sphere with spiny pseudopods will occur with additional stimulation. This alteration in cellular shape is triggered by an increase in the level of cytoplasmic calcium. Such changes in shape accompanied by internal cellular contractions can result in the release of many of the internal organelles. A loss of viability is associated with this change to a spiny sphere.

Cellular Ultrastructure of a Mature Platelet

Examination of a platelet with the electron microscope reveals a variety of structures. These structures are fundamental to the functioning of the platelet.

TABLE 26.4	Developmental Characteristics of Mature Megakaryocytic Cells	
	Megakaryocyte	**Platelet**
Size	30–160 μm	2–4 μm
Nucleus-cytoplasm ratio	1:1–1:12	
Nucleus		
Shape	Lobulated (2 or more lobes)	(Anuclear)
Chromatin color	Blue-purple	—
Chromatin clumping	Granular	—
Nucleoli	Not visible	—
Cytoplasm		
Color	Pinkish-blue	Light-blue fragments
Shape	Occasional pseudopods Irregular border	
Amount	Abundant	
Granules	Abundant near the borders of the cytoplasm	Scattered

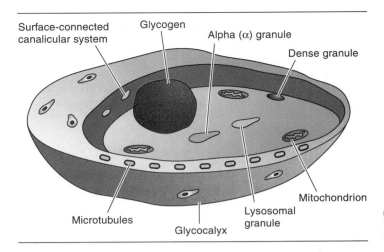

FIGURE 26.2 Platelet ultrastructure. (Adapted from A. R. Thompson and L. A. Harker, *Manual of Hemostasis and Thrombosis* [3rd ed]. Philadelphia: F. A. Davis, 1983.)

The Glycocalyx

Ultrastructure examination of the platelet (Fig. 26.2) reveals that the cellular membrane is surrounded externally by a fluffy coat or **glycocalyx.** This glycocalyx is unique among the cellular components of the blood. It is composed of plasma proteins and carbohydrate molecules that are related to the coagulation, complement, and fibrinolytic systems. The glycoprotein receptors of the glycocalyx mediate the membrane contact reactions of platelet adherence, change of cellular shape, internal contraction, and aggregation.

Cytoplasmic Membrane

Adjacent to the glycocalyx is the cytoplasmic membrane whose chemical composition and physical structure is described in Chapter 3. Extending through the plasma membrane and into the interior of the platelet is an open canalicular or surface-connecting system. It is this system that forms the invaginated, spongelike portion of the cell that provides an expanded reactive surface to which plasma clotting factors are selectively adsorbed. Contact activation of the membrane phospholipids also generates procoagulant activity and arachidonic acid to the blood-clotting process. The cytoplasmic membrane and open canalicular membrane system articulate with the dense tubular system that is not surface-connected.

Although the canaliculi penetrate the cytoplasm in a random manner, they are generally in close proximity to granules and other organelles. Therefore, products released by the granules or cytoplasm can be transported to the exterior environment through the canaliculi. In addition to the movement of extracellular materials against the concentration gradient through the canaliculi, phagocytosis is also likely to occur through these channels. Additionally, the channels of the open canalicular system and dense tubular system appear to constitute the calcium-regulating mechanism of the cell.

Microfilaments and Microtubules

Directly beneath the cell membrane is a series of submembrane filaments and microtubules that form the cellular cytoskeleton. In addition to providing the structure for maintaining the circulating discoid shape of the cell, the cytoskeleton also maintains the position of the organelles. A secondary system of microfilaments is functional in internal organization and secretion of blood coagulation products, such as fibrinogen. The microfilaments interact with the dense tubular system in sequestering calcium, which initially causes centralization of internal organelles. These subcellular and cytoplasmic filaments make up the contractile system (sol gel zone) of the platelet.

Granules

Three different types of storage granules related to hemostasis are present in the mature platelet. These granules are **alpha granules, dense** or **delta granules,** and **lysosomes.** The alpha granules are the most abundant. Alpha granules contain heparin-neutralizing platelet factor 4 (PF 4), beta thromboglobulin, platelet-derived growth factor, platelet fibrinogen, fibronectin, von Willebrand factor (vWF), and thrombospondin. Dense bodies, named because of their appearance when viewed by electron microscopy, contain serotonin, ADP, ATP, and calcium. Lysosomes, the third type of granule, store hydrolase enzymes. Extrusion of the contents of these storage granules requires internal, cellular contraction. Secretions from the granules are released into the open canalicular system.

Other Cytoplasmic Constituents

In addition to containing substantial quantities of the contractile proteins, including actomyosin (thrombosthenin), myosin, and filamin, the cytoplasm of the platelet contains glycogen and enzymes of the glycolytic and hexose pathways. Energy for metabolic activities and cellular contraction is derived from aerobic metabolism in the mitochondria and anaerobic glycolysis-utilizing glycogen stores. The platelet is a very high-energy cell with a metabolic rate 10 times that of an erythrocyte. Based on energy availability and endogenous constituents, the platelet is effectively equipped to fulfill the role of protecting the body against vascular trauma.

Platelet Kinetics, Life Span, and Normal Values

An average megakaryocyte produces about 1000 to 2000 platelets. Marrow transit time, or the maturation period of the megakaryocyte, is about 5 days.

It is believed that platelets initially enter the spleen, where they remain for 2 days. Following this period, platelets are in either the circulating blood or the active splenic pool. At all times, approximately two thirds of the total number of platelets are in the systemic circulation, while the remaining one third exist as a pool of platelets in the spleen that freely exchange with the general circulation. A normal person has an average of $250 \times 10^9/L$ (range $150 \times 10^9/L$ to $450 \times 10^9/L$) platelets in the systemic circulation. Platelet turnover or "effective thrombopoiesis" averages $350 \times 10^9/L \pm 4.3 \times 10^9/L/$day.

The life span of a mature platelet is 9.0 days ± 1 day. At the end of their life span, platelets are phagocytized by the liver and spleen and other tissues of the mononuclear phagocytic system.

PLATELET FUNCTION IN HEMOSTASIS

Platelets normally move freely through the lumen of blood vessels as components of the circulatory system. Maintenance of normal vascular integrity involves nourishment of the endothelium by some platelet constituents or the actual incorporation of platelets into the vessel wall. This process requires less than 10% of the platelets normally in the circulating blood. For hemostasis to occur, platelets not only must be present in normal quantities but also must function properly. In this section, the hemostatic functions of platelets, including platelet adherence and aggregation, are discussed.

The Overall Functions of Platelets

Following damage to the endothelium of a blood vessel, a series of events occur, including adhesion to the injured vessel, shape change, aggregation, and secretion. Each structural and functional change is accompanied by a series of biochemical reactions that occur during the process of platelet activation. The platelet plasma membrane is the focus of interactions between extracellular and intracellular environments. Agonists that lead to platelet activation are varied and include a nucleotide (ADP), lipids (thromboxane A_2, platelet-activating factor), a structural protein (collagen), and a proteolytic enzyme (thrombin).

One of the distinct activities associated with platelet activity in response to vascular damage is the continued maintenance of vascular integrity by the rapid adherence of platelets to exposed endothelium. In addition, platelets spread, become activated, and form large aggregates. Formation of a "platelet plug" initially arrests bleeding.

The adherence and aggregation of platelets at the sites of vascular damage allow for the release of molecules involved in hemostasis and wound healing and provide a membrane surface for the assembly of coagulation enzymes that lead to fibrin formation. Vascular healing is promoted by stimulating the migration and proliferation of endothelial cells and medial smooth muscle cells through the release of the mitogen, platelet-derived growth factor.

Platelet Adhesion

If vascular injury exposes the endothelial surface and underlying collagen (Fig. 26.3), platelets *adhere* to the subendothelial collagen fibers, spread pseudopods along the surface, and clump together (**aggregate**). Platelet adhesion to subendothelial connective tissues, especially collagen,

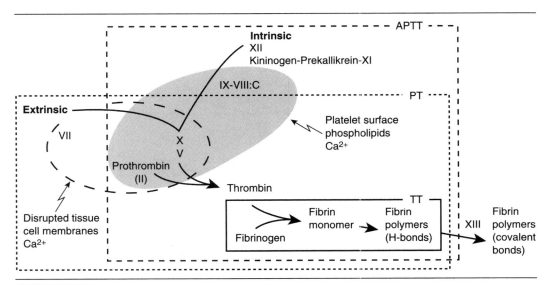

FIGURE 26.3 Coagulation mechanisms. Shaded areas ("platelet surface phospholipids") enclose the intrinsic coagulation reactions that occur on the surface membranes of platelets. Dashed lines enclose the extrinsic coagulation reactions that occur on disrupted tissue cell phospholipoprotein membranes intruded into the circulation. APTT = activated partial thromboplastin time; PT = prothrombin time; TT = thrombin time. (From P. R. Reich, *Hematology* [2nd ed]. Boston: Little, Brown & Co., 1984.)

occurs within 1 to 2 minutes after a break in the endothelium.

Epinephrine and serotonin promote vasoconstriction. ADP increases the adhesiveness of platelets. Considerable evidence indicates that the adhesion and aggregation of platelets are mediated by the binding of large soluble macromolecules to distinct glycoprotein receptors anchored in the platelet membrane. This increase in adhesiveness causes circulating platelets to adhere to those already attached to the collagen. The result is a cohesive platelet mass that rapidly increases in size to form a platelet plug.

The transformation of the platelet from a disc to a sphere with pseudopods produces surface membrane reorganization. Internal contraction of the platelet results in release of granular contents of the alpha and dense granules and the lysosomal contents. This process resembles the secretory activities of other cells.

Platelets adhere at sites of mechanical vascular injury and then undergo activation and express functional glycoprotein IIb/IIIa receptors (also referred to as integrin alpha$_{IIb}$beta$_3$) for circulating adhesive ligand proteins (primarily fibrinogen). These functional glycoprotein IIb/IIIa receptors mediate the recruitment of local platelets by forming fibrinogen bridges between platelets—a process called platelet cohesion. Although functional glycoprotein IIb/IIIa receptors bind with other circulating adhesive molecules in plasma (including von Willebrand's factor, fibronectin, vitronectin, and thrombospondin), fibrinogen is the predominant ligand because of its relatively high concentration. The peptide recognition sequence arginine-glycine-aspartic acid present in these different adhesive molecules mediates binding with expressed glycoprotein IIb/IIIa receptors. Glycoprotein IIb/IIIa is specific for platelets. Platelet recruitment depends almost exclusively on the final phase of glycoprotein IIb/IIIa-dependent platelet cohesion. Glycoprotein IIb/IIIa is the most abundant platelet membrane protein (with approximately 50,000 receptors per platelet).

Platelet Aggregation

A variety of agents are capable of producing platelet aggregation, an energy-dependent process. These agents include particulate material such as collagen, proteolytic enzymes such as thrombin, and biological amines such as epinephrine and serotonin.

It is believed that bridges formed by fibrinogen in the presence of calcium produce a sticky surface on platelets. This results in aggregation. If these aggregates are reinforced by fibrin, they are referred to as a thrombus.

Aggregation of platelets by at least one pathway can be blocked by substances such as prostaglandin E (PG E), adenosine, and nonsteroidal antiinflammatory agents (e.g., aspirin). Aspirin induces a long-lasting functional defect in platelets (Fig. 26.4). It is clinically detectable as a prolongation of the bleeding time. The mechanism of aspirin appears to be primarily, if not exclusively, the permanent inactivation of prostaglandin G/H synthase, which catalyzes the first step in the synthesis of the prostaglandins, the conversion of arachidonate to prostaglandin H$_2$. Reduced formation of various eicosanoids (thromboxane A$_2$, prostaglandin E$_2$, and prostacyclin) in various tissues probably accounts for the

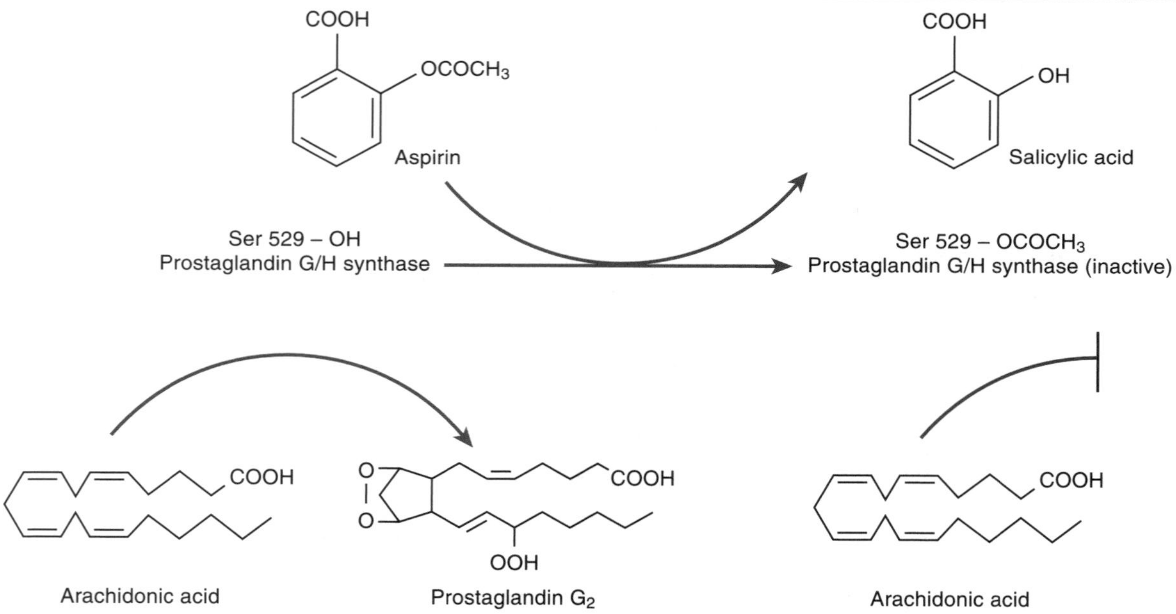

FIGURE 26.4 Mechanism of the antiplatelet action of aspirin. Aspirin acetylates the hydroxyl group of a serine residue at position 529 (Ser529) in the polypeptide chain of human platelet prostaglandin G/H synthase, resulting in the inactivation of cyclooxygenase catalytic activity. Aspirin-induced blockade of prostaglandin synthesis will result in decreased biosynthesis of prostaglandin H$_2$ and thromboxane A$_2$. (From C. Patrono, "Aspirin as an Antiplatelet Drug." *N. Engl. J. Med.*, Vol. 330, No. 18, May 5, 1994, pp. 1288.)

variety of pharmacologic effects of aspirin that form the basis of its therapeutic use and its toxicity.

Because platelets lack the biosynthetic mechanisms needed to synthesize new protein, the defect induced by aspirin cannot be repaired during their life span (approximately 8 to 10 days). Therefore, after treatment with aspirin is stopped, cyclooxygenase activity recovers slowly, as a function of platelet turnover. This explains the apparent paradox of how a drug with a 20-minute half-life in the systemic circulation can be fully effective as an antiplatelet agent when administered once daily.

Because of the permanent nature of aspirin-induced inactivation of platelet prostaglandin G/H synthase, the inhibitory effect of repeated daily doses below 100 mg is cumulative. Daily administration of 30 to 50 mg of aspirin results in virtually complete suppression of platelet thromboxase biosynthesis after 7 to 10 days. These changes in platelet biochemistry are associated with maximal inhibition of thromboxane-dependent platelet aggregation, and prolongation of the bleeding time accounts for the antithrombotic effects of aspirin.

Platelet Plug Consolidation and Stabilization

The permanently anchored platelet plug requires additional consolidation and stabilization. Fibrinogen, under the influence of small amounts of thrombin, provides the basis for this consolidation and stabilization. This process involves the precipitation of polymerized fibrin around each platelet. The result is a fibrin clot that produces an irreversible platelet plug (Table 26.5).

Laboratory Assessment of Platelets

A platelet count is a fundamental component in the evaluation of a patient. Examination of the peripheral blood smear for platelet number and morphology is critical because many clinical clues may be obtained from an evaluation of platelet quantity and morphology.

Quantitative Determination of Platelets

The circulating platelet count can be accurately determined in a blood sample using an electronic particle counter (see Chapter 25) or by manual methods (see Chapter 24). Examination of a stained blood film provides a rapid estimate of platelet numbers. Normally, there are 8 to 20 platelets per $100\times$ (oil) immersion field in a properly prepared smear (where the erythrocytes barely touch or just overlap). At least 10 different fields should be carefully examined for platelet estimation. The average number (e.g., 14) can be multiplied by a factor of 20,000 to arrive at an approximation

---

TABLE 26.5 Summary

Vascular injury → exposes subendothelium and vasoconstriction → platelet adhesion → platelet aggregation → platelet plug formation → consolidation of platelets → fibrin stabilization

---

TABLE 26.6 Laboratory Assessment of Platelet Function

Peripheral blood smear
Platelet count
Template bleeding time
Petechiometer
Platelet aggregation
   Adenosine diphosphate (ADP)
   Epinephrine
   Collagen
   Ristocetin
   Arachidonate
   Thrombin
Platelet lumiaggregation (release)
Platelet antibodies (IgM and IgG)
Platelet membrane glycoproteins (flow cytometry)
Platelet factor IV
(Beta)-thromboglobulin
Thromboxanes

---

of the quantitative platelet concentration. If an average number of 14 platelets is multiplied by 20,000, the approximate platelet concentration would be 280,000 or $280 \times 10^9/L$. Although the estimation of platelets from a blood smear does *not* replace an actual quantitative measurement, it should be done as a cross-check of the quantitative measurement.

Qualitative Assessment of Platelets

If a platelet count is normal but a patient has a suggestive bleeding history, an assessment of platelet function should be conducted. Methods of evaluation (Table 26.6) include bleeding time, aggregating agents, and lumiaggregation.

Bleeding Time With and Without Aspirin

The bleeding time test (see Chapter 24) is an in vivo measurement of platelet adhesion and aggregation on locally injured vascular subendothelium. This test provides an estimate of the integrity of the platelet plug and thereby measures the interaction between the capillaries and platelets. Platelet adhesiveness is the process of the sticking of platelets to the vessel wall, whereas platelet aggregation is the sticking or clumping of platelets to each other. The bleeding time reflects these aspects of platelet function.

As the platelet count drops below $100 \times 10^9/L$, the bleeding time increases progressively from a normal of 3 to 8 minutes to more than 30 minutes. A prolonged bleeding time in a patient with a platelet count above $100 \times 10^9/L$ indicates either impaired platelet function or a defect of subendothelial factor. Results between 8 and 11 minutes are usually not clinically significant. With borderline results, the aspirin tolerance test is often useful and is repeated 2 hours after aspirin challenge.

Clot Retraction

The contractile abilities of platelets also result in the contraction of formed clots (see Chapter 24).

Clot retraction reflects the number and quality of platelets, fibrinogen concentration, fibrinolytic activity, and packed red cell volume. Since the fibrin clot enmeshes the cellular elements of the blood, primarily erythrocytes, the degree of clot retraction is limited to the extent that fibrin contracts by the volume of erythrocytes (hematocrit). Therefore, the smaller the hematocrit, the greater the degree of clot retraction.

The degree of clot retraction is directly proportional to the number of platelets and inversely proportional to the hematocrit and the level of the blood coagulation factor fibrinogen. When clot dissolution (fibrinolysis) is very active, the fibrin clot may be dissolved almost as quickly as it is formed, and clot retraction will be impaired.

Platelet Aggregation

Most platelet aggregation procedures (see Chapter 25) are based on some variation of Born's method. Agents such as ADP, collagen, epinephrine, snake venom, thrombin, and ristocetin can be used to aggregate platelets. The principle of the test is that platelet-rich plasma is treated with a known aggregating agent. If aggregated, cloudiness or turbidity can be measured using a spectrophotometer. Depending on the type of aggregating agent used, a curve that can be used to assess platelet function is obtained.

In vivo, platelets participate in primary hemostasis by first adhering, then aggregating at the site of an injured blood vessel. In vitro, platelet aggregation assays use various platelet activators to identify abnormal platelet function and to monitor antiplatelet drug therapy. ADP, collagen, epinephrine, ristocetin, and arachidonic acid are reagents commonly used to induce platelet aggregation.

The platelet aggregation procedure is performed on a turbidimetric aggregometer as first described by Born. Changes in aggregation are recorded as platelet-rich plasma and aggregating reagents are stirred together in a cuvette. The aggregometer serves as a standardized spectrophotometer. As aggregation proceeds, more light passes through the sample.

Epinephrine is usually used in two doses, as is ADP. A monophasic curve is elicited with ADP. A biphasic curve is usually elicited with epinephrine. Ristocetin and arachidonic acid also usually induce a monophasic curve. Lumiaggregation is an extension of aggregation.

Platelet Adhesion

Platelet adhesion in vivo occurs as platelets attach either to a damaged vessel wall or to each other. Methods of in vitro analysis rely on the adherence of platelets to glass surfaces. The amount of adherence of platelets in a blood sample to a glass surface can be measured by counting the number of platelets before and after exposure to glass beads. The reliability of this methodology has been questioned, therefore, use of the method is not universal.

Antiplatelet Antibody Assays

Antibodies against platelets may appear in the plasma of patients in certain clinical conditions, although it may be difficult to demonstrate these antibodies in cases of immune thrombocytopenia. Available techniques can include complement fixation methods, lysis of chromium 51–labeled platelets, assays of platelet-bound immunoglobulins, and competitive inhibition assays.

BLOOD COAGULATION FACTORS

Bleeding from small blood vessels may be stopped by vasoconstriction and the formation of a platelet plug, but the formation of a clot (thrombus) usually occurs as part of the normal process of hemostasis. The soluble blood coagulation factors are critical components in the formation of a thrombus.

Hepatic cells are the principal site of the synthesis of coagulation factors. However, other cells, such as the endothelial cells, also play an important role in the normal process of hemostasis and thrombosis. Classically, the coagulation factors have been described as reacting in a cascading sequence. Modifications of this sequence are now known to occur as the blood factors interact to form the final insoluble gelatinous thrombus.

The Basic Concepts of Blood Coagulation

Blood coagulation is a sequential process of chemical reactions involving plasma proteins, phospholipids, and calcium ions. Most of the circulating factors (Table 26.7) that participate in the coagulation process are designated by Roman numerals. The activated form of an enzymatic factor appears as a Roman numeral followed by the suffix -a, while the inactive enzymatic factors, zymogens, are indicated by the Roman numeral alone. For example, factor II, prothrombin, is designated as factor II; however, in the active state, it is IIa, thrombin. Nonenzymatic factors have no such designations. It is important to note that the Roman numeric designation does *not* indicate the sequence of reactions in the clotting process. For example, factor X precedes factor II in the coagulation pathway.

Common Characteristics of Coagulation Factors

Proteins that are clotting factors have four characteristics in common. These characteristics are as follows:

1. A deficiency of the factor generally produces a bleeding tendency disorder with the exception of factor XII, prekallikrein (Fletcher factor), and high-molecular-weight kininogen.
2. The physical and chemical characteristics of the factor are known.
3. The synthesis of the factor is independent of other proteins.
4. The factor can be assayed in the laboratory.

In order to develop an understanding of the theory of coagulation as well as the underlying principles of related laboratory procedures, it is helpful to compare the characteristics (Table 26.8) of various coagulation factors. Three groups of factors exist: the fibrinogen group, the prothrombin group, and the contact group.

TABLE 26.7 Proteins in Blood Coagulation

Factor	Name	Alternate Terms
Coagulation Factors		
I	Fibrinogen	
II	Prothrombin	
V	Proaccelerin	Labile factor, Ac globulin
VII	Proconvertin	Stabile factor, SPCA
VIII	Antihemophilic factor (AHF)	Antihemophilic globulin (AHG), antihemophilic factor A
IX	Plasma thromboplastin component (PTC)	Christmas factor, antihemophilic factor B
X	Stuart factor	Stuart-Prower factor
XI	Plasma thromboplastin antecedent	PTA, antihemophilic factor C
XII	Hageman factor	Glass or contact factor
XIII	Fibrin stabilizing factor	FSF
Others	Prekallikrein	Fletcher factor
	High-molecular-weight (HMW) kininogen	HMW kininogen, Fitzgerald factor
	von Willebrand factor	Factor VIII–related antigen
	Fibronectin	
	Antithrombin III	
	Heparin cofactor II	
	Protein C	
	Protein S	

The fibrinogen group consists of factors I, V, VIII, and XIII. These factors are consumed during the process of coagulation. Factors V and VIII are known to decrease during blood storage in vitro. These factors are known to increase during pregnancy, in the presence of conditions of inflammation, and subsequent to the use of oral contraceptive drugs.

The **prothrombin group** consists of factors II, VII, IX, and X. All of these factors are dependent on vitamin K during their synthesis. Vitamin K is available to the body through dietary sources and intestinal bacterial production. This group is inhibited by warfarin. The group is considered to be stable and remains well preserved in stored plasma.

The **contact group** consists of factors XI, XII, prekallikrein (Fletcher factor), and high-molecular-weight kininogen (Fitzgerald factor). These factors are involved in the intrinsic coagulation pathway. They are moderately stable and are not consumed during coagulation.

TABLE 26.8 Characteristics of Coagulation Factors

Characteristic	Group		
	I[a]	II[b]	III[c]
Molecular weight	High	Low	?
Plasma	Present	Present	Present
Serum	Absent	Present, except II	Present
Absorption (BaSO$_4$)	No	Yes	None or partial
Destruction	Thrombin, plasmin		
Stability	Factors V, VIII unstable	Heat-stable	Stable
Increase	Inflammation, pregnancy, stress and fear, oral contraceptives	Pregnancy, oral contraceptives	
Decrease		Oral anticoagulants	

[a]Group I: fibrinogen group (factors I, V, VIII, XIII).

[b]Group II: prothrombin group (factors II, VII, IX, X).

[c]Group III: contact group (factors XI, XII, Fletcher factor, Fitzgerald factor).

Characteristics of Individual Factors

Each of the individual coagulation factors has some unique characteristics. These characteristics include the following.

Factor I (Fibrinogen)

Fibrinogen is a large, stable globulin protein (mol wt 341,000). It is the precursor of fibrin, which forms the resulting clot. When fibrinogen is exposed to thrombin, two peptides split from the fibrinogen molecule, leaving a fibrin monomer. These monomers aggregate together to form the final polymerized fibrin clot product.

$$\text{Fibrinogen—thrombin} \rightarrow \text{fibrin monomers} \longrightarrow \text{fibrin clot}$$

Factor II (Prothrombin)

Prothrombin is a stable protein (mol wt 63,000). In the presence of ionized calcium, prothrombin is converted to thrombin by the enzymatic action of thromboplastin from both extrinsic and intrinsic sources. Prothrombin has a half-life of almost 3 days with 70% consumption during clotting.

$$\text{Prothrombin} + \text{Ca}^{2+}\text{—extrinsic or intrinsic thromboplastin} \rightarrow \text{thrombin}$$

Factor IIa (Thrombin)

Thrombin (mol wt 40,000) is the activated form of prothrombin, which is normally found as an inert precursor in the circulation. This proteolytic enzyme, which interacts with fibrinogen, is also a potent platelet-aggregating substance. A large quantity of thrombin is consumed during the process of converting fibrinogen to fibrin. A unit of thrombin will coagulate 1 mL of a standard fibrinogen solution in 15 seconds at 28°C.

$$\text{Fibrinogen—thrombin} \rightarrow \text{fibrin monomer} + \text{peptides}$$

Tissue Thromboplastin (Formerly Factor III)

Tissue thromboplastin is the term given to any nonplasma substance containing lipoprotein complex from tissues. These tissues can be from the brain, lung, vascular endothelium, liver, placenta, or kidneys; these tissue types are capable of converting prothrombin to thrombin.

Ionized Calcium (Formerly Factor IV)

The term *ionized calcium* has replaced the term factor IV. Ionized calcium is necessary for the activation of thromboplastin, and for conversion of prothrombin to thrombin. Ionized calcium is the physiologically active form of calcium in the human body and only small amounts are needed for blood coagulation. A calcium deficiency would not be expressed as a coagulation dysfunction, except in cases of massive transfusion.

Factor V (Proaccelerin)

Factor V is an extremely labile globulin protein. It deteriorates rapidly, having a half-life of 16 hours. Factor V is consumed in the clotting process and is essential to the later stages of thromboplastin formation.

Factor VII (Proconvertin)

Factor VII, a beta globulin, is not an essential component of the intrinsic thromboplastin-generating mechanism. It is not destroyed or consumed in clotting and is found in both plasma and serum, even in serum left at room temperature for up to 3 days. The action of factor VII is the activation of tissue thromboplastin and the acceleration of the production of thrombin from prothrombin. This factor is reduced by vitamin K antagonists.

Factor VIII (Antihemophilic Factor)

This factor is consumed during the clotting process and is not found in serum. Factor VIII is extremely labile, with a 50% loss within 12 hours at 4°C in vitro and a similar 50% loss in vivo within 8 to 12 hours after transfusion.

Factor VIII can be subdivided into various functional components. The total molecule, consisting of both a high-molecular-weight fraction and a low-molecular-weight fraction, is described by the nomenclature VIII/vWF. Factor VII/vWF consists of two major moieties. The high-molecular-weight moiety consists of the vWF, VIIIR:RCo, and VIIIR:Ag components. The low-molecular-weight moiety consists of the VIII:C and VIIIC:Ag components.

Factor VIII:C has procoagulant activity as measured by clotting assay techniques. Factor VIII/vWF multimers form ionic bonds with factor VIII:C and transport VIII:C in the circulation.

Factor VIIIC:Ag is a procoagulant antigen as measured by immunological techniques using antibodies for factor VIII:C. Factor VIIIR:Ag is a related factor VIII antigen that has been identified using immunological techniques employing heterologous antibodies to VIII/vWF.

Factor VIIIR:RCo demonstrates ristocetin-cofactor activity, which is required for the aggregation of human platelets induced by the antibiotic ristocetin.

Factor VIII/vWF is factor VIII—von Willebrand factor. Endothelial cells are known to synthesize and secrete VIII/vWF multimers.

Factor IX (Plasma Thromboplastin Component)

Factor IX is a stable protein factor that is neither consumed during clotting nor destroyed by aging at 4°C for 2 weeks. It is an essential component of the intrinsic thromboplastin-generating system, where it influences the amount rather than the rate of thromboplastin formation.

Factor X (Stuart Factor)

This alpha globulin is a relatively stable factor that is not consumed during clotting. Together with factor V, factor X in the presence of calcium ions forms the final common pathway through which the products of both the extrinsic and intrinsic thromboplastin-generating systems merge to form the ultimate thromboplastin that converts prothrombin to thrombin. The activity of factor X appears to be related to factor VII.

Factor XI (Plasma Thromboplastin Antecedent)

Factor XI, a beta globulin, can be found in serum because it is only partially consumed during the clotting process.

This factor is essential to the intrinsic thromboplastin-generating mechanism.

Factor XII (Hageman Factor)

Factor XII is a stable factor that is not consumed during the coagulation process. Adsorption of factor XII and kininogen (with bound prekallikrein and factor XI) to negatively charged surfaces such as glass or subendothelium (collagen) exposed by blood vessel injury initiates the intrinsic coagulation pathway. Surface absorption alters and partially activates factor XII to factor XIIa by exposing an active enzyme (protease) site. Because of a feedback mechanism, kallikrein (activated Fletcher factor) cleaves partially activated factor XIIa molecules adsorbed onto the subendothelium to produce a more kinetically effective form of XIIa.

Factor XIII (Fibrin-Stabilizing Factor)

Fibrin-stabilizing factor in the presence of ionized calcium produces a stabilized fibrin clot.

Fine fibrin clots—factor XIII + calcium ions
$\rightarrow$ stable fibrin clot

The Mechanism of Coagulation

Many chemical reactions occur in hemostasis, from the initial stimulus that triggered bleeding to the final formation of a stable clot. In order to more easily understand the process, portions of the normal coagulation sequence are artificially segregated into smaller sections such as the extrinsic and intrinsic pathways. These pathways are not actual physiological pathways of hemostasis, but allow for the grouping of factor defects and the focusing of laboratory assays.

The initiation of the coagulation process may occur via one of two pathways: the extrinsic pathway and the intrinsic pathway. Regardless of the initiating pathway, the two pathways converge into a final common pathway. The outcome of this process is the conversion of circulating insoluble coagulation factors into a gelatinous fibrin clot with entrapped blood cells, a blood clot. As repair of damaged tissue takes place, the clot is lysed and the particulate matter is removed by the mononuclear phagocytic system.

Coagulation Pathways

Initiation of clotting begins with either the extrinsic or the intrinsic pathway. Factor X activation is the point of convergence. Factor X can be activated by either of the two pathways and subsequently catalyzes the conversion of prothrombin to thrombin.

The Extrinsic Coagulation Pathway

The extrinsic pathway (Fig. 26.5) is initiated by the entry of tissue thromboplastin into the circulating blood. Tissue thromboplastin is derived from phospholipoproteins and organelle membranes from disrupted tissue cells. These membrane lipoproteins, termed **tissue factors,** are normally extrinsic to the circulation. Platelet phospholipids are not necessary for activation of the extrinsic pathway because tissue factor supplies its own phospholipids.

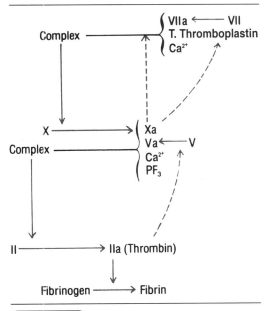

FIGURE 26.5 Extrinsic pathway of coagulation. PF$_3$ = platelet factors 3. (From "Hemostasis Pathways," Dade Thromboplastin IS. Miami: Baxter Diagnostics, 1990, p. 4.)

Factor VII binds to these phospholipids in the tissue cell membranes and is activated to factor VIIa, a potent enzyme capable of activating factor X to Xa in the presence of ionized calcium. The activity of the tissue factor–factor VII complex seems to be largely dependent on the concentration of tissue thromboplastin. The proteolytic cleavage of factor VIIa by factor Xa results in inactivation of factor VIIa. Factor VII participates *only* in the extrinsic pathway. Membranes that enter the circulation also provide a surface for the attachment and activation of factors II and V. The final step is the conversion of fibrinogen to fibrin by thrombin.

The Intrinsic Coagulation Pathway

The intrinsic pathway (Fig. 26.6) involves the contact activation factors prekallikrein, high-molecular-weight kininogen, factor XII, and factor XI. These factors interact on a surface to activate factor IX to IXa. Factor IXa reacts with factor VIII, PF 3, and calcium to activate factor X to Xa. In the presence of factor V, factor Xa activates prothrombin (factor II) to thrombin, which in turn converts fibrinogen to fibrin.

Strong negatively charged solids that can participate in the activation of factor XII include glass and kaolin in vitro, and elastin, collagen, platelet surfaces, kallikrein, plasmin, and high-molecular-weight kininogen in vivo. Collagen exposed by blood vessel injury greatly influences the rate of reaction.

Factor XIIA interacts in a feedback loop to convert prekallikrein to additional kallikrein. This reaction is facilitated by the action of high-molecular-weight kininogen. In the absence of prekallikrein, factor XIIA is generated more slowly.

Ionized calcium plays an important role in the activation of certain coagulation factors in the intrinsic pathway. Calcium is not required for the activation of factor XII, prekalli-

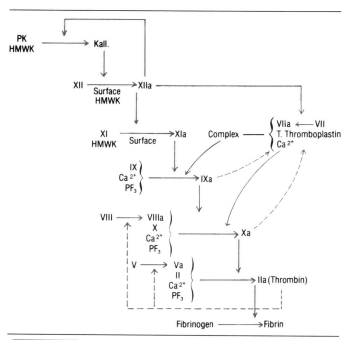

FIGURE 26.6 Intrinsic pathway of coagulation. PK HMWK = prekallikrein, high-molecular-weight kinonogen; Kall. = kallikrein; PF$_3$ = platelet factor 3. (From C. R. Hillman, "The Intrinsic Clotting System." In Techniques for One-Stage Factor VIII Assay. Miami: Baxter Healthcare, 1989, p. 21.)

krein, or factor XI, but it is necessary for the activation of factor IX by factor XIa.

Final Common Pathway

Once factor X is activated to Xa, the extrinsic and intrinsic pathways enter a common pathway. Factor II, prothrombin, is activated to thrombin (factor IIa), which normally circulates in the blood as an inactive factor.

Following the activation of factor Xa, it remains platelet-bound and activates factor V. The complex of factors Xa and Va on the platelet surface is formed near platelet-bound factor II molecules. In turn, the platelet-bound Xa/Va complex cleaves factor II into thrombin, factor IIa. The stage is accelerated by factor V and ionized calcium.

Fibrin Formation

Clotting is the visible result of the conversion of plasma fibrinogen into a stable fibrin clot. Thrombin plays a major role in converting factor XIII to XIIIa and in converting fibrinogen to fibrin. Fibrin formation occurs in three phases: proteolysis, polymerization, and stabilization.

Initially, thrombin, a protease enzyme, cleaves fibrinogen, which results in a fibrin monomer, fibrinopeptide A, and fibrinopeptide B fragments. In the second step, the fibrin monomers spontaneously polymerize end-to-end due to hydrogen bonding. Finally, the fibrin monomers are linked covalently by factor XIIIa into fibrin polymers. These polymers form a meshy network and the final fibrin solution is converted to a gel when more than 25% of the fibrinogen is converted to fibrin.

Factor XIII is converted to the active form, factor XIIIa, in two steps. In the first step, thrombin cleaves a peptide from each of the two alpha chains of factor XIII with formation of an inactive intermediate form of factor XIII. In the second step, calcium ions cause factor XIII to dissociate forming factor XIIIa.

Fibrinogen is normally present in the plasma as a soluble molecule. Subsequent to the action of thrombin, fibrinogen is transformed into fibrin, an insoluble gel. This conversion of fibrinogen to a cross-linked gel occurs in several stages.

Factor XIIIa introduces peptide bonds within the polymerized fibrin network. This cross-linking makes the fibrin more elastic and less susceptible to lysis by fibrinolytic agents.

Fibrin forms a loose covering over the injured area, reinforces the platelet plug, and closes off the wound. After a short period of time, the clot begins to retract and becomes smaller and more dense. This retraction process is thought to be due to the action of platelets trapped along with erythrocytes and leukocytes in the clot. As the fibrin filaments gather around the aggregated platelets, the platelets send out cytoplasmic processes that attach to the fibrin and pull the fibers closer together. When a clot forms in a test tube, clot retraction can be observed (refer to the procedure in Chapter 24). The fluid squeezed from this clot is **serum.**

Fibrinolysis

Fibrin clots are temporary structures that seal off a damaged area until healing can take place. Fibrinolysis is the physiological process that removes insoluble fibrin deposits by enzymatic digestion of the stabilized fibrin polymers. As healing occurs, the clots themselves are dissolved by plasmin. Plasmin digests fibrin and fibrinogen by hydrolysis to produce progressively smaller fragments. This slow-acting process gradually dissolves away the clot as tissue repair is taking place, with the particulate matter being phagocytized by the mononuclear phagocytic system.

Inactive **plasminogen** circulates in the plasma until an injury occurs. The activators of plasminogen consist of endogenous and exogenous groups (Table 26.9). Plasminogen activation to plasmin is the result of the activity of a number of proteolytic enzymes. These enzymes, the kinases, are referred to as the **plasminogen activators.** Plasminogen activators are found in various sites, such as the vascular endothelium or lysosomal granules, and biological fluids. At least

TABLE 26.9 Components of the Plasma Fibrinolytic System

Plasminogen activators
  Endogenous
    Tissue-type plasminogen activator (tPA)
    Urokinase
  Exogenous
    Streptokinase
    Acyl-plasminogen streptokinase activator complex (APSAC)
Inhibitors
  Alpha-2 plasmin inhibitor
  Tissue plasminogen activator inhibitor

two forms of tissue activators have been described: those that seem related to urokinase, a urinary activator of plasminogen, and those unrelated to urokinase. The activators unrelated to urokinase include thrombin, bacterial products such as streptokinase from beta-hemolytic streptococci, and staphylokinase. Plasma activators of plasminogen include plasma kallikrein, activated plasma thromboplastin antecedents (factor XI) and activated Hageman factor (factor XIIa).

It is estimated that 1.5 million Americans suffer a heart attack each year. Most are caused by clots that cut off blood flow to the heart muscle. Tissue-type plasminogen activator (tPA) is present in minute quantities in the vascular endothelium. When tPA encounters a blood clot, tPA transforms plasminogen to plasmin, and plasmin then degrades the clot's fibrin network. As a result of biotechnology (recombinant DNA), a synthetic tissue-type plasminogen has been developed and is used clinically to treat postmyocardial infarction and pulmonary emboli. tPA is considered by many to be more specific and twice as effective as streptokinase in dissolving clots, and has exhibited fewer side effects.

Through its lysis of fibrin or fibrinogen, plasmin is responsible for forming degradation or fibrin split products consisting of intermediate fragments X and Y, and fragments D and E. These fragments exert an antithrombin effect, inhibit the hemostasis system through interference with fibrin monomer polymerization, and interfere with platelet aggregation.

Small amounts of plasmin become trapped in the clot. The specificity of plasmin ensures that clot dissolution occurs without widespread proteolysis of other proteins. Plasmin also activates the complement system; liberates kinins from kininogen; and can hydrolyze coagulation factors V, VIII, and XII. Further clot formation is impeded by antiplasmins and naturally occurring inhibitors, some of which prevent the activation of plasminogen. The naturally occurring inhibitors include antithrombin III, alpha-2 macroglobulin inhibitor, and alpha-1 antitrypsin. Plasmin is not normally found in plasma because it is neutralized by an excess of inhibitors.

Laboratory Assessment of Blood Coagulation Factors

The intrinsic and extrinsic pathways are now thought to function in an interrelated manner in vivo, and previously established in vitro methods are valid to screen for abnormalities.

A variety of laboratory procedures (see Chapter 24) are of value in assessing coagulation factors. General procedures include the activated partial thromboplastin time (APTT), the prothrombin time (PT), the thrombin time, and quantitative fibrinogen concentration assay. More specialized or classic procedures include the ethanol gelation test, the euglobulin lysis test, the fibrin split products test, the Hicks-Pitney modification of the thromboplastin generation time test, the partial thromboplastin substitution test, the plasma recalcification test, protamine sulfate assays, the prothrombin consumption time test, the thromboplastin generation test (TGT), specific factor assays, and various tests for inhibitors and circulating anticoagulants. Preoperative screening tests usually include a bleeding time, platelet count, APTT, and PT.

The Activated Partial Thromboplastin Time

The **APTT** procedure measures the time required to generate thrombin and fibrin polymers via the intrinsic and common pathway. Although a partial thromboplastin time test can be performed, contact factors can be activated through the addition of substances such as kaolin. In the APTT, calcium ions and phospholipids that substitute for platelet phospholipids are added to blood plasma. In vitro, the activation of factor XII to XIIa, prekallikrein to kallikrein, and factor XI to XIa occurs on the negatively charged glass surface. The generation of fibrin is the end point.

The APTT assay reflects the activity of prekallikrein, high-molecular-weight kininogen, and factors XII, XI, IX, VIII, X, V, II, and I. APTT may be prolonged due to a factor decrease, such as fibrinogen (factor I), or the presence of circulating anticoagulants. The normal APTT is less than 35 seconds (depending on the activator used).

Prothrombin Time

The PT procedure evaluates the generation of thrombin and the formation of fibrin via the extrinsic and common pathway. With calcium ions present, the tissue thromboplastin forms complexes with and activates factor VII. This provides surfaces for the attachment and activation of factors X, V, and II. Thromboplastin, derived from tissues that supply phospholipoprotein, and calcium are added to the blood plasma. The time required for the fibrin clot to form is measured.

Normal values range from 10 to 13 seconds. Prolonged results can indicate a deficiency of one or more factors in the extrinsic pathway: factors VII, X, V, and II or I. Prolonged values will be seen if an oral anticoagulant such as coumarin or a coumarin-containing substance (e.g., rat poison) is ingested.

International Normalized Ratio (INR)

INR values are preferable to the PT because different thromboplastin reagents have different sensitivities to warfarin-induced changes in levels of clotting factors. The use of the INR corrects for most, but not all, of reagent differences, expressed as the ISI, the international sensitivity index (a correction factor assigned by the manufacturer), of the thromboplastin reagent.

The INR is not without problems. A major problem is that the concept and reasons for use are poorly understood and the value is generally misused. Some ISI values reported by manufacturers have been found to be inaccurate. In fact, the ISI values reported by manufacturers vary markedly, depending on the instrument used to perform the PT.

Oral Anticoagulants

Oral anticoagulants are of two types: the warfarins and the indanedione derivatives. Indanedione derivatives no longer are generally used but remain useful for individuals sensitive to the warfarin drugs.

Warfarin drugs are vitamin K antagonists that interfere with the normal synthesis of factors II, VII, IX, and X and proteins C and S. These drugs cause incomplete coagulation because they lack calcium-binding sites and cannot form enzyme substrate complexes. Thus, these factors are unable to function as procoagulants or anticoagulants.

Biological activity is markedly decreased, as revealed by the prothrombin time. The onset of action of most warfarin derivatives is between 8 and 12 hours. The maximum effect occurs in approximately 36 hours and the duration of action is approximately 72 hours.

The prothrombin time, utilized to adjust the dose of oral anticoagulation, should be reported according to the INR, not the prothrombin time ratio or the prothrombin time expressed in seconds. The INR is essentially a "corrected" prothrombin time that adjusts for the several dozen assays used in North America and Europe.

$$INR = \frac{PT \ patient^{ISI}}{PT \ normal}$$

When the INR is used to guide anticoagulant therapy, there are fewer bleeding events compared with use of the prothrombin time ratio. There is also a trend toward fewer thromboembolic complications. The target INR for pulmonary embolism treatment is 3.0, for the duration of anticoagulation. Periods of treatment have also lengthened: first-time deep venous thrombosis (DVT) patients are treated for 3 to 6 months, and first-time pulmonary embolism (PE) patients are treated for 6 to 12 months with Coumadin. Anticoagulation is called treatment, but it really constitutes secondary prevention of recurrent PE.

Three regimens are currently used for oral anticoagulant therapy: low-intensity, fixed-dose therapy (usually 1.0 to 2.0 mg/day); moderate-intensity therapy (PT ratio of approximately 1.3 to 1.5, INR of 2.0 to 3.0); and high-intensity therapy (PT ratio of approximately 1.5 to 1.8, INR of 2.5 to 3.5). INR is used only for patients receiving stable, orally administered anticoagulant therapy. It does not substantially contribute to the diagnosis or the treatment of patients whose PT is prolonged for other reasons.

Heparin

Heparin anticoagulation is the mainstay of immediate therapy for acute PE. Heparin helps prevent new thrombus formation and buys time for endogenous fibrinolytic mechanisms to lyse the clot. Heparin can cause bleeding, thrombocytopenia, and osteopenia. Before initiating heparin, patients should be screened for clinical evidence of active bleeding. The baseline laboratory evaluation should include CBC, platelets, PTT, PT, stool analysis for occult blood, and urine dipstick for hematuria.

Low-molecular-weight heparin (LMWH), a new family of compounds produced by the controlled fragmentation of heparin, is available for clinical use. These heparins react with the regulatory protein antithrombin III to inhibit activated factor X (factor Xa), but not thrombin (factor IIa). Unfractionated heparin, by contrast, is active against both procoagulants. LMWH is less capable than standard heparin of activating resting platelets so that they release platelet factor 4, and it binds less well to platelet factor 4. Newly developed solid-phase assays that use complexes of heparin and platelet factor 4 as targets for the detection of heparin-induced antibodies are much more sensitive than the serotonin-release test.

New Thromboplastins

The new types of thromboplastins for measuring the PT are mixtures of phospholipids and recombinantly derived human tissue factor. Because the new thromboplastins are more sensitive (typical ISI = 1.0) than the traditional North American ones (ISIs = 1.8 to 3.0), the PTs for patients with inherited or acquired deficiencies of coagulation factors will be much more prolonged with use of the new reagents, although normal values may change minimally. However, the therapeutic range (in seconds) of the PTs in patients receiving orally administered anticoagulant agents is wider with the sensitive thromboplastins than with the traditional ones. The INR, however, will be the same, as will the recommended ranges of the INR for intensity of anticoagulation.

Recombinant thromboplastin has the following advantages:

1. It is made from a human protein, not from the protein of a different species.
2. The material is pure, and the concentration can be readily adjusted, unlike currently available rabbit brain thromboplastins. Adjustment will minimize variation between different lots of the reagent, thus, the normal and therapeutic ranges of the PT will remain the same.
3. The reagent is free of contamination with noxious viruses because it is a recombinant product.
4. When the ISI is approximately 1.0, the PTs will be the same as those obtained with use of the WHO reference thromboplastin. Therefore, the PT ratio (PT of patient/mean normal PT) will be the same as the INR.
5. The new reagents are more sensitive to mild deficiencies of coagulation factors than are the traditional thromboplastins. Patients with hemostatically adequate levels of coagulation factors II, V, VII, or X (30% to 40% of mean normal activity) will have INRs of 1.4 or less.

Thrombin Time

The thrombin time test determines the rate of thrombin-induced cleavage of fibrinogen to fibrin monomers and the subsequent polymerization of hydrogen-bonded fibrin polymers. The normal value is less than 20 seconds. Prolonged results will be seen if the fibrinogen concentration is less than 100 mg/dL. Abnormal results will also be encountered in the presence of thrombin inhibitors or substances that interfere with fibrin formation (e.g., heparin, fibrin degradation products), or high concentrations of immunoglobulins that interfere with fibrin monomer polymerization such as in cases of multiple myeloma.

Fibrinogen Levels

Fibrinogen assays are useful in detecting deficiencies of fibrinogen and alterations in the conversion of fibrinogen to fibrin. The normal value of 200 to 400 mg/dL may be decreased in liver disease or the consumption of fibrinogen owing to accelerated intravascular clotting. Fibrinogen titers may be useful. The normal titer of fibrinogen is 1:128 to 1:256; a titer below 1:64 is abnormal.

Normal Protective Mechanisms Against Thrombosis

In the blood circulation, the predisposition to thrombosis depends on the balance between procoagulant and anticoagulant factors. Several important biological activities normally protect the body against thrombosis. These activities include the following:

1. The normal flow of blood
2. The removal of activated clotting factors and particulate material
3. Natural anticoagulant systems known to be operative in vivo:
    A. Antithrombin III (AT-III)
    B. Heparin cofactor II (HC-II)
    C. Protein C and its cofactor, protein S
4. Cellular regulators

The Normal Blood Flow

The normal flow of blood prevents the accumulation of procoagulant material. This mechanism reduces the chance of local fibrin formation.

Removal of Activated Clotting Factors and Particulate Material

Another normal mechanism against inappropriate thrombosis is the removal from the blood of activated clotting factors by hepatocytes. This process, along with the naturally occurring inhibitors, limits intravascular clotting and fibrinolysis by inactivation of such factors as XIa, IXa, Xa, and IIa. Removal of particulate material by the cells of the mononuclear phagocytic system is also important in preventing the initiation of coagulation.

The Natural Anticoagulant Systems

The in vivo existence of natural anticoagulant systems is essential to prevent thrombosis. These natural anticoagulant systems include antithrombin III, heparin cofactor II, and protein C and its cofactor, protein S. AT-III and HC-II are serine-protease inhibitors. When activated, protein C is capable of degrading activated factors V (Va) and VIII (VIIIa) in the presence of the cofactor protein S.

Antithrombin III

Antithrombin III (AT-III) is considered the major inhibitor of coagulation. AT-III is one of the "serpin" superfamily of *serine proteinase inhibitors* that also includes alpha-1 antitrypsin, C1 inhibitor, alpha-2 antiplasmin, heparin cofactor II, and plasminogen activator inhibitor.

AT-III is an alpha-2 globulin glycoprotein that circulates in the plasma. It is synthesized by hepatocytes, megakaryocytes, and vascular endothelium. AT-III is the principal phys-

iological inhibitor of thrombin that slowly and irreversibly inhibits thrombin by forming a stable one-to-one complex with thrombin. This complex is devoid of any thrombotic or antithrombotic activity. AT-III is also the principal physiological inhibitor of factor Xa. In addition, it is known to inhibit factors IXa, XIa, and XIIa.

AT-III is normally a slow inhibitor, but in the presence of heparin it rapidly inhibits activated serine proteases such as activated factors II, IX, X, XI, and XII. The binding of AT-III and thrombin is increased 1000-fold or greater in the presence of heparin. Initially, AT-III was designated heparin cofactor. The enhancement of the activity of AT-III is considered to be the primary mechanism of heparin's anticoagulation effects. Normally, AT-III accounts for the majority of the thrombin inhibitory activity in plasma. The concentration of AT-III at the endothelial surface is rate-limiting for inactivation of thrombin and factor Xa when the plasma level of AT-III falls below 50%.

AT-III is rapidly removed from the circulation following one-to-one binding with an activated coagulation factor. The half-life of AT-III in plasma is approximately 70 hours.

Heparin Cofactor

Heparin is produced endogenously by mast cells, and heparin-like molecules are found in the endothelium. Two heparin-dependent thrombin inhibitors are present in human plasma: AT-III heparin cofactor and heparin cofactor II, previously referred to as heparin cofactor A. The inhibitory activity of heparin cofactor II is accelerated by heparin. The inhibition of thrombin by heparin cofactor II is not limited to the activity of thrombin or fibrinogen; also inhibited are thrombin-induced platelet aggregation and release. In addition to thrombin, heparin cofactor II inhibits chymotrypsin. It does not significantly inhibit blood coagulation factors IXa, Xa, and XIa or plasmin.

Protein C

Protein C and protein S are involved in one of the major natural anticoagulation systems in the body. Deficiency and/or alteration in either protein has been clearly associated with predisposition to thrombosis.

Protein C, a vitamin K–dependent plasma protein **synthesized in the liver**, represents a natural anticoagulant formed in response to thrombin generation. Protein C circulates in the blood as a **zymogen,** an inactive precursor form. The majority of plasma protein C exists as a two-chain zymogen (mol wt 62,000) before activation. A single-chain form and a minor beta form have also been demonstrated.

Protein C requires proteolytic cleavage to become active. It is converted by thrombin to its enzymatically active form. All forms can be activated. Thrombin activates protein C in the presence of the endothelial cell–associated lipoprotein cofactor **thrombomodulin.** This reaction converts the zymogen form into the serine protease, activated protein C **(APC).** Thrombin activation of PC is also enhanced by activated factor V, though considerably less efficiently.

The protein C anticoagulant pathway is recognized as a major blood coagulation regulatory mechanism. Activated protein C is a potent plasma anticoagulant. Once activated, protein C (APC), in the presence of its cofactor protein S (S), proteolytically cleaves factors Va (V-Vi) and VIIIa (VIII-VIIIi). This cleavage dramatically decreases the conversion of prothrombin to thrombin and is one of the regulatory feedback mechanisms of coagulation. Thrombin thus acts not only as a procoagulant, but also activates natural anticoagulation.

Protein C requires a second vitamin K–dependent factor, protein S, to function as an anticoagulant. APC is also believed to promote fibrinolysis by neutralizing the inhibitor of tissue plasminogen activator (TPA). TPA inhibitor (TPA-I) functions by inhibiting TPA, an enzyme responsible for the conversion of plasminogen to plasmin.

Protein C is involved in each stage of the anticoagulant pathway. This pathway can be divided into three stages:

1. Protein C activation
2. Expression of activated protein C anticoagulant activity
3. Inhibition of activated protein C

Protein C can be activated by thrombin, but the rate of activation is too slow to be physiologically relevant. Thrombomodulin (Table 26.10) is expressed in a functional form on the surface of the vascular endothelium. Rapid protein C activation occurs when thrombin binds to thrombomodulin. The interaction of thrombin with thrombomodulin is characterized by the formation of a reversible, high-affinity complex between thrombin and thrombomodulin. Protein C is inhibited slowly in human plasma. An identified plasma protease inhibitor may be the major mechanism for the clearance of activated protein C, but it has been demonstrated to have a half-life of approximately 8 minutes. Direct cell-mediated clearance of activated protein C cannot be excluded as an important secondary mechanism.

The normal plasma concentration of protein C is 4 to 5 μg/mL. Many cases of familial thrombotic disease (e.g., deep venous thrombosis) associated with decreased levels of protein C have been described in the last decade. In addition, their production is impaired in vitamin K deficiency, liver disease, and warfarin therapy.

Oral anticoagulants can reduce the levels of protein C and protein S. Protein C levels decrease dramatically in patients with DIC. Patients with impaired liver function or those in a postoperative period may also experience decreased levels of protein C.

Laboratory Findings

The ability to detect decreased protein C activity depends on the type of assay used (Table 26.11). Plasma is evaluated for lupus anticoagulant (LA) prior to performing the protein C assay, to be sure that LA is not the cause of thrombosis. The plasma concentration of purified protein C is 4 μg/mL.

Laboratory diagnosis of protein C and protein S deficiency involves functional and antigenic assays. Diagnosis of a deficiency is best made using functional assays for screening and a combination of functional and antigenic assays for confirmation and characterization of the deficiency.

Protein C Testing

Functional protein C assays can be either clot-based or chromogenic. The clot-based method involves a snake venom that specifically activates protein C. The resulting activated protein C inhibits factors Va and VIIIa, and thus prolongs the activated partial thromboplastin time (APTT) of a system in which all the coagulation factors are constantly present and in excess.

Chromogenic protein C assay involves the same venom to activate protein C. The quantity of activated protein C formed is measured by its amidolytic activity on a specific chrombenic substrate.

Antigenic protein C can be assessed by ELISA or Laurell technologies, which have been well defined.

Protein S

Protein S is another vitamin K–dependent plasma protein that is an essential cofactor in order for activated protein C to express an anticoagulant effect. Protein S does not require proteolytic modification to function, but it can be regulated by proteolysis.

Protein S circulates to C4b-binding protein (C4b-BP) in two forms, free and bound, in a ratio of 40% free to 60% bound. Only the free protein molecule supports the functional activity. Elevation of C4b-binding protein (which is

---

TABLE 26.10 **Properties of Thrombomodulin**

Molecular weight	~74,000, single chain
Cellular location	Endothelium
Function	Accelerates protein C activation by thrombin
Mechanism	Forms 1:1 complex with thrombin; functions as a cofactor
Role of Ca²⁺ in protein C activation	Ca²⁺ is required
Role of Ca²⁺ in complex formation between thrombin and thrombomodulin	Ca²⁺ is not required
Control of protein C activation	Thrombin can be inhibited by AT-III when bound to thrombomodulin
Other functions of thrombomodulin	Reduces thrombin's ability to clot fibrinogen, activate factor V, and trigger platelet activation
Vitamin K–dependent	No

AT-III = antithromboplastin III.

Source: C. T. Esmon, *The Protein C Anticoagulant Pathway.* Miami: Baxter Healthcare, 1990.

TABLE 26.11 **General Assay Types for Determination of Protein C in Plasma**

Antigenic	Measures amount of material present Does not measure function
Chromogenic	Measures some but not all of the functions
Clotting	Measures all functions of the protein C molecule

an acute-phase reactant protein) results in an acquired decrease of free protein S.

Relevant properties and functions of protein S are summarized in Table 26.12. Basic science research studies suggest that free, functional protein S forms a one-to-one complex with activated protein C on synthetic membrane surfaces, which increases the affinity of activated protein C for membrane surfaces approximately 10-fold.

Protein S increases the rate of inactivation of factor Va by activated protein C by enhancing the binding of activated protein C to phospholipids, thereby stimulating the inactivation of factor Va. Protein S has been found within platelets, suggesting that these cells may also be responsible for limiting coagulation by the protein S-enhanced inactivation of factors Va and VIIIa by activated protein C. Similar interactions occurring in vivo may be localized on the surface of platelets, peripheral blood cells, and endothelial cells. An increase in activated protein C mediated by thrombin necessitates an increase in protein S levels to attain maximum protein C activity.

Protein S Testing

The principle of a protein S functional assay is based on the cofactor activity of protein S, which enhances the anticoagulation action of activated protein C (APC). This enhancement is reflected by the prolongation of the clotting time of a system enriched with factor Va, which is a physiological substrate of APC.

Like antigenic protein C, antigenic protein S can be measured by ELISA or Laurell technologies. More recently, a rapid technology has been developed involving agglutination of antibody-coated microlatex particles. This agglutination is read spectrophotometrically.

Both total and free protein S antigen can be assessed by these techniques. The measurement of free (versus total) forms of protein S is done on 25% polyethylene glycol–treated plasma.

The association of C4b-binding protein and protein S necessitates C4b-binding protein evaluation to exclude acquired free protein S deficiency. C4b-binding protein can be measured by the Laurell technique or microlatex agglutination.

TABLE 26.12 **Protein S Structure, Function, and Regulation**

Protein S structure	Single chain, Mr = 69,000 Accelerate factor Va and factor VIIIa inactivation by activated protein C (functions as a cofactor)
Vitamin K–dependent	Yes
Binds to membranes	Yes: forms a 1:1 complex with activated protein C on membrane surfaces
Forms in plasma	Free and in reversible complex with C4b binding protein
Regulation	Inactivated by thrombin; not active when complexed to C4b binding protein

Source: T. Esmon, *The Protein C Anticoagulant Pathway.* Miami: Baxter Healthcare, 1990.

Cellular Regulators

Cellular activities related to thrombosis are becoming recognized as essential to the maintenance of hemostasis and thrombosis.

Cellular Proteases

Plasma possesses, in addition to plasmin, another powerful mechanism to limit the formation or spread of clotting and the reliquification of clots. This mechanism consists of the cellular proteases derived from the lysosomes of granulocytes that may be trapped within a thrombus. These proteases block the activation or action of plasmin. Of particular interest is alpha-2 plasmin inhibitor, which rapidly neutralizes the fibrinolytic properties of plasmin.

Cells That Regulate Coagulation

Synthesis of blood coagulation proteins was once thought to be the domain of the hepatic cells; however, it is now known that other cells are capable of synthesizing some of the coagulation factors and cofactors. Monocytes and macrophages have been demonstrated to synthesize factor VII. Platelets and endothelial cells are now known to be the principal components in the initiation, propagation, and suppression of hemostasis and thrombosis.

Platelets store and release high-molecular-weight kininogen, vWF, and factor V, all of which are involved in clot formation. Endothelial cells are known to synthesize vWF, factor VIII, factor V, high-molecular-weight kininogen, and protein S.

The production of protein S cofactor by endothelial cells is believed to play a significant regulatory role in the initiation, propagation, and suppression of hemostasis and thrombosis. Endothelial cells synthesize and secrete protein S and internalize this molecule in a dynamic manner. Once low levels of activated protein C are formed by thrombin on the endothelial surface, it may be in proximity to protein S (receptor), resulting in the formation of an active, stable inactivator complex for factors VIIIa and Va.

SUMMARY

Blood Vasculature: Structure and Function

Arteries have the thickest walls of the vascular system. Veins are larger and have a more irregular lumen than the arteries. In comparison to arteries, veins are relatively thin-walled with a weaker middle coat. Arterioles are the microscopic continuation of arteries. Microscopically sized veins are referred to as venules. Venules connect the capillaries to the veins. Blood passes from the arterial to the venous system via the capillaries. Capillaries are the thinnest-walled and most numerous of the blood vessels.

Vascular injury to a large or medium-size artery or vein requires rapid surgical intervention in order to prevent exsanguination. When a smaller blood vessel is injured, contraction occurs in order to control bleeding. This contraction of the blood vessel wall is called **vasoconstriction.**

The endothelium is involved in the metabolism and clearance of molecules such as serotonin, angiotensin, and bradykinin that affect blood pressure regulation, the movement of fluid across the endothelium, and inflammation. With respect to blood coagulation, one of the basic characteristics of normal, intact endothelium is its nonreactivity with platelets and inability to initiate surface contact activation of clotting factor XII. Endothelin-1 is the only family member produced in endothelial cells. Endothelin-2 has no unique physiological functions, as compared with endothelin-1. Endothelin-3, like endothelin-1, circulates in the plasma, but its source is not known. Endothelium is highly active metabolically and is involved in the clotting process by producing or storing clotting components. It is also rich with plasminogen activator, which, if appropriately stimulated, is released and activates plasminogen, which ensures rapid lysis of fibrin clots. Additionally, the endothelium elaborates prostacyclin, which is synthesized by the endothelium from prostaglandin precursors and strongly inhibits platelet aggregation and adhesion.

Minimal interactions leading to platelet activation or clot formation occur between the circulating blood and intact endothelial surfaces. However, disrupted endothelial cells release thromboplastic substances that can initiate coagulation. Collagen, in particular, initiates contact activation of factor XII, thereby initiating blood coagulation. Disruption of the endothelium directly activates all four components of hemostasis.

The Megakaryocytic Cell Series

Mature **platelets (thrombocytes),** metabolically active cell fragments, are the second critical component in the maintenance of hemostasis. These anuclear cells circulate in the peripheral blood after being produced from the cytoplasm of bone marrow **megakaryocytes,** the largest cells found in the bone marrow.

Bone marrow megakaryocytes are derived from pluripotential stem cells. The sequence of development from megakaryocytes to platelets is thought to progress from the proliferation of progenitors to polyploidization, that is, nuclear endoreduplication, and finally to cytoplasmic maturation and the formation of platelets.

Platelet Kinetics, Life Span, and Normal Values

An average megakaryocyte produces about 1000 to 2000 platelets. Marrow transit time, or the maturation period of the megakaryocyte, is about 5 days.

It is believed that platelets initially enter the spleen where they remain for 2 days. Following this period, platelets are in either the circulating blood or the active splenic pool. At all times, approximately two thirds of the total number of platelets are in the systemic circulation, whereas the remaining one third exist as a pool of platelets in the spleen that freely exchange with the general circulation. A normal person has an average of $250 \times 10^9/L$ (range $150 \times 10^9/L$ to $450 \times 10^9/L$) platelets in the systemic circulation. Platelet turnover or "effective thrombopoiesis" averages $350 \times 10^9/L \pm 4.3 \times 10^9/L/day$.

The life span of a mature platelet is 9.0 days ± 1 day. At the end of their life span, platelets are phagocytized by the liver and spleen and other tissues of the mononuclear phagocytic system.

Platelets normally move freely through the lumen of blood vessels as components of the circulatory system. For hemostasis to occur, platelets not only must be present in normal quantities but also must function properly. Following damage to the endothelium of a blood vessel, a series of events occur, including adhesion to the injured vessel, shape change, aggregation, and secretion. Each structural and functional change is accompanied by a series of biochemical reactions that occur during the process of platelet activation. The platelet plasma membrane is the focus of interactions between extracellular and intracellular environments. Agonists that lead to platelet activation are varied and include a nucleotide (ADP), lipids (thromboxane A_2, platelet-activating factor), a structural protein (collagen), and a proteolytic enzyme (thrombin).

A platelet count is a fundamental component in the evaluation of a patient. Examination of the peripheral blood smear for platelet number and morphology is critical because many clinical clues may be obtained from an evaluation of platelet quantity and morphology. If a platelet count is normal but a patient has a suggestive bleeding history, an assessment of platelet function should be conducted.

Blood Coagulation Factors

Bleeding from small blood vessels may be stopped by vasoconstriction and the formation of a platelet plug, but the formation of a clot (thrombus) usually occurs as part of the normal process of hemostasis. The soluble blood coagulation factors are critical components in the formation of a thrombus.

Blood coagulation is a sequential process of chemical reactions involving plasma proteins, phospholipids, and calcium ions.

The **prothrombin group** consists of factors II, VII, IX, and X. All of these factors are dependent on vitamin K during their synthesis. The **contact group** consists of factors XI, XII, prekallikrein (Fletcher factor), and high-molecular-weight kininogen (Fitzgerald factor). These factors are involved in the intrinsic coagulation pathway. Each of the individual coagulation factors has some unique characteristics.

The initiation of the coagulation process may occur via one of two pathways: the extrinsic pathway and the intrinsic pathway. Regardless of the initiating pathway, the two pathways converge into a final common pathway. The outcome of this process is the conversion of circulating insoluble coagulation factors into a gelatinous fibrin clot with entrapped blood cells, a blood clot. As repair of damaged tissue takes place, the clot is lysed and the particulate matter is removed by the mononuclear phagocytic system.

The intrinsic and extrinsic pathways are now thought to function in an interrelated manner *in vivo,* and previously established *in vitro* methods are valid to screen for abnormalities. A variety of laboratory procedures are of value in assessing coagulation factors. General procedures include the activated partial thromboplastin time (APTT), the prothrombin time (PT), the thrombin time, and quantitative fibrinogen concentration assay. More specialized or classic procedures include the ethanol gelation test, the euglobulin lysis test, fibrin split products test, the Hicks-Pitney modification of the thromboplastin generation time test, the partial thromboplastin substitution test, the plasma recalcification test, protamine sulfate assays, the prothrombin consumption time test, the thromboplastin generation test (TGT), specific factor assays, and various tests for inhibitors and circulating anticoagulants.

Normal Protective Mechanisms Against Thrombosis

In the blood circulation, the predisposition to thrombosis depends on the balance between procoagulant and anticoagulant factors. The normal flow of blood prevents the accumulation of procoagulant material. This mechanism reduces the chance of local fibrin formation. Another normal mechanism against inappropriate thrombosis is the removal from the blood of activated clotting factors by hepatocytes. This process, along with the naturally occurring inhibitors, limits intravascular clotting and fibrinolysis by inactivation of such factors as XIa, IXa, Xa, and IIa. Removal of particulate material by the cells of the mononuclear phagocytic system is also important in preventing the initiation of coagulation.

The in vivo existence of natural anticoagulant systems is essential to prevent thrombosis. These natural anticoagulant systems include antithrombin III, heparin cofactor II, and protein C and its cofactor, protein S. AT-III and HC-II are serine-protease inhibitors. When activated, protein C is capable of degrading activated factors V (Va) and VIII (VIIIa) in the presence of the cofactor protein S.

BIBLIOGRAPHY

Bick, Rodger L. "Oral Anticoagulants in Thromboembolic Disease." *Lab. Med.*, Vol. 26, No. 3, March, 1995, pp. 188–193.

Bode, Arthur P., A. Pattison, and H. Ridgway. *Evaluation of Platelet Function*, Beaumont, TX: Helena Laboratories, 1993.

Carrol, James J. "Role of Endothelial Cells in Coagulation." *Adv. for Med. Lab. Prof.*, Vol. 8, No. 1, January 8, 1996, pp. 10–11, 18.

Cohen, Annabelle and Martin H. Rosen. *Handbook of Microscopic Anatomy for the Health Sciences*. St. Louis: Mosby, 1975, pp. 45–46.

Colman, Robert W. "Platelet Receptors." *Hematol. Oncol. Clin. North Am.*, Vol. 4, No. 1, February, 1990, pp. 27–42.

Creager, Joan G. *Human Anatomy and Physiology*. Belmont, CA: Wadsworth, 1983, pp. 431–435, 468–469.

D'Angelo, A. et al. "Comparison of Mean Normal Prothrombin Time with PT of Fresh Normal Pooled Plasma or of a Lyophilized Control Plasma (R82A) as Denominator to Express PT Results: Collaborative Study of the International Federation of Clinical Chemistry." *Clinical Chem.*, Vol. 43, No. 11, 1997, pp. 2169–2174.

deFouw, Nanneke J. et al. "The Cofactor Role of Protein S in the Acceleration of Whole Blood Clot Lysis by Activated Protein C In Vitro." *Blood*, Vol. 67, No. 4, April, 1986, pp. 1189–1192.

Esmon, Charles T. "The Protein C Anticoagulant Pathway." Miami: Baxter Healthcare, 1990.

Fair, Daryl S. et al. "Human Endothelial Cells Synthesize Protein S." *Blood*, Vol. 67, No. 4, April, 1986, pp. 1168–1171.

FDP News, Vol. 1, No. 3, June, 1984. Research Triangle Park, NC: Wellcome Diagnostics, A Division of Burroughs Wellcome.

FDP News, Vol. 1, No. 2, March, 1984. Research Triangle Park, NC: Wellcome Diagnostics, A Division of Burroughs Wellcome.

Francis, Charles W. and Victor J. Marder. "Concepts of Clot Lysis." *Annu. Rev. Med.*, Vol. 37, 1986, pp. 187–204.

Gewirtz, Alan M. and Ronald Hoffman. "Human Megakaryocyte Production." *Hematol. Oncol. Clin. North Am.*, Vol. 4, No. 1, February, 1990, pp. 43–64.

Gimbrone, Michael. "Endothelium in Health and Disease," in *Intensive Review of Internal Medicine*, Boston: Harvard University, 1995, pp. 891–900.

Ginsburg, David. "The von Willebrand Factor Gene and Genetics of von Willebrand's Disease." *Mayo Clin. Proc.*, Vol. 66, 1991, pp. 506–515.

Gralnick, Harvey R. et al. "Platelet von Willebrand Factor." *Mayo Clin. Proc.*, Vol. 66, 1991, pp. 634–640.

Greenberg, Charles S. et al. "Cleavage of Blood Coagulation Factor XIII and Fibrinogen by Thrombin During In Vitro Clotting." *J. Clin. Invest.*, Vol. 75, May, 1985, pp. 1463–1470.

Hassell, K. L. "A Practical Guide to Hypercoagulability Testing." *Int. Med.*, July, 1996, pp. 55–60.

Hole, John W. *Human Anatomy and Physiology* (3rd edition). Dubuque, IA: Wm. C. Brown, 1984, pp. 672–673.

Hillis, L. B. "Low Molecular Weight Heparins." *Adv. for Med. Lab. Prof.*, December 1, 1997, pp. 32–34.

Jandl, James H. *Blood*. Boston: Little, Brown & Co., 1987, pp. 1147–1150.

Kaatz, Scott S. et al. "Accuracy of Laboratory and Portable Monitor International Normalized Ratio Determinations." *Arch. Intern. Med.*, Vol. 155, September 25, 1995, pp. 1861–1865.

Kitchens, Craig S. "Vascular Aspects of Hemostasis." *Coagulation Education*. T. Hirsch (ed.). Miami: American Dade, 1983, pp. 99–105.

Kjeldsen, J. et al. "Biological Variation of International Normalized Ratio for Prothrombin Times, and Consequences in Monitoring Oral Anticoagulant Therapy: Computer Simulation of Serial Measurements with Goal-Setting for Analytical Quality." *Clin. Chem.*, Vol. 43, No. 11, 1997, pp. 2175–2182.

Koepke, J. A. "Von Willebrand Profile." *MLO*, March, 1996, p. 16.

Leung, Lawrence and Ralph Nachman. "Molecular Mechanisms of Platelet Aggregation." *Annu. Rev. Med.*, Vol. 37, 1986, pp. 179–186.

Levin, Ellis R. "Mechanisms of Disease." *New Engl. J. Med.*, Vol. 333, No. 6, August 10, 1995, pp. 356–363.

Lollar, Pete. "The Association of Factor VIII with von Willebrand Factor." *Mayo Clin. Proc.*, Vol. 66, 1991, pp. 524–534.

McEver, Rodger P. "The Clinical Significance of Platelet Membrane Glycoproteins." *Hematol. Oncol. Clin. North Am.*, Vol. 4, No. 1, February, 1990, pp. 87–105.

Miller, Jonathan L. "Blood Coagulation and Fibrinolysis," in *Clinical Diagnosis and Management by Laboratory Methods* (18th edition). John B. Henry (ed.). Philadelphia: Saunders, 1991, pp. 738–739.

Nichols, W. L. and E. J. W. Bowie. "Standardization of the Prothrombin Time for Monitoring Orally Administered Anticoagulant Therapy With Use of the International Normalized Ratio System." *Mayo Clin. Proc.*, Vol. 68, September, 1993, pp. 897–898.

O'Connor, Barbara H. *A Color Atlas and Instruction Manual of Peripheral Blood Cell Morphology*. Baltimore: Williams & Wilkins, 1984, pp. 101–112.

Patrono, C. "Aspirin as an Antiplatelet Drug." *New Engl. J. Med.*, Vol. 330, No. 18, May 5, 1994, pp. 1287–1294.

Statland, Bernard E. (ed.). "Skin Bleeding Time Test." *Med. Lab. Observer*, Vol. 15, October, 1985, p. 14.

The Le, D. et al. "The International Normalized Ratio (INR) for Monitoring Warfarin Therapy: Reliability and Relation to Other

Monitoring Methods.'' *Ann. Intern. Med.*, Vol. 120, No. 7, April 1, 1994, pp. 552–558.

Thomas, Clayton L. (ed.). *Taber's Cyclopedic Medical Dictionary* (13th edition). Philadelphia: F. A. Davis, 1977, p. 173.

Turco, Salvatore J. ''Biotechnology.'' *Parenterals*, Vol. 4, No. 5, October–November, 1986, pp. 1–5.

Van De Graft, Kent. *Concepts of Human Anatomy and Physiology.* Dubuque, IA: Wm. C. Brown, 1986, p. 618.

Wheater, Paul R. et al. *Functional Histology.* Edinburgh: Churchill-Livingstone, 1979, pp. 76–86.

Warwick, Roger and Peter L. Williams (ed.). *Gray's Anatomy* (35th British edition). Philadelphia: Saunders, 1973, pp. 590–593.

REVIEW QUESTIONS

1. Normal hemostasis depends on all of the following *except:*
   A. An intact vascular system.
   B. Inadequate numbers of platelets.
   C. Appropriate coagulation factors.
   D. Fibrinolysis.

Questions 2 through 6: the sequence of events following injury to a small blood vessel is: *(2)* ___ to *(3)* ___ to *(4)* ___ to *(5)* ___ to *(6)* ___.

   A. Contact between damaged blood vessel, blood platelets, and coagulation proteins.
   B. Formation of a platelet plug.
   C. Fibrinolysis and reestablishment of vascular integrity.
   D. Development of a blood clot around the injury.
   E. Blood vessel spasm (vasoconstriction).

7. Which blood vessels have the thickest walls?
   A. Veins.   C. Capillaries.
   B. Arteries.   D. Arterioles.

8. All blood and lymphatic vessels are lined with:
   A. Endothelium.
   B. Nerve endings.
   C. Stratified epithelial cells.
   D. Simple squamous epithelium.

9. Blood passes from the arterial to the venous system via:
   A. Arterioles.   C. Veins.
   B. Capillaries.   D. Arteries.

10. The *initiating* stimulus to blood coagulation following injury to a blood vessel is:
   A. Contact activation with collagen.
   B. Vasoconstriction.
   C. Stenosis.
   D. Release of serotonin.

11. Endothelium is involved in the metabolism and clearance of molecules such as:
   A. Serotonin.   C. Bradykinin.
   B. Angiotensin.   D. All of the above.

12. Which of the following is *not* correct?
   A. Vasoconstriction reduces blood flow and promotes contact activation of platelets and coagulation factors.
   B. Platelets adhere to exposed endothelial connective tissues.
   C. Aggregation of platelets releases thromboxane A_2 and vasoactive amines (serotonin and epinephrine).
   D. None of the above.

13. Which of the following are true of endoreduplication?
   A. Duplication of DNA without cell division.
   B. Results in cells with ploidy values of $4n$, $8n$, $16n$, and $32n$.
   C. Is unique to the megakaryocytic type of blood cell.
   D. All of the above are true.

14. Which of the following is true of thrombopoietin?
   A. Thought to stimulate the production and maturation of megakaryocytes.
   B. Is influenced by various cytokines, which increase megakaryocyte size.
   C. Is influenced by various cytokines, which impact maturational stage and ploidy.
   D. All of the above.

15. Which of the following is *not* a characteristic of platelets?
   A. The presence of a nucleus.
   B. Size of 2 to 4 μm.
   C. Cytoplasm is light blue with fine red-purple granules.
   D. A discoid shape as an inactive cell.

16. The cellular ultrastructural component(s) unique to the platelet is (are):
   A. Cytoplasmic membrane.   C. Mitochondria.
   B. Glycocalyx.   D. Microtubules.

17. Choose the *incorrect* statement regarding storage granules related to hemostasis in the mature platelet:
   A. Alpha granules contain platelet factor 4, beta thromboglobulin, and platelet-derived growth factor.
   B. Alpha granules contain platelet fibrinogen and von Willebrand factor (vWF).
   C. Dense bodies contain serotonin and ADP.
   D. Lysosomes contain actomyosin, myosin, and filamin.

18. At all times, approximately ___ of the total number of platelets are in the systemic circulation.
   A. One fourth.   C. One half.
   B. One third.   D. Two thirds.

19. The normal range of platelets in the systemic circulation is:
   A. 50 to 150 $\times$ 10^9/L.   C. 150 to 350 $\times$ 10^9/L.
   B. 100 to 200 $\times$ 10^9/L.   D. 150 to 450 $\times$ 10^9/L.

20. The functions of platelets in response to vascular damage include:
   A. Maintenance of vascular integrity by sealing minor defects of the endothelium.
   B. Formation of a platelet plug.
   C. Promotion of fibrinolysis.
   D. All of the above.

Questions 21 and 22: if vascular injury exposes the endothelial surface and underlying collagen, platelets ___ (21) to the collagen fibers and ___ (22).

    A. Adhere.   B. Aggregate.

23. Agents that are capable of aggregating platelets include:

    A. Collagen.   C. Serotonin.
    B. Thrombin.   D. All of the above.

24. Examination of a Wright-stained peripheral blood smear provides an estimate of platelet numbers. Using 100× (oil) immersion in the areas of erythrocytes just touching each other, the upper limit of the number of platelets seen per field should *not* exceed:

    A. 10–15.   C. 20–25.
    B. 15–20.   D. 25–30.

25. If 10 platelets are seen per oil immersion field, what is the approximate platelet count?

    A. $50 \times 10^9/L$.   C. $150 \times 10^9/L$.
    B. $100 \times 10^9/L$.   D. $200 \times 10^9/L$.

26. Aspirin ingestion has the following hemostatic effect in a normal person:

    A. Prolongs the bleeding time.
    B. Prolongs the clotting time.
    C. Inhibits factor VIII.
    D. No effect.

27. The bleeding time test measures:

    A. The ability of platelets to stick together.
    B. Platelet adhesion and aggregation on locally injured vascular subendothelium.
    C. The quantity and quality of platelets.
    D. Antibodies against platelets.

28. The clot retraction test is:

    A. A visible reaction to the activation of platelet actomyosin (thrombosthenin).
    B. A reflection of the quantity and quality of platelets and other factors.
    C. A measurement of the ability of platelets to stick to glass.
    D. A measurement of the cloudiness of blood.

Questions 29 through 31: match the following.

29. ___ Fibrinogen group.   A. Factors II, VII, IX, and X.
30. ___ Prothrombin group.   B. Factors I, V, VIII, and XIII.
31. ___ Contact group.   C. Factors XI, XII, prekallikrein, and high-molecular-weight kininogen.

32. The fibrinogen group of coagulation factors is:

    A. Known to increase during pregnancy.
    B. Known to increase in conditions of inflammation.
    C. Known to increase subsequent to the use of oral contraceptives.
    D. All of the above.

33. The prothrombin group of coagulation factors is:

    A. Dependent on vitamin K for production.
    B. Considered to be stable.
    C. Well preserved in stored plasma.
    D. All of the above.

34. Warfarin acts by:

    A. Neutralizing the effects of thrombin.
    B. Interfering with fibrin monomer formation.
    C. Interfering with the synthesis of vitamin K–dependent factors.
    D. Inducing hypercoagulation.

Questions 35 through 38: match the name of the coagulation factor with the appropriate symbolic designation.

35. ___ Thrombin.   A. III.
36. ___ Tissue thromboplastin.   B. XII.
                                  C. VIII.
37. ___ Antihemophilic factor.   D. IIa.
38. ___ Hageman factor

Questions 39 through 42: arrange the four stages of coagulation in their proper sequence.

39. ___   A. Fibrinolysis.
40. ___   B. Formation of thrombin from prothrombin.
41. ___
42. ___   C. Generation of plasma thromboplastin.

                                  D. Formation of fibrin from fibrinogen.

43. The extrinsic pathway of coagulation is triggered by the entry of ___ into the circulation:

    A. Membrane lipoproteins (phospholipoproteins).
    B. Tissue thromboplastin.
    C. Ca^{2+}
    D. Factor VII.

44. The intrinsic pathway of coagulation begins with the activation of ___ in the early stage:

    A. Factor II.   C. Factor XII.
    B. Factor I.   D. Factor V.

45. The final common pathway of the intrinsic-extrinsic pathway is:

    A. Factor X activation.   C. Factor I activation.
    B. Factor II activation.   D. Factor XIII activation.

46. Prothrombin is converted to thrombin by:

    A. A complex of activated factors IX and VII.
    B. Calcium ions only.
    C. A complex of phospholipids and factor VII.
    D. A complex of activated factors X and V.

47. Fibrinogen is converted to fibrin monomers by:

    A. Prothrombin.   C. Calcium ions.
    B. Thrombin.   D. Factor XIIIa.

48. The inactive plasminogen is activated to ___ by proteolytic enzymes.

    A. Prothrombin.
    B. Plasmin.
    C. Plasma kallikrein.
    D. Plasma thromboplastin antecedent.

49. Which of the following statements are true of the fibrinolytic system?

    A. Plasmin digests fibrin and fibrinogen.
    B. The active enzyme of the system is plasmin.
    C. Plasminogen circulates in the plasma until an injury occurs.
    D. All of the above.

50. If a pediatric preoperative patient has a family history of bleeding but has never had a bleeding episode herself, what test should be included in a coagulation profile in addition to the prothrombin time (PT), activated partial thromboplastin time (APTT), and platelet count?

    A. Lee-White clotting time.   C. Bleeding time.
    B. Clot retraction.   D. Fibrin split products.

51. A patient with a severe decrease in factor X activity would demonstrate normal:

    A. APTT.   C. Thrombin time.
    B. PT.   D. Bleeding time.

52. Neither the APTT nor the PT detects a deficiency of:

    A. Platelet factor 3.   C. Factor VIII.
    B. Factor VII.   D. Factor IX.

53. The function of thromboplastin in the prothrombin test is to provide ___ to the assay:

    A. Kaolin.   C. Phospholipoprotein.
    B. Fibrinogen.   D. Thrombin.

54. An abnormally prolonged APTT may indicate:

    A. A severe depletion of fibrinogen.
    B. The presence of a circulating anticoagulant.
    C. Factor VIII deficiency.
    D. All of the above.

55. If a child ingested rat poison, which of the following tests should be performed to test the effect of the poison on the child's coagulation mechanism:

    A. APTT.   C. Fibrinogen assay.
    B. PT.   D. Thrombin time.

56. Which of the following conditions can cause an increased thrombin time?

    A. Fibrin split products.
    B. High concentrations of immunoglobulins.
    C. Heparin therapy.
    D. All of the above.

57. Heparin inhibits the clotting of blood by neutralizing the effect of:

    A. Thrombin.   C. Platelets.
    B. Calcium ions.   D. Factor VIII.

58. A patient has a prolonged APTT and a normal PT. The APTT is *not* corrected by factor VIII–deficient plasma but is corrected by factor IX–deficient plasma. Which factor does the patient appear to be deficient in?

    A. Factor II.   C. Factor VIII.
    B. Factor V.   D. Factor IX.

59. The normal protective mechanisms against thrombosis include:

    A. The flow of blood.
    B. The action of antithrombin III.
    C. Protein C and protein S.
    D. All of the above.

60. If heparin therapy is initiated in a patient, a decreased anticoagulant response can be caused by decreased levels of:

    A. Platelet factor 3.   C. Antithrombin III.
    B. Platelet factor 4.   D. Factor XIII.

61. Which of the following are characteristic of protein C?

    A. It is not vitamin K–dependent.
    B. It is formed in response to thrombin generation.
    C. It inactivates factors Va and VIIIa.
    D. Both B and C.

62. Which of the following characteristics are true of protein S?

    A. It is a cofactor of protein C.
    B. It increases the rate of inactivation of factor Va.
    C. It enhances the binding of activated protein C to phospholipids.
    D. All of the above.

63. Antithrombin III is the principal physiological inhibition of:

    A. Thrombin.   C. Factor XIa.
    B. Factor Xa.   D. Both A and B.

64. Which of the following *is not correct* regarding cellular proteases?

    A. They block the activation or action of plasmin.
    B. They include alpha-2 inhibitor.
    C. They rapidly neutralize the fibrinolytic properties of plasmin.
    D. They participate in clot formation.

27 Disorders of Hemostasis and Thrombosis

Vascular disorders
Abnormal platelet morphology
Quantitative platelet disorders
Thrombocytopenia
Thrombocytosis
Qualitative characteristics of platelets: thrombocytopathy
Types of platelet dysfunction

Bleeding disorders related to blood clotting
Defective production
Disorders of destruction and consumption
Disorders related to elevated fibrin split products
The hypercoagulable state
General features

Impaired fibrinolysis
Protein C deficiencies
Antithrombin III
Laboratory assessment of hypercoagulation
Summary
Case studies
Bibliography
Review questions

OBJECTIVES

Vascular disorders
- Define the term **purpura,** and describe various vascular conditions that can produce this condition.

Abnormal platelet morphology
- Name and compare four types of disorders in which abnormal platelet morphology can be observed.

Quantitative platelet disorders
- Cite at least two symptoms of thrombocytopenia.
- List the three major mechanisms that produce thrombocytopenias.
- Summarize the major characteristics of each of the three thrombocytopenic categories, including examples of disorders within each of the categories or subcategories.
- List and summarize the characteristics of the two categories of thrombocytosis, including examples of disorders within each category.

Qualitative characteristics of platelets: thrombocytopathy
- Compare the four categories of platelet dysfunctions, including examples of disorders within each category.

Bleeding disorders related to blood clotting factors
- Give examples and describe conditions that contribute to the defective production of blood coagulation factors.

- Describe the physiology of the destruction and consumption of coagulation factors, including the role of factor VIII, protein C, and thrombin in the process of fibrinolysis.
- Compare the laboratory test results in conditions of disseminated intravascular coagulation and fibrinolysis.
- Name and describe the factors that contribute to the pathological inhibition of coagulation.

The hypercoagulable state
- Explain the role of vascular damage and blood flow in the hypercoagulable state.
- Detail how platelets contribute to hypercoagulation.
- Describe the activity of blood coagulation factors in increasing the tendency toward thrombosis.
- Describe the relationship between impaired fibrinolysis and protein C, antithrombin III, and plasminogen.
- Describe the laboratory assessments that illustrate the condition of hypercoagulation.

Case studies
- Apply the laboratory data to the stated case studies and discuss the implications of these cases to the study of hematology.

VASCULAR DISORDERS

Disorders of the microcirculation, platelets, or plasma proteins may cause abnormal bleeding. Abnormal bleeding involving the loss of red blood cells from the microcirculation expresses itself as the condition of **purpura,** which is characterized by hemorrhages into the skin, mucous membranes, and internal organs.

Purpura may be produced by a variety of vascular abnormalities. These abnormalities include:

1. Purpura associated with direct endothelial cell damage. Endothelial damage may result from physical or chemical injury to the tissue caused by microbial agents such as in rickettsial disease or immunological antibody-mediated injury. Bacterial toxins produce de-endothelialization induced by an endotoxin. Antibody vascular injury, vasculitis, may be induced by drug reactions, insect bites, or the activation of complement.
2. Purpura associated with an inherited disease of the connective tissue. Alterations of the vascular supportive framework can occur in disorders such as diabetes.
3. Purpura associated with decreased mechanical strength of the microcirculation. Decreased strength can be seen in conditions such as scurvy and amyloidosis.
4. Purpura associated with mechanical disruption of small venules. The principal cause of this type of purpura is increased intraluminal pressure. This condition can be observed around the ankles with prolonged standing, and may be due to the presence of abnormal proteins in macroglobulinemias or hyperviscosity disorders.
5. Purpura associated with microthrombi (small clots). This type of disorder is associated with abnormal intravascular coagulation conditions.
6. Purpura associated with vascular malignancy. Purpura of this origin is observed in Kaposi's sarcoma and vascular tumors.

ABNORMAL PLATELET MORPHOLOGY

When examining a peripheral blood smear for platelets, the morphology of the platelets should be observed. Abnormal variations in size should be noted. Disorders of platelet size include:

1. Wiscott-Aldrich syndrome, which demonstrates the smallest platelets seen.
2. May-Hegglin anomaly, which is characterized by the presence of large platelets and the presence of Döhle-like bodies (see Chapter 6) in the granulocytic leukocytes.
3. Alport's syndrome, a disorder that exhibits giant platelets and thrombocytopenia.
4. Bernard-Soulier syndrome, which demonstrates the largest platelets seen and is also referred to as giant platelet syndrome. In this disorder, it has been demonstrated that the giant platelets are probably an artifact of the slide preparation. Actual measurement of the platelets reveals that their mean platelet volume (MPV) is normal.

QUANTITATIVE PLATELET DISORDERS

The normal range of circulating platelets is $150 \times 10^9/L$ to $450 \times 10^9/L$. When the quantity of platelets decreases to levels below this range, a condition of thrombocytopenia exists. If the quantity of platelets increases, thrombocytosis is the result. Disorders of platelets can be classified as quantitative (thrombocytopenia or thrombocytosis) or qualitative (thrombocytopathy).

Thrombocytopenia

A correlation exists between severe thrombocytopenia and spontaneous clinical bleeding. If platelets are absent or severely decreased below $100 \times 10^9/L$, clinical symptoms usually include the presence of **petechiae** or **purpura.** Petechiae appear as small, purplish hemorrhagic spots on the skin or mucous membranes; purpura is characterized by extensive areas of red or dark-purple discoloration.

Thrombocytopenia can result from a wide variety of conditions, such as following the use of extracorporeal circulation in cardiac bypass surgery or in alcoholic liver disease. Heparin-induced thrombocytopenia and associated thrombotic events, relatively common side effects of heparin therapy, can cause substantial morbidity and mortality. Thrombocytopenia in itself rarely poses a threat to affected patients, but disorders associated with it, which include deep venous thrombosis, disseminated intravascular coagulation (DIC), pulmonary embolism, cerebral thrombosis, myocardial infarction, and ischemic injury to the legs or arms, can produce severe morbidity and mortality. Serum from patients with heparin-induced thrombocytopenia contains IgG that, in the presence of small amounts of heparin, activates normal platelets and causes them to aggregate and release the contents of their granules, including serotonin. Platelet-activating antibodies are specific not for heparin but for complexes formed between heparin and platelet factor 4, a heparin-binding protein normally found in the alpha granules of platelets. IgG and IgM also react with endothelial cells coated with platelet factor 4 (Fig. 27.1). This suggests a mechanism of antibody-mediated vascular injury that could predispose a patient to thrombosis or DIC when challenged with heparin. In order to prevent these complications, it has become standard medical practice to monitor platelet counts in patients receiving heparin for any extended period.

Most thrombocytopenic conditions can be classified into major categories. These categories are:

1. Disorders of production
2. Disorders of destruction, including decreased megakaryocytopoiesis and ineffective platelet production, and disorders of utilization
3. Disorders of platelet distribution and dilution

Disorders of Production

Decreased production of platelets may be due to hypoproliferation of the megakaryocytic cell line or ineffective thrombopoiesis caused by acquired conditions or hereditary factors (Table 27.1). A hypoproliferative state frequently affects other normal cell lines of the bone marrow as well as platelets. Thrombocytopenia due to hypoproliferation can result from acquired damage to hematopoietic cells of the bone marrow caused by factors such as irradiation, drugs (e.g., chloramphenicol and chemotherapeutic agents), chemicals (e.g., insecticides), and alcohol. Infiltration of the bone mar-

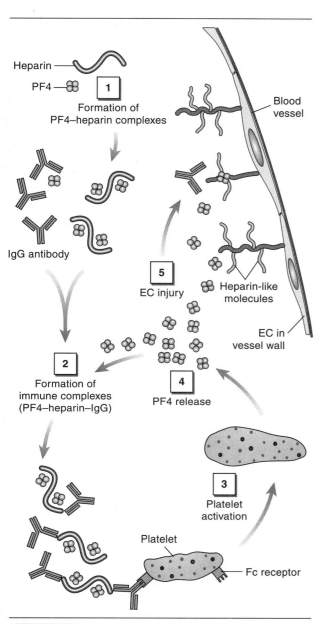

TABLE 27.1 Hereditary Platelet Function Defects

Adhesion defects
　Bernard-Soulier syndrome
　Impaired adhesion to collagen

Aggregation defects: primary
　Glanzmann's thrombasthenia
　Essential athrombia

Aggregation defects: secondary
　Storage pool diseases
　Aspirin-like defects
　Release reaction defects

Isolated platelet factor III deficiency

Severe coagulation factor deficiencies
　Afibrinogenemia
　Factor VIII: C deficiency
　Factor IX: C deficiency

FIGURE 27.1 Proposed explanation for the presence of both thrombocytopenia and thrombosis in heparin-sensitive patients who are treated with heparin. Researchers believe that injected heparin reacts with platelet factor 4 (PF4) that is normally present on the surface of endothelial cells or released in small quantities from circulating platelets to form PF4–heparin complexes (**1**). Specific IgG antibodies react with these conjugates to form immune complexes (**2**) that bond to Fc receptors on circulating platelets. Fc-mediated platelet activation (**3**) releases PF4 from alpha granules in platelets (**4**). Newly released PF4 binds to additional heparin, and the antibody forms more immune complexes, establishing a cycle of platelet activation. PF4 released in excess of the amount that can be neutralized by available heparin binds to heparin-like molecules (glycosaminoglycans) on the surface of endothelial cells (EC) to provide targets for antibody binding. This process leads to immune-mediated EC injury (5) and heightens the risk of thrombosis and disseminated intravascular coagulation. (From R. H. Aster, "Heparin-Induced Thrombocytopenia and Thrombosis," *N. Engl. J. Med.,* Vol. 332, No. 20, March 18, 1995, p. 1375.)

row by malignant cells in conditions of metastatic cancer, leukemia, and Hodgkins's disease can produce a hypoproliferative state. Hypoproliferation may also result from nonmalignant conditions, such as infections, lupus erythematosus, granulomatous disease such as **sarcoidosis,** and idiopathic causes.

Ineffective thrombopoiesis may result in decreased platelet production. Thrombocytopenias of this type may be the manifestation of a nutritional disorder, such as a deficiency of vitamin B_{12} or folic acid. In these megaloblastic anemias caused by deficiencies of vitamin B_{12} or folic acid, the defect in thymidine and DNA synthesis affects megakaryocytes and causes decreased or ineffective thrombopoiesis. Another disorder related to ineffective thrombopoiesis is iron deficiency anemia, which usually results in a decrease in megakaryocyte size and the suppression of megakaryocyte endoproliferation and size. Hereditary thrombocytopenias include Fanconi's syndrome, constitutional aplastic anemia and its variants, ameiosis thrombocytopenia (TAR syndrome), X-linked amegakaryocytic thrombocytopenia, Wiskott-Aldrich syndrome, May-Hegglin anomaly, and hereditary macrothrombocytopenia (e.g., Alport's syndrome).

Disorders of Destruction or Utilization

Increased destruction or utilization of platelets may result from a number of mechanisms.

Destruction Due to Immune Mechanisms: Antigens, Antibodies, or Complement Activities

Drugs or foreign substances can produce platelet destruction. These drugs include quinidine, sulfonamide derivatives, heroin, morphine, and snake venom. Sulfonamide derivative reactions involve the interaction of platelet antigens with drug antibodies. Morphine reactions involve the activation of complement.

Bacterial sepsis causes increased destruction of platelets due to the attachment of platelets to bacterial antigen-antibody immune complexes. Certain microbial antigens may attach initially to platelets followed by specific antibodies to the microorganism. This mechanism has been reported to cause the thrombocytopenia that frequently complicates the *Plasmodium falciparum* type of malaria.

Antibodies of either autoimmune or isoimmune origin may produce increased destruction of platelets. An example of an autoimmune thrombocytopenia is neonatal autoimmune thrombocytopenia. This condition occurs in infants born to mothers with chronic immune thrombocytopenia following transplacental passage of maternal IgG platelet autoantibodies.

Examples of thrombocytopenias of isoimmune origin include posttransfusion purpura and isoimmune neonatal thrombocytopenia. Posttransfusion purpura is a rare form of isoimmune thrombocytopenia. Isoimmune neonatal thrombocytopenia results from the immunization of a pregnant female by a fetal platelet antigen. The antigen is inherited by the fetus from the father and is absent on maternal platelets.

Increased Utilization of Platelets

Accelerated consumption of platelets is another cause of thrombocytopenia. One of the most important and frequently encountered forms of increased consumption of platelets is idiopathic thrombocytopenic purpura (ITP). This antibody-related response, which may be preceded by infection, is believed to have a devastating effect on platelet survival. ITP may complicate other antibody-associated disorders such as **systemic lupus erythematosus** (SLE). Patients with immunological thrombocytopenic purpura usually demonstrate petechiae, bruising, menorrhagia, and bleeding after minor trauma.

Idiopathic Thrombocytopenic Purpura

Idiopathic thrombocytopenic purpura, also known as immunological thrombocytopenic purpura, is characterized by a low platelet count, normal bone marrow, and the absence of other causes of thrombocytopenia.

Typically, adult ITP is a chronic disease. ITP in children is a clinically distinct disorder and is usually acute. Among adults, ITP is most common in young women (about 70% of patients are 10 to 40 years old). ITP in children is more common than the adult disease. Forty percent of all patients with ITP are younger than 10 years old, and both sexes are equally affected. In children, the onset is typically abrupt, with severe thrombocytopenia. Spontaneous, permanent remissions occur in about 80% of children.

The unusual occurrence of chronic thrombocytopenia in children is associated with features reminiscent of the adult disease, affecting more women than men, typically over 10 years of age, and with a longer history of purpura and a higher platelet count at presentation. Chronic idiopathic thrombocytopenic purpura is a destructive thrombocytopenia caused by an autoantibody. About 80% of patients have remissions after either corticosteroid therapy or splenectomy. Some patients respond to other therapy; a substantial group of patients are refractory to therapy.

Clinical Signs and Symptoms. Onset is often insidious. Purpura, epistaxis, and gingival bleeding are common. Hematuria and gastrointestinal bleeding are less common, and intracerebral hemorrhage is rare. Serious bleeding does not occur in most patients.

Laboratory. Isolated thrombocytopenia is the essential abnormality. Antibodies to specific platelet-membrane glycoproteins can be detected in most patients, but neither these assays, which are performed only in investigational laboratories, nor measurements of platelet IgG, which are often erroneously referred to as antiplatelet-antibody tests, are important for diagnosis or management. Diagnosis requires the exclusion of other causes of thrombocytopenia.

Pathophysiology. ITP is principally a disorder of increased platelet destruction mediated by autoantibodies to platelet-membrane antigens. Relative marrow failure, perhaps mediated by an effect of antiplatelet antibodies on megakaryocytes, also contributes to the thrombocytopenia, since platelet production is not appropriately increased in most patients. Autoantibodies that are reactive with major membrane glycoproteins can be identified in about 80% of patients. Most autoantibodies are directed against epitopes on glycoprotein IIb/IIIa, the most abundant and immunogenic platelet-surface glycoprotein.

Treatment. Platelet transfusions are seldom indicated. Survival time of transfused platelets is short, but they are important for controlling severe hemorrhage. The efficacy of platelets may improve immediately after an infusion of intravenous immune globulin. Intravenous immune globulin is an important agent in managing acute bleeding as well as in preparing for procedures, such as delivery. Treatment of pregnant women with ITP is a complex problem.

Splenectomy was a well-recognized treatment for ITP for more than 30 years before glucocorticoids were introduced in 1950, and its success in achieving complete responses in two thirds of patients has been remarkably consistent for more than 60 years. A response to splenectomy typically occurs within several days; responses after 10 days are unusual. When treatment is considered for patients with more severe thrombocytopenia and symptoms, it must be with the understanding that complete and permanent correction of thrombocytopenia is infrequent with any therapy.

Thrombocytopenic Purpura

Intravascular coagulation, vascular injury or occlusion, and tissue injury can all contribute to the increased utilization of platelets. Intravascular coagulation or DIC rapidly consumes platelets. Trauma, obstetrical complications, and microbial sepsis are examples of disorders that can trigger the accelerated consumption of platelets. In the case of bacterial sepsis, thrombin-induced platelet aggregation in vivo contributes to the thrombocytopenia. Vascular injury (vasculitis) causes a decrease in platelets due to the direct consumption of platelets at the sites of endothelial loss without appreciable depletion of clotting factors such as fibrinogen. Thrombotic thrombocytopenic purpura is an example of a disorder that is a combination of fluctuating ischemic vascular occlusion, hemolytic anemia, and thrombocytopenia. Direct injury to tissues, such as trauma or surgery, produces a combined destruction of platelets and fibrinogen that is localized at the site of injury.

Disorders of Platelet Distribution

A platelet distribution disorder can result from a pooling of platelets in the spleen, which is frequent if splenomegaly is present. This type of thrombocytopenia develops when more than a double or triple increase in platelet production is required to maintain the normal quantity of circulating platelets. Disorders that may produce splenomegaly with resultant splenic pooling or delayed intrasplenic transit include alcoholic or posthepatic cirrhosis with portal hypertension, lymphomas and leukemias, and lipid disorders such as Gaucher's disease.

Thrombocytosis

Thrombocytosis is generally defined as a substantial increase in circulating platelets over the normal upper limit of $450 \times 10^9/L$. Thrombocytosis is usually grouped according to cause: reactive or benign etiologies, versus platelet elevations linked to a specific hematological disorder.

Reactive thrombocytosis may be observed in a variety of disorders and conditions, including chronic blood loss, chronic inflammatory diseases, chronic infections, drugs, asplenic states and splenectomy, malignancies, rebound thrombocytosis following treatment of immunologic thrombocytopenic purpura, pernicious anemia, discontinuance of myelosuppressive drugs, acute blood loss, exercise, and myelodysplastic and hemolytic anemias. After a splenectomy, increases are noted because of the loss of the spleen. As the bone marrow adjusts to new requirements, platelet numbers progressively return to normal.

Thrombocytosis related to specific hematological disorders may demonstrate increased platelet counts. Thrombocytosis is seen in association with myeloproliferative disorders. Due to a poorly understood mechanism of stimulation associated with the hemolytic process, thrombocytosis may also be seen in **autoimmune hemolytic anemia.**

QUALITATIVE CHARACTERISTICS OF PLATELETS: THROMBOCYTOPATHY

If platelets are normal in number but fail to perform effectively, a platelet dysfunction exists. In addition to both an individual and family medical history, laboratory tests are critical in determining a platelet dysfunctional diagnosis.

TABLE 27.2 Categories of Platelet Dysfunctions

Type	Etiology	Typical Disorders
Acquired	Blood plasma inhibitor	Uremia, pernicious anemia, liver disease
Drug-induced	Aspirin	
Hereditary	Defect of connective tissue or coagulation factors	von Willebrand's disease
	Structural or biochemical defects of platelets	Bernard-Soulier syndrome Glanzmann's thrombasthenia

Laboratory tests of platelet function include bleeding time, clot retraction, platelet aggregation, platelet adhesiveness, and antiplatelet antibody assay.

Types of Platelet Dysfunction

Three separate categories of platelet dysfunction can be identified based on etiology (Table 27.2). These include the more common acquired and less frequent hereditary causes. Disorders within these categories can be identified using specific laboratory tests (Table 27.3). Hyperactive platelets associated with hypercoagulability and thrombosis make up an additional category of abnormal platelet function.

Acquired

Acquired platelet function defects can be due to a blood plasma inhibitory substance. Examples of disorders or diseases that may exhibit this dysfunction include infused dextran, uremia, liver disease, and pernicious anemia. Laboratory testing reveals the presence of fibrinolytic degradation or split products (discussed later in this chapter).

The most common acquired platelet defects are summarized in Table 27.4. Many patients with these platelet function disorders are candidates for surgery and may bleed profusely as a result of surgery or trauma.

Myeloproliferative Syndromes

Acquired platelet dysfunction is commonly seen in the myeloproliferative syndromes. Platelet aggregation patterns are often not characteristic, and could represent any combination of platelet aggregation defects.

TABLE 27.3 Selected Laboratory Tests for Platelet Dysfunctions

Disorder	Clot Retraction	Bleeding Time	Adhesion	Aggregation		Release of ADP
				ADP	ristocetin	
von Willebrand's disease	Decreased	Usually prolonged	Decreased	Normal	Decreased or normal	Normal
Glanzmann's thrombasthenia	Absent	Prolonged	Decreased	Absent	Normal	Normal
Storage disease	Normal	Prolonged	Decreased	Usually normal	Normal	Decreased

ADP = adenosine diphosphate.

TABLE 27.4 Acquired Platelet Function Defects

Myeloproliferative syndromes
    Essential thrombocythemia
    Chronic myelogenous leukemia
    Polycythemia vera
    Paroxysmal nocturnal hemoglobinuria
    Agnogenic myeloid metaplasia
    Myelofibrosis
    RAEB syndrome
    Sideroblastic anemia
Paraprotein disorders
    Multiple myeloma
    Waldenstrom's macroglobulinemia
    Essential monoclonal gammopathy
Autoimmune diseases
    Collagen vascular disease
    Antiplatelet antibodies
    Immune thrombocytopenias
Fibrinogen degradation products
    Disseminated intravascular coagulation
    Primary fibrinolytic syndromes
    Liver disease
Anemia
    Severe iron deficiency
    Severe B_{12} or folate deficiency
Uremia
Drug-induced

Uremia

Uremia is commonly accompanied by bleeding caused by platelet dysfunction. It is proposed that circulating guanidinosuccinic or hydroxyphenolic acids interfere with platelet function. Dialysis often corrects or improves platelet function. Other mechanisms of altered platelet function in uremia, including altered prostaglandin metabolism, have been proposed.

Paraprotein Disorders

Paraprotein disorders including malignant or benign paraprotein, such as multiple myeloma, Waldenstrom's macroglobulinemia, or other monoclonal gammopathies harbor platelet dysfunction. Dysfunction results from the paraprotein coating the platelet membranes but does not depend on the type of paraprotein present. Almost all patients with malignant paraprotein disorders will demonstrate clinically significant bleeding as well as abnormal platelet function by aggregation.

Cardiopulmonary Bypass and Platelet Function

These conditions demonstrate severe platelet function deficit that assumes major importance in surgical bleeding after bypass.

Miscellaneous Disorders Associated With Platelet Dysfunction

Acquired defects are seen in autoimmune disorders, such as systemic lupus erythematosus (SLE), rheumatoid arthri-

tis (RE), idiopathic thrombocytopenic purpura (ITP), and scleroderma. Fibrinogen degradation products (FDPs) including the later degradation products, fragments D and E, have a high affinity for the platelet membrane and produce a severe platelet function defect. Patients with severe iron, folate, or cobalamin deficiency may also have platelet function defects.

Drug-Induced

Many drugs can induce platelet function defects, resulting in hemorrhage. A typical example of this dysfunction is the ingestion of aspirin. One or two aspirin tablets are sufficient to extend the bleeding time to twice the normal value.

The most common mechanisms of interference involve drug interference with platelet membrane or membrane receptor sites, drug interference with prostaglandin biosynthetic pathways, and drug interference with phosphodiesterase activity.

Platelet Membrane Receptors

Platelet membrane receptors can be altered by drugs, such as chlorpromazine (Thorazine), cocaine, xylocaine, cephalothin (Keflin), ampicillin, penicillin, and alcohol. In addition, prostaglandin pathways are inhibited by aspirin, ibuprofen, hydrocortisone, and cyclosporine (Cyclosporine A).

The arachidonic acid platelet aggregation assay is the only practical way to monitor the effects of aspirin therapy, now widely used to prevent stroke and heart attacks.

Hereditary

Hereditary platelet dysfunctions are due to an inherited platelet defect that is either structural or biochemical (Table 27.5). Examples of adhesion disorders include Bernard-Soulier syndrome, a collagen receptor defect, Glanzmann's thrombasthenia, and storage granule abnormalities. Secondary aggregation disorders include hereditary storage pool defect and hereditary aspirin-like defects.

Also included among hereditary disorders are defects of connective tissue, such as collagen, and failure of platelets to adhere to the subendothelium due to a decrease or defect in plasma coagulation factors. An example of a defect of platelet plug formation due to decreased platelet adhesion to the subendothelium is von Willebrand's disease (see the discussion of von Willebrand's disease later in this chapter).

Bernard-Soulier Syndrome

Bernard-Soulier syndrome, **an autosomal** hereditary bleeding disorder, is a platelet adhesion disorder in which platelet membrane glycoproteins Ib, V, and IX are missing. Heterozygotes are often asymptomatic. The condition is characterized by the presence of giant platelets. In this syndrome there is a mild thrombocytopenia, but the predominant abnormality is of the membrane glycoprotein Ib. This abnormal platelet membrane lacks the receptor site for von Willebrand factor (vWF), which is necessary for platelets to adhere to vascular subendothelium. A blood film from a patient with Bernard-Soulier syndrome may resemble that for a patient with immunological thrombocytopenic purpura. Platelet aggrega-

TABLE 27.5 Examples of Inherited Platelet Dysfunction

Surface membrane defects
    Bernard-Soulier syndrome
    Glanzmann's thrombasthenia
    Collagen receptor defect
    Platelet-type von Willebrand's disease
Defects of granule storage
    Alpha granule deficiency
        Gray platelet syndrome
    Dense granules
        Wiskott-Aldrich syndrome
        Hermansky-Pudlak syndrome
        Chédiak-Higashi syndrome
        TAR baby syndrome

tion is normal with all agents except ristocetin. Clinical features include easy bruising, epistaxis, hypermenorrhagia, and petechiae (Table 27.6).

Glanzmann's Thrombasthenia and Essential Athrombia

Glanzmann's thrombasthenia and **essential athrombia** are similar, rare, primary aggregation disorders. Glanzmann's thrombasthenia is an autosomal recessive disorder. Clinical features involve platelet dysfunction, easy and spontaneous bruising, subcutaneous hematomas, and petechiae. Intra-articular bleeding with hemarthrosis may occur in some patients but tends to diminish with age.

This disorder involves an abnormality of the surface membrane glycoprotein complex IIb/IIIa. On a peripheral blood film, platelets from patients with this disorder remain isolated and do not exhibit the clumping that is normally seen. Epinephrine, collagen, and thrombin fail to induce aggregation. This results in a prolonged bleeding time in the presence of a normal platelet count, decreased platelet retention in glass bead columns, and an absence of a primary wave of aggregation in response to ADP. Clot retraction is also decreased.

Hereditary Storage Pool Defect

Hereditary storage pool defect is a secondary aggregation disorder. Overall, Hereditary storage pool disorders are more common than primary aggregation disorders of the hereditary platelet function defects. In rare instances, storage pool defects are seen in patients with other diseases, including Wiskott-Aldrich syndrome, TAR baby syndrome, Hermansky-Pudlak syndrome, and Chédiak-Higashi syndrome. Clinical features of secondary aggregation disorders are mucocutaneous hemorrhages and hematuria, peristasis, and easy and spontaneous bruising. Petechiae are less common than in other qualitative platelet disorders.

Hereditary aspirin-like defects are a rarer form of secondary aggregation defect. Clinical features are similar to other platelet function defects.

Storage granule abnormalities, primarily an absence of the dense granules, exist in conjunction with other clinical disorders, such as Chédiak-Higashi syndrome, Wiskott-Aldrich syndrome, and Hermansky-Pudlak syndrome. In these disorders, platelet aggregation with weaker agents, such as ADP and epinephrine, is diminished.

BLEEDING DISORDERS RELATED TO BLOOD CLOTTING FACTORS

Vascular response and platelet plug formation are responsible for the initial phases of hemostasis. Subsequent to these activities, the clotting factors are initiated to form the fibrin clot. Fibrin formation can occur if the activity of various factors is at least 30% to 40% of normal.

TABLE 27.6 Laboratory Profiles of Disorders of Platelet Function

Disorder	Laboratory Profile
Bernard-Soulier syndrome	Giant platelets, borderline platelet count, abnormal adhesion, abnormal ristocetin aggregation, normal or decreased thrombin aggregation, other aggregation responses normal
von Willebrand's disease	Abnormal adhesion, abnormal ristocetin aggregation (type IIB—increased, exhibits increased sensitivity to low concentrations)
Glanzmann's thrombasthenia	Clot retraction abnormal, bleeding time prolonged, primary aggregation absent with ADP, thrombin, collagen, epinephrine; pf3 abnormal, ADP primary and secondary, epinephrine primary and secondary, ristocetin not diagnostic
Storage pool defect	Bleeding time prolonged; ADP and epi primary and secondary responses decreased; arachidonic acid normal or decreased, collagen decreased, thrombin and ristocetin not diagnostic
Aspirin-like disorder or aspirin ingestion; aspirin (aspirin-like disorder); deficiency of cyclo-oxygenase inhibitor; or thromboxane	Bleeding time prolonged; aggregation primary and secondary ADP and epinephrine decreased; arachidonic acid decreased, collagen decreased, thrombin and ristocetin not diagnostic

TABLE 27.7 Clinical Comparison of Disorders

Observation	Disorders of Platelets or Vessels ("Purpuric" Disorders)	Disorders of Coagulation
Petechiae	Characteristic	Rare
Deep dissecting hematomas	Rare	Characteristic
Superficial ecchymoses	Characteristic; usually small and multiple	Common; usually large and solitary
Hemarthrosis	Rare	Characteristic
Delayed bleeding	Rare	Common
Bleeding from superficial cuts and scratches	Persistent; often profuse	Minimal
Sex of patient	Relatively more common in females	80%–90% of hereditary forms occur in females
Positive family history	Rare	Common
Site of bleeding	Skin, mucous membranes, gums, nose, etc.	Deep in soft tissue, e.g., joints, muscles
Bleeding after surgery	Immediate, usually mild	Delayed (usually 1 to 2 days), often severe

Bleeding and defective fibrin clot formation are frequently related to a coagulation factor. Disorders of the blood coagulation factors (Table 27.7) can be grouped into three categories:

1. Defective production
2. Excessive destruction
3. Pathological inhibition

Defective Production

Vitamin K Deficiency

A condition of defective production may be related to a deficiency of vitamin K. The synthesis of vitamin K–dependent factors can be disrupted due to prolonged periods of inadequate nutrition or prolonged use of broad-spectrum antibiotics. Vitamin K deficiencies are also encountered in neonates, malabsorption syndrome, biliary obstruction, and patients taking oral anticoagulants. Factors II, VII, IX, and X are vitamin K–dependent.

Severe Liver Disease

Because the liver is the primary site of synthesis of coagulation factor, severe liver disease can cause defective production of coagulation factors. Severe liver disease may produce decreased plasma levels of fibrinogen, although low levels of fibrinogen rarely produce hemorrhage. In patients with liver disease, the prothrombin time (PT) is noticeably prolonged, while the activated partial thromboplastin times (APTTs) are variable.

Hereditary Clotting Defects

Classic hemophilia (hemophilia A) and von Willebrand's disease are examples of hereditary disorders that represent functionally inactive factor VIII.

Hemophilia

Etiology. Hemophilia has been used as a paradigm for understanding the molecular pathological processes that underlie hereditary disease. The cloning of factor VIII facilitated the identification of mutations that lead to hemophilia A, an inherited deficiency of factor VIII coagulant activity that causes severe hemorrhage. Two types of mutations dominate the defects identified so far: gene deletions and point mutations. Gene deletions are associated with severe hemophilia A in which no factor VIII circulates in the blood. To date, approximately 50 deletion mutations in the gene for factor VIII have been characterized at the molecular level, and about 34 independent deletion mutations in the factor IX gene have been found to be the cause of hemophilia B. Point mutations, in which a single base in DNA is mutated to another base, represents a second type of mutation that causes hemophilia.

Epidemiology. Individuals with hereditary clotting defects may be either genetically homozygous or heterozygous carriers of the trait. The level of factor activity ranges from 0 to 25% in homozygotes and 15% to 100% in persons heterozygous for the trait. Defects of this origin may result from the decreased production of a clotting factor, factor VIII, or the production of functionally inactive molecules of the clotting factor. Hemophilia A, a sex-linked homozygous disorder expressed in males, occurs in 1 in 10,000 males.

Pathophysiology. Classic hemophiliacs have an intact high-molecular-weight moiety and a deficient low-molecular-weight procoagulant portion. This disorder of procoagulant synthesis expresses itself by decreased factor VIII clotting activity in laboratory assay and a normal bleeding time. Conversely, severe von Willebrand's disease has both a decreased high-molecular-weight portion and a decreased low-molecular-weight portion.

Plasma levels of factor VIII can be temporarily corrected and the bleeding tendency reversed in most patients following infusion of factor VIII in appropriate blood products. One would expect that correction of the hemostatic defect would place a patient at the same risk of thromboembolism as an unaffected individual, but thromboembolic events in patients with hemophilia A are distinctly uncommon.

Von Willebrand's Disease

In 1926, Erik von Willebrand first described a hemorrhagic disorder characterized by a prolonged bleeding time and an autosomal inheritance pattern that distinguished the disease from classic hemophilias. In the early 1950s, an additional

TABLE 27.8 Nomenclature of the Factor VIII–von Willebrand Factor (vWF) Complex

Term	Description
VIII:C	Factor VIII procoagulant activity
VIII:CAg	Antigenic expression of VIII:C
vWF:Ag	Antigenic expression of vWF
Ristocetin cofactor	A property of vWF that promotes agglutination of platelets in the presence of the antibiotic ristocetin
Factor VIII–vWF complex	The form in which VIII:C and vWF usually circulate in plasma

component of the disease was identified: a deficiency of factor VIII procoagulant activity (Table 27.8). These and other observations distinguish von Willebrand's disease (vWD) from classic factor VIII:C deficiency (hemophilia A). In addition, evaluation of the multimeric structures of vWF has aided in the classification of the variant forms of vWD.

Etiology. Von Willebrand's disease may be an acquired or inherited disorder. The congenital disorder is autosomally dominant in most cases. Inherited abnormalities in von Willebrand's disease are associated with a defect of the vWF gene on chromosome 12, but in some patients the coexistence of an impaired response of plasminogen activator and telan-

giectasia suggests the presence of a regular defect or more extensive endothelial abnormalities. In several families, a large vWF gene deletion has been identified as the basis for von Willebrand's disease.

More than 20 distinct clinical and laboratory subtypes of von Willebrand's disease have been described (Table 27.9). Three broad types of von Willebrand's disease are recognized. In addition, a platelet-type von Willebrand's disease (pseudo–von Willebrand's disease) is due to an abnormal platelet receptor for vWF. In addition, acquired von Willebrand's disease may complicate other diseases such as lymphoproliferative and autoimmune disorders, and proteolytic degradation of vWF complicates myeloproliferative disorders. Variant forms of von Willebrand's disease can be identified by their patterns of genetic transmission and the vWF abnormalities in the plasma and the cellular compartment. Distinguishing between various subtypes of von Willebrand's disease is important in determining appropriate therapy (Table 27.10).

Epidemiology. Von Willebrand's disease is recognized as one of the most common hereditary bleeding disorders in humans. The exact incidence is difficult to determine because milder forms are often not clinically recognized, but it has been estimated to have a prevalence as high as 1% in the general population.

No racial or ethnic predisposition has been determined. Both sexes are affected but there is a higher frequency of clinical manifestation in women.

TABLE 27.9 Classification of von Willebrand's Disease

Type	Features
IA	All vWF multimers are present in plasma in normal relative proportion No evidence of intrinsic functional abnormality of vWF Subgroups: platelet concentration and activity may be normal, low, or discordant
IB	All vWF multimers are present in plasma but the larger ones are relatively decreased vWF has less ristocetin cofactor activity than normal
IC	All vWF multimers are present in plasma in normal relative proportion but a structural abnormality of individual multimers is present vWF has less ristocetin cofactor activity than normal
Miscellaneous: I-1, I-2, I-3, I New York, undesignated types	Variable deficiencies of vWF:Ag in plasma and/or platelets, and other abnormalities
IIA	Large and intermediate vWF multimers are absent in plasma and platelets Increased proteolysis of vWF; some variability in size of multimer present; few cases show recessive inheritance
IIA-1, IIA-2, and IIA-3	Subtypes demonstrate variable concentrations of plasma and/or platelet vWF:Ag
IIB	Hyperresponsiveness to low doses of ristocetin; Large vWF multimers are absent in plasma; all multimers are preset in platelets Increased proteolysis of vWF; few cases demonstrate recessive inheritance
IIC, IID	Large vWF multimers are absent; unique structural abnormality of individual multimers Decreased proteolysis of vWF
IIE	Large vWF multimers are appreciably decreased; structural abnormality of individual multimers Recessive inheritance Decreased proteolysis of vWF
IIF, IIG, IIH, type B	Rare examples of a variety of abnormalities
III	Severe form of the disease; also called severe type I by some

vWF = von Willebrand factor.

TABLE 27.10 Characteristics of Various Types of von Willebrand's Disease

Feature	Type I	Type IIA	Type IIB	Platelet	Type IIC	Type III
Platelet count	N	N	N or ↓	low N or ↓	N	N
Bleeding time	↑ or N	↑	↑	↑	↑	↑
Factor VIII:C	N or ↓	N or ↓	N or ↓	N or ↓	N	N
vWF:Ag	↓	N or ↓	N or ↓	N or ↓	N	
vWF:RCoF	↓	↓	N or ↓	N or ↓		
RIPA	N or ↓	↓ or absent	↑	↑	↓	Absent

vWF = von Willebrand factor; vWF:RCoF = ristocetin cofactor; RIPA = ristocetin-induced platelet aggregation; N = normal.

Pathophysiology. Von Willebrand's disease is characterized by abnormal platelet function, expressed as a prolonged bleeding time. This is a consistent finding and may be accompanied by decreased factor VIII procoagulant activity.

vWF circulates in the blood in two distinct compartments, with two types of cells being responsible for vWF production. Vascular endothelium is the primary source of the synthesis and release of plasma vWF; the other type of cell that synthesizes vWF is the megakaryocyte. Approximately 15% of circulating vWF is produced in the megakaryocyte. vWF circulates in platelets, being stored primarily in the alpha granules, in association with factor VIII procoagulant protein (VIII:Ag). Platelet vWF is released from the alpha granules by various agonists and subsequently rebinds to the glycoprotein IIb/IIIa complex. The site synthesis of VIII:Ag remains unknown, although the liver is thought to play an important role.

vWF is a large, adhesive, multimeric glycoprotein present in plasma, platelets, and subendothelium. It is synthesized as a large precursor that consists of a signal peptide, a propeptide (von Willebrand antigen II), and the vWF subunit. It has the two main functions of regulating coagulant activity (VIII:C) and aiding in adhesion of platelets to subendothelial cell walls following vessel damage. In circulating blood, vWF is part of a noncovalent bimolecular complex with the factor VIII procoagulant protein. This complex stabilizes factor VIII and protects it from rapid removal from the circulation. The vWF portion represents over 95% of the mass of the complex and therefore controls the molecular stereochemistry. The vWF consists of repeating multimers with the smallest circulating multimer thought to be a dimer or tetramer.

Circulating vWF undergoes proteolytic cleavage under physiological conditions; thus, it can be distinguished from platelet vWF, which is not proteolyzed. The pathogenesis of von Willebrand's disease is based on quantitative or qualitative abnormalities, or both, of vWF. When an abnormality is present, the decreased factor VIII procoagulant activity is attributable to the reduced concentration of vWF.

vWF is essential in providing the basis for formation of a normal platelet thrombus. vWF binds to specific sites on the platelet, namely glycoprotein Ib and glycoprotein IIb/IIIa, while concurrently binding to the subendothelium of damaged vessel walls, forming a bridge. Patients with decreased levels of vWF, especially the larger multimeric forms, will lack adequate "bridging action" that produces prolonged bleeding times. Qualitative or quantitative abnormalities of vWF result in decreased adhesion and are responsible for the bleeding associated with vWD.

The significance of vWF in the regulation of VIII:C remains unclear. The increase in VIII:C following infusion of purified vWF suggests a possible role of vWF in the synthesis, release, or stabilization of VIII:Ag. Therefore, decreased levels of vWF may prolong the rate of blood clotting.

Clinical Signs and Symptoms. The severity of symptoms among patients with vWD varies greatly. Severe cases are not easily distinguishable clinically from severe hemophilia A, in which bleeding occurs into the joints and fascial planes. Characteristically, in patients with vWD the bleeding is mucosal in origin, with epistaxis, menorrhagia, and gastrointestinal bleeding being the most common. Bleeding associated with surgical procedures and oral surgery is a particular problem. Homozygous patients may experience severe bleeding including hemarthrosis or potentially lethal gastrointestinal tract or central nervous system hemorrhage.

Inherited Classification of vWD. Type I is the most common variant of von Willebrand's disease and appears to be based on a quantitative deficiency of vWF. It is expressed as an autosomal dominant trait and is presumed to be due to an inheritance of one normal and one deficient allele. Patients with severe type III may have homozygous type I (or compound heterozygous) disease. The molecular basis for type I and type III disease is unclear but is characterized by decreased circulating levels of vWf. Factor VIII:C is decreased proportionally with respect to vWF.

Most patients with von Willebrand's disease (50% or more) have quantitative abnormalities and no evidence of a functional abnormality of vWF, which corresponds to type I von Willebrand's disease and its subtypes. The genetic transmission of the disease is dominant, except possibly for subtype I-3. Most patients have low plasma levels of vWF antigen (usually between 5% and 30% of normal) and correspondingly low levels of ristocetin cofactor activity (the assay reflects the property of vWF to bind to glycoprotein Ib and mediate platelet agglutination). The factor VIII procoagulant protein is also decreased in proportion to the decrease in vWF. In these cases, the bleeding is due to insufficient levels of circulating vWF and factor VIII. Bleeding manifestations are less severe in patients who have a normal concentration of platelet vWF than in others (Table 27.11).

TABLE 27.11 von Willebrand Factor (vWF) Requirements for Primary Hemostasis

Activity	Interaction	Reaction
Plasma vWF	Subendothelial deposition interaction with glycoprotein Ib	Platelet contact
Platelet vWF	Binding to glycoprotein IIB/IIIa subendothelial surface	Platelet spreading
	Platelet-platelet interaction	Platelet aggregation

In all patients whose vWF shows low ristocetin cofactor activity, except for those designated as having type B disease, the vWF has an abnormal multimeric structure and there is a decrease in or absence of the large multimers.

Type II is characterized by structurally abnormal vWF. The circulating levels of vWF may be decreased or normal and VIII:C may be affected similarly. Type IIA and type IIB are autosomally dominant, whereas type IIC is recessive.

Patients with type III, the most severe form of von Willebrand's disease, are likely to have a major episode of bleeding early in life because markedly decreased amounts of vWF and VIII:C are produced. Genetically they are thought to be homozygous or double heterozygous. These patients probably comprise a separate group because of the typically recessive modality of genetic transmission (Table 27.12).

Acquired von Willebrand's Disease. Von Willebrand's disease is occasionally seen as an acquired condition. Associations have been made with lupus erythematosus and other autoimmune disorders, and myeloproliferative disorders. The presence of a circulating antibody to vWF may be implicated in some cases. Another mechanism responsible for decreased amounts of vWF in acquired states is the absorption of the coagulation component onto abnormal cell surfaces. Hemorrhagic complications are generally more severe in patients with acquired vWD. Bleeding from mucous membranes is more common and reflects the much lower levels of vWF activity in these individuals. vWF activity is typically 20% or less of normal.

Pseudo–von Willebrand's Disease. This is a rare disorder in which patients resemble those with vWD due to low levels or absence of large multimeric forms of vWF in the plasma. Patients with "pseudo" vWD have a platelet abnormality in which spontaneous platelet aggregation occurs. Low lev-

els of larger multimers result from increased consumption during platelet aggregation.

Increased Levels of vWF. Increased levels of vWF have been associated with stress, inflammation, postsurgical states, pregnancy, renal disease, diabetes, rheumatoid disorders, scleroderma, and Raynaud's phenomena. vWF may be an indicator of vascular endothelial status. Drugs such as 1-deamino-8-D-arginine vasopressin (DDAVP), steroids, and hormones may also result in elevated levels of vWF.

Laboratory Findings. The following laboratory results are typical of vWD:

- Bleeding time: mildly to moderately prolonged
- Platelet retention: typically decreased
- Platelet agglutination: ristocetin—abnormal
- Platelet aggregation: normal with all but ristocetin
- von Willebrand factor function (ristocetin cofactor activity)

Quantitation of vWF antigen (VWF:Ag) can be determined by Laurell rocket immunoelectrophoresis as well as ELISA and RIA methods. These assays measure total amounts of vWF protein, independent of its ability to function. Finally, von Willebrand factor multimeric analysis is useful in distinguishing between subtypes and in determining therapeutic management. vWF multimeric analysis uses SDS agarose gel electrophoresis and radiolabeled antibody to visualize the different molecular weight multimers.

Other Hereditary Deficiencies

A deficiency of factor IX is known as **hemophilia B** or **Christmas disease.** This form of hemophilia is non–sex-linked and occurs at a rate of 1/50,000 in the general population, with a defective molecule being the usual cause. It is clinically indistinguishable from hemophilia A and must be differentiated by laboratory testing. A deficiency of factor XI is referred to as **hemophilia C.** This genetic defect is an autosomal recessive trait that occurs almost exclusively in people of Jewish descent. It is usually a mild disorder characterized by easy bruising, epistaxis, and hemorrhage in conjunction with trauma. The laboratory results in this defect, as well as those of other hemophilias and von Willebrand's disease, are presented in Table 27.13.

Fibrinogen deficiency as a genetic disorder may represent a defect of production or dysfunctional molecules. Hereditary deficiencies of the other coagulation factors are relatively rare. Examples of rare defects include **factor XII deficiency,** in which no clinical bleeding tendencies are apparent, and **factor XIII deficiency,** which is associated with spontaneous abortion and poor wound healing.

TABLE 27.12 Clinical Features of Various Types of von Willebrand's Disease

Type	Bleeding Time	Bleeding Tendency	Petechiae	Hemarthroses
I	Normal or increased	Mild	None	Rare
II	Increased	Moderate	Usually none	Rare
III	Increased	Often severe	Occasionally	Occur

TABLE 27.13　Laboratory Test Results in Hereditary Coagulation Defects

Test	Hemophilia A	von Willebrand's Disease	Hemophilia B	Hemophilia C
Bleeding time	Normal	Increased	Normal	Normal
Clot retraction	Normal	Normal	Normal	Normal
Platelet count	Normal	Normal	Normal	Normal
Platelet aggregation	Normal	Decreased	Normal	Normal
PT*	Normal	Normal	Variable	Normal
APTT	Increased	Increased	Increased	Increased
PT consumption	Decreased	Decreased	Decreased	Decreased
Fibrinogen	Normal	Normal	Normal	Normal
Factor VIII	Decreased	Decreased		
Factor VIII:C	Decreased 2% or less	Decreased 10–30%		
Factor VIIIC:Ag	Normal	Decreased		
Factor VIII/vWF	Normal	Decreased or absent		
Factor IX assay			Decreased	Normal
Factor XI assay			Normal	Decreased

PT = prothrombin time; APTT = activated partial thromboplastin time.

*This test is normal when performed with human brain thromboplastin, but in a variant of the disease, the PT is prolonged if bovine brain thromboplastin is used. This variation is produced by a molecular abnormality of factor IX that inhibits the thromboplastin–factor VII reaction of the extrinsic pathway.

Disorders of Destruction and Consumption

Enhanced fibrin deposits can result in thrombosis and damage to organs due to impeded blood flow and ischemia. The fibrinolytic system serves as a protective mechanism against excessive fibrin deposits by lysing both fibrin and fibrinogen.

Blood coagulation factors can be destroyed in vivo by enzymatic degradation or by pathological activation of coagulation with excessive utilization of the clotting factors. Enzymatic destruction can result from bites by certain species of snakes whose venom contains an enzyme that degrades fibrinogen to a defective fibrin monomer. In vivo activation of coagulation by tissue thromboplastin-like materials can produce excessive utilization of clotting factors. Conditions associated with this consumption of coagulation factors include obstetrical complications, trauma, burns, prostatic and pelvic surgery, shock, advanced malignancy, septicemia, and intravascular hemolysis.

General Features of Fibrinolysis

Primary and secondary fibrinolysis are recognized as extreme complications of a variety of intravascular and extravascular disorders and may have life-threatening consequences. Primary fibrinolysis is associated with conditions in which gross activation of the fibrinolytic mechanism with subsequent fibrinogen and coagulation factor consumption occurs. The important characteristic of primary fibrinolysis is that no evidence of fibrin deposition occurs. Primary fibrinolysis occurs when large amounts of plasminogen activator enter the circulatory system as a result of trauma, surgery, and malignancies.

Although the same clinical conditions may also induce secondary fibrinolysis or DIC, the distinction between the

two is essentially in the demonstration of fibrin formation. In secondary fibrinolysis, excessive clotting and fibrinolytic activity occur. Increased amounts of fibrin split (degradation) products (FSPs) and fibrin monomers are detectable because of the action of thrombin on the fibrinogen molecule. This fibrinolytic process is only due to excessive clotting; therefore, it is a secondary condition. Distinguishing between primary and secondary fibrinolysis (Table 27.14) is important in the treatment of the patient.

Disseminated Intravascular Coagulation

Etiology

DIC is actually a complication or intermediary phase of many diseases and does not constitute a disorder in itself. It is also known as consumptive coagulopathy or defibrination syndrome. Triggering events that may predispose patients to DIC include alterations in the endothelium, direct activation of fibrinogen, release of thromboplastin-like substances, and erythrocyte or platelet destruction. Extravascular trauma, abruptio placentae, advanced malignancy, leuke-

TABLE 27.14　Selected Characteristics of Primary and Secondary Fibrinolysis

Laboratory Test	Primary Fibrinolysis	Secondary Fibrinolysis
Platelet count	Normal	Decreased
Protamine sulfate test	Negative	Positive
Fibrin split products	Increased	Increased
Fibrinogen	Decreased	Decreased

mia, and retained fetal syndrome are examples of clinical situations in which tissue thromboplastin can activate co-agulation.

Infections, most commonly gram-negative microorganisms, can trigger DIC by producing endotoxins that expose collagen. Stasis, shock, or tissue necrosis can have the same effect. Snake bites may introduce substances which initiate coagulation by direct activation of fibrinogen to form fibrin. Red blood cell or platelet injury may contribute to the consumptive coagulopathy by releasing phospholipids that accelerate coagulation. Red cell injury may be a result of intravascular hemolysis due to malaria, incompatible transfusion products, and other clinical states. Platelet destruction also releases coagulation factors V, VIII, XII, and XIII.

Other causes can include liver disease, lymphoproliferative disorders, and renal disease. In addition, DIC can also be triggered by trauma including shock, hypothermia, and extensive tissue damage, such as in myocardial infarction and eclampsia. It has been associated with multiple surgical, obstetrical and medical disorders. Coma and convulsions can result.

Pathophysiology

The overall DIC process involves coagulation factors, platelets, vascular endothelial cells, fibrinolysis, and plasma inhibitors. This major breakdown of the hemostatic mechanism occurs when the procoagulant factors outweigh the anticoagulant mechanisms.

Initiation of DIC can be caused by a number of factors. If vascular endothelial damage results in the exposure of collagen and basement membrane, collagen can activate factor XII. Factor XII has multiple roles in the direct or indirect activation of coagulation including:

1. Initiation of the intrinsic clotting cascade resulting in thrombin formation
2. Participation as a cofactor for the conversion of prekallikrein to kallikrein
3. Initiation of fibrinolysis

Regardless of the initiating event, DIC is characterized by excess thrombin formation, conversion of fibrinogen to fibrin, and platelet consumption and deposition. Secondary fibrinolysis occurs as a result of fibrin deposition and can decrease plasma coagulation factors, leading to a hemorrhagic diathesis.

Thrombin is central to the mechanism of consumptive coagulopathy. The action of thrombin on the coagulation systems includes:

1. Proteolytic cleavage of fibrinogen to fibrin monomer, releasing fibrinopeptides A and B (fibrin monomer may form soluble complexes with fibrinogen or form fibrin thrombi which entrap platelets during thrombus formation.
2. Activation of factor XIII, which stabilizes fibrin by cross-linking.
3. Stimulation of platelets, resulting in decreased circulating platelets. These stimulated platelets undergo shape change, adhesion, aggregation, and secretion. The contents of the dense and alpha granules are released, leading to

an acquired storage pool deficiency. If, during perhaps a 3-hour span, platelet counts and fibrinogen levels decrease significantly on a critically ill patient, DIC should be the prime suspect as the cause of this change.
4. Activation of factor V and VIII; however, thrombin activation results in unstable end products that have decreased factor V and VIII activity.
5. Activation of protein C, which degrades factors V and VIII.

The deposition of fibrin thrombi in the vasculature, primarily in the microvasculature, initiates fibrinolysis. This secondary fibrinolysis is responsible for the hemorrhagic complication of DIC.

When the fibrinolytic system is activated, plasminogen is converted to plasmin. Alpha-2 antiplasmin is the fibrinolytic inhibitor uniquely designed to cope with plasmin. The more plasmin generated, the more alpha-2 antiplasmin the patient consumes. This produces a vicious cycle in which increased activation leads to decreased inhibitors; this, in turn, allows more increased activation to continue. This is known as a positive feedback loop and leads to a situation incompatible with life.

Damaged tissue, especially renal cells, releases plasminogen activators that convert plasminogen to plasmin. Plasmin is a proteolytic enzyme that destroys fibrin, fibrinogen, and clotting factors V and VIII. Circulating plasmin may lead to systemic fibrinolysis, causing increased hemorrhagic events.

In the microcirculation, plasmin's action is primarily directed against fibrin. In the circulation, the breakdown of fibrin results in fibrin split products, labeled X, Y, D, and E, which inhibit thrombin and normal platelet function.

As fibrinogen is degraded by plasmin, FSPs form. Degradation occurs whether the plasmin comes from DIC or primary fibrinogenolysis. Fibrin split products compete with regular fibrinogen molecules for thrombin molecules. This competitive binding makes the thrombin unavailable for the conversion of fibrinogen to fibrin. In this situation, patients with high FSP levels have a circulating anticoagulant behaving like heparin. If the FSP level is high, the thrombin clotting time is markedly prolonged and fibrinogen quantitation is low. The second effect is on platelets. These split products coat the platelet surface, blocking the receptor site needed for further platelet activation.

When pathological fibrinolysis occurs, not only are factors destroyed, but through the destruction of fibrinogen, a profound anticlotting effect inhibits secondary hemostasis and platelets.

If the fibrinolytic system is activated, it will contribute to the consumption of many clotting factors. Plasmin, the primary proteolytic enzyme of fibrinolysis, directly attacks and destroys them. This becomes another form of "consumptive coagulopathy" originating from an entirely different source with the same end result.

When systemic clotting activation begins, the body usually attempts to stop it. The two major inhibitor systems of coagulation are antithrombin and the protein C and S systems. These inhibitors are consumed in the DIC process. Therefore, the compensatory mechanisms are often unable to stabilize the consumptive process. Coagulation factors and platelets are consumed more rapidly than they can be replaced, antithrombin III (AT-III) levels are depleted, and the impaired mononuclear phagocytic system cannot effectively remove the activated coagulation proteins.

Alternate Forms of DIC. DIC is one of several forms of an acute state in which a patient's clotting and/or fibrinolytic system is suddenly activated throughout the body. In essence, it is a systemic pathological process. Because two types of systems are involved, the clotting and/or the fibrinolytic system, several types of this consumptive coagulopathy can be clinically identified:

1. DIC: Clotting and lysis strongly activated (most common type)
2. DIC: Clotting predominates with little or no lysis (poor prognosis)
3. Primary fibrinogenolysis: Only lysis activated, but many clotting factors consumed

In the usual form of DIC, the patient's clotting system and the fibrinolytic system are activated. Patients are systemically forming thrombin, which, in turn, converts fibrinogen to fibrin. In most instances, the simultaneous generation of plasmin will dissolve the fibrin. Both the clotting and fibrinolytic states are performing at abnormally high rates. If clot lysis does not occur, a different form of DIC exists. In this case, the prognosis is very poor. A third type is represented by a state in which the patient predominantly has fibrinolysis-disseminated intravascular fibrinogenolysis. Coagulation factors are degraded by the excess plasmin being generated.

The Role of Factor VIII. A very close relationship exists between factor VIII:C (procoagulant) and factor VIII:CAg (procoagulant antigen). In DIC, it is believed that the VIII:CAg is inactivated to a lesser extent than VIII:C by enzymes released during the process. It is known that factor VIII:C activity is destroyed by minute amounts of thrombin, plasmin, and activated protein C.

It is strongly suspected that the in vivo inactivation of VIII:C found in DIC is related to the degree of severity of DIC. Furthermore, low values of factors VIII:C and VIIIR:Ag and factors VIII:C and VIIIR:CoF found in patients with irreversible shock indicate a grave clinical outcome. Discrepancies are also known to exist between VIII:C and VIIIR:Ag in patients with thromboembolic disease. Such ratios are useful indicators for assessing the severity of DIC. Current thinking indicates that data on the factor VIII complex show that the dogma of a characteristic decrease of the factor VIII procoagulant activity in DIC formulated in the past is not generally valid.

The Role of Protein C. Protein C is one of the major regulatory mechanisms of hemostasis. This system decreases the rate of thrombin formation by controlling factors Va and VIII:C, both of which are involved in the rate-limiting steps of coagulation. Protein C also functions as a profibrinolytic enzyme, increasing the rate of fibrin degradation.

The induction of fibrinolytic activity by the protein C system may facilitate the clearance of excess thrombi and generation of fibrin split products. If activated protein C is being consumed too rapidly, the regulatory ability of the protein C system is sharply reduced, which results in uncontrollable thrombosis.

In patients with hereditary deficiencies of protein C (levels of 60% or less of normal), thromboembolic complications are known to occur. Individuals born with a homozygous protein C deficiency develop fatal neonatal purpura. The stimuli that can induce DIC may ultimately result in abnormal levels of protein C. Both normal and abnormal levels of protein C antigen can be found, depending on the sample time relative to the onset of DIC. Plasma levels of protein C antigen and activity have been found to be decreased in patients with DIC. Whereas three fourths of DIC patients have a decrease in protein C antigen, almost all DIC patients have a decreased level of protein C activity. Monitoring patients reveals that protein C antigen and activity decrease progressively during the initial stages of DIC and remain at a low level for 24 to 48 hours before gradually returning toward normal in nonfatal cases.

The Role of Thrombin. Mechanisms involved in DIC result in the generation of thrombin in the circulating blood. Among its many feedback reactions, thrombin participates indirectly in the activation of the fibrinolytic system secondary to DIC and activates protein C. The latter reaction is accelerated by the presence of the endothelial cell cofactor, protein S.

Besides cleaving fibrinogen and performing its other procoagulant functions, some of the excess thrombin binds to protein S on the endothelial cell surface. This event leads to increased levels of activated protein C in the plasma. Once the generation of excess thrombin is decreased by the action of activated protein C and other regulatory mechanisms, the coagulation process can return to normal. This negative feedback mechanism has the potential to slow down the formation of excess thrombin and to stop DIC.

Clinical Signs and Symptoms. The DIC phenomenon can have varied clinical and laboratory manifestations due to the many physiological abnormalities associated with the syndrome. DIC may be acute or subacute (chronic). Chronic DIC is more common than the acute form but is often more difficult to diagnose. Chronic DIC can covert to acute consumption if the balance of procoagulant-anticoagulant is lost.

Either form may initially be seen with varying degrees of thrombosis and hemorrhage, but bleeding is usually the major symptom, particularly in acute cases. Both hemorrhagic and thrombotic complications may accompany DIC, often being manifested in the same patient. In chronic or low-grade DIC, thrombosis may predominate. Thrombotic complications can include deep venous thrombosis.

Acute DIC is severe and often life threatening. Its onset is rapid and both fibrinogen and platelets may be depleted. Patients with chronic DIC may have mild manifestations of the disorder or be recognizable only by laboratory data. Hemorrhagic complications are also seen but are generally milder than in acute DIC.

Clinical manifestations of DIC include petechiae, purpura, hemorrhagic bullae, surgical wound bleeding, trau-

TABLE 27.15 Significant Laboratory Findings in Disseminated Intravascular Coagulation

- Peripheral blood smear—fragmented RBC
- Platelet count—decreased
- Fibrinogen levels—decreased
- Thrombin time—prolonged
- Reptilase time—prolonged
- APTT and PT—prolonged
- Fibrin split products (FSPs)—present
- Ethanol gel or protamine sulfate test—positive
- Other tests—euglobulin clot lysis time, antithrombin III, coagulation factor assays, and plasminogen level

matic wound bleeding, venipuncture site bleeding, arterial line oozing, and subcutaneous hematomas.

A condition that is similar to DIC is thrombotic thrombocytopenia purpura (TTP) (Table 27.15). In addition, pediatric respiratory distress syndrome (PRDS), adult respiratory distress syndrome (ARDS), hemolytic uremic syndrome, preeclampsia or frank eclampsia, circulating immune complex, cavernous hemangiomas, and Rocky Mountain spotted fever can resemble DIC.

Laboratory Findings

Although the quantitative measurement of FSPs cannot distinguish between primary and secondary fibrinolysis, such measurement plays the major role in diagnosing and monitoring these conditions. Laboratory diagnosis of DIC requires the availability of tests that are rapid and simple to perform. There is no single test that confirms the diagnosis, but rather a combination of tests (Table 27.16). Because DIC is a dynamic process, values from tests performed a single time, whether normal or abnormal, cannot be used as diagnostic indicators. Sequential testing is necessary to provide an accurate diagnosis and effectively manage therapy. The most important consideration in the treatment of DIC is the resolution of the underlying disease or triggering event.

Tests for Fibrinolysis and DIC. Because the manifestations of fibrinolysis and DIC are extremely variable, diagnosis depends on laboratory testing. Coagulation assays such as the platelet count, fibrinogen levels, fibrin split product test, factor V assay, ethanol gelation test, and thrombin time–reptilase test can all be useful. Prekallikrein and AT-III have

also been suggested to be of prognostic value. The key feature is an elevation of circulating fibrinogen-FSPs (Table 27.17).

Typical results in DIC include prolonged APTT, PT, and thrombin time. Fibrinogen levels and the total platelet count may vary, although thrombocytopenia and a decrease in fibrinogen are common. The platelet count decreases earlier than fibrinogen in endotoxin-induced DIC. The reverse is true when tissue factor release is responsible, such as in obstetrical accidents or trauma. Excessive fibrinolysis with the release of FSPs occurs secondary to intravascular fibrin formation. Although the presence of fibrin split products is characteristic, the finding is not specific for DIC and cannot be used as the sole criterion for diagnosis.

Disorders Related to Elevated Fibrin Split Products

The normal level of serum FSPs is less than 10 μg/mL. Serum values can vary owing to exercise or stress. Elevated urinary levels are always indicative of a disease state. High levels of fibrin split products indicate renal dysfunction. Normal urinary FSP values are generally less than 0.25 μg/mL but may rise to as high as 50 μg/mL in certain kidney disorders.

Elevated levels of FSPs can be found in diseases of the neonate, in sepsis, or in the DIC that these conditions may generate. In cases of pulmonary embolism, levels can exceed 100 μg/mL; however, in rare cases, values can reach more than 400 μg/mL. These excessively high levels return to near normal within 24 hours after the cessation of the disorder (e.g., sepsis). FSP levels are elevated, frequently as high as 80 μg/mL, in cases of mild chronic intravascular coagulation, which occurs when the placenta slowly releases thromboplastic substances into the circulation. The FSP test can help distinguish between eclampsia and hypertension and edema associated with pregnancy.

THE HYPERCOAGULABLE STATE

Thrombi may form because coagulation is enhanced or because protective devices such as fibrinolysis are impaired. An increase in the likelihood of blood to clot is referred to as the **hypercoagulable state.**

Thrombosis is promoted by vascular damage, by retarded blood flow, and by alterations in the blood that increase the

TABLE 27.16 Comparative Test Results in Diagnosing Various Forms of Acute Consumptive Coagulopathy

Test	Clotting & Lysis	Clotting	Lysis
Fibrinogen	Decreased	Decreased	Decreased
Platelets	Decreased	Decreased	Decreased or normal
Fibrin split products	Positive	Negative	Positive
Fibrin monomers	Positive	Positive	Negative
D-dimer	Positive	Negative	Negative

TABLE 27.17 Disseminated Intravascular Coagulation (DIC) Versus Thrombotic Thrombocytopenia Purpura (TTP)

	Clinical Manifestations	Laboratory Abnormalities	Micropathological Findings
TTP	Unexplained fever; central nervous system dysfunction; renal failure in 11%	Thrombocytopenia; FDP mildly elevated in 50%; hemolytic anemia with schistocytes and fragmented red cells	Microvascular thrombosis with impaired fibrinolysis
DIC	Fever; hypotension; hemorrhage; thrombosis; shock. Wide variety of underlying illnesses; all ages.	Thrombocytopenia; anemia; schistocytes and fragmented red cells; elevated FDP	Microvascular thrombosis; fibrin deposition; active fibrinolysis

likelihood of clotting. A number of factors may contribute to hypercoagulation.

Hypercoagulable states include various inherited as well as acquired clinical disorders characterized by an increased risk for thromboembolism. Primary hypercoagulable states (Table 27.18) include relatively rare inherited conditions that lead to disordered endothelial cell thromboregulation. These conditions include decreased thrombomodulin-dependent activation of activated protein C, impaired heparin binding of AT-III, or down-regulation of membrane-associated plasmin generation.

The major inherited inhibitor disease states include AT-III deficiency, protein C deficiency, and protein S deficiency. These conditions should be considered in patients who have recurrent, familial, or juvenile deep-vein thrombosis or occlusion in an unusual location such as a mesenteric, brachial, or cerebral vessel.

Secondary hypercoagulation states may be seen in a number of heterogeneous disorders. In many of these conditions, endothelial activation by cytokines leads to the loss of normal vessel-wall anticoagulant surface functions, with conversion to a proinflammatory thrombogenic phenotype. Important clinical syndromes associated with substantial thromboembolic events include the antiphospholipid syndrome, heparin-induced thrombopathy, the myeloproliferative syndromes, and cancer.

General Features

Vascular Damage and Blood Flow

Vascular endothelial damage exposes circulating blood to subendothelial structures that initiate thrombosis. Constriction of blood vessels additionally creates stasis. Thrombosis can begin in areas of low blood flow or in situations in which the viscosity of blood is increased. In patients with a high risk of thrombosis, the concentration of fibrinogen is often elevated. High concentrations of fibrinogen may induce aggregation of circulating erythrocytes, which produces increased blood viscosity. This may encourage thrombosis by decreasing the blood flow at critical sites with the accumulation of activated clotting factors.

Platelets

Stasis makes it easier for platelets to be detached from flowing blood. An increase in the number of circulating platelets may create a tendency toward thrombosis. Platelets accumulate at the site of vascular damage, where they can furnish phospholipid for the intrinsic pathway, and also promote thrombin formation by adsorbing activated factor X from plasma to their surfaces. High platelet counts additionally foster thrombosis.

Another possibility is that a thrombotic tendency may be caused by qualitative alterations in platelets. These alter-

TABLE 27.18 Primary and Secondary Hypercoagulable States

Primary Hypercoagulable States	Secondary Hypercoagulable States
Antithrombin II deficiency	Cancer
Protein C deficiency	Pregnancy
Protein S deficiency	Oral contraceptives
Fibrinolytic abnormalities	Nephrotic syndrome
Hypoplasminogenemia	Myeloproliferative disorders
Dysplasminogenemia	Hyperlipidemias
Tissue plasminogen activator release deficiency	Diabetes mellitus
Increased levels of plasminogen activator inhibitor	Paroxysmal nocturnal hemoglobinuria
Dysfibrinogenemia	Postoperative states
Homocystinuria	Vasculitis
Heparin cofactor II deficiency	Antiphospholipid syndrome
Increased levels of histidine-rich glycoprotein	Increased levels of factor VII and fibrinogen
	Anticancer drugs
	Heparin thrombocytopenia
	Obesity

ations may be caused by intrinsic platelet defects or by changes in the surrounding plasma. Qualitative abnormalities may result in spontaneous aggregation, enhanced sensitivity to aggregating agents, or increased adhesiveness.

Blood Clotting Factors

A tendency toward abnormal thrombosis may be caused by qualitative alterations in blood clotting factors. Another possibility is that an increased titer of activated clotting factors can create a tendency toward thrombosis. These factors might contribute to thrombosis in that activated factors might reach critical levels in the circulating blood.

Multiple abnormalities in the levels of coagulation factors and platelets have been observed in patients with proteinuria. These patients are known to have repeated thrombotic attacks. It is known that Orientals are less prone to thromboembolic disease than American whites; the titer of factor XII in Orientals is half the titer found in white Americans. Women who use oral contraceptives have titers of factor XII that are twice as high as the average titer in other women; it is known that thromboembolism can occur as a consequence of this medication. These relationships may be correlational rather than causal because patients with a hereditary deficiency of factor XII have sustained thrombosis and myocardial infarction. In other cases, rare examples of a familial tendency for recurrent thrombosis have been correlated with excessively high titers of factor V or VIII.

One way in which activated factors within the circulation may induce thrombus formation has been demonstrated. These experiments demonstrate that factors X, IX, and IXa and thrombin bind to cultured vascular endothelial cells. Additionally, factor Xa binds to platelets and thrombin binds to monocytes.

Circulating Anticoagulants

Acquired inhibitors of clotting proteins, also known as circulating anticoagulants, inactivate or inhibit the usual procoagulant activity of coagulation factors. Inhibitors are frequently characterized as specific, those directed against a coagulation factor, or nonspecific, those directed against a complex of factors, such as the lupus anticoagulant.

The majority of these inhibitors exhibit biochemical properties, suggesting that they are immunoglobulins. Inhibitors may arise following transfusion of blood products or in patients with no previous hemostatic disorders. Acquired inhibitors can be a significant cause of hemorrhage.

Specific inhibitors against factors II, V, VII, VIII, IX, XII, XIII and vWF have been detected in patients with individual factor deficiencies. However, some inhibitors of factors II, V, VII, IX, XII and vWF have been observed in patients having no deficiencies of coagulation factors. Patients with acquired specific inhibitors may exhibit hemorrhagic episodes, whereas nonspecific inhibitors are not generally associated with bleeding tendencies.

Etiology

The incidence of circulating anticoagulants has been benchmarked at 0.75% of the general population. Certain patient populations have a higher incidence of inhibitor development. Inhibitors, found in both serum and plasma, are not inactivated by heating at 56° C for 30 minutes and remain stable when stored at −20° C. Inhibitors are more stable than clotting factors and more tolerant of changes in pH and temperature. Inhibitors may remain in the circulation for months and in some instances have been found in patients years after development.

Specific Inhibitors

Lupus Anticoagulant

Lupus anticoagulant occurs in approximately 10% of patients with systemic lupus erythematosus (SLE). Lupus anticoagulant is the most common coagulation inhibitor found in SLE patients, although these patients may have other acquired inhibitors as well. Lupus anticoagulant, also known as antiphospholipid antibody, occurs in the presence of disease states other than SLE, such as acquired immunodeficiency syndrome (AIDS) and malignancy, and in procainamide, hydralazine, or chlorpromazine therapy. Distinct from the specific inhibitors, antiphospholipid antibody is believed to have inhibitor activity directed against the in vitro phospholipid component of the coagulation mechanism.

Factor VIII Inhibitor

Factor VIII inhibitors are the most common specific factor inhibitors. Inhibitors of factor VIII develop in 10% to 15% of patients with factor VIII deficiency (hemophilia A), and the majority occur in patients with severe hemophilia (those having less than 1% factor VIII activity). Inhibitors have developed in patients exposed to factor VIII after as few as 10 exposure days, but may develop after several hundred days. Approximately 65% of patients with hemophilia who develop inhibitors do so before the age of 20. Nonhemophiliac women have been reported to develop factor VIII inhibitors during the postpartum period, most frequently after the birth of the first child. Patients with underlying immunological disorders such as rheumatoid arthritis, SLE, drug allergies, ulcerative colitis, and bronchial asthma also have an increased tendency to develop factor VIII inhibitors. Many patients have been observed to develop factor VIII inhibitors with no underlying disease. The majority of these patients are middle-aged or older, and both sexes are affected.

Inhibitors against vWF occur in patients with von Willebrand's disease, underlying diseases such as malignancy or SLE, and in previously healthy persons. A familial tendency for the development of vWF inhibitors has been noted.

Factor IX Inhibitor

Inhibitors are found in about 2% to 3% of factor IX–deficient (hemophilia B) patients, but the incidence of inhibitors in severe hemophilia B may be as high as 12%. Although these inhibitors are predominantly a result of transfusion of blood products, spontaneous inhibitor formation has been reported.

Factor V Inhibitor

Factor V inhibitors are rare and are not generally associated with hereditary factor V deficiency. Some patients have had exposure to streptomycin but no causal relationship has been established.

Fibrinogen, Fibrin, and Factor XIII Inhibitors

Inhibitors of fibrinogen, fibrin, and factor XIII have been reported. These inhibitors have occurred following plasma transfusions or appeared spontaneously. Some patients have a common denominator of taking isoniazid, an antituberculosis drug.

Factor II, VII, IX, and X Inhibitors

Factor II, VII, IX, and X inhibitors are rare. The causes for factor inhibitor development are varied and include congenital deficiencies, immune disorders, and amyloidosis.

Factor XI and XII Inhibitors

Inhibitors of factors XI and XII have been reported infrequently in patients with SLE, Waldenstrom's macroglobulinemia, and other disorders, and with chlorpromazine administration.

Clinical Presentation

The lupus anticoagulant is the most commonly acquired and has an interesting presentation in patients that demonstrate its presence. In the absence of other hemostatic abnormalities, the lupus anticoagulant is rarely associated with bleeding tendencies, even with surgical procedures. Bleeding episodes in these patients are usually the result of thrombocytopenia or another anomaly. Paradoxically, patients with lupus anticoagulant are at increased risk for arterial and venus thromboembolism. Venous thrombosis involving the leg veins, with associated pulmonary emboli, is the most frequent complication. Spontaneous abortion and intrauterine deaths are also increased in patients with lupus anticoagulant.

The presence of a specific factor inhibitor can be suspected in patients with no history of bleeding episodes who experience hemorrhage from various sites or in hemophiliac patients not responsive to their usual dosage of blood product infusion. Bleeding episodes in hemophiliac patients with inhibitors do not appear to be any more frequent or severe than in patients without inhibitors. When hemorrhagic events do occur, treatment of a patient with inhibitor is difficult.

Nonhemophiliac patients with acquired inhibitors of factor VIII can have major bleeding requiring transfusion. Patients with inhibitors to vWF, factor XI, and factor XII do not generally exhibit a hemorrhagic tendency. However, therapy for these patients can be complicated by the presence of the inhibitor. Patients with acquired factor IX inhibitors have clinical courses similar to hemophilia A patients with inhibitors. Factor V inhibitors may cause clinical bleeding, although the degree of hemorrhage varies considerably. Inhibitors of factors XIII, II, VII, IX, and X; fibrin; or fibrinogen can result in serious hemorrhagic events for patients.

Laboratory Findings

Prolonged PT or APTT are classic laboratory findings. Incubation of patient's plasma with normal plasma at 37°C (mixing study) and determination of APTT and PT may detect the presence of an inhibitor. The mixing study will be prolonged in the presence of an inhibitor. Inhibitors are more time- and temperature-stable than their specific clotting factors. To quantitate the levels of inhibitors, the Bethesda assay is most commonly used in the United States. One Bethesda unit is defined as the amount of antibody that will neutralize 50% of the inhibitor activity in a mixture of equal parts of normal plasma and antibody containing plasma that has been incubated for 2 hours at 37°C.

Detection of antiphospholipid antibody is based on prolongation of phospholipid-dependent coagulation assays. Antiphospholipid antibody is considered one of the most common causes of a prolonged APTT. Assays include the Russell viper venom time, kaolin clotting time, platelet neutralization procedure, and tissue thromboplastin inhibition test.

Impaired Fibrinolysis

Impaired fibrinolytic mechanisms have been noted to be both genetic and acquired in their origin. Impairment of fibrinolysis may predispose an individual to thrombosis. Patients with type II hyperlipoproteinemia due to familial hypercholesterolemia demonstrate impairment of fibrinolysis. A high incidence of recurrent thrombosis has been noted in patients with hereditary deficiencies of protein C or AT-III. Protein S deficiency also joins the group of other plasma protein deficiencies associated with inherited thrombophilia (Table 27.19). Deficiencies of inhibitors to factors VIII and V have also been correlated with recurrent thrombosis.

Protein C Deficiencies

Protein C activity has been demonstrated to be related to the commonly occurring thrombotic episodes in patients with an inherited deficiency of protein C and protein S. However, the hypercoagulable state in patients with proteinuria is not caused by decreased levels of protein C. Elevated protein C levels may represent a protective mechanism to the hypercoagulable state in patients with proteinuria because the anticoagulant activities of AT-III and protein C are probably complementary.

Deficiencies of protein C and protein S can be acquired or congenital. Acquired deficiencies occur in DIC, severe liver disease, vitamin K deficiency, and oral anticoagulation therapy. Congenital deficiencies are transmitted in an autosomal dominant fashion. Thrombotic complications usually involve the venous system, although more recently protein S has been associated with arterial thrombosis as well.

Several types of protein C defects have been reported (Table 27.20). Type I protein C deficiency is characterized by low antigenic and functional levels of the protein. In those with type II deficiency, the antigenic level of protein C is

TABLE 27.19 Prevalence of Congenital Deficiencies

Deficient Protein	All Patients	Patients With Recurrent Thrombosis
Protein C	4–8%	12–18%
Protein S	2–8%	15–18%

TABLE 27.20 Classification of Congenital Protein C Deficiency

Classification	Functional	Antigenic
Type I	Decreased	Decreased
Type IIa	Decreased*	Normal
Type IIb	Normal/Abnormal†	Normal

*Chromogenic and functional

†Chromogenic is normal; clotting is abnormal

normal, but the function of the molecule is impaired. Two subtypes of the type II defect have been described: the classic type IIa, in which both chromogenic and clotting functional assays are abnormal, and the type IIb, in which only the clotting functional method is abnormal. Protein C deficiencies should, accordingly, be screened by using a protein C functional assay (clot-based or chromogenic), since this will detect both types I and II. Once a low level of protein C activity is determined, an immunological assay should be performed to distinguish type I from type II protein C deficiency.

Activated Protein C Resistance

Activated protein C (APC) resistance, a new discovery, has been added to the list of causes of thrombotic disease. APC resistance may be caused by an inherited deficiency of an anticoagulant factor that functions as a cofactor to APC. APC resistance appears to be inherited as an autosomal dominant trait, suggesting that a single gene is involved. It is possible that patients with severe APC resistance are homozygous for the genetic defect, whereas an APC response closer to the normal range indicates heterozygosity. The genetically determined defect in anticoagulation characterized by resistance to APC is highly prevalent in patients with venous thrombosis. This defect appears to be at least 10 times more common in such patients than any of the other known inherited deficiencies of anticoagulant proteins. The anticoagulant cofactor that corrects inherited APC resistance is identical to unactivated factor V. APC-resistant plasma contains normal levels of factor V procoagulant, which suggests that APC resistance may be due to a selective defect in an anticoagulant function of factor V (Fig. 27.2).

Protein S Deficiency

Familial studies indicate that patients with a deficiency of protein S have an increased incidence of thrombosis. Early descriptions indicate that protein S deficiency is much more common than either protein C or AT-III deficiency.

The congenital deficiency of protein S is associated with an increased risk of recurrent juvenile venous and arterial thromboembolism. The association of a thrombotic diathesis with acquired protein S deficiency is less clear-cut.

Congenital Protein S Deficiency

Diagnosis of protein S deficiency differs significantly from that of vitamin K–dependent plasma proteins owing to pro-

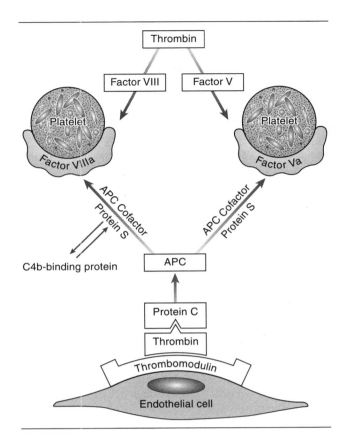

FIGURE 27.2 The protein C anticoagulant pathway. Thrombin converts factor VIII and factor V to their activated forms, factor VIIIa and factor Va. A complex of thrombin with the endothelial-cell receptor thrombomodulin activates protein C. APC inactivates factor VIIIa and factor Va on the platelet surface, and this reaction is accelerated by APC cofactor and free protein S. (From K. A. Bauer, "Hypercoagulability–A New Cofactor in the Protein C Anticoagulant Pathway," *N. Engl. J. Med.,* Vol. 330, No. 8, Feb. 24, 1994, p. 566.)

tein S binding with C4b-BP and repartitioning between free (functional) and bound (nonfunctional) forms. The classification of congenital protein S is based on the comparison of functional and antigenic (free and total) as well as C4b-BP levels (Table 27.21). Currently, three types of congenital deficiencies have been identified: type I, low functional and antigenic protein S levels; type II, low functional protein S levels with a normal antigenic repartition (molecule dysfunctional); and type III, low functional protein S levels corresponding to a decrease in free antigenic protein S along with a normal C4b-BP. However, it needs to be noted that a decrease in free/functional protein S due to increased synthesis of C4b-BP can occur transiently during acute phase reactions.

A protein S functional assay should be used to screen for all types of protein S deficiencies. Antigenic levels of both free and total forms of protein, as well as C4b-BP, will then be determined to differentiate type I, II, and III.

Antithrombin III Deficiency

Hereditary defects of AT-III may be due to quantitative or qualitative defects. Quantitative deficiency of AT-III is trans-

TABLE 27.21 Classification of Congenital Protein S Deficiency

Classification	Functional Clotting	Free PS Antigen	Total PS Antigen	C4b-BP
Type I	Decreased	Decreased	Decreased	—
Type II	Decreased	Normal	Normal	—
Type III	Decreased	Decreased	Normal	Normal
Acute phase reaction	Decreased	Decreased	Normal	Increased

mitted as an autosomal dominant disorder. Type I (quantitative) deficiencies represent the majority of cases. Familial studies reveal that severe thromboembolic problems usually begin to be manifested in late adolescence or early adulthood. Manifestations of AT-III deficiency are rare in infancy. Women with the deficiency have a much higher incidence of thrombosis because pregnancy, delivery, and oral contraceptives are causative factors.

Defects of a qualitative nature (type II deficiency) are often characterized by decreased heparin cofactor activity. This functional manifestation of defective AT-III is not associated with a reduction in molecular concentration. More than half of patients with type II deficiency develop recurrent deep venous thrombosis.

Decreased AT-III Levels: Congenital

The relative incidence of congenital AT-III deficiency is between 1:2000 and 1:5000. AT-III deficiency is inherited as an autosomal dominant disorder. Homozygotes have not been reported in AT-III deficiency. Patients manifest signs and symptoms between 10 and 30 years of age, with their first thrombotic event. An initial event is spontaneous in about one half of patients. Women frequently experience manifestations during pregnancy or because of oral contraceptive use. Decreased levels of AT-III usually correlate with the severity of venous thrombosis. Arterial thrombosis is a less common finding in AT-III deficiency.

Decreased AT-III Levels: Acquired

Acquired AT-III deficiency can be due to decreased synthesis, increased consumption, or other disorder, or it can be drug-induced. The associated disorders are:

Decreased synthesis: arteriosclerosis; cardiovascular disease; chronic hepatitis; cirrhosis; diabetes mellitus, type II
Increased consumption: DIC, homocystinuria, nephrotic syndrome, postoperative, postpartum, protein-losing enteropathy, pulmonary embolism, stroke, thrombophlebitis
Drug-induced: fibrinolysin, heparin, L-asparginase, oral contraceptives
Other disorders: burns, malignancies

Heparin Cofactor Deficiency

Although deficiency of AT-III is the most common, recurrent thrombotic complications have been associated with a defi-ciency of heparin cofactor II. The latter defect has been observed to be inherited in an autosomal dominant manner. Sympathetic heterozygous patients exhibit about half the normal plasma levels of heparin cofactor II activity. This deficiency results from defective protein synthesis rather than from a qualitative abnormality. Heparin cofactor II deficiency can also be demonstrated in patients with DIC. In these situations, both AT-III and heparin cofactor II levels are diminished in parallel.

Clinical Signs and Symptoms

Clinical presentation of patients with deficiencies of naturally occurring anticoagulants is similar. Deficiencies of 50% of normal for protein C, protein S, and AT-III may lead to serious thrombotic events. Frequent presentations include thrombophlebitis, deep vein thrombosis, and pulmonary emboli. The frequency of protein deficiencies correlated with recurrent thromboembolic disease is as follows:

Protein S: 5% to 10%
Protein C: 7%
AT-III: 2% to 4%

Venous Thromboembolism. Venous thromboembolism has a reported incidence of 300,000 episodes per year in the United States, and the complication of pulmonary embolism causes 5% to 10% of all deaths in the hospital. Venous thrombosis can result from hereditary or acquired factors or both.

Patients with venous thromboembolism can be divided into two groups. The first group includes patients with a disease such as cancer, a predisposing factor such as recent surgery, or an acquired abnormality such as the lupus anticoagulant that is known to increase the risk of thrombosis. The pathophysiology is poorly understood (Table 27.22).

A second category consists of patients without the usual risk factors that predispose people to venous thrombosis. In some of these patients, it is possible to identify a deficiency of AT-III, protein C, or protein S and family studies show hereditary defects. APC resistance occurs in about one third of patients. Precipitating factors for thrombosis, such as pregnancy and the use of oral contraceptives, are identified in 60% of these patients. APC resistance appears to be 5 to 10 times more common than a deficiency of AT-III, protein C, or protein S in patients with venous thrombosis.

Laboratory Assessment of Hypercoagulation

The hypercoagulable state can be detected at an early age. The increased sensitivity of platelets to ADP seen in patients with type II hyperlipoproteinemia can result in platelet aggregation in vivo under conditions in which none would occur in normal persons.

Originally, the thromboelastograph (TEG) was introduced as an instrument that measured coagulation from the fluid plasma state until a solid clot was formed and continued to the clot lysis state. Hypercoagulability detected by TEG could be correlated to the amount of fibrinogen formation.

Proof of hypercoagulability can be demonstrated only by the presence of activated clotting factors such as VIIa or Xa.

TABLE 27.22 Hypercoagulable States Associated With Venous Thrombosis

Hypercoagulable State	Comments
Mutation in factor V gene	Replaces arginine 506 with glutamine, rendering factor V resistant to inactivation by activated protein
Mutation in protein C gene	Associated with protein C deficiency
Protein S deficiency	Protein S is a cofactor for protein C
Antithrombin III deficiency	Autosomal dominant inheritance
Antiphospholipid antibodies	Encompasses anticardiolipin antibodies and lupus anticoagulant; associated with venous and arterial thrombosis
Elevated concentration of factor VIII	Relative risk of venous thrombosis is 5-fold higher among patients with factor V concentrations >1500 IU/L

Frequency in Venous Thrombosis
Protein C 2%–4%
Protein S 2%–5%
Antithrombin 1%–3%
Plasminogen 0.5%–2%

Source: S. Z. Goldhaber, "Deep Vein Thrombosis and Pulmonary Embolism." *Intensive Review of Internal Medicine,* Boston: Harvard University, August, 1995, p. 75.

Activated factors may additionally be present in cases of severely abnormal liver function which results in a temporary decrease of coagulation factors. Other tests that draw attention to hypercoagulability include the APTT, FSP, protamine sulfate, and ethanol gel tests; cryofibrinogen, fibrinogen, and factor assays; and tests for protein C and AT-III.

SUMMARY

Vascular Disorders

Abnormal bleeding involving the loss of red blood cells from the microcirculation expresses itself as **purpura,** which is characterized by hemorrhages into the skin, mucous membranes, and internal organs.

Purpura may be associated with a variety of vascular abnormalities including direct endothelial cell damage, an inherited disease of the connective tissue, decreased mechanical strength of the microcirculation, mechanical disruption of small venules, microthrombi (small clots), and vascular malignancy.

Abnormal Platelet Morphology

When examining a peripheral blood smear for platelets, the morphology of the platelets should be observed. Abnormal variations in size should be noted. Disorders of platelet size include Wiscott-Aldrich syndrome, May-Hegglin anomaly, Alport's syndrome, and Bernard-Soulier syndrome.

Quantitative Platelet Disorders

The normal range of circulating platelets is 150×10^9/L to 450×10^9/L. When the quantity of platelets decreases to levels below this range, a condition of thrombocytopenia exists. If the quantity of platelets increases, thrombocytosis is the result.

Thrombocytopenia can result from a wide variety of conditions, such as following the use of extracorporeal circulation in cardiac bypass surgery or in alcoholic liver disease. Heparin-induced thrombocytopenia and associated thrombotic events, relatively common side effects of heparin therapy, can cause substantial morbidity and mortality. Most thrombocytopenic conditions can be classified into the major categories of disorders of production, disorders of destruction, and disorders of platelet distribution and dilution.

Decreased production of platelets may be due to hypoproliferation of the megakaryocytic cell line or ineffective thrombopoiesis caused by acquired conditions or hereditary factors. Thrombocytopenia due to hypoproliferation can result from acquired damage to hematopoietic cells of the bone marrow caused by factors such as irradiation, drugs and cancer chemotherapeutic agents, chemicals, and alcohol. Hypoproliferation may also result from nonmalignant conditions, such as infections, lupus erythematosus, granulomatous disease such as **sarcoidosis,** and idiopathic causes. Ineffective thrombopoiesis may result in decreased platelet production. Thrombocytopenias of this type may be the manifestation of a nutritional disorder, such as a deficiency of vitamin B_{12} or folic acid. Another disorder related to ineffective thrombopoiesis is iron deficiency anemia, which usually results in a decrease in megakaryocyte size and the suppression of megakaryocyte endoproliferation and size. Hereditary thrombocytopenias include Fanconi's syndrome, constitutional aplastic anemia and its variants, amegakaryocytic thrombocytopenia (TAR syndrome), X-linked amegakaryocytic thrombocytopenia, Wiskott-Aldrich syndrome, May-Hegglin anomaly, and hereditary macrothrombocytopenia (e.g., Alport's syndrome).

Increased destruction or utilization of platelets may result from a number of mechanisms. It can be due to antigens, antibodies, drugs, or foreign substances. Bacterial sepsis causes increased destruction of platelets owing to the attachment of platelets to bacterial antigen-antibody immune complexes. Antibodies of either autoimmune or isoimmune origin may produce increased destruction of platelets.

Accelerated consumption of platelets is another cause of thrombocytopenia. One of the most important and frequently encountered forms of increased consumption of platelets is idiopathic thrombocytopenic purpura (ITP). This antibody-related response, which may be preceded by infection, is believed to have a devastating effect on platelet survival. ITP may complicate other antibody-associated disorders such as **systemic lupus erythematosus** (SLE). Patients with immunologic thrombocytopenic purpura usually demonstrate petechiae, bruising, menorrhagia, and bleeding after minor trauma.

Disorders of Platelet Distribution

A platelet distribution disorder can result from a pooling of platelets in the spleen, which is frequent if splenomegaly is present. This type of thrombocytopenia develops when more than a double or triple increase in platelet production is required to maintain the normal quantity of circulating platelets.

Thrombocytosis is generally defined as a substantial increase in circulating platelets over the normal upper limit of $450 \times 10^9/L$. Thrombocytosis is usually grouped according to cause: reactive or benign etiologies versus platelet elevations linked to a specific hematological disorder.

Qualitative Platelet Disorders

If platelets are normal in number but fail to function properly one of four separate categories of platelet dysfunction can exist. These include the more common acquired and less frequent hereditary causes. Hyperactive platelets associated with hypercoagulability and thrombosis make up an additional category of abnormal platelet function.

Acquired platelet function defects can be due to a blood plasma inhibitory substance. In addition, acquired platelet dysfunction is commonly seen in the myeloproliferative syndromes and uremia. Miscellaneous disorders can be associated with platelet dysfunction. Many drugs can induce platelet function defects, resulting in hemorrhage.

Hereditary disorders include adhesion disorder; Bernard-Soulier syndrome; primary aggregation disorders, such as Glanzmann's thrombasthenia and essential athrombia; and secondary aggregation disorders, such as hereditary storage pool defect and hereditary aspirin-like defects.

Bleeding Disorders Related to Blood Clotting Factors

Bleeding and defective fibrin clot formation are frequently related to a coagulation factor. Disorders of the blood coagulation factors can be grouped into three categories: defective production, excessive destruction, and pathological inhibition.

A condition of defective production may be related to a deficiency of vitamin K. Severe liver disease may produce decreased plasma levels of fibrinogen, although low levels of fibrinogen rarely produce hemorrhage. Hereditary clotting defects including classic hemophilia (hemophilia A) and von Willebrand's disease are examples of hereditary disorders that represent functionally inactive factor VIII.

Hemophilia has been used as a paradigm for understanding the molecular pathological processes that underlie hereditary disease. The cloning of factor VIII facilitated the identification of mutations that lead to hemophilia A, an inherited deficiency of factor VIII coagulant activity that causes severe hemorrhage. Von Willebrand's disease may be an acquired or inherited disorder. The congenital disorder is autosomally dominant in most cases. Three broad types of von Willebrand's disease are recognized. In addition, a platelet-type von Willebrand's disease (pseudo–von Willebrand's disease) is due to an abnormal platelet receptor for vWF. Acquired von Willebrand's disease may complicate other diseases such as lymphoproliferative and autoimmune disorders, and proteolytic degradation of vWF complicates myeloproliferative disorders.

A deficiency of factor IX is known as **hemophilia B** or **Christmas disease.** A deficiency of factor XI is referred to as **hemophilia C. Fibrinogen deficiency** as a genetic disorder may represent a defect of production or dysfunctional molecules. Hereditary deficiencies of the other coagulation factors are relatively rare. Examples of rare defects include **factor XII deficiency** where no clinical bleeding tendencies are apparent and **factor XIII deficiency,** which is associated with spontaneous abortion and poor wound healing.

Disorders of Destruction and Consumption

Blood coagulation factors can be destroyed in vivo by enzymatic degradation or by pathological activation of coagulation with excessive utilization of the clotting factors. Enzymatic destruction can result from bites by certain species of snakes whose venom contains an enzyme that degrades fibrinogen to a defective fibrin monomer. In vivo activation of coagulation by tissue thromboplastin-like materials can produce excessive utilization of clotting factors. Conditions that can cause this consumption of coagulation factors include obstetrical complications, trauma, burns, prostatic and pelvic surgery, shock, advanced malignancy, septicemia, and intravascular hemolysis.

Primary and secondary fibrinolysis are recognized as extreme complications of a variety of intravascular and extravascular disorders and may have life-threatening consequences. Primary fibrinolysis is associated with conditions in which gross activation of the fibrinolytic mechanism with subsequent fibrinogen and coagulation factor consumption occurs. The important characteristic of primary fibrinolysis is that no evidence of fibrin deposition occurs. Primary fibrinolysis occurs when large amounts of plasminogen activator enter the circulatory system as a result of trauma, surgery, and malignancies.

Although the same clinical conditions may also induce secondary fibrinolysis or **disseminated intravascular coagulation (DIC),** the distinction between the two is essentially in the demonstration of fibrin formation. In secondary fibrinolysis, excessive clotting and fibrinolytic activity occur. Increased amounts of fibrin split (degradation) products (FSPs) and fibrin monomers are detectable because of the action of thrombin on the fibrinogen molecule. This fibrinolytic process is only due to excessive clotting; therefore, it is a secondary condition. This distinguishes between primary and secondary fibrinolysis.

The Hypercoagulable State

Thrombi may form because coagulation is enhanced or because protective devices such as fibrinolysis are impaired. An increase in the likelihood of blood to clot is referred to as the **hypercoagulable state.**

Hypercoagulable states include various inherited as well as acquired clinical disorders characterized by an increased risk for thromboembolism. Primary hypercoagulable states include relatively rare inherited conditions that lead to disordered endothelial cell thromboregulation. These conditions include decreased thrombomodulin-dependent activation of activated protein C, impaired heparin binding of AT-III, or down-regulation of membrane-associated plasmin generation.

The major inherited inhibitor disease states include AT-III deficiency, protein C deficiency, and protein S deficiency. Secondary hypercoagulation states may be seen in many heterogeneous disorders.

Acquired inhibitors of clotting proteins, also known as circulating anticoagulants, inactivate or inhibit the usual procoagulant activity of coagulation factors. Inhibitors are frequently characterized as specific, those directed against a coagulation factor, or nonspecific, those directed against a complex of factors, such as the lupus anticoagulant. The majority of these inhibitors exhibit biochemical properties, suggesting they are immunoglobulins. Inhibitors may arise following transfusion of blood products or in patients with no previous hemostatic disorders. Acquired inhibitors can be a significant cause of hemorrhage.

Specific inhibitors against factors II, V, VII, VIII, IX, XII, and XIII and vWF have been detected in patients with individual factor deficiencies. However, some inhibitors of factors II, V, VII, IX, and XII and vWF have been observed in patients having no deficiencies of coagulation factors.

CASE STUDIES

CASE 1 A 2-year-old boy fell from a backyard gym set. His shoulder and upper arm became very swollen shortly after the fall. The boy's mother took him to the emergency room a few hours after the incident because he was complaining of pain. On physical examination, the emergency room physician noted that a large hematoma had formed in the upper part of the boy's right arm. There was no history of surgery (he had not been circumcised), injury, or illness. The boy was receiving no medication.

Emergency room treatment consisted of aspirating the hematoma. Subsequent to this treatment, the boy began to bleed extensively. He was admitted to the hospital.

The following stat laboratory tests were ordered: a hemoglobin and hematocrit, platelet count, and bleeding time. Because the bleeding continued, a type and crossmatch for 2 units of fresh blood were ordered on a standby basis.

Additional information from the mother revealed that the boy's cousin had a "bleeding problem."

Laboratory Data
Hemoglobin 8.0 gm/L
Hematocrit 0.26 L/L
Platelet count 200 × 10⁹/L (normal: 150 to 450 × 10⁹/L)
Bleeding time 5 minutes (normal: 3 to 8 minutes)

Subsequent coagulation profile tests were ordered prior to the transfusion of 2 units of fresh whole blood. The results of these tests were as follows:

PT 12 seconds (normal: 11 to 15 seconds)
APTT 60 seconds (normal: 28 to 35 seconds)
Thrombin time–reptilase method 20 seconds (normal: 18 to 22 seconds)

Questions
1. Do the laboratory data support a diagnosis of a disorder of hemostasis?
2. What types of disorders can be preliminarily identified by the tests that were performed?
3. What confirmatory tests must be done in this case?

Discussion
1. Yes, the abnormal results of the APTT suggest that a coagulation defect may be the cause of this child's bleeding.
2. A normal platelet count and bleeding time suggest that platelets are not the causative agent in this bleeding disorder. Because the thrombin time was normal, a decrease or abnormality of fibrinogen and the presence of a circulating anticoagulant can be excluded.

   By comparing the APTT and PT, certain blood coagulation factors can be isolated as being deficient.

Test		
APTT	PT	Deficient factor(s)
Increased	Normal	VIII, IX, XI, or XII
Increased	Increased	II, V, X, or anticoagulant
Normal	Increased	VII

   In this case, an increased APTT with a normal PT suggests that the patient is deficient in any of these factors: VIII, IX, XI, or XII.
3. Factor substitution testing or a thromboplastin generation time (TGT) might be of value before a specific factor assay is performed. These screening tests are useful in isolating either specific factors or groups of factors that are deficient in a patient's plasma. In order to confirm a specific factor deficiency, a factor assay must be performed. In this case, a factor VIII assay revealed that the boy was deficient in factor VIII.

☞ Diagnosis: Factor VIII deficiency (hemophilia type A)

CASE 2 A 21-year-old black prison inmate was admitted to the hospital for the repair of an abdominal hernia. His physician was concerned that strangulation of the hernia could oc-

(continued)

CASE STUDIES (*continued*)

cur. The patient was in extremely good physical condition. He did not remember having any unusual illnesses. His family history did include minor bleeding problems among some of his relatives.

Laboratory Data

On admission the hemoglobin and hematocrit were 15.0 gm/L and 0.44 L/L, respectively. The PT was 13 seconds (normal: 10 to 15 seconds), and the APTT 55 seconds (normal: 28 to 35 seconds).

Because of the results obtained on the original and a repeat specimen of the APTT in conjunction with a vague family history of bleeding, this patient's surgery was postponed until a bleeding disorder could be ruled out.

Questions

1. What coagulation deficiencies might be present in this patient?
2. What supplementary laboratory assays would be appropriate?
3. How could this be distinguished from other similar disorders?

Discussion

1. As in Case 1, a prolonged APTT with a normal PT suggests the presence of a deficiency of factor VIII, IX, XI, or XII. Because deficiencies of factors XI and XII are rare, it is unlikely that they would be responsible for the prolonged APTT. Either a deficiency of factor VIII or IX would be more common.
2. Factor substitution studies would be of value. If the substitution studies reveal an abnormality, a specific factor assay should be conducted.
3. In this case, factor VIII activity was found to be decreased (patient 30% activity, normal 50 to 150%). This finding and the lack of a bleeding history in the patient suggest that the patient may not have a classic factor VIII deficiency. Further testing was performed. The results were as follows: bleeding time increased, platelet aggregation decreased, factor VIII decreased, and factor VIII/vWF decreased. Based on these findings, the diagnosis of classic hemophilia was excluded. The laboratory findings support a diagnosis of von Willebrand's disease.

✏ Diagnosis: von Willebrand's disease

CASE 3 A 62-year-old white man with a history of abnormal bleeding was admitted to the hospital for a medical workup prior to dental surgery. A brother had died at age 19 of traumatic bleeding after being injured in a car accident.

The patient had his first bleeding episode at 7 years of age following a lymph node resection. He reported having had marked hemorrhaging as a teenager following mild trauma. At age 30, the patient had a tooth extraction followed by 3 weeks of bleeding, at which time he received a blood transfusion. At age 31, he was given a blood transfusion prior to an appendectomy and on that occasion had no bleeding whatsoever. Two years before admission the patient suffered from gastrointestinal bleeding following surgery for a hiatal hernia. At that time he was given 2 units of bank blood and 2 units of fresh blood. Bleeding subsided and his subsequent recovery was good.

Laboratory Data

The laboratory findings were as follows:

Hemoglobin 7.0 gm/L
Hematocrit 0.23 L/L
Platelet count = 498×10^9/L
Bleeding time (Ivy) 2 minutes (normal: less than 8 minutes)
Whole blood clotting time averaged 188 minutes (normal: less than 70 minutes)
Platelet aggregation normal
APTT 53 seconds (control: 39 seconds)
PT 13.8 seconds (control: 13.3 seconds)

Specific assays for factors VIII and IX were performed. The level of activity of factor IX was less than 5%.

Questions

1. What is the diagnosis in this case?
2. Can this patient safely undergo surgery?
3. What is the role of the laboratory in a surgical case of this type?

Discussion

1. The diagnosis in this case is factor IX deficiency.
2. Yes, but the patient received a factor IX concentrate rather than whole or fresh blood to correct the deficiency. He did receive 2 units of blood because of his low red cell volume.
3. Because factor IX has a half-life of 8 to 24 hours, it is important that the patient receive appropriate amounts of concentrates. A minimum static level of 20 to 30% must be achieved before and during surgery. The level of factor activity must be sustained until healing is sufficient to prevent breakthrough bleeding.

TABLE 27.23 Factor IX Activity Levels

Assay	Date	Time	Units of Factor IX Complex (Konyne*)	Activity (%)
Admission				
1	10/6	A.M.	0	5
2	10/6	2 P.M.	2 units of blood	30
3	10/7	11 A.M.	5	93
4	10/8	7 P.M.	0	35
5	10/8	9 A.M.	2	72
Surgery				
6	10/8	2 P.M.	2	72
7	10/9	7 A.M.	0	22
8	10/9	2 P.M.	2	49
9	10/10	8 A.M.	2	46
10	10/11	8 A.M.	4	38
11	10/11	2 P.M.	4	55
12	10/12	8 A.M.	4	52
13	10/13	3 P.M.	4	62
14	10/14	8 A.M.	4	55
15	10/15	9 A.M.	0	40
16	10/16	9 A.M.	0	20
Discharged				

*Konyne, Cutter Laboratories, Berkeley, CA, 1 unit = 1 bottle of 500 units.

(*continued*)

Table 27.23 and the following figure represent how the patient was monitored preoperatively and postoperatively. Each specimen was drawn within 30 minutes of the administration of the concentrate. The solid line denotes assay values; the broken line denotes therapeutic factor IX.

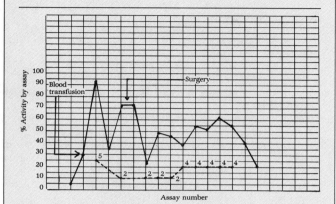

✏ Diagnosis: Hemophilia type B (Christmas disease)

CASE 4 A 22-year-old white woman had recently graduated from college and relocated to accept her first professional job. She was being seen for the first time by a local gynecologist because of prolonged menstrual bleeding. Her medical history included several episodes of severe nosebleeds during childhood that required cauterization to arrest. She reported that her menses lasted from 8 to 12 days. When questioned about family illnesses or disorders, she reported that her mother and two sisters also had long menstrual periods, and that one of her two brothers needed several blood transfusions after an appendectomy.

Physical examination revealed an essentially normal patient. However, she appeared pale and several large bruises were noted on her extremities. The patient was referred to the outpatient laboratory for a hemoglobin, hematocrit, and coagulation profile.

Laboratory Data
Hemoglobin 10.0 gm/L
Hematocrit 0.27 L/L

Her coagulation profile results were as follows:

Bleeding time 7 minutes (normal: 1 to 3 minutes)
PT 11 seconds (control: 12.2 seconds)
APTT 29 seconds (control: 34 seconds)
Clot retraction decreased

Questions
1. What additional tests would be suggested based on the initial laboratory results?
2. What would the Wright-stained blood film look like?
3. What is the most likely diagnosis and prognosis?

Discussion
1. A platelet count and qualitative platelet studies would be appropriate follow-up procedures in view of the prolonged bleeding time and poor clot retraction.
2. If a platelet disorder is suspected, the peripheral blood smear may be of value. Obviously decreases in platelets would support the quantitative assay and an abnormality in platelet size could be detected. In this case, both the distribution and morphology of the platelets appeared normal.
3. Further testing for platelet function revealed a deficiency in both platelet aggregation and adhesion. The diagnosis of Glanzmann's thrombasthenia was made. This autosomal recessive disorder usually becomes less severe as a patient ages. In this woman's case, severe bleeding or future surgical interventions would need to be supported by the use of platelet concentrates.

✏ Diagnosis: Glanzmann's thrombasthenia

CASE 5 A woman was admitted in labor to the obstetrical unit at 11 P.M. Her history and physical examination revealed no significant abnormalities. At the time of admission, she was having irregular contractions.

In the delivery room, bleeding became extensive. A stat hemoglobin, hematocrit, type and crossmatch for 4 units of blood, and coagulation profile were ordered.

Laboratory Data
The patient's laboratory data were as follows:

Hemoglobin 10.0 gm/L
Hematocrit 0.27 L/L
Platelet count 75 × 10⁹/L
Bleeding time 10 minutes
APTT 65 seconds (control: 29 seconds)
PT 19 seconds (control: 11 seconds)
Thrombin time 24 seconds (normal: 18 to 22 seconds)
Fibrinogen 90 mg/dL (normal: 200 to 400 mg/dL)
Fibrin split product screen positive
Protamine sulfate test positive

Questions
1. What is the most probable cause of the extensive bleeding in this case?
2. What is the etiology of this disorder?
3. Will the transfusion of whole or fresh blood repress the bleeding?

Discussion
1. The laboratory test results support the condition of fibrinolysis, specifically DIC. In secondary fibrinolysis as compared with primary fibrinolysis, the platelet count is decreased and the protamine sulfate test result is positive.
2. The release of placental tissue into the maternal circulation can trigger the coagulation mechanism. When this stimulation supersedes the body's natural protective mechanism, secondary bleeding occurs. In this case, the consumption of coagulation factors is evident in the laboratory findings.

(continued)

> **CASE STUDIES** (*continued*)
>
> 3. Although transfusions may temporarily replace the blood volume lost through bleeding, they will not alleviate the problem. Overwhelming fibrinolysis can be fatal. In many cases, heparin is administered to stop the cyclical process that is in progress.
>
> ✐ **Diagnosis: Disseminated intravascular coagulation (DIC)**

BIBLIOGRAPHY

Abrams, Charol. "Knowing Assay Limitations Helpful in Detecting Thrombotic Disorders," *ADVANCE for Medical Laboratory Professionals*, Vol. 7, No. 25, December 18, 1995, pp. 18–19.

Aledort, Louis M. "Treatment of von Willebrand's Disease." *Mayo Clin. Proc.*, Vol. 66, 1991, pp. 841–846.

Aster, Richard H. "Heparin-Induced Thrombocytopenia and Thrombosis." *New Engl. J. Med.*, Vol. 332, No. 20, March 18, 1995, pp. 1374–1376.

Bauer, K. A. "Hypercoagulability—A New Cofactor in the Protein C Anticoagulant Pathway." *New Engl. J. Med.*, Vol. 330, No. 8, February 24, 1994, pp. 566–567.

Bick, Rodger L. and Steven M. Scates. "Qualitative Platelet Defects." *Lab. Med.*, Vol. 23, No. 2, February 1992, pp. 95–103.

Bick, Roger L. and Lori Kunkel. "Hypercoagulability and Thrombosis." *Lab. Med.*, Vol. 23, No. 4, April, 1992, pp. 233–238.

Bick, Rodger L. "Oral Anticoagulants in Thromboembolic Disease." *Lab. Med.*, Vol. 26, No. 3, March, 1995, pp. 188–193.

Bloom, Arthur L. "von Willebrand Factor: Clinical Features of Inherited and Acquired Disorders." *Mayo Clin. Proc.* Vol. 66, 1991, pp. 743–751.

Boral, Leonard I. "Platelet Transfusion Therapy." *Lab. Med.*, Vol. 16, No. 4, April, 1985, pp. 221–227.

Burrows, R. F. and John G. Kelton, M. D. "Fetal Thrombocytopenia and Its Relation to Maternal Thrombocytopenia." *New Engl. J. Med.*, Vol. 329, No. 20, November 11, 1993, pp. 1463–1466.

Bussel, J. B. et al. "Fetal Alloimmune Thrombocytopenia." *New Engl. J. Med.*, Vol. 337, No. 1, July 3, 1997, pp. 22–26.

Cosio, F. G. et al. "Plasma Concentrations of the Natural Anticoagulants Protein C and Protein S in Patients with Proteinuria." *J. Lab. Clin. Med.*, Vol. 106, No. 2, 1985, pp. 218–222.

Epstein, Murray. "Thrombocytopenia and the Neglected Megakaryocyte." *New Engl. J. Med.*, Vol. 327, No. 25, December 17, 1992, pp. 1812–1813.

Ewenstein, B. M. "Antithrombotic Agents and Thrombolytic Disease." *New Engl. J. Med.*, Vol. 337, No. 19, November 6, 1997, pp. 1383–1384.

Figueroa, Michael et al. "Combination Chemotherapy in Refractory Immune Thrombocytopenic Purpura." *New Engl. J. Med.*, Vol. 328, No. 17, April 29, 1993, pp. 1226–1229.

Fritsma, G. A. and L. A. Quarles. "Top 10 Problems in Coag." *Adv. Med. Lab. Prof.*, Vol. 9, No. 24, December 1, 1997, pp. 8–13.

George, James N., Mayez A. El-Harake. "Chronic Idiopathic Thrombocytopenic Purpura." *New Engl. J. Med.*, Vol. 331, No. 18, Nov. 3, 1994, pp. 1207–1215.

Gimbrone, Michael. "Endothelium in Health and Disease." *Intensive Review of Internal Medicine.* Boston: Harvard University, 1995, pp. 891–900.

Glueck, Helen I. et al. "Thrombosis in Systemic Lupus Erythematosus." *Arch. Intern. Med.*, Vol. 145, August, 1985, pp. 1389–1394.

Goldhaber, Samuel Z. "Deep Vein Thrombosis and Pulmonary Embolism." *Intensive Review of Internal Medicine*, Boston: Harvard University. August, 1995, p. 75.

Hajjar, K. A. "Factor V Leiden—An Unselfish Gene." *New Engl. J. Med.*, Vol. 330, No. 23, December 8, 1994, pp. 1585–1586.

Harker, Laurence A. "Platelets and Vascular Thrombosis." *New Engl. J. Med.*, Vol. 330, No. 14, April 7, 1994, pp. 1006–1007.

Hudson, Pat et al. "Troubleshooting Coagulation Screening Test Results." Miami: Baxter Healthcare, 1988.

Hutchison, Doug. "Platelet Function, Disorders and Testing," in *Coagulation Education.* T. Hirsch (ed.). Miami: American Dade, 1983, pp. 78–96.

Ingram, G. I. C. "The History of Haemophilia." *J. Clin. Pathol.*, Vol. 29, No. 6, 1976, pp. 469–479.

Intensive Review of Internal Medicine. Boston: Harvard University, August, 1995.

Jameson, C. "Hemostasis During Open-Heart Surgery." *Laboratory Medicine*, Vol. 28, No. 10, October, 1997, pp. 632–633.

Marlar, Richard A. et al. "Serial Studies of Protein C and Its Plasma Inhibitor in Patients With Disseminated Intravascular Coagulation." *Blood*, Vol. 66, No. 1, July, 1985, pp. 59–63.

Meyer, Dominique et al. "von Willebrand Factor: Structure and Function." *Mayo Clin. Proc.*, Vol. 66, 1991, pp. 516–523.

Morgan, Charles and John A. Penner. "Bleeding Complications During Surgery: Part II. Acquired Hemorrhagic Disorders." *Lab. Med.*, Vol. 17, No. 5, May, 1986, pp. 262–270.

Moroose, Rebecca and Leon W. Hoyer. "von Willebrand Factor and Platelet Function." *Annu. Rev. Med.*, Vol. 37, 1986, pp. 157–163.

Nachman, R. L. and R. Silverstein. "Hypercoagulable States." *Ann Intern Med.*, Vol. 119, No. 8, October 15, 1993, pp. 819–827.

Patrono, C. "Aspirin as an Antiplatelet Drug." *New Engl. J. Med.*, Vol. 330, No. 18, May 5, 1994, pp. 1287–1294.

Pitcher, Pamela M. "The Detection of Fibrinogen Degradation Products (FDP) in Serum and Urine." *Can. J. Med. Technol.*, Vol. 10, October, 1972, pp. 3–15.

Ratnoff, Oscar D. "Thrombosis and the Hypercoagulable State." *Circulation*, Vol. 70, Suppl. III, November, 1984, pp. III-72–76.

Reich, Paul R. *Hematology—Physiopathologic Basis for Clinical Practice* (2nd edition). Boston: Little, Brown & Co., 1984, pp. 439–486.

Ridker, P. M. et al. "Ethnic Distribution of Factor V Leiden in 4047 Men and Women." *New Engl. J. Med.*, Vol. 277, No. 16, April 23/30, 1997, pp. 1305–1307.

Rothenberger, S. S. and L. J. McCarthy. "Neonatal Alloimmune Thrombocytopenia." *Lab. Med.*, Vol. 28, No. 9, September, 1997, pp. 592–596.

Ruggeri, Azverio M. "Structure and Function of von Willebrand Factor: Relationship to von Willebrand's Disease." *Mayo Clin. Proc.*, Vol. 66, 1991, pp. 847–861.

Schick, Barbara P. "Clinical Implications of Basic Research." *New Engl. J. Med.*, Vol. 331, No. 13, September 29, 1994, pp. 875–876.

Schwarz, Hans P. et al. "Plasma Protein S Deficiency in Familial Thrombotic Disease." *Blood*, Vol. 64, No. 6, December, 1984, pp. 1297–1300.

Starrett, Dawn. "Applications of a Thromboelastograph." *Am. Clin. Products Rev.*, Vol. 23, April, 1985, pp. 34–42.

Svensson, P. J. and V. Dahlback. "Resistance to Activated Protein C as a Basis for Venous Thrombosis." *New Engl. J. Med.*, Vol. 330, No. 8, February 24, 1994, pp. 517–522.

Triplett, Douglas A. "Laboratory Diagnosis of von Willebrand's Disease." *Mayo Clin. Proc.*, Vol. 66, 1991, pp. 832–840.

Wagner, Denisa D. and Roberta Bonfanti. "von Willebrand Factor and the Endothelium." *Mayo Clin. Proc.*, Vol. 66, 1991, pp. 621–627.

Zondag, A. C. P. et al. "Simple Screening Techniques for the Detection of Hypercoagulation." *Haemostasis*, Vol. 14, 1984, pp. 445–452.

REVIEW QUESTIONS

1. Which of the following is a condition associated with purpura:
   A. Direct endothelial damage.
   B. Inherited disease of the connective tissue.
   C. Mechanical disruption of small venules.
   D. All of the above.

Questions 2 through 4: match the following platelet disorders with the appropriate morphology (use only one answer).

2. ___ Wiscott-Aldrich syndrome.
3. ___ May-Hegglin anomaly.
4. ___ Bernard-Soulier syndrome.

   A. Giant platelets.
   B. Smallest platelets seen.
   C. Large platelets.

Questions 5 through 7: match the etiologies of these platelet dysfunctions with the appropriate associated disorder. Use each answer once.

5. ___ Acquired.
6. ___ Drug-induced.
7. ___ Hereditary.

   A. Aspirin.
   B. von Willebrand's disease.
   C. Uremia.

8. Which of the following parameters is usually abnormal in classic von Willebrand's disease Type I?
   A. Bleeding time.
   B. Prothrombin time.
   C. Platelet count.
   D. All of the above.

9. The most common form of von Willebrand's disease is:
   A. Type I.
   B. Type II.
   C. Type III.
   D. All have about the same incidence.

10. Laboratory results in acute disseminated intravascular coagulation reflect abnormalities in which of the following coagulation components?
    A. Platelet function.
    B. Excessive clotting and fibrinolysis.
    C. Accelerated thrombin formation.
    D. Fibrin formation.

11. Primary fibrinolysis is characterized by:
    A. Gross activation of the fibrinolytic mechanism.
    B. Consumption of fibrinogen.
    C. Consumption of coagulation factors.
    D. All of the above.

12. The hallmark of secondary fibrinolysis is the presence of:
    A. Fibrin split products.
    B. Fibrin degradation products.
    C. Fibrin monomers.
    D. All of the above.

13. DIC is characterized by:
    A. Excess thrombin formation.
    B. Conversion of fibrinogen to fibrin.
    C. Platelet consumption and deposition.
    D. All of the above.

14. Which of the following factors can contribute to hypercoagulation?
    A. Vascular endothelial damage.
    B. Increased blood flow.
    C. Decreased platelets.
    D. Decreased titers of clotting factors.

Questions 15 through 19: match the following.

15. ___ Antithrombin III deficiency.
16. ___ Oral contraceptives.
17. ___ Protein C deficiency.
18. ___ Cancer.
19. ___ Pregnancy.

    A. Primary hypercoagulable state.
    B. Secondary hypercoagulable state.

Questions 20 through 22: match the following terms with the appropriate description.

20. ___ Circulating anticoagulants.
21. ___ Lupus anticoagulant.
22. ___ Factor VIII inhibitor.

    A. The most common specific factor inhibitor.
    B. Acquired inhibitors of clotting proteins.
    C. Also known as antiphospholipid or anticardiolipin antibody.

absolute lymphocytosis An increase in the total number of lymphocytes in the circulating blood. Seen in viral infections such as infectious mononucleosis and rubella (German measles).

absolute polycythemia See *secondary polycythemia*.

absolute reticulocyte count See *corrected reticulocyte count*.

absorbance Optical density.

accuracy Describes how close a test result is to the true value.

actomyosin (thrombosthenin) A contractile protein found in platelets.

acute Severe and of short duration.

adenopathy Swelling of the lymph nodes.

adhesiveness In coagulation, the process of platelets sticking to the blood vessel wall.

ADP Adenosine diphosphate.

agammaglobulinemia The absence or severe decrease of the gamma globulin protein fraction in the blood.

agglutination Clumping of cells.

agglutinin An antibody produced in response to a specific antigen (foreign substance).

aggregation In blood coagulation, the process in which platelets stick or clump together.

Alder-Reilly inclusions Abnormal purple-red particles representing precipitated mucopolysaccharides that are seen primarily in neutrophilic, eosinophilic, and basophilic leukocytes.

aleukemic leukemia A form of leukemia in which little change is seen in the total leukocyte count or cellular maturity in the peripheral blood. An increased number of immature cells can be found in the bone marrow.

alkaline A basic solution (pH 7.1 to 14.0) with the ability to neutralize acids.

ALL Acute lymphoblastic leukemia.

allele One of two or more genes that occur at the same locus on homologous chromosomes

amplitude Height or magnitude.

amyloidosis The abnormal deposition of amyloid, a protein, in various tissues.

anaphase A stage in cellular division (mitosis).

anaphylaxis A severe and often life-threatening reaction to a foreign protein.

anaplasia Highly pleomorphic and bizarre cytologic features associated with malignant tumors that are poorly differentiated.

anemia A condition of decreased or dysfunctional erythrocytes.

angina Any condition characterized by spasmodic feelings of suffocation.

anisochromia Variation of the color of erythrocytes due to unequal hemoglobin concentration.

anisocytosis A general term used to denote an increased variation in cell size.

ANLL Acute nonlymphoblastic leukemia.

anomaly A marked deviation from normal.

anorexia Loss of appetite.

anoxia Without oxygen. The reduction of oxygen in the tissues below physiological levels.

antibody An immunoglobulin produced in response to an antigen.

antihemophilic factor Factor VIII.

anti–human globulin test (AHG) Previously referred to as the Coombs' test. May be either a direct or an indirect test to detect the presence of antibodies on erythrocytes (direct test) or the presence of antibodies capable of coating erythrocytes (indirect test).

antithrombin III An alpha-2 globulin that circulates in the plasma.

apoferritin A protein that combines with iron to form ferritin.

appendicular skeleton The bones of the limbs of the body.

APTT Activated partial thromboplastin time.

argon An inert gas used in lasers.

arteries Distributing blood vessels that leave the heart.

arterioles Microscopic continuations of arteries that give off branches called metarterioles, which in turn join the capillaries.

arthritide An eruption of the skin due to gout.

arthrocentesis Entry into a joint cavity to aspirate fluid.

arthrography Radiographic (x-ray) study of a joint.

artifact Any artificial particles seen in stained preparations, diluting fluids, etc.

aspirate The process of physically removing, usually with a syringe, fluid from a body cavity or space.

assay The determination of the purity of a substance or the amount of a particular substance in a mixture or compound.

ATP Adenosine triphosphate.

atrophy A decrease in the number or size of cells that produces a reduction in the size of a normal organ or tissue.

atypical antibody An antibody not usually found in the blood plasma. Also referred to as an alloantibody.

Auer rods or Auer bodies These cellular inclusions are aggregates of cytoplasmic granules that appear as red, elongated structures. They may occur alone or in groups in myeloblasts and occasionally monoblasts.

autoantibody Antibodies capable of reacting with one's own cells. In autoimmune hemolytic anemia, patients develop antibodies that produce hemolysis of the patient's own cells.

autosomal dominant A genetic trait that expresses itself, if present, and is carried on one of the chromosome pairs 1 through 22.

axial skeleton The bones of the head and trunk of the body.

azurophilic granules Granules that stain red due to azure dyes.

B cell disease Disorders associated with B-type lymphocytes such as CLL.

B cells or B lymphocytes The primary source of cells responsible for antibody responses.

bacteremia A bacterial infection of the blood.

base pair A nucleotide (either adenine, guanine, cytosine, thymidine, or uracil) and its complementary base on the opposite strand.

basic calcium phosphate (BCP) A type of crystal that can be seen in joint (synovial) fluid.

basophilia An abnormal increase in the number of erythrocytes with a blue appearance. The presence of fine, evenly distributed basophilic granules is referred to as polychromatophilia in Wright-stained blood smears.

basophilic granules Blue-staining granules.

BCP See *basic calcium phosphate*.

Bence Jones protein The abnormal protein frequently found in the urine of patients with multiple myeloma. It precipitates at 50°C, disappears at 100°C, and reappears on cooling to room temperature.

benign Nonmalignant or noncancerous.

Bernard-Soulier syndrome A disorder characterized by the largest platelets seen in a platelet disorder.

beta-thalassemia A form of anemia in which beta chain synthesis is impaired.

bilirubin A breakdown product of heme from hemoglobin.

biliverdin A breakdown product arising from the oxidation of bilirubin.

bit map A polygonal figure with as many as 16 sides drawn around the cells to be analyzed or sorted in flow-cell cytometry.

blast The most immature form of a cell.

blast crisis The dominance of immature blood cells in the blood or bone marrow of patients with a treated leukemia previously in remission.

blood-brain barrier Walls of blood vessels of the central nervous system that prevent or delay the entry of certain blood substances into the brain tissue.

blotting Transfer or fixation of nucleic acids onto a solid matrix, such as nitrocellulose, so that they may be hybridized with a probe.

bone marrow The material in the cavities of bones. Red marrow is the site of hematopoiesis.

buffer solution A solution that will resist sudden changes in acidity or alkalinity.

buffy coat The interface layer in a tube of anticoagulated blood between the plasma and erythrocytes. This layer contains leukocytes and thrombocytes.

burst-forming unit-erythroid The most primitive identifiable unipotent erythroid stem cell in primitive fetal cells.

Cabot rings Ring-shaped, figure-eight, or loop-shaped inclusions seen in stained erythrocytes.

calcium pyrophosphate dihydrate An abnormal crystal found in joint (synovial) fluid.

calibration The comparison of an instrument measurement or reading to a known physical constant.

CAP College of American Pathologists.

capillaries A unit of the microcirculation that functions as the link between the arterial and venous blood circulation.

capillary blood Blood obtained from the capillaries of sites such as the fingertip, toe, or heel.

catecholamines Biologically active amines such as epinephrine that are derived from the amino acid tyrosine.

CDC Centers for Disease Control and Prevention.

cDNA Complementary DNA, produced from mRNA using reverse transcriptase.

celiac disease An uncommon malabsorption syndrome (also known as nontropical sprue) characterized by an inability to digest and utilize fats, starches, and sugars.

cell coincidence error More than one cell passing through the aperture of an impedance cell-counting instrument at the same time.

centrioles A pair of central spots inside the centrosome.

centrosome The area of the cell where the cytoplasm is homogeneous, where there are no mitochondria, and where there are two tiny spots at the center.

cerebrospinal fluid A fluid formed continuously in the choroid plexus of the cerebral ventricles. It is found in the subarachnoid space, four ventricles of the brain, and the central canal of the spinal cord.

CFU-E Colony-forming units-erythroid.

CH Constant region of the immunoglobulin heavy chain gene locus.

channel analyzer A device in which individual pulses are categorized into specific-sized channels forming a histogram, with size on the x axis and frequency on the y axis.

Charcot-Leyden crystals Colorless, hexagonal, needle-like crystals derived from disintegrating eosinophils. Found in sputum, bronchial secretions, and feces.

Chédiak-Higashi anomaly A rare inherited autosomal recessive trait that is characterized by the presence of large granules and inclusion bodies in the cytoplasm of leukocytes. The leukocytic neutrophils display impaired chemotaxis and delayed killing of ingested bacteria.

chemotaxis The release of substances that attract phagocytic cells as the result of traumatic or microbial damage.

chloroma A malignant tumor arising from myeloid tissue.

chromatid Half of a chromosome pair bound together in duplicate during cell division.

chromatin The network of small fibers in the nucleus of a cell.

chromoprotein A conjugated protein having respiratory functions (e.g., hemoglobin).

chromosomes Structures consisting of DNA wrapped around a protein core that are visible in the nucleus of a cell during cell division.

chronic Gradual or of long duration.

chronic granulomatous disease A sex-linked autosomal recessive genetic disorder that produces defective phagocytosis because the cells are unable to destroy previously engulfed bacteria.

circulating anticoagulants Abnormal substances that can produce bleeding.

CLL Chronic lymphocytic leukemia.

clone Daughter cells descended from the same single cell, all having identical phenotypes and growth characteristics as the original precursor cell.

coefficient of variation A statistical term denoting the precision of results.

coincidence In automated impedance cell counting, if more than one cell is within the boundaries of the aperture at the same time, only a single pulse is counted.

cold agglutinins Antibodies in the plasma that react best at 0° to 20°C.

collagen A protein found in skin, tendons, bone, and cartilage.

collagen disease Diseases of the skin, tendons, bone, and cartilage, such as systemic lupus erythematosus and rheumatoid arthritis.

colony-stimulating growth factor A soluble substance that promotes cell growth.

combined scatter histogram A type of histogram that includes both forward- and right-angle scatter information.

contact group Blood coagulation factors XI and XII, prekallikrein, and high-molecular-weight kininogen.

control (*n.*) A specimen for which the value is known that is used for comparison with the unknown specimen.

control (*v.*) To keep within limits.

Cooley's anemia Thalassemia major is usually equivalent to beta thalassemia in a homozygous form and is sometimes called Cooley's anemia.

Coombs' test See *anti–human globulin test.*

coproporphyrin A porphyrin formed in the intestine from bilirubin. Abnormal amounts may be found in the urine in some forms of anemia.

cord blood Blood obtained from the umbilical vessels at birth.

corrected reticulocyte count A mathematical adjustment of the reticulocyte count to account for variations due to erythrocyte quantity.

Coulter principle A method of cell counting and volumetric sizing based on the detection and measurement of changes in electrical resistance produced by a particle, suspended in a conductive liquid, traversing a small aperture.

counterstain A stain used to enhance a previously applied primary stain.

CPPD See *calcium pyrophosphate dihydrate*.

cryoglobulin A serum globulin that precipitates, gels, or crystallizes spontaneously at low temperatures. May be found in multiple myeloma and collagen disease.

crystalline inclusions Rod-shaped deposits of IgG.

CSF (A) Refers to colony-stimulating factor, a specific glycoprotein macromolecule that stimulates the growth of granulocytes and macrophage cells; or (B) is an abbreviation for cerebrospinal fluid.

curve-fitting In computerized automated instruments, the instrument's computer process of fitting a log-normal curve to the platelet raw data.

cytochemical stains Staining reactions that produce a colored precipitate from a specific insoluble compound in a cell.

cytochemistry The identification of specific types of molecules in a cell.

cytogenetics The branch of genetics concerned with the cellular elements of heredity.

cytokinesis Cytoplasmic division during cellular division (mitosis).

cytological Refers to cells.

cytology The study of cells.

cytomegalovirus infection A herpes-family virus that can cause congenital infections in the newborn and a clinical syndrome resembling infectious mononucleosis.

degranulation The loss of granules such as in the basophil when an antigen binds to two adjacent IgE antibody molecules located on the surface of mast cells.

deletion A chromosomal aberration in which a segment of a chromosome is lost.

denaturation The process of treating a protein with agents such as heat or acid and causing it to lose its native properties due to disruption of secondary and tertiary bonding such as hydrogen bonds.

de novo A newly presented, primary case of a disorder or disease.

deoxyhemoglobin Reduced hemoglobin.

denatured DNA Double-stranded helix separates into two single strands, breaking hydrogen bonds; caused by changes in temperature, pH, or nonphysiological concentrations of salt, detergents, or organic solvents.

DH Diversity region of the immunoglobulin heavy chain gene locus.

diabetes mellitus A disorder of carbohydrate metabolism due to an insufficiency of insulin.

diagnosis Determination of the nature of a disorder or disease.

dialysate The soluble materials and fluids (e.g., water) that pass through a semipermeable membrane.

diapedesis ameboid Movement of cells.

DIC Disseminated intravascular coagulation. This is a serious coagulation disorder that consumes platelets and blood coagulation factors, and is an example of a major breakdown of the hemostatic mechanism that occurs when the procoagulant factors outweigh the anticoagulant system.

diverticulitis Inflammation of the small blind pouches that form in the lining or wall of the colon.

DNA Deoxyribonucleic acid.

Döhle bodies (Amato bodies) Abnormal inclusion bodies that appear as light-blue–staining vacuoles predominantly in neutrophils in viral diseases and other toxic conditions.

Downey cells An early classification system of certain forms of variant lymphocytes. Downey I types have many vacuoles in the cytoplasm; Downey II types resemble plasma cells; Downey III types are an immature form of lymphocyte.

Down syndrome A chromosomal abnormality. Also referred to as mongolism.

DPG Diphosphoglycerate (2,3-DPG) combines with the beta chains of deoxyhemoglobin and diminishes the molecule's affinity for oxygen.

drumsticks An appendage of nuclear material attached to the nucleus of a segmented neutrophil. May be seen in some cells in women.

DsDNA Double-stranded DNA.

dyscrasia An abnormal or pathological condition of the blood.

dyserythropoiesis Defective red blood cell maturation.

dysgranulopoiesis Defective white blood cell maturation.

dysmegapoiesis karyocyte Defective platelet maturation.

dysplasia (*adj.* dysplastic) Abnormal development (e.g., defective cellular development). Abnormal cytological features and tissue organization, often is a premalignant change.

dyspnea Difficulty in breathing.

dyspoiesis An abnormality in the development of blood cells.

dyspoietic syndrome A combination of defective and disrupted cell line development.

EAC Erythrocyte-antibody-complement rosette test.

eclampsia A toxic condition of pregnancy.

edema An abnormal accumulation of fluid in the body's intercellular spaces.

EDTA (K3 EDTA) Tripotassium ethylenediaminetetraacetate. A commonly used anticoagulant in blood collection.

electrical impedance principle A method of cell counting and sizing based on the detection and measurement of changes in electrical resistance.

elution Removal of antibodies from the erythrocytes that they are coating or bound to.

Embden-Meyerhof glycolytic pathway The major, anaerobic, energy-yielding pathway associated with the breakdown of glucose in erythrocytes (glycolysis).

embryonic hemoglobin Primitive hemoglobins such as Gower I, Gower II, and Portland that are formed in the yolk sac.

endocarditis An inflammation of the lining membrane of the heart.

endocytosis The process in which specialized cells engulf particles and molecules, with the subsequent formation of membrane-bound vacuoles within the cytoplasm.

endoplasmic reticulum (ER) An extensive, lacelike network composed of pairs of membranes enclosing interconnecting cavities or cisternae.

endoreduplication (endomitosis) The process that occurs in the megakaryocyte during early maturation. In this process, chromosomal materials (DNA) and the other events of mitosis occur without subsequent division of the cytoplasmic membrane into identical daughter cells.

endothelial cells or endothelium Simple squamous epithelium that lines blood and lymphatic vessels and the heart.

enzyme-linked immunosorbent assay (ELISA) Technique in which an enzyme is complexed to an antigen or antibody and a substrate added that generates a color proportional to the amount of binding.

enzymopathy A pathological enzyme deficiency.

eosin An acidic stain that stains some cytoplasmic structures of the cell an orange-red color. The red-staining structures are acidophilic or eosinophilic substances.

eosinophilic granules Orange-staining granules found in a specific leukocyte type.

ependyma The membrane lining the cerebral ventricles and the central canal of the spinal cord.

epidemiology The study of infectious diseases or conditions in many individuals in the same geographical location at the same time.

epinephrine A hormone produced by the adrenal medulla that acts as a vasoconstrictor.

Epstein-Barr virus The virus associated with the development of infectious mononucleosis in western countries and Burkitt's lymphoma in Africa.

erythrocyte Refers to red blood cells.

erythroleukemia A form of leukemia that is usually acute and represents the overproliferation of both immature granulocytic and erythrocytic cell types.

erythropoiesis The process of red blood cell (erythrocyte) production.

erythropoietin A glycoprotein hormone (mol wt 46,000) that stimulates erythropoiesis. It is produced mainly by the kidneys in response to tissue hypoxia.

ESR Erythrocyte sedimentation rate. Also referred to as sed rate.

etiology The study of the cause(s) of disease.

euchromatin Chromatin that is rich in nucleic acid, is genetically active, and stains lightly. It is considered to be partially or fully uncoiled.

extramedullary hematopoiesis The formation and development of blood cells outside of the bone marrow in sites such as the liver and spleen.

extravascular destruction The destruction of an erythrocyte through phagocytosis and digestion by macrophages of the mononuclear phagocyte system.

extrinsic pathway The initiation of blood clotting begins with either the extrinsic or the intrinsic pathway. The extrinsic pathway is activated by the entry into the blood of phospholipoproteins and organelle membranes from disrupted tissue cells.

FAB Abbreviation for the French-American-British classification.

ferritin A storage form of iron.

fibrin A meshy protein clot formed by the action of thrombin on fibrinogen.

fibrinogen Blood coagulation factor I.

fibrinogen group Factors I, V, VIII, and XIII.

fibrinolysis The dissolution of a fibrin clot.

fibrin-stabilizing factor Factor XIII.

filamin A contractile protein found in platelets.

Fitzgerald factor High-molecular-weight kininogen.

Fletcher factor Prekallikrein.

folic acid One of the vitamins of the B complex.

folic acid antagonists Substances that inhibit the synthesis of folic acid.

French-American-British classification FAB classification.

frequency distribution The grouping of data in classes and determination of the number of observations that fall in each of the classes.

G phase The gap period in cellular division referred to as a part of interphase (e.g., G_1, G_2, G_0).

gastric mucosa The lining membrane of the stomach.

Gaucher's disease A monocytic disorder that represents a deficiency of the enzyme beta-glucosidase, which normally splits glucose from its parent sphingolipid, glucosylceramide.

gaussian distribution A symmetrical bell-shaped curve.

gene The functional unit of the chromosome that is usually responsible for the structure of a single protein or polypeptide.

genetics The study of the transmission of inherited characteristics.

genotype The total genetic composition of an individual.

Giemsa stain A Romanowsky-type blood stain.

gingival hyperplasia Excessive proliferation of gum tissue, often producing a white appearance.

Glanzmann's thrombasthenia A blood coagulation disorder characterized by a failure of platelets to aggregate in response to all aggregating agents.

glycocalyx A fluffy outer coat that surrounds the platelet's cellular membrane.

glycogen A long-chain polysaccharide composed of repeating units of glucose.

glycosylated hemoglobin A subfraction of normal hemoglobin that is formed during the maturation of the erythrocyte.

Golgi apparatus A horseshoe-shaped or hook-shaped cellular organelle with an associated stock of vesicles or sacs.

gout A form of arthritis characterized by excessive quantities of uric acid in the blood, with possible deposition in the joints and other tissues.

granulocytes Segmented neutrophils, band neutrophils, metamyelocytes, basophils, and eosinophils.

grape cell (Mott's cell) A plasma cell whose cytoplasm contains inclusions that are transparent blue sacs or crystal-like in nature.

Hageman factor Factor XII.

haptoglobin A plasma globulin that binds with the alpha-beta dimers of hemoglobin.

Hb Hemoglobin.

Hct Hematocrit or packed cell volume (PCV).

Heinz bodies An accumulation in the erythrocyte of oxidized glutathione that forms an insoluble complex with hemoglobin because of the absence of NADPH.

hemagglutination inhibition The prevention of erythrocyte clumping.

hematology The study of blood.

hematoma Accumulation of blood in the tissues or space in the body.

hematopoiesis (*adj.* hematopoietic) The formation and development of blood cells, chiefly in the bone marrow.

hematopoietic dysplasia See myelodysplastic syndrome.

hematuria Blood in the urine.

heme An iron-bearing compound that is the nonprotein pigment portion of hemoglobin.

hemochromatosis A disorder of iron metabolism characterized by the deposition of excessive iron in the tissues.

hemoglobin A The major form of normal adult hemoglobin.

hemoglobin electrophoresis A separation method of hemoglobin fractions based on the principle that hemoglobin molecules in an alkaline solution have a net negative charge and move toward the anode in an electrophoretic system.

hemoglobinemia The presence of free hemoglobin (not membrane-enclosed) in the blood plasma.

hemoglobin F Fetal hemoglobin. The predominant hemoglobin variety in the fetus and neonate.

hemoglobinopathies Inherited (genetic) defects related to hemoglobin. These defects may result in an abnormal structure of the hemoglobin molecule or a deficiency in the synthesis of normal adult hemoglobin.

hemoglobin S Sickle-type hemoglobin found in sickle cell anemia and/or sickle cell trait.

hemoglobinuria Free hemoglobin in the urine.

hemolysin A substance that liberates hemoglobin from erythrocytes.

hemolytic disease of the newborn A disorder seen in unborn and newborn infants if maternal antibodies that correspond to fetal erythrocytes pass through the placental barrier.

hemophilia A Classic hemophilia is a hereditary disorder that produces factor VIII deficiency.

hemophilia B Christmas disease. A hereditary disorder that produces factor IX deficiency.

hemophilia C A hereditary disease that produces factor XI deficiency.

hemosiderin Granular, iron-rich, brown pigment found in body tissues.

hemosiderinuria The presence of granular, iron-rich, brown pigment in the urine.

hemostasis The stoppage of bleeding from a blood vessel.

heparin An anticoagulant that acts as an antithrombin.

hepatomegaly Excessive enlargement of the liver.

hepatosplenomegaly An enlarged liver and spleen.

Hermansky-Pudlak syndrome A blood coagulation disorder characterized by storage granule abnormalities of the platelets (thrombocytes).

heterochromatin A type of chromatin that is tightly coiled, assumes a dark stain, and is genetically inactive.

heterogeneous Dissimilar.

heterozygous In genetics, possessing the alternate characteristics on a pair of homologous chromosomes.

hexose monophosphate shunt This ancillary energy-yielding system is also referred to as the oxidative pathway. The system couples oxidative metabolism with pyridine nucleotide and glutathione reduction.

high-molecular-weight kininogen Fitzgerald factor.

histogram A pictorial display of frequency and class limits of a sample.

Hodgkin's disease A major form of malignant lymphoma.

hof The area of the cell cytoplasm encircled by the concavity of the nucleus.

homeostasis The tendency of a biological system to maintain equilibrium or balance.

homogeneous Uniform or same.

homozygous In genetics, when the genes for a trait on homologous chromosomes are the same.

Howell-Jolly bodies Very coarse, round, solid-staining dark-blue to purple abnormal granules seen in erythrocytes.

HTLV (human T cell leukemia virus) This virus family is associated with T cell leukemia, hairy cell leukemia, and acquired immunodeficiency syndrome (AIDS).

hybridization Interaction between two single-stranded nucleic acid molecules to form a double-stranded molecule.

hydrophilic Water-attracting.

hydrophobic Water-repelling.

hypercoagulable state An increase in the likelihood of blood to clot in vivo.

hyperplasia Excessive tissue growth or cellular multiplication.

hypersegmentation An abnormal condition in which more than five nuclear segments are observed in segmented neutrophils.

hypertension Increased blood pressure.

hypertrophy Increase in the size of cells that produces an enlargement of tissue mass or organ size.

hypervolemia An increased total blood volume.

hypochromia When the central pallor of erythrocytes exceeds one third of the cell's diameter.

hypolobulation A condition of neutrophils in which normal segmentation fails to occur.

hypoproliferative disorders A term that may be substituted for the reduced growth or production of cells, particularly erythrocytes.

hypothyroidism Decreased thyroid activity.

hypoxia A decrease of oxygen in the body tissues.

idiopathic A disorder or disease without an identifiable external etiology, or self-originated.

immune deficiency disease A defect in the ability to detect antigens and/or to produce antibodies against foreign antigens.

immunity The process of being protected against foreign antigens.

immunocompetent The ability to recognize and respond to a foreign antigen.

immunodeficiency A dysfunction in the body defense mechanism that detects foreign antigens and produces antibodies against them.

immunoglobulin A protein belonging to the gamma globulin fraction. Immunoglobulins are divided into five classes, with IgG being the most abundant.

immunological dysfunction Refers to immune deficiency disease.

incidence The frequency of an occurrence, for example, a disease.

infarct An area of necrosis in a tissue due to obstruction of the blood circulation.

infectious mononucleosis A benign lymphoproliferative disorder.

inflammation Tissue reaction to injury caused by physical or chemical agents, including microorganisms. Symptoms include redness, tenderness, pain, and swelling.

intravascular destruction An alternate pathway for erythrocyte breakdown that normally accounts for less than 10% of red cell destruction.

intrinsic factor (IF) Substance secreted by the parietal cells of the mucosa in the fundus region of the stomach.

intrinsic pathway The initiation of blood clotting begins with either the intrinsic or the extrinsic pathway. In the intrinsic pathway, coagulation begins with the activation of factor XII to XIIa.

in vitro In the test tube or outside the body.

in vivo Within the living organism.

iso Equal. Isotonic saline solution has a concentration of 0.85%, which is equal to the concentration of sodium chloride in cellular cytoplasm.

isoimmune Possessing antibodies to antigens of the same system.

isolation technique Precautions used to prevent the transmission of disease either to or from a patient or patient specimen.

jaundice A yellow appearance of the skin, sclerae, and body excretions.

JCAHO The Joint Commission on Accreditation of Healthcare Organizations.

JH Joining region of the immunoglobulin heavy chain gene locus.

kallikrein Activated Fletcher factor.

karyokinesis The division of the nuclear membrane during cellular division.

karyorrhexis A stage of cellular degeneration when chromatin is distributed irregularly throughout the cytoplasm.

karyotype The full complement of chromosomes in an organism.

kb Kilobase pairs, 1000 bases.

kinins Small biologically active peptides.

Kleihauer-Betke test A semiquantitative test for fetal hemoglobin.

krypton An inert gas used in lasers.

Kupffer's cells Cells in the liver that have the ability to engulf or phagocytize foreign particles as part of the mononuclear phagocytic system.

kwashiorkor A severe protein deficiency seen in infants and children.

labile Unstable.

lambda Equivalent to microliter (μL) or 1/1000 of a milliliter (mL).

LAP Leukocyte alkaline phosphatase cytochemical stain.

laparotomy Incision in the abdomen.

Laser *L*ight *a*mplification by *s*timulated *e*mission of *r*adiation.

LDH Lactic dehydrogenase.

leukemia A neoplastic proliferative disease characterized by an overproduction of immature or mature cells of various leukocyte types in the bone marrow or peripheral blood.

leukocyte White blood cell.

leukocytosis A significant increase in the total white cell count.

leukopenia A severe decrease in the total white cell count.

leukotrienes A newly identified class of compounds that mediate the inflammatory functions of leukocytes.

Levy-Jennings chart A quality control chart used to graphically display the assay values of controls versus time.

LIF Leukocytosis-inducing factor. A regulator that influences the release of neutrophils from the bone marrow into the circulatory system.

lipids One of the three major biochemical classes. This class includes the fatty acids and steroids.

lipophilic dyes Stains with an affinity for fatty substances.

liquefaction The process of conversion into liquid form.

Luebering-Rapaport pathway An important oxygen-carrying pathway of erythrocytes that permits the accumulation of 2,3-DPG.

lymphadenopathy Disease of the lymph nodes.

lymphoblastic leukemia A major form of leukemia characterized by the presence of increased numbers of immature lymphocytes in the peripheral blood, bone marrow, and lymph nodes.

lymphocytes A type of leukocyte.

lymphocytopenia A severe decrease in the total number of lymphocytes in the peripheral blood.

lymphocytosis A significant increase in the total number of lymphocytes in the peripheral blood.

lymphoma Solid, malignant tumors of the lymph nodes and associated tissues or bone marrow.

lymphoproliferative disorders A group of diseases characterized by the proliferation of lymphoid tissues and/or lymphocytes.

lymphosarcoma Malignant neoplastic disorders of the lymphoid tissues, excluding Hodgkin's disease.

lyse To break apart or dissolve.

lysosomes Cytoplasmic organelles that contain lytic enzymes.

M phase The phase of cellular division in which the cell actually divides.

macroglobulin A high-molecular-weight protein of the globulin type.

macrophage A large mononuclear phagocytic cell of the tissues that exists either as a fixed type that lines the capillaries and sinuses of organs such as the bone marrow, spleen, and lymph nodes, or as a wandering type.

malabsorption syndrome Impaired absorption of nutrients in the intestine.

malaise A general feeling of tiredness or discomfort.

malignant Cancerous.

manifestation The display of symptoms of a disease or disorder.

marginating pool The granulocytes that adhere to the vascular endothelium.

mast cells Tissue basophils.

Maurer's dots Red dots seen in stained erythrocytes infected with the malaria parasite *Plasmodium falciparum.*

May-Hegglin anomaly An abnormal genetic condition characterized by the presence of Döhle body–like inclusions in neutrophils, eosinophils, and monocytes. Abnormally large platelets and thrombocytopenia frequently coexist in this condition.

MCH Mean corpuscular hemoglobin of an erythrocyte.

MCHC Mean corpuscular hemoglobin concentration of an erythrocyte.

MCV Mean corpuscular volume of an erythrocyte.

MDS See *myelodysplastic syndrome.*

mean The arithmetic average.

median The middle value of a set of numbers arranged according to size.

megakaryocytes Blood platelets or precursors.

megaloblastic dyspoiesis Uneven development of the nucleus and cytoplasm during erythrocyte maturation.

megalocyte An extremely large erythrocyte with a diameter exceeding 12 μm. This cell is larger than a macrocyte.

meiosis The process in which ova or sperm with half the normal number of chromosomes ($1n$) are produced.

mesenteric thrombosis A condition of clotting in the membranous tissues attaching the small intestine to the posterior abdominal wall.

metaphase A period in cellular division (mitosis).

metaplasia Change from one adult cell type to another, e.g., glandular epithelium to squamous epithelium metaplasia.

metarubricyte Normoblasts (acidophilic) or nucleated red blood cells.

metastatic carcinoma A malignancy that has spread from its original focal point.

metastatic disease See *metastatic carcinoma*.

methemoglobin reductase pathway An erythrocytic metabolic pathway that functions to prevent the oxidation of heme iron.

methylene blue A basic stain that stains the nucleus and some cytoplasmic structures of a cell a blue color. The blue-stained structures are basophilic substances.

microfilaments Cellular ultrastructures consisting of the protein actin.

microtubules Small, hollow cellular ultrastructures composed of polymerized, macromolecular protein subunits, tubulin.

mitochondria Cellular ultrastructures composed of an outer, smooth membrane and an inner, folded membrane, the cristae. These organelles are associated with cellular energy-yielding activities.

mitogen A substance that stimulates cell division (mitosis).

mitosis The process of body cellular division.

mode The number of values that occur with the greatest frequency.

monoclonal antibodies Immune globulins directed against antigens derived from a single cell line.

monocyte A large mononuclear type of leukocyte.

mononuclear cells Cells with a single large nucleus such as monocytes, promyelocytes, myelocytes, and blasts.

mononuclear phagocyte system The body defense system that consists of a variety of types of cells that have the ability to engulf or phagocytize substances such as foreign particles.

monosodium urate An abnormal crystal that may be observed in synovial fluid.

morphology The visual appearance, form, and shape of a cell.

MPD Myeloproliferative disorders.

MPV Mean platelet volume. A measure of the average volume of the platelet population contained within the platelet curve.

MSU Monosodium urate.

mtDNA Mitochondrial DNA.

mRNA Messenger RNA; final processed transcript of the structural gene, present in the cytoplasm, from which a protein is produced.

multiple myeloma A malignant disorder of plasma cells that is also known as plasma cell myeloma.

myeloblastic A major form of leukemia characterized by large numbers of immature or mature granulocytes or related cells such as monocytes in the peripheral blood and/or bone marrow.

myelodysplasia See *MPD*.

myelodysplastic syndrome (MDS) A group of disorders associated with abnormalities of erythrocytes, platelets, granulocytes, and monocytes.

myelogenous Refers to the myeloid or granulocytic type cell line.

myocardial infarction Necrosis of the muscular tissue of the heart.

myosin A contractile protein.

NCCLS The National Committee for Clinical Laboratory Standards.

Neisseria gonorrhoeae A gram-negative bacteria that causes gonorrhea.

neoplasm A new growth.

nephropathy A disease of the kidneys.

neutropenia A severe decrease in the number of neutrophilic granulocytes in the peripheral blood.

neutrophilia A significant increase in the number of neutrophilic granulocytes in the peripheral blood.

neutrophilic reaction When both the basic and the acidic stains stain the cytoplasmic structures, a pink or lilac color develops.

Niemann-Pick disease A monocytic disorder that represents the deficiency of an enzyme that normally cleaves phosphorylcholine from its sphingolipid, sphingomyelin.

northern blot. Hybridization technique similar to the Southern blot, using RNA instead of DNA as a target.

NRBC/100 WBC The number of nucleated erythrocytes counted during a 100-cell leukocyte count.

NRF Neutrophil-releasing factor. A regulator that influences the release of neutrophils from the bone marrow into the circulatory system.

nucleoli The region of the nucleus rich in RNA.

nucleotide Basic building block of nucleic acids, consisting of a nitrogenous base, a pentose sugar, and phosphoric acid.

null cells A type of lymphocyte without either T or B cell surface markers.

ochronosis A peculiar discoloration of body tissue.

oncogenes Transforming genes of cellular origin that are contained in retroviruses and associated with acute leukemias.

opportunistic infections Microbial diseases that infect a debilitated host.

organelles Small cellular ultrastructures that are the functional units of a cell.

OSHA Occupational Safety and Health Administration.

osmotic fragility The ability or flexibility of the cellular membrane to withstand pressure.

osteoarthritis Degenerative joint disease characterized by degeneration of the articular cartilage.

osteoarthropathy Any disease of the joints and bones.

oxidant stress A decrease in the level of oxygen available to the tissues due to agents such as drugs.

oxidative pathway See *hexose monophosphate shunt*.

oxyhemoglobin Oxygenated hemoglobin.

pallor Paleness of the skin and mucous membranes.

pancytopenia A severe decrease in all of the blood cells.

Papanicolaou stain A cytological stain used most commonly to detect uterine and cervical cancer.

Pappenheimer bodies (siderotic granules) Abnormal basophilic iron-containing granules seen in erythrocytes.

parameter Any numerical value that describes an entire population.

PAS stain The periodic acid–Schiff stain reaction for cellular carbohydrates.

pathogenesis The origin of disease.

PDW Platelet distribution width.

Pelger-Huët anomaly An autosomal dominant genetic disorder that produces hyposegmentation of neutrophils.

pericardial fluid Watery liquid in the sac surrounding the heart.

peripheral blood Blood in the extremities (e.g., capillary blood).

peritoneal fluid Watery liquid in the abdominal cavity.

pernicious anemia An erythrocytic disorder associated with defective vitamin B_{12} uptake.

petechiae Small purple hemorrhagic spots on the skin or mucous membranes.

pH A numerical value expressing acid, neutral, or alkaline (basic) conditions of a solution. A pH of 7.0 is neutral. Values from 0 to 6.9 are acidic and values from 7.1 to 14.0 are alkaline.

phagocyte Any cell that is capable of engulfing and destroying foreign particles such as bacteria.

phagocytosis A form of endocytosis. This important body defense mechanism is the process by which specialized cells engulf and destroy foreign particles.

pharyngitis An inflammation of the throat.

phenotype The outward or physical expression of an inherited characteristic.

Philadelphia chromosome The Philadelphia chromosome (Ph^1) is a translocation involving chromosomes 22 and 9. This translocation is present in the precursors and megakaryocytes of patients with chronic myelogenous leukemia.

phlebotomy The collection of venous blood or venipuncture.

photon A basic unit of radiation.

pia mater The innermost of the three meninges covering the brain and spinal cord.

pinocytosis A form of endocytosis. This is the process in which specialized cells engulf fluids.

plasma The straw-colored fluid component of blood.

plasmacyte A mature plasma cell that is not normally found in the circulating blood.

plasma thromboplastin antecedent Factor XI.

plasma thromboplastin component Factor IX.

plasmid Small, circular, self-replicating molecule of DNA in bacteria; foreign genetic material can be introduced into the plasmid and amplified as the plasmid replicates; a cloning vector.

plasmin A proteolytic enzyme with the ability to dissolve formed fibrin clots.

plasminogen The inactive precursor of plasmin that is converted to plasmin by the action of substances such as urokinase.

platelet plug The meshing together of platelets into a solid mass.

pleocytosis The presence of a greater-than-normal number of cells.

pleural fluid Watery liquid in the chest cavity.

PLT Platelet count.

PNH Paroxysmal nocturnal hemoglobinuria. A rare, acquired chronic hemolytic anemia.

poikilocytosis Alterations or variations in the shape of erythrocytes.

point mutation A change that affects a single base in DNA.

polychromasia See *polychromatophilia*.

polychromatophilia Fine, evenly distributed basophilic (blue) granules that impart a blue color to Wright-stained erythrocytes.

polycythemia vera A blood dyscrasia in which the erythrocytes, leukocytes, and thrombocytes are all increased above normal.

polymerase chain reaction (PCR) Method for synthetically amplifying known DNA sequences in vitro using many cycles of denaturation and polymerization with synthetic oligonucleotide primer extension employing Taq polymerase.

polysaccharide A carbohydrate containing 10 or more monosaccharides.

porphyrin Any of a group of iron- or magnesium-free cyclic tetrapyrrole derivatives which form the basis of the respiratory pigments of animals and plants. Porphyrins in combination with iron form *hemes*.

precision The closeness of test results when repeated analyses of the same material are performed.

prefix The beginning portion of a medical term.

prekallikrein Fletcher factor.

preleukemia An older term for a condition preceding acute leukemia.

primary lymphoid tissues The bone marrow and thymus gland are classified as primary or central lymphoid tissue.

primer Short nucleic acid sequence that pairs with ssDNA and provides a free 3'-OH end to "prime," or begin, polymerase synthesis of a complimentary polynucleotide chain.

proaccelerin Factor V.

probe A known, labeled sequence of DNA or RNA used to detect complementary sequences in target polynucleotides by hybridization.

proconvertin Factor VII.

prognosis A forecast of the probable outcome of a condition, disorder, or disease.

prophase The first stage in cellular division (mitosis).

prorubricyte Basophilic normoblast.

prostaglandins Naturally occurring fatty acids that stimulate the contraction of uterine and other smooth muscle tissues.

prostatitis Inflammation of the male gland, the prostate.

prostatovesiculitis Inflammation of the prostate and seminal vesicle.

proteases Enzymes that digest proteins.

protein C A plasma protein that functions as a potent natural anticoagulant.

protein S A plasma protein that functions as a potent natural anticoagulant.

prothrombin Factor II.

prothrombin group Blood coagulation factors II, VII, IX, and X.

pseudo–Pelger-Huët anomaly A false form of this anomaly. See *Pelger-Huët anomaly*.

pseudopods Cytoplasmic extrusions that resemble false feet.

PT Prothrombin time.

purines An organic family that forms the nucleic acid bases.

purpura Extensive areas of red or dark-purple discoloration of the skin.

pyknosis Contraction of a cell's nucleus that produces a dark, dense appearance.

pyrimidine analog A compound that can be substituted for a pyrimidine base to interrupt protein synthesis in actively mitotic cells.

pyrimidines An organic family that forms the nucleic acid bases.

qualitative A difference in type rather than quantity.

quality control A process that monitors the accuracy and reproducibility of patient results through the use of control specimens.

RA See *rheumatoid arthritis*.

ragocytes Cells of the body fluid.

range The difference between the highest and lowest measurements in a series.

RCMI Red cell morphology index. Derived from a comparison of the patient's measured red cell volume distribution with a distribution representing the average patient population served by the laboratory. The calculation of RCMI relates to a statistical function called z, which measures the difference between a random variable and the mean under the curve. If the RCMI is outside the −2.0 to +2.0 range, this indicates a significant number of abnormal red cells.

RDW Red cell distribution width. An index of the variation in red cell size. It is computed from the red cell histogram by dividing the standard deviation by the mean and multiplying by 100.

reactive eosinophilia An increase in eosinophils due to inflammation or allergic reaction.

refractive index A measurement of the passage of light.

refractory anemia A deficiency of red blood cells that does not readily yield to treatment.

regimen A schedule of treatment.

Reiter's disease A disease of males characterized in part by migratory polyarthritis.

remission A period of time in which the signs and symptoms of a disease, such as leukemia, subside.

restriction endonuclease Bacterial enzyme that recognizes short palindromic sequences of DNA and cleaves the DNA near this "restriction site"; each enzyme is named for the bacteria from which it has been isolated.

restriction fragment length polymorphism (RFLP) Alteration in DNA fragment size due to a change such as a deletion; relatively stable and can be detected with nucleic acid probes; if close on the chromosome to a disease-producing gene, it can be used as a marker for this disease.

reticulocyte The last stage of the immature erythrocyte. This cell lacks a nucleus and is found in both the bone marrow and peripheral blood.

reticuloendothelial system (RES) See mononuclear phagocyte system.

reticuloendotheliosis Increased growth and development (hyperplasia) of the reticuloendothelial system.

rheumatoid arthritis A form of arthritis most commonly seen in young adults.

ribosomes Cellular organelles that occur both on the surface of the rough endoplasmic reticulum and free in the cytoplasm. They are associated with cellular protein synthesis.

Rieder cells Cells that are similar to lymphocytes.

RNA Ribonucleic acid.

Romanowsky stain Any stain containing methylene blue and/or its products of oxidation, and a halogenated fluorescein dye, usually eosin B or eosin Y.

root term The part of a medical term that usually refers to an anatomical structure.

rouleaux formation The appearance of erythrocytes that resembles a stack of coins.

RPI Reticulocyte production index. A measurement of erythropoietic activity when "stress" reticulocytes are present.

rRNA Ribosomal RNA; component of ribosomes that serve as scaffolding for polypeptide synthesis.

rubriblast The earliest specific red blood cell precursor. Also referred to as pronormoblast.

rubricyte Polychromatophilic normoblast.

Russell bodies Round, glassy, transparent bodies that may be seen in plasma cells.

S phase The period during the cellular division cycle in which DNA is replicated.

sample A subset of a population.

Schuffner's dots Red particles seen in erythrocytes containing malarial (Plasmodium vivax) parasites.

scleroderma A chronic disorder characterized by progressive collagenous fibrosis of many organs and systems.

secondary lymphoid tissue Lymph nodes, spleen, and Peyer's patches in the intestine.

secondary polycythemia An increased concentration of erythrocytes in the blood.

sed rate Erythrocyte sedimentation rate.

seminal fluid Liquid produced by the male reproductive system.

septic arthritis Joint inflammation caused by microorganisms.

septicemia The presence of pathogenic microorganisms in the blood.

serotonin A vasoconstrictor produced from tryptophan that stimulates smooth muscle.

serous fluid Producing or containing serum.

serum Straw-colored fluid that is present after blood clots.

serum electrophoresis Separation of serum proteins by electrical methods.

Sézary cell A large lymphocyte with a nucleus that occupies most of the cell.

sickle cell disease Results from the substitution of a valine for glutamic acid at the sixth position on the beta chain of the hemoglobin molecule. In homozygous form (SS), causes sickle cell anemia.

sideroblastic anemia A disorder of iron utilization in which the body has adequate iron but is unable to incorporate it in hemoglobin synthesis.

siderotic granules Pappenheimer bodies.

Singer and Nicholson's fluid mosaic model This model explains the arrangement of the components of the cell membrane into a bilaminar layer of phospholipids, with protein molecules interspersed as either integral or peripheral units.

sinusoids Specialized capillaries found in locations such as the bone marrow, spleen, and liver.

size distribution histogram A display of the distribution of cell volume and frequency. Each channel on the x axis represents size in femtoliters (fL). The y axis represents the relative number of cells.

SLE Abbreviation for systemic lupus erythematosus.

Small-bowel stricture A narrowing of the intestine.

Smoldering leukemia See MPD.

smudge cells A natural artifact seen on peripheral blood smears that represents the bare nuclei of leukocytes (e.g., lymphocytes). Increased numbers are seen in CLL.

sodium citrate A blood anticoagulant that is frequently used in a concentration of 3.2% for coagulation studies.

Southern blot. Hybridization technique invented by E. M. Southern in which DNA is digested with restriction enzymes, separated by electrophoresis, transferred to a solid matrix, and hybridized to a labeled probe.

spermatozoa Male reproductive cells, sperm.

splenic infarction Tissue necrosis of the spleen.

splenomegaly An extremely enlarged spleen.

sprue A chronic form of malabsorption syndrome.

ssDNA Single-stranded DNA.

standard A highly purified substance of a known composition.

standard deviation The square root of the variance.

stasis Stopping of bleeding.

stat Immediately.

statistic Any numerical value describing a sample.

stem term Root term.

stenosis The narrowing of a vessel. In a blood vessel, the lumen decreases the flow of blood if stenosis exists.

stercobilinogen Fecal urobilinogen.

sterile body fluid Watery fluids in the body that lack microorganisms.

stroma The structural protein of an erythrocyte. Remains after the erythrocyte has been washed free of hemoglobin and appears as a ghost cell or shadow when viewed under the microscope.

Stuart factor Factor X.

subacute leukemia See *MPD*.

subarachnoid space The space between the arachnoid and pia mater layers of the meninges of the brain.

subsets Subgroups of a sample.

sudanophilic Having an affinity for Sudan stain.

suffix The ending of a medical term.

supernatant The fluid above the solid portion in a centrifuged or settled mixture.

symptomatic A deviation from usual function or appearance.

syndrome A set or group of symptoms that occur together.

synovial fluid Joint fluid.

systemic circulation Blood circulation throughout the body.

systemic lupus erythematosus (SLE) A multisymptom disorder that can affect practically every organ of the body.

T lymphocytes or T cells Cells responsible for the cellular immune response and involved in the regulation of antibody reactions.

tanycytes Body fluid cells.

Taq DNA polymerase Thermostable DNA polymerase used to polymerize new DNA strands; used in the PCR procedure.

telophase The final stage in cellular division (mitosis).

thoracentesis Piercing of the thorax (chest cavity) for the purpose of removing fluid.

thrombin A blood coagulation factor (factor IIa) that is the activated form of prothrombin.

thrombocytes Blood platelets.

thrombocytopenia A severe decrease in circulating platelets.

thrombocytosis An increase in the number of circulating platelets (thrombocytes).

thromboplastin Blood coagulation factor III.

thrombopoietin A hormone believed to be of renal origin that is secreted in response to the need for platelets.

thrombosis Clotting or the presence of a clot.

thrombosthenin Actomyosin.

thromboxane A2 A short-lived substance that facilitates the release of platelet granular contents, induces other platelets to aggregate, and stimulates vasoconstriction.

thrombus A clot.

TIBC Total iron-binding capacity.

titer The strength or concentration of a solution.

toxic granulation Abnormally dark granulation seen in band and segmented neutrophils or monocytes.

transcobalamin A specific globulin protein that is involved in the physiological mechanism of vitamin B_{12}.

transferrin A beta globulin protein that binds iron and transports it back to the bone marrow for hemoglobin synthesis.

transcription Process in which mRNA translates DNA into RNA nucleotide sequences.

translocation A kind of chromosomal aberration in which a segment of one chromosome breaks away from its normal location and attaches to another, nonhomologous, chromosome.

trisomy A chromosomal alteration in which a third chromosome exists with a homologous pair of chromosomes.

tRNA Transfer RNA; small RNA molecules that interact with amino acids and mediate their correct insertion into a growing polypeptide chain.

trophoblasts The peripheral cells of the blastocyst.

tunica adventitia The layer of a blood vessel that consists of fibrous connective tissue innervated with automatic nerve endings.

tunica intima The smooth surface of endothelium in a blood vessel.

tunica media The thickest layer of a blood vessel. It is composed of smooth muscle and elastic fibers.

turbidity Cloudiness.

ultrastructure Cellular organelles that can be viewed with electron microscopy.

unconjugated bilirubin Bilirubin not bound to protein.

vacuolated lymphocytes Vacuolation may be seen in variant lymphocytes or as a reaction to radiation and chemotherapy.

variance The position of each observation (test) in relationship to the mean.

variant lymphocytes Atypical lymphocytes. Downey cells, reactive or transformed lymphocytes, lymphocytoid or plasmacytoid lymphocytes, and virocytes. These cells may be found in infectious mononucleosis, viral pneumonia, and viral hepatitis.

vasa vasorum Small networks of blood vessels that supply nutrients to the tissues of the wall of a blood vessel.

vascular integrity The resistance to vessel disruption.

vasoconstriction Contraction of the blood vessel wall.

veins Collecting vessels that return blood to the heart.

ventricles Cerebral ventricles are hollow spaces in the brain.

venules Microscopically sized veins.

VH Variable region of the immunoglobulin heavy chain gene locus.

viscosity Thickness.

von Willebrand's disease A genetic disorder producing a deficiency and defect of blood coagulation factor VII and defective platelet function.

Waldenstrom's primary macroglobulinemia A neoplastic proliferation of the lymphocyte plasma cell system.

western blot Hybridization technique similar to the Southern blot in which the electrophoresed sample is protein and the detector is immunoglobulin.

Wiscott-Aldrich syndrome A blood coagulation disorder characterized by extremely small platelets (thrombocytes).

Wright stain A Romanowsky-type blood stain.

xanthochromia Yellow color.

CHAPTER 1

1. D	10. B	19. B
2. A	11. D	20. D
3. A	12. A	21. C
4. C	13. A	22. A
5. A	14. B	23. C
6. A	15. C	24. A
7. C	16. B	25. D
8. B	17. C	26. D
9. D	18. A	27. B

CHAPTER 2

1. B	12. C	23. B
2. B	13. A	24. D
3. D	14. C	25. D
4. B	15. B	26. C
5. D	16. D	27. A
6. C	17. D	28. B
7. A	18. D	29. A
8. E	19. D	30. A
9. B	20. D	31. A
10. A	21. D	32. B
11. D	22. D	33. C

CHAPTER 3

1. B	14. C	26. A
2. B	15. D	27. D
3. B	16. A	28. B
4. D	17. B	29. C
5. E	18. D	30. D
6. E	19. D	31. D
7. A	20. B	32. D
8. C	21. E	33. B
9. B	22. A	34. B
10. D	23. C	35. D
11. C	24. B	36. C
12. A	25. E	37. A
13. B		

CHAPTER 4

1. C	6. B	11. D
2. C	7. A	12. C
3. D	8. A	13. B
4. B	9. B	14. A
5. B	10. E	

CHAPTER 5

1. B	7. D	13. D
2. D	8. D	14. C
3. A	9. C	15. C
4. A	10. A	16. C
5. D	11. C	17. D
6. D	12. B	18. C

19. D	34. A	49. B
20. A	35. B	50. D
21. A	36. C	51. A
22. C	37. A	52. A
23. B	38. D	53. D
24. D	39. B	54. D
25. D	40. C	55. D
26. B	41. D	56. D
27. D	42. D	57. D
28. B	43. C	58. A
29. B	44. D	59. C
30. B	45. D	60. B
31. B	46. D	61. C
32. C	47. B	62. B
33. C	48. B	63. A

CHAPTER 6

1. C	14. C	27. D
2. B	15. A	28. A
3. C	16. D	29. B
4. A	17. B	30. C
5. D	18. D	31. D
6. D	19. C	32. D
7. A	20. A	33. A
8. C	21. D	34. B
9. B	22. B	35. C
10. A	23. D	36. B
11. C	24. C	37. D
12. B	25. A	38. A
13. D	26. B	39. C

CHAPTER 7

1. D	3. A	5. D
2. D	4. C	

CHAPTER 8

1. B	4. B	6. C
2. A	5. B	7. D
3. A		

CHAPTER 9

1. D	4. D	7. C
2. B	5. D	8. B
3. D	6. A	

CHAPTER 10

1. D	8. C	15. A
2. D	9. C	16. A
3. E	10. D	17. D
4. A	11. A	18. A
5. B	12. B	19. D
6. D	13. D	20. C
7. C	14. B	

CHAPTER 11

1. D	6. C	11. B
2. D	7. D	12. C
3. D	8. C	13. C
4. D	9. A	14. D
5. B	10. A	15. C

CHAPTER 12

1. A	10. E	18. A
2. B	11. D	19. C
3. A	12. B	20. C
4. B	13. A	21. D
5. A	14. B	22. C
6. C	15. D	23. C
7. B	16. B	24. C
8. C	17. B	25. A
9. A		

CHAPTER 13

1. D	6. B	10. C
2. D	7. B	11. D
3. A	8. B	12. C
4. A	9. B	13. D
5. D		

CHAPTER 14

1. A	11. D	21. A
2. B	12. D	22. D
3. A	13. D	23. D
4. B	14. A	24. A
5. B	15. D	25. A
6. C	16. B	26. D
7. C	17. B	27. C
8. B	18. D	28. A
9. B	19. D	29. A
10. D	20. A	30. B

CHAPTER 15

1. D	9. C	16. A
2. D	10. C	17. B
3. D	11. A	18. B
4. D	12. B	19. A
5. D	13. B	20. A
6. B	14. D	21. A
7. A	15. C	22. D
8. D		

CHAPTER 16

1. B	8. A	15. B
2. C	9. C	16. B
3. B	10. D	17. A
4. A	11. B	18. B
5. A	12. B	19. A
6. B	13. C	20. B
7. D	14. C	21. A

22. C	25. A	28. A
23. D	26. C	29. D
24. D	27. D	

CHAPTER 17

1. D	7. B	12. A
2. B	8. A	13. C
3. B	9. A	14. D
4. A	10. A	15. B
5. B	11. C	16. D
6. A		

CHAPTER 18

1. D	3. B	5. C
2. B	4. D	6. A

CHAPTER 19

1. A	11. A	21. C
2. B	12. D	22. C
3. C	13. D	23. B
4. A	14. B	24. A
5. D	15. C	25. A
6. C	16. A	26. B
7. D	17. A	27. B
8. C	18. B	28. A
9. E	19. B	29. C
10. B	20. A	30. C

CHAPTER 20

1. B	5. C	9. C
2. C	6. D	10. D
3. B	7. D	11. B
4. C	8. B	

CHAPTER 21

1. C	13. C	24. B
2. A	14. A	25. D
3. B	15. D	26. C
4. A	16. B	27. D
5. C	17. C	28. A
6. B	18. D	29. C
7. B	19. D	30. C
8. D	20. A	31. D
9. C	21. D	32. D
10. C	22. A	33. B
11. D	23. D	34. C
12. D		

CHAPTER 22

1. A	7. A	13. D
2. B	8. B	14. B
3. D	9. C	15. A
4. B	10. C	16. A
5. E	11. D	17. B
6. C	12. D	18. C

CHAPTER 22 (Cont'd)

19. A	23. A	27. B
20. B	24. E	28. A
21. B	25. D	29. D
22. C	26. D	

CHAPTER 23

1. A	30. D	59. A
2. B	31. D	60. B
3. D	32. D	61. C
4. E	33. B	62. D
5. C	34. B	63. A
6. C	35. A	64. B
7. A	36. C	65. D
8. B	37. D	66. C
9. A	38. B	67. A
10. C	39. D	68. D
11. B	40. E	69. B
12. A	41. A	70. D
13. B	42. C	71. D
14. D	43. C	72. E
15. C	44. C	73. B
16. B	45. D	74. A
17. A	46. D	75. D
18. D	47. B	76. C
19. B	48. C	77. B
20. C	49. D	78. D
21. A	50. A	79. C
22. D	51. A	80. C
23. A	52. D	81. A
24. E	53. D	82. B
25. B	54. D	83. D
26. C	55. A	84. A
27. A	56. C	85. B
28. B	57. B	86. C
29. A	58. A	

CHAPTER 24

1. C	22. A	43. A
2. A	23. D	44. C
3. C	24. B	45. B
4. D	25. B	46. D
5. B	26. C	47. B
6. B	27. D	48. D
7. A	28. A	49. C
8. C	29. B	50. A
9. B	30. C	51. D
10. A	31. A	52. B
11. C	32. D	53. C
12. B	33. D	54. A
13. A	34. C	55. B
14. E	35. D	56. A
15. D	36. D	57. D
16. C	37. D	58. C
17. B	38. D	59. B
18. A	39. D	60. A
19. D	40. B	61. D
20. C	41. A	62. C
21. C	42. C	63. B

64. C	89. D	114. C
65. A	90. B	115. A
66. B	91. A	116. B
67. D	92. D	117. C
68. A	93. C	118. A
69. B	94. B	119. D
70. C	95. D	120. D
71. A	96. C	121. A
72. D	97. E	122. B
73. D	98. A	123. C
74. B	99. B	124. B
75. B	100. C	125. A
76. D	101. C	126. A
77. A	102. E	127. D
78. A	103. B	128. E
79. B	104. D	129. B
80. C	105. A	130. C
81. D	106. E	131. A
82. A	107. B	132. D
83. A	108. C	133. D
84. B	109. D	134. D
85. B	110. C	135. D
86. B	111. B	136. D
87. C	112. A	137. D
88. A	113. D	

CHAPTER 25

1. B	12. A	23. C
2. B	13. D	24. B
3. A	14. B	25. D
4. C	15. A	26. D
5. C	16. C	27. D
6. B	17. B	28. C
7. D	18. D	29. C
8. D	19. B	30. D
9. A	20. B	31. C
10. C	21. C	32. D
11. D	22. C	

CHAPTER 26

1. B	20. B	39. C
2. E	21. A	40. B
3. B	22. B	41. D
4. A	23. D	42. A
5. D	24. C	43. B
6. C	25. D	44. C
7. B	26. A	45. A
8. A	27. B	46. D
9. B	28. B	47. B
10. A	29. B	48. B
11. D	30. A	49. D
12. D	31. C	50. C
13. D	32. D	51. D
14. D	33. D	52. A
15. A	34. C	53. C
16. B	35. D	54. D
17. D	36. A	55. B
18. D	37. C	56. D
19. D	38. B	57. A

58. C
59. D
60. B

61. D
62. D

63. D
64. D

CHAPTER 27

1. D
2. B
3. C
4. A
5. C
6. A
7. B
8. A

9. A
10. B
11. D
12. D
13. D
14. A
15. A

16. B
17. A
18. B
19. B
20. B
21. C
22. A

Medical terminology encompasses many of the words used in the biological sciences; however, terms that are unique to medical applications are also included. Latin and Greek terms form the basis of many of these words. The Romance languages (French, Spanish, Portuguese, and Italian) continue to reflect their Latin origins. Many terms are encountered in modern English.

The reader should be able to:

- Name the three basic components of a medical term.
- Define the listed prefixes, root terms, and suffixes.

A medical term is ideally composed of three principal parts: a **prefix**, a **stem** or **root term**, and a **suffix**. A prefix is located at the beginning of the term. The root term, which commonly refers to a body part or anatomical structure, is found in the middle of the term. The suffix is located at the end of the term.

The word **thrombocytopenia** is an example of a hematological term. This term can be divided into three basic components: **thrombo-** (the prefix), **-cyto-** (the root), and **-penia** (the suffix). By combining the meanings of each of these components, the definition of the word emerges. **Thrombo-** means clot, **-cyto-** means cell, and **-penia** means a severe decrease. Hence, the term **thrombocytopenia** is defined as a severe decrease in the cells that are associated with clotting (platelets).

Prefixes may also serve as coupling forms. In this case, a term may have only two components: a prefix and a suffix. An example of this is the word **anemia.** The two components are: **an-** and **-emia. An-** means no, not, or without, and **-emia** means blood. Literally translated, the term **anemia** means "without blood." Two-part terms may also be composed of a root term and a suffix such as the word **appendectomy.** The root term **appendico** refers to the appendix and the suffix, **-ectomy,** refers to surgical removal. Therefore, an appendectomy is the surgical removal of the appendix.

Many new terms are introduced within the text of this book. Some of these terms describe conditions such as leukocytosis, whereas other terms relate to an overall patient diagnosis such as aplastic anemia. Definitions of newly introduced terms are included either within the text or in the Glossary; however, a basic working knowledge of commonly used prefixes, roots, and suffixes is essential. The following short list of prefixes and suffixes should be mastered.

PREFIXES

a-, an-, no, not, without
ab-, away from
acantho-, spiny
aniso, unequal
ante-, before
anti-, against
auto-, self
baso-, basic
bi-, two
bili-, bile

blast-, germ cell
chromo-, color
crena-, wrinkled
cryo-, extreme cold
di-, two
dys-, difficult, painful
eosin-, orange-red
erythro-, red
gen-, precursor, producer
granulo-, granular
hema-, hemato-, blood
hyper-, increased
hypo-, decreased
intra-, within
iso-, equal
leuk-, white
macro-, large
megalo-, extremely large
micro-, small
mono-, one, single
morpho-, appearance
multi-, many
neo-, new
neutro-, neutral
ortho-, normal
pan-, all
para-, next to
path-, disease
peri-, around
phago-, to eat
poikilo-, irregular
poly-, many
post-, after
pre-, before
pro-, before
pykno-, dense
reticulo-, netlike
rubri-, red
sidero-, iron
sphero-, round
thrombo-, clot
trans-, across

SUFFIXES

-algia, pain along a nerve
-ase, an enzyme
-cide, the killer of
-crit, to separate
-cyte, a cell
-ectomy, incision and removal
-emia, blood
-itis, an inflammation
-logy, the study of
-lysis, to break up
-oma, a tumor
-osis, a condition

-penia, a severe decrease
-phil, love of
-plasia, growth
-poiesis, cell growth
-rhage, -rhagia, to flow
-rhea, discharge, to flow
-scopy, to visually examine
-tomy, to cut
-uria, urine

MEDICAL TERM QUIZ

Match the prefix with the term.

1. Endo-
2. Card-
3. Ex-
4. Hemo-
5. A-, an-
6. Hypo-
7. Mal-
8. Path-
9. Phleb-
10. Trans-

A. Heart
B. No, not
C. Disease
D. Inner
E. Vein
F. Out of
G. Decreased
H. Bad, growing worse
I. Across
J. Blood
K. Increased

Match the suffix with the term.

1. -algia
2. -ectomy
3. -otomy
4. -oscopy
5. -ostomy

A. Incision and formation of an opening
B. To examine visually
C. Respiration
D. Incision
E. Pain
F. To remove

Explain these general terms:

1. Hematoma
2. Hematuria
3. Erythrocyte
4. Cardiogram
5. Dyspnea
6. Cytoscopy
7. Pathology
8. Calculus
9. Dermatitis
10. Thrombophlebitis

SI units have been recommended for the standardization of clinical laboratory data. This system is based on an international system of units (Système International) proposed in 1967 and is supported by the International Committee for Standardization in Hematology. It is expected that these units will be adopted worldwide for reporting clinical laboratory data.

The SI units consist of seven dimensionally independent base units:

Quantity	Name	Symbol
Length	meter	m
Mass	kilogram	kg
Time	second	s
Electrical current	ampere	A
Temperature	Kelvin	K
Luminous intensity	candela	cd
Amount of substance	mole	mol

There are two kinds of derived units: coherent units, which are derived directly from base units without the use of conversion factors, and noncoherent units, which are constructed from the base units and which contain a numerical factor to make the numbers more convenient to use.

Examples of prefixes to denote fractions of multiple bases and derived SI units are as follows: deci 10^{-1}, centi 10^{-2}, milli 10^{-3}, micro 10^{-6}, nano 10^{-9}, pico 10^{-12}, and femto 10^{-15}.

The expression of SI units in hematology is usually straightforward, for example:

	Conventional Units	Factor	SI Units
Erythrocytes	$4.6 \times 10^6/\mu L$	10^6	$4.6 \times 10^{12}/L$

However, occasionally the conversion will result in a new appearing value, as in the following:

	Conventional Units	Factor	SI Units
Hemoglobin	13.5 gm/dL	0.155	2.09 mmol/L

Index